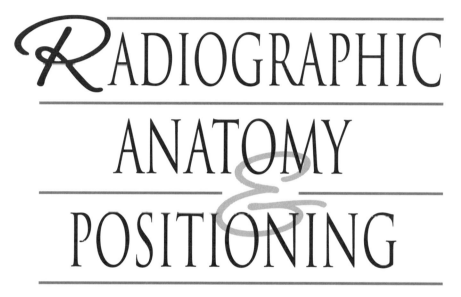

RADIOGRAPHIC ANATOMY & POSITIONING

An Integrated Approach

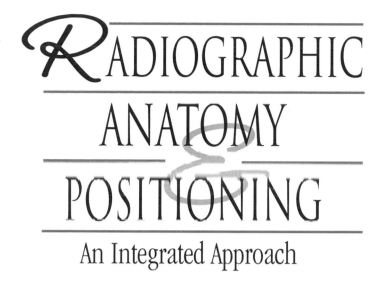

RADIOGRAPHIC ANATOMY & POSITIONING

An Integrated Approach

Andrea Gauthier Cornuelle, MS, RT(R)
Associate Professor
Radiologic Technology Program
Department of Allied Health,
Human Services & Social Work
Northern Kentucky University
Highland Heights, Kentucky

Diane H. Gronefeld, MEd, RT(R)
Associate Professor
Radiologic Technology Program
Department of Allied Health,
Human Services & Social Work
Northern Kentucky University
Highland Heights, Kentucky

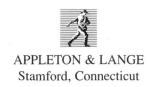

APPLETON & LANGE
Stamford, Connecticut

98 99 00 01 02   / 10 9 8 7 6 5 4 3 2 1

Prentic Hall International (UK) Limited, *London*
Prentice Hall of Australia Pty. Limited, *Sydney*
Prentice Hall Canada, Inc., *Toronto*
Prentice Hall Hispanoamericana, S.A., *Mexico*
Prentice Hall of India Private Limited, *New Delhi*
Prentice Hall of Japan, Inc., *Tokyo*
Simon & Schuster Asia Pte. Ltd., *Singapore*
Editora Prentice Hall do Brasil Ltda., *Rio de Janeiro*
Prentice Hall, *Upper Saddle River, New Jersey*

Cornuelle, Andrea Gauthier.
    Radiographic anatomy & positioning: an integrated approach/
Andrea Gauthier Cornuelle, Diane H. Gronefeld.
        p.   cm.
    Includes bibliographical references and index.
    ISBN 0-8385-8238-9 (case : alk. paper)
    1. Radiography, Medical—Positioning.   2. Radiography, Medical—
Positioning—Atlases.   I. Gronefeld, Diane H.   II. Title.
    [DNLM: 1. Technology, Radiologic,   2. Anatomy.   WN 160 C819r
1997]
RC78.4.C67   1997
616.07'572—dc21
DNLM/DLC
for Library of Congress   96-46591
                                                                            CIP

Editor In Chief: Cheryl L. Mehalik
Editor: Kimberly A. Davies
Editorial Assistant: Nicole Cooper
Production Editor: Karen W. Davis
Designer: Janice Barsevich Bielawa

ISBN 0-8385-8238-9
90000

PRINTED IN THE UNITED STATES OF AMERICA

To our students, past and present, and to the radiographers
who have donated their talents and time
to make contributions to this text,
and most of all,
to our families, friends, and colleagues
who have supported us throughout this process.

CONTENTS

CONTENTS
IN DETAIL

CONTENTS IN DETAIL

CONTRIBUTORS

Trina L. Koscielicki, MEd, RT(R)
Assistant Professor
Radiologic Technology Department of Allied Health,
Human Services & Social Work
Northern Kentucky University
Highland Heights, Kentucky

MaryAnn Nestheide, BS, RT(R)(CV)
Cardiovascular Technologist
Cardiovascular Catheterization Lab
St. Elizabeth Medical Center
Edgewood, Kentucky

Angela M. Pickwick, MS, RT(R)(M)
Department Chair
Biology & Health Sciences & Physical Education
Montgomery College
Radiologic Technology
Takoma Park, Maryland

Dorothy A. Saia, BS, RT(R)
Director Radiography Program
The Stamford Hospital
Stamford, Connecticut

PREFACE

Although an excellent atlas of radiographic positioning is available to students, we, as radiography educators, felt an atlas may not be the best resource available from which students can learn radiographic positioning and procedures. This textbook was designed for the learner. It includes pedagogical elements found in traditional textbooks: chapter outlines, objectives, summaries, review questions, and film critiques. Tables and charts are used throughout the text to summarize anatomy and other important information.

The sections on anatomy are easy to read and are presented at a level appropriate for the radiographer. The *Curriculum Guide for Radiography* by the American Society of Radiologic Technologists was used to ensure that all required procedural content was included in this text. Contributing authors with appropriate credentials were selected to write the specialized chapters on mammography and cardiovascular imaging.

To promote critical thinking skills, the Questions for Critical Thinking and Application at the end of each chapter were written to require students to take the information presented a step further—they must apply the information learned and solve problems, using higher levels of thinking, rather than simply recall facts. Many of these questions have no single correct answer and can, therefore, be used as a basis for group discussion. The reader is also asked to apply learned knowledge by answering specific questions relative to one or more radiographs. The Film Critiques require the student to use critical thinking skills to answer the questions.

While other texts present separate chapters on pediatric and geriatric patients, students are exposed to a variety of age groups throughout their clinical experience. Because students learn in an integrated fashion, information regarding pediatric and geriatric patients is introduced in appropriate chapters throughout this text. Following a similar approach, mobile and trauma radiography have been included in relevant chapters. In addition, radiographic procedures cannot be completed without basic knowledge of equipment and exposure factors. Basic information and guidelines are included relative to needed equipment and recommendations for exposure factors.

Although many radiography programs require their students to complete a medical terminology course, this information is not always retained or reinforced after the course has ended. Medical terminology related to specific systems is incorporated into Chapters 2, 3, 4, 14, 15, 16, 17, and 18. Most of the terms included are those that might be seen in a patient's chart or on an examination request form; they may also be part of patient history. Pronunciations are included for terms, anatomical structures, and procedures that may be difficult to pronounce. While this text was not meant to replace traditional medical terminology courses or textbooks, inclusion of medical terminology reinforces these terms and places them into context.

This text also includes an innovative illustration program. In addition to using color to highlight numerous diagrams, side-by-side radiographs are included with the projections—a traditional radiograph and an identical radiograph with the anatomy outlined. Anatomical structures are numbered with a key placed beside the image. Students have the opportunity to quiz themselves on radiographic anatomy as they review the appearance of accurately positioned structures. Critical anatomy, or those structures best seen on each projection, is highlighted in color.

Several supplements have been developed to complement this textbook. The *Applications Manual* by Diane H. Gronefeld and Mary L. Madigan is a unique radiographic anatomy and positioning workbook. Drawings which represent radiographic projections and positions are presented for the student to color and label. This tactile approach will aid the student in visualizing the critical anatomy demonstrated on various positions and projections, and reinforce how the exams should be performed. Study questions are written in a "fill-in-the-blank" format and are intended to reinforce the student's knowledge of basic anatomy and positioning, as well as present more complex situations requiring thoughtful answers. Case studies involving atypical patients are included in the workbook to encourage the student to think about how he or she might adapt routine positioning skills to perform an examination under unusual circumstances.

The *Competency Manual,* by Andrea Gauthier Cornuelle, is designed for use in the laboratory or clinical setting. It is a mechanism for evaluating positioning competency prior to the student performing the examination on a patient. It presents routine radiographic positions or projections in a logical, sequential method that the student can follow or modify as needed. The laboratory or clinical instructor can assess the student's competency as he or she performs the procedure.

The *Pocket Manual,* by Mary L. Madigan, Andrea Gauthier Cornuelle, and Diane H. Gronefeld, condenses the radiographic positioning sections of the textbook into a concise, easy-to-read format in a convenient pocket size. Important tables, such as grid-conversion factors, are also included.

The *Instructor's Resource Manual,* by Mary L. Madigan and Diane H. Gronefeld, is a valuable resource for the course instructor, offering chapter outlines, suggested schedules, sample test questions, transparency masters, and a more comprehensive list of objectives than those presented in this textbook. A chart comparing subject matter and relevant page numbers conveniently directs the instructor to the material of interest. This manual is also the source of the answers to the study questions found in the *Applications Manual.* In addition, a computerized test bank (IBM compatible) with more than 1400 questions was created by Michele G. Miller and can be used by instructors to assess mastery of the content of this text.

In lieu of traditional slides, we are developing a CD ROM image bank for use in the classroom by the instructor. This CD ROM will enable the instructor to customize his or her own presentation, and it will contain anatomical line art, radiographic images with critical anatomy overlays, numerous images for film critiques, and sectional images. For more information on this new supplement, please contact your local Appleton & Lange representative.

While we have invested countless hours researching, writing, and reviewing the manuscript to ensure accuracy and comprehensiveness, it is entirely possible that you as the reader may identify omissions or errors. Constructive comments that may contribute to an improved version are certainly welcome and appreciated.

Andrea Gauthier Cornuelle & Diane H. Gronefeld

ACKNOWLEDGMENTS

No project of this magnitude can be completed without the support of many others. Dorothy Saia, BS, RT(R), and Trina Koscielicki, MEd, RT(R), wrote the professionalism and technical considerations sections of the introductory chapter, respectively. Angela M. Pickwick, MS, RT(R)(M), authored, "Mammography" and worked diligently to locate appropriate films for that chapter. MaryAnn Nestheide, BS, RT(R)(CV) shared her years of experience working in cardiovascular imaging by writing the chapter on the "Cardiovascular System." We were also very fortunate to have excellent reviewers who spent many hours reviewing the manuscript and offered numerous ideas and suggestions.

The completion of this book would not have been possible without the support of Cheryl Mehalik, Kim Davies, Ginny Rosow, Karen Davis, and Jennifer Sinsavich of Appleton & Lange. While Cheryl helped us develop the initial proposal, Kim helped us pull things together at the end. As editorial assistant, Ginny kept us on track by giving us gentle reminders of work outstanding.

Many others contributed their expertise in the way of suggestions, radiographs, photographs, or products and are owed special thanks. Dr. Richard Laib, Dr. Jim Barnes, and Dr. James Schmitt served as resources and provided encouragement during the process. Linda Winkler, RT(R)(N), Terri Gosney, RT(R)(CT), Peggy Neal, RT(R), RDMS, Stephanie Wetherell, RT(R), Debbie Kruetzkamp, RT(R)(N), Amy Arnold, RT(R), and Jane Greenwell, RT(R) provided many of the nuclear medicine, ultrasound, and CT images in this text. Numerous other radiographers and students contributed various radiographs throughout the text. Colleagues Carol Thiemann, RT(R) and Trina Koscielicki, MEd, RT(R) and some of our students helped by searching through barrels of purged films for textbook-quality radiographs. Our affiliate hospitals in the Cincinnati/Northern Kentucky area served as resources for radiographs and photography sites. Donna Pellegrino of LoRad, Kathy Sullivan of Bennett, Gini Wentz of Agfa, Adrienne Palmer of American Mammographics, and Jennifer Ebner of Broadwest Corporation deserve special thanks for contributing the photographs for the mammography chapter. Dean Rindlisbach and Paul Kellogg of Philips Medical and Duncan McGrew of General Electric helped by providing photographs of various types of equipment. Martin Ratner of Nuclear Associates, Inc. and Gil Welman of Alcraft–Welman Products graciously provided photographs of several products. We owe Chris Geiger of Bracco Diagnostics and Gregg Kamp of E-Z-Em special thanks for providing contrast media and supplies for photographs included in Chapters 1 and 13.

Last, but not least, we want to thank our families for their patience and support during the past 3+ years. We realize the added responsibilities our spouses, Paul and Tony, had to carry while we kept writing, reviewing, and editing the many pages of manuscript. Although Jeffrey and Daniel Cornuelle missed spending a number of Saturdays, Sundays, and evenings with their mom, they were troopers. Thank you for your support, your patience, and your encouragement; without it we could not have completed this project.

Andrea Gauthier Cornuelle
Diane H. Gronefeld

A GUIDE TO KEY FEATURES

Icons are used in chapters to identify the following special sections:

Pediatric   **Geriatric**   **Mobile Radiography**

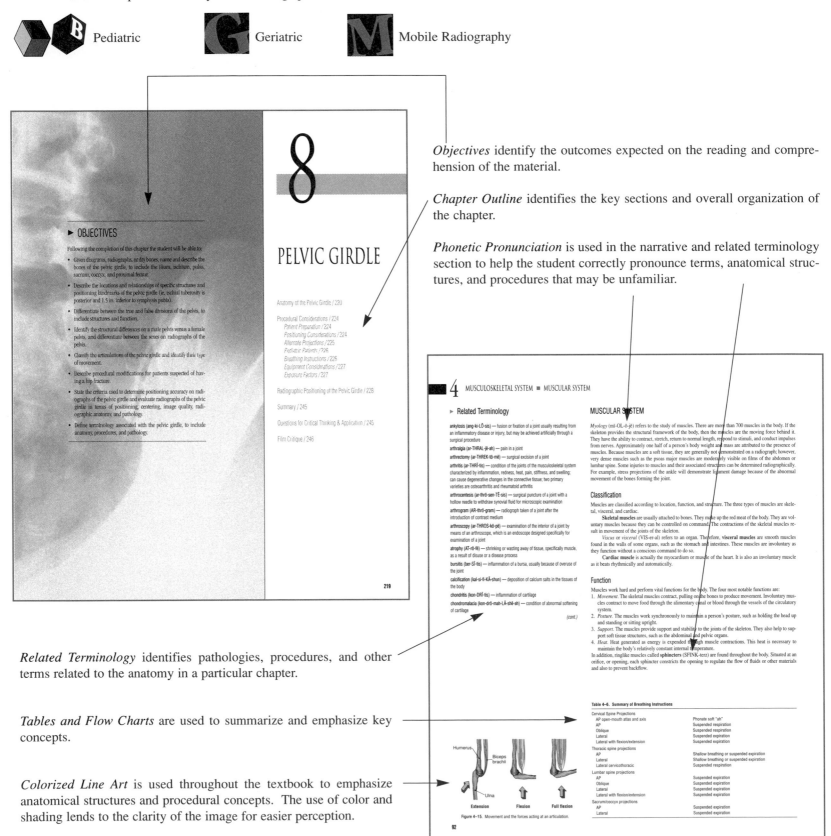

Objectives identify the outcomes expected on the reading and comprehension of the material.

Chapter Outline identifies the key sections and overall organization of the chapter.

Phonetic Pronunciation is used in the narrative and related terminology section to help the student correctly pronounce terms, anatomical structures, and procedures that may be unfamiliar.

Related Terminology identifies pathologies, procedures, and other terms related to the anatomy in a particular chapter.

Tables and Flow Charts are used to summarize and emphasize key concepts.

Colorized Line Art is used throughout the textbook to emphasize anatomical structures and procedural concepts. The use of color and shading lends to the clarity of the image for easier perception.

Cassette Size and Orientation are included for each of the radiographic projections.

AEC Cells (if appropriate) are suggested for the radiographic projections.

Collimation Guidelines provide more specific instructions for entry-level radiographers.

Central Ray is highlighted to better illustrate direction.

Radiographs of high quality are used with each projection. Adjacent radiographs include a traditional image and an identical image with the critical anatomy outlined in color.

Chapter Summary concisely lists important procedural information.

Questions for Critical Thinking & Application promote cognitive skills by asking the student to apply learned information to solve a variety of situations.

Film Critiques Intentionally flawed radiographs are provided at the end of each chapter to faciliate critical thinking skills and group discussion.

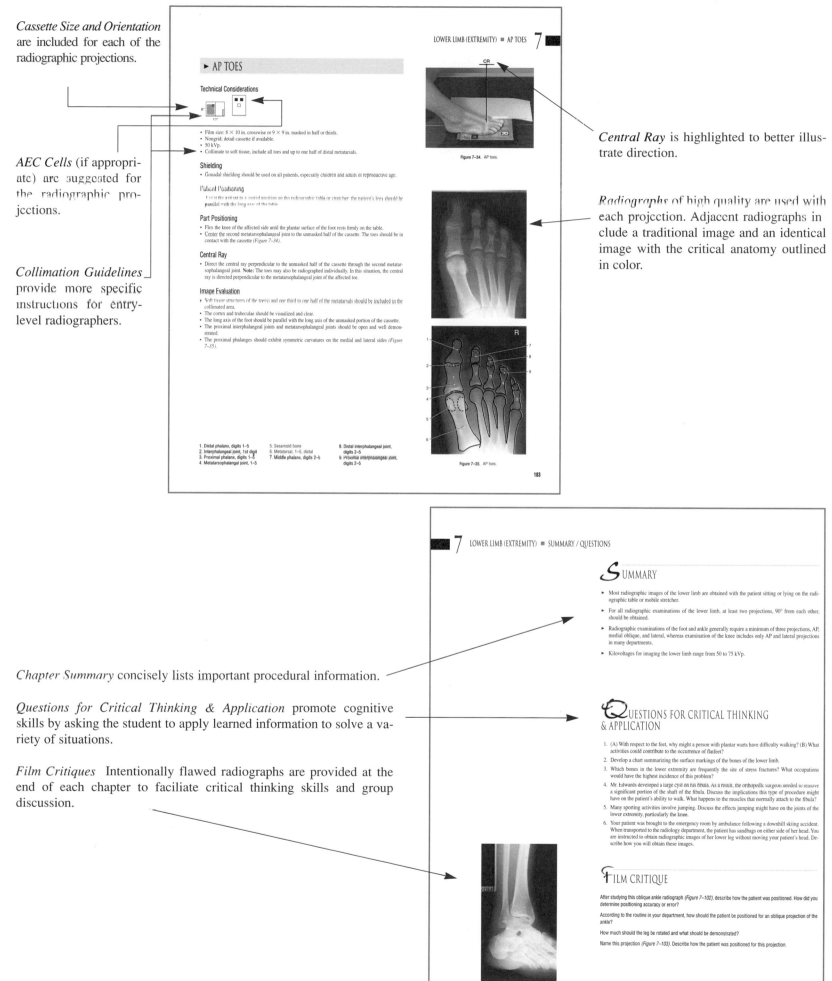

1

INTRODUCTION TO RADIOGRAPHY

► OBJECTIVES

Following the completion of this chapter the student will be able to:

- Discuss the Code of Ethics and professionalism as they relate to the radiologic technologist.

- Describe factors relative to effective communication with patients of all ages.

- Describe appropriate infection control procedures and the radiographer's role in prevention of disease transmission.

- Identify and describe the four basic types of body habitus and explain how they may affect patient centering and positioning.

- Define sectional anatomy and differentiate between sagittal, coronal, and transverse/axial images.

- Define terminology related to patient/part positioning.

- Describe the appropriate steps for completion of a radiographic examination.

- Identify and describe the factors that contribute to image quality.

- Briefly describe the radiographic and accessory equipment used in the radiology department.

- Describe appropriate methods of radiation protection for the radiographer and patient.

- Identify and describe five general components of a systematic film evaluation.

- Briefly describe computed tomography, diagnostic medical sonography, nuclear medicine, and magnetic resonance imaging.

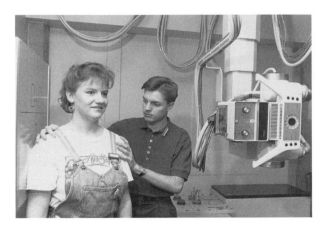

Radiography is more than positioning a patient and pushing a button to make the exposure. The radiographer must be able to communicate effectively with all patients, provide appropriate patient care, complete radiographic examinations following prescribed procedures, use radiation wisely, and evaluate radiographic quality.

► PROFESSIONAL ETHICS

CODE OF ETHICS

Every profession has a set of ethical rules or standards that all members of that profession are expected to follow. The Code of Ethics for the radiologic technologist, which forms the first part of the *Standards of Ethics,* has been adopted by the American Society of Radiologic Technology and the American Registry of Radiologic Technology and addresses professional conduct, patient care, utilization of equipment that produces ionizing radiation, appropriate application of theoretical knowledge with regard to procedures and technique, radiation protection, and continued professional education *(Table 1–1).* The Rules of Ethics form the second part of the *Standards of Ethics* and include mandatory, specific standards of minimally acceptable professional conduct for registered technologists and applicants and can be the basis for sanctions with regard to professional certification.

PROFESSIONALISM

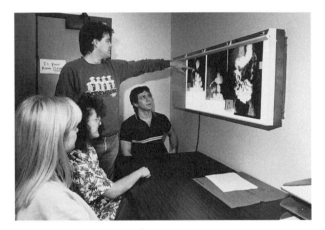

It is difficult to pick up any radiologic science literature today without finding at least one article or letter to the editor about professionalism. Some radiographers associate the terms *professional* and *professionalism* with procurement of an academic degree. Others claim it is gained through the endorsement of a certification board and documentation of continuing education. Still others associate it with officially recognized status gained through the passage of state licensure.

All these things have something to do with professionalism because they represent the attainment of the required knowledge and skills, but being a professional requires more than just knowledge and skills. Certain attitudes, behaviors, and morals are needed to complete the picture.

Table 1–1. The Code of Ethics

1. The Radiologic Technologist conducts himself/herself in a professional manner, responds to patient needs, and supports colleagues and associates in providing quality patient care.
2. The Radiologic Technologist acts to advance the principal objective of the profession to provide services to humanity with full respect for the dignity of mankind.
3. The Radiologic Technologist delivers patient care and service unrestricted by the concerns of personal attributes or the nature of the disease or illness, and without discrimination regardless of sex, race, creed, religion, or socioeconomic status.
4. The Radiologic Technologist practices technology founded upon theoretical knowledge and concepts, utilizes equipment and accessories consistent with the purposes for which they have been designed, and employs procedures and techniques appropriately.
5. The Radiologic Technologist assesses situations, exercises care, discretion, and judgment, assumes responsibility for professional decisions, and acts in the best interest of the patient.
6. The Radiologic Technologist acts as an agent through observation and communication to obtain pertinent information for the physician to aid in the diagnosis and treatment management of the patient, and recognizes that interpretation and diagnosis are outside the scope of practice for the profession.
7. The Radiologic Technologist utilizes equipment and accessories, employs techniques and procedures, performs services in accordance with an accepted standard of practice, and demonstrates expertise in minimizing the radiation exposure to the patient, self, and other members of the health care team.
8. The Radiologic Technologist practices ethical conduct appropriate to the profession and protects the patient's right to quality radiologic technology care.
9. The Radiologic Technologist respects confidences entrusted in the course of professional practice, respects the patient's right to privacy, and reveals confidential information only as required by law or to protect the welfare of the individual or the community.
10. The Radiologic Technologist continually strives to improve knowledge and skills by participating in educational and professional activities, sharing knowledge with colleagues, and investigating new and innovative aspects of professional practice. One means available to improve knowledge and skill is through professional continuing education.

Adopted by the ASRT and ARRT, 1994.

As we observe physicians, technologists, nurses, aides, and others in the health care team treating and caring for patients, we have surely seen some that merely "go through the motions." That is, they do what is necessary and required; they could not be taken to task for not being efficient and thorough. Yet, there are others in the health care team that "go the extra mile" for their patients. These individuals try to understand and address the patient's concerns and anxieties; they make pleasant conversation with the patient as they go about their work; they treat each patient with the dignity and respect they deserve; they emanate a certain warmth. In short, they are just the sort of individual that we would like to care for us, should we require health care. These are the professionals.

Your observations of members of the health care team should also include moments that are not involved in direct patient care. For example, while a patient is being transported from his room to a department for testing, one transporter may converse loudly, or joke with friends he passes in the hallway, or actually stop to chat with other personnel. Another transporter focuses on his patient, makes an attempt at appropriate conversation, and delivers his patient to the department in a timely manner. This is professionalism.

What about appearance and tone of voice? Do you think these make a difference in the delivery of health care? Imagine you are the patient and the nurse comes to your room to deliver your next medication. You notice the soiled cuffs of her "white" pants above dirty, rundown sneakers. As she comes closer, you get a better view of greasy looking hair hanging to her shoulders. She greets you with a booming "How are 'ya doin', dearie? Roll up on your side, it's time for your shot." Making no effort to preserve your modesty, she pulls away your gown just in time to reveal your derriere to squads of visitors marching down the hall! Another nurse delivers your next medication. She appears clean, tidy, and nicely groomed. As she approaches you she addresses you by name, speaking in a well-modulated tone. She explains that it is time for medication and draws the curtain around your bed for privacy. This is professionalism.

Another example is that of two newly graduated radiographers just hired by your radiology department. One of them has a know-it-all-attitude that annoys everyone. All the students try to avoid working with this person because he seems to take pleasure in intimidating and demeaning students. The other radiographer enjoys helping the students, explaining new procedures and encouraging them throughout the day. This is professionalism.

The above examples, then, appear to indicate that professionalism is largely an "inner" thing, a feeling of fellowship with the human race, an intangible. Another aspect of professionalism, however, is making an effort to "give back" some of what radiologic technology has given you. Radiographers, new and experienced, who share their knowledge with students, helping and encouraging them, "give back" some of the experiences they found helpful as students. Other radiographers, as their way of "giving back," choose to play an active role in their local and regional societies that function to help technologists continue their education and represent the interests of the membership to the public and government.

So, more important than simply *attaining* professionalism is *retaining* professionalism. Professionalism, then, seems to be a long road that we travel, beginning with study and practice to gain our initial certification. As we continue along the road, we document our continuing education, whether it is studying for advanced certification, pursuing one or more academic degrees, doing committee work in our local and regional societies, conducting research, or publishing. Regardless of the direction we travel, we continue to encounter and interact with patients. Here we must realize that all our activities and pursuit of greater things are almost meaningless unless we continue to monitor our attitudes and behavior toward our patients. As long as we continue to "go that extra mile," we can consider ourselves professionals.

► *A Patient's Rights*

The patient has the right

- *to care that is respectful and considerate*

- *to privacy regarding his care and condition*

- *to refuse treatment*

- *to be informed of the nature, probable length of recovery time, and the risks involved prior to the start of any procedure*

- *to receive, in understandable terms, current information regarding diagnosis, treatment, and prognosis from a physician*

- *to confidentiality with respect to all records and communication related to his care*

From "A Patient's Bill of Rights," the American Hospital Association, 1975.

► COMMUNICATION & PATIENT CARE

Patient care encompasses a patient's physical, psychological, and emotional needs. Although most individuals feel more comfortable tending to a patient's physical needs—providing warmth, easing pain, assisting the patient to the restroom—it is often the psychological and emotional needs that have a greater impact on a patient's quality of health care and recovery.

The radiographer is perceived by patients as an educated professional who is expected to act in a responsible and safe manner. One responsibility of the radiographer is effective communication with the patient and with other members of the health care team for the relay of vital information regarding the patient's care. A patient who is ill or acutely injured may become aggressive, demanding, or withdrawn. The radiographer must assess the patient's needs and communicate appropriately, to reassure and comfort the patient while providing care.

Effective communication is central to good health care and is as important to the radiographer as knowing how to use complex radiographic equipment. In addition to receiving, interpreting, and carrying out directions, the radiographer must also give instructions and offer consolation and reassurance to the pa-

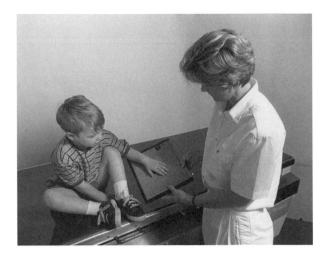

Figure 1–1. Preschool children may like to examine the equipment.

tient. Communication includes both spoken and unspoken messages. Unfortunately, the message the communicator sends may be misinterpreted by the person receiving the message. Any problem with communication can have an impact on patient care. A patient who leaves the department feeling confused or misunderstood may discontinue future health care. It is important for the radiographer to assess his or her communication skills by listening and observing the patient. The response received, either verbally or visibly, will let the radiographer know whether the intended message was received; misunderstandings can be clarified at the time and communication continued.

Unfortunately, nonverbal communication often says more than verbal communication. The radiographer who speaks with an uncaring tone of voice, never looks at the patient while communicating, maintains a long distance from the patient, and does not offer the patient an opportunity to ask questions is telling the patient that he or she is not important. Conversely, the radiographer has the opportunity to observe the patient for signs the patient is in pain, confused, insecure, or distrustful. Nonverbal messages provide the radiographer with the opportunity to clarify instructions or comfort the patient.

An individual's feelings and attitudes can lead to bias or discrimination toward others. Attitudes are a set of beliefs an individual holds regarding specific issues or persons and are learned as a result of exposure to family and friends who, throughout life, let their preferences be known. Attitudes lead to biases, which can affect behavior and impact patient care. The radiographer must understand her or his own feelings and attitudes to be successful as a professional who can provide compassionate care to all patients.

Because an informed patient is more compliant, patient communication and education are integral to a successful examination. Patient cooperation can reduce the amount of time it takes to complete the procedure, can improve radiographic quality by minimizing patient motion, and can reduce the number of repeat radiographs.

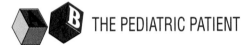 THE PEDIATRIC PATIENT

The pediatric patient can present some rather unique challenges to the radiographer. Depending on their age, children may have a limited understanding of what is happening to them. They may be sick, hurt, tired, and/or uncooperative. Young children cannot be trusted to sit alone on the radiographic table or refrain from touching equipment that could be potentially harmful to them. The approach the technologist takes toward the pediatric patient can be a significant factor in obtaining the child's cooperation.

Pediatric patients can be divided into groups by age: neonates, infants, toddlers, preschool children, school-age children, and adolescents. Each group has different needs, limitations, and concerns.

Neonates

Neonates (birth to 4 weeks) require the basic needs of warmth, food, and love. When possible, swaddling a baby in a blanket will provide a feeling of warmth and security. During the first 4 weeks of life, neonates can become hypothermic very quickly. Limiting the amount of time a neonate is uncovered and placing radiolucent sheeting between the baby and table or cassette will help prevent hypothermia; care must be taken to ensure there are no wrinkles in the sheet that may cause artifacts on the radiographs. When fasting is required for an examination, limited use of a pacifier may appease the neonate; prolonged use may cause an air-filled stomach and a stomachache. If the neonate is hungry and able to eat, feeding the child may result in drowsiness, contentedness, and cooperativeness.

Infants

Because an infant (4 weeks to 12 months) increasingly develops an awareness of people and surroundings, crying is a normal response when he or she is taken from the mother in an unfamiliar place. It is usually more helpful, therefore, to allow at least one parent to remain with an infant during the examination; to eliminate the possible exposure of a pregnant mother, the father is often chosen for this purpose.

Toddlers

The group of children least likely to be cooperative is toddlers (12 months to 3 years). Early in this period, children learn to walk and love to explore; they do not like to be restrained or limited. During this stage, they also learn the word "no"—and like to use it! Because the radiographic procedures and the equipment are strange to them, they need a lot of reassurance. Communication should be firm, quiet, and calm. Whispering into the ear of crying, thrashing toddlers may capture their curiosity and attention and calm them. A special toy and the presence of a parent may also help in obtaining the necessary cooperation.

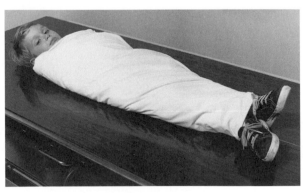

Figure 1–2. The octagon board **(A)** can be used to immobilize small children for abdominal radiography. Using a sheet to mummy wrap a child **(B)** can also be an effective immobilization technique *(continued).*

Preschool Children

Preschool children (3 to 6 years) are able to communicate verbally and exhibit increasing levels of independence. They can understand radiographic procedures on a basic level—they are "going to have a picture taken with a special camera." They may want to touch the equipment *(Figure 1–1.)* Because they are very trusting, it is important to be honest with them. If a procedure is going to hurt, explain what it will feel like and offer encouragement: "You're doing great!" "It won't last long." "Squeeze my hand as tightly as you'd like." "We'll work as quickly as possible." Because preschoolers take things literally, the radiographer should avoid using the words *dye* and *shot,* which could have negative connotations and invoke unnecessary fear in the patient. Coaching by the radiographer and bribery, such as a sticker or band-aid, are helpful; because many children are on special diets, candy is not recommended.

School-age Children

Because a 4-year-old child may look more like a 7-year-old child, it is important to assess the developmental age and needs of the school-age child (6 to 12 years). Additionally, an older child may appear younger because of an illness. The radiographer must also be sensitive to a child who may have endured a chronic or debilitating illness that may have had a negative effect on the child's social life.

Children in this age group are usually capable of communicating and are helpful and friendly. They can understand the basic explanations of the procedure. Six- and seven-year-old patients will probably be very interested in watching the radiographer; pictures of animals or other images strategically placed on the wall or ceiling will help them maintain their position. Following appropriate instruction and practice, these children can also hold their breath.

During the preteen years, children are generally very modest. The radiographer should respect their modesty by keeping them covered and giving them the same privacy afforded an adult. Considering the cognitive level of the child, preparation for examination should include an explanation of the procedure, including the child's role with respect to pain, shots, holding still, and breathing instructions, and a tour of the room to be used.

Adolescents

Appearance is very important to adolescents (13 years and older). Dress or debilitating illness that sets them apart from the social norm may make teenagers feel insecure. Because adolescent patients tend to have chronic illness, traumatic injuries, or serious diseases requiring prolonged hospitalization, they may be unable to maintain normal activities, including schoolwork, sports, and social events. The inability to function at a normal level may cause the adolescent patient to be unfriendly, sassy, or childish. Although these patients may look like adults, they are not adults and will respond differently to knowledge of their illness. They may know a little about radiation and be concerned about the effect it might have on their sexuality; they may try to distance themselves from what is being done; they may fuss, cry, or be withdrawn. Teenagers of any age should be informed about the procedure and should participate in decisions relative to their care.

Because pregnancy may be an issue, the radiographer should take appropriate precautions in determining whether a female patient is pregnant. Individual states and health care centers may have specific guidelines and requirements relative to assessing the possibility of pregnancy; the radiographer should be familiar with these guidelines. Because some patients under age 18 live away from home and are financially independent, they may be able to make their own decisions regarding health care, depending on state law. Parents under age 18 have the responsibility for making decisions about health care and treatment for their children, even though they are not of legal age.

General Comments

Because children do not develop at the same rate and may regress emotionally due to illness and unfamiliar surroundings, the radiographer must assess each child individually. Immobilization devices and techniques, such as sandbags, sponges, tape, mummy wrap, plexiglass, and head clamps, should be age appropriate *(Figure 1–2).* To relieve anxiety, parents, or legal guardians, should be educated about the procedures and offered the opportunity to ask questions. Children can sense when their parents are anxious and afraid, causing the children to have the same feelings. The health care worker should communicate with the child at the child's eye level, which may require the radiographer to sit, stoop, or kneel *(Figure 1–3).* It is the radiographer's responsibility to provide an understanding, supportive, and compassionate environment which will ultimately contribute to better patient care and radiographic quality.

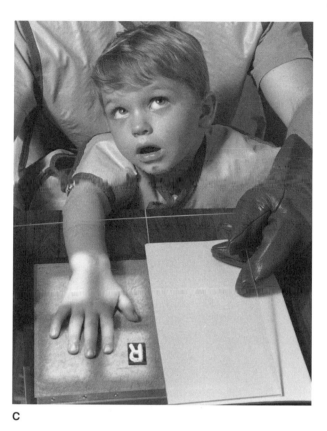

C

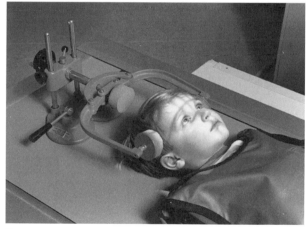

D

Figure 1–2 *(continued).* Plexiglass **(C),** used to immobilize hands and feet, and head clamps **(D)** are other valuable tools for immobilization.

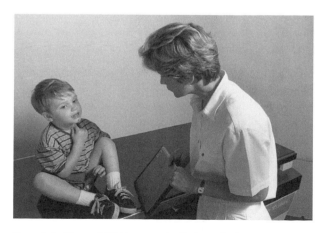

Figure 1–3. When establishing rapport with the pediatric patient, the technologist should make all attempts to talk to the patient at eye level.

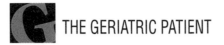

THE GERIATRIC PATIENT

As the average age of the general population is increasing, the average age of patients seen in the radiology department is also rising. This population of patients is often looked at negatively because they cannot move as quickly or as well as younger patients, they may not be able to hear or see as well, and they often represent a stage in life that many people fear. Some older patients have never been to the hospital, may be afraid of the unknown, and may not understand the requirements of the procedure. After all, these older patients were born when radiography was in its infancy!

The older patient is often stereotyped. Do not assume that the 80-year-old patient lying on the stretcher cannot hear what is said. Communication should be slow and clearly articulated; speak in a normal voice level near the patient's ear, rather than yell. Patient assessment is important in determining ability. The 90-year-old may be more agile than the 60-year-old. As with all patients, respect, understanding, and empathy are requirements for providing the best patient care for the geriatric patient.

Physical changes, such as loss of calcium in the bones, loss of elasticity of body tissues, and diminished muscle strength, are responsible for many of the health problems of elderly patients. They are more likely to have respiratory problems, hypertension, coronary artery disease, strokes, malignant neoplasms, and arthritis than their younger counterparts. Because of some of these problems, they may not be able to attain the positions necessary for quality radiographs. In addition, care should be taken when moving elderly patients to prevent bruising and damage to the skin. The radiographer should be alert to potential problems and provide appropriate care at all times.

▶ INFECTION CONTROL

Hospitals are havens for the sick and are, therefore, often the source for transmission of disease. Because patients who are sick have a weakened resistance, they are more susceptible to disease. It is the responsibility of all health care workers to do everything within their means to prevent the transmission of disease. Cleanliness measures, which include proper cleaning of equipment with a disinfectant, use of fresh linens for each patient, appropriate disposal of used linens, and handwashing before and after each patient, should be taken by all health care workers.

Disease can be transmitted by *direct contact,* in which an infected person comes in contact with a susceptible person, or by *indirect contact,* where transmission occurs by way of a fomite, vector, or airborne droplets or dust *(Table 1–2).* Practicing aseptic techniques can help prevent the transmission of disease. To accomplish this, the radiographer should stay at home when ill, cover the mouth when sneezing or coughing, wear a clean uniform daily, follow thorough handwashing techniques consistently, wear disposable gloves and gowns when appropriate, and practice good housekeeping techniques. When cleaning the radiographic table, for example, clean from the least to most contaminated area and from the top down.

▶ *Aseptic Handwashing Technique*

1. *Consider sink contaminated; avoid contact with clothing.*

2. *With hands lower than elbows, wet hands thoroughly.*

3. *Apply soap (liquid preferred).*

4. *Using a firm, circular motion, rub hands and fingers together for at least 20 seconds.*

5. *Rinse by allowing the water to run over the hands.*

6. *Repeat the steps to cleanse from elbows to fingertips.*

7. *Dry thoroughly.*

8. *Using toweling, turn the water off.*

Table 1–2. Infection Control Terminology

Nosocomial infection	An infection acquired in the hospital
Medical asepsis	Reducing the number of infectious organisms in the environment; decreasing the probability that an infectious organism will be transmitted to a susceptible individual
Microbial dilution	Process of reducing the total number of infectious organisms
Disinfection	Destruction of pathogens through use of chemicals
Fomite	An object that has been contaminated by an infectious person (eg, dressings, radiographic table, linens)
Vector	Insect or animal carriers of disease (eg, mosquitoes that transmit malaria; fleas that carry bubonic plague; rabid dogs, bats, or squirrels)
Surgical asepsis	Sterilization; complete removal of all organisms and their spores through the use of chemicals, boiling, gas, or steam (autoclaving)
Disease-specific isolation	Certain practices are defined for each communicable disease, depending on the route of transmission (eg, strict isolation used for chickenpox)
Category-specific isolation	Diseases requiring similar isolation techniques are grouped together based on their common route of transmission (eg, hepatitis B and AIDS are grouped together because they require "universal blood and body fluid" precautions)

Soiled linens should be folded from the outside in and properly disposed; grossly contaminated linens should be placed in a separate bag and clearly labeled. Any equipment coming in contact with the patient (eg, cassette, stethoscope) should be cleaned after use. Needles and syringes should be placed in designated containers without recapping the needle; recapping needles places the health care worker at risk of a needle prick and contamination *(Figure 1–4)*.

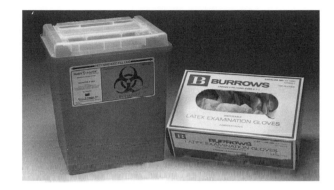

Figure 1–4. Sharps container for used needles and syringes; disposable gloves.

UNIVERSAL PRECAUTIONS

The Centers for Disease Control and Prevention established *Universal Precautions* in 1987 in response to concerns about HIV and hepatitis B. Universal Precautions were developed to protect health care workers and have been identified by the Occupational Safety and Health Administration (OSHA) as the minimum standard for safety. According to these precautions, all patients are considered to be carriers of bloodborne pathogens. Any time there is a chance for contact with blood or body fluids, the health care worker is required to wear disposable gloves. Masks/face shields and eye protection should be used whenever there is a possibility of splashes or droplets of blood or body fluid touching the face or eyes. Gowns and impermeable aprons must be worn when clothing may be soiled by blood or body fluids.

ISOLATION PROCEDURES

Although infection control measures should be used with all patients, special precautions are initiated when a patient is known or suspected of having a communicable disease. *Isolation precautions* are used to help control the spread of pathogens that cause disease, either from patient to staff or from staff to patient; the latter was formerly called *reverse* or *protective isolation* (those patients requiring reverse isolation include burn victims and others who have a compromised immune system). Currently, several different types of isolation precaution systems are used, including *disease-specific isolation* and *category-specific isolation* (defined in *Table 1–2*); the category-specific isolation system is used most frequently in health care institutions *(Table 1–3)*. It is each radiographer's responsibility to learn specific guidelines followed at his or her facility.

When radiographing an isolation patient, two radiographers usually work together. One radiographer remains *clean,* or *uncontaminated,* and touches only the cassette and the radiographic equipment, which is often difficult to clean thoroughly. The second radiographer is considered *dirty,* or *contaminated,* and has the responsibility of positioning the patient; when performing a mobile examination, the contaminated radiographer handles the cassette after it has been placed in a protective plastic cover. Protective mask, gown, and/or gloves should be used as appropriate for the specific type of isolation; lead aprons should be worn under the protective gown.

Because isolation patients often remain in solitude for long periods and may feel neglected, communication here is a vitally important part of patient care. The radiographer should take time to explain the procedure to the patient and answer any questions the patient might have. It is important to treat the patient with dignity and respect, regardless of the reason for isolation.

Table 1–3. Category-specific Isolation

Category	Necessary Protection
Drainage–secretion Examples: burn infection, conjunctivitis, wound infection	Gloves, gown (if necessary) Handwashing (2 minutes)
Enteric (fecal material) Examples: coxsackievirus, viral meningitis, gastroenteritis	Gloves and gown if possible contact with infectious material Thorough handwashing
Acid-fast bacillus (AFB) Example: tuberculosis	Mask Handwashing Gown if gross contamination possible
Respiratory Examples: measles, mumps, bacterial meningitis	Mask Handwashing
Contact Examples: herpes simplex, influenza in young children	Mask, gloves, gown Handwashing
Strict Examples: chickenpox, pneumonic plague	Mask, gloves, gown Handwashing

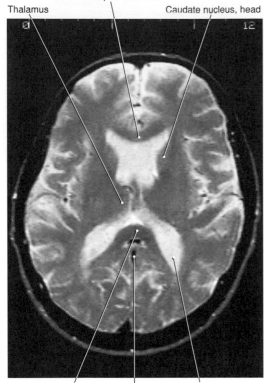

Genu of corpus callosum

Thalamus   Caudate nucleus, head

Splenium of corpus callosum | Posterior horn, lateral ventricle
Straight sinus

A

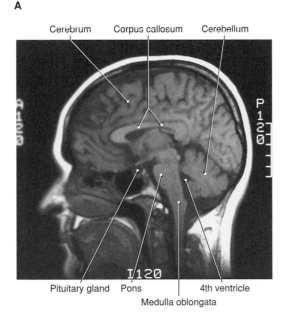

Cerebrum   Corpus callosum   Cerebellum

Pituitary gland   Pons   4th ventricle
Medulla oblongata

B

Figure 1–5. Magnetic resonance images can be obtained in transverse **(A)**, sagittal **(B)**, and coronal **(C)** planes *(continued)*.

Table 1–4. Classification of Body Habitus

Hypersthenic
Approximately 5% of population
Deep, broad thorax
Ribs nearly horizontal
Short thoracic cavity
Short, wide heart
Elevated diaphragm
Stomach and gallbladder very
   high and almost horizontal
Gallbladder away from midline
Colon high and wide, traveling
   around periphery of abdomen

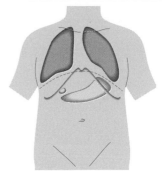

Hypersthenic habitus

Sthenic
Approximately 50% of population
Modification of hypersthenic type
Thorax slightly longer and narrower
Ribs more vertical
Thoracic cavity longer
Heart narrower and longer
Diaphragm not as high
Stomach and gallbladder lower and not as transverse
Colon slightly lower and more centrally located

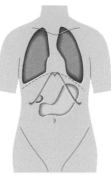

Sthenic habitus

Hyposthenic
Approximately 35% of population
Thorax longer; diaphragm lower
Stomach and gallbladder lower and closer to midline
Colon lower and closer to middle of abdomen

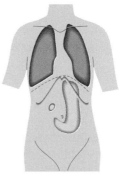

Hyposthenic habitus

Asthenic
Approximately 10% of population
Exaggeration of hyposthenic type
Thorax narrow and shallow
Lungs broader superiorly and narrower at bases
Heart long and narrow
Diaphragm very low
Short abdomen
Stomach and gallbladder very low, vertical, and near midline
Colon low, folds on itself, and lies near midline

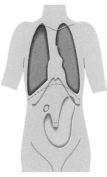

Asthenic habitus

▶ INTRODUCTION TO ANATOMY

To determine whether a patient was accurately positioned for any given radiograph, the radiographer must know what anatomical structures should be demonstrated based on the patient's physical position. In-depth knowledge of anatomical structures and their location, therefore, is required. Unfortunately, people come in different shapes, sizes, and levels of fitness. Although this may not be much of a problem when imaging the extremities, it can be a problem when radiographing the structures of the thorax and abdomen.

BODY HABITUS

The term *habitus* refers to the physical characteristics of the body, including shape, size, muscle tone, and position of internal organs. Because an individual's body habitus determines the location of specific organs within the abdomen, the radiographer must be able to assess body habitus for accurate patient centering. People are generally classified as having one of four different types of body habitus. Knowing the classification helps determine the location of internal structures *(Table 1–4)*

SECTIONAL ANATOMY

Routine diagnostic radiographic images of anatomy result in the anatomy appearing "flattened" because various structures are superimposed on one another, giving no depth perception. Radiographers become accustomed to identifying anatomy on these two-dimensional images of three-dimensional structures. The widespread use of computed tomography, magnetic resonance imaging, and ultrasonography, however, has presented the radiographer with the need to look at anatomy differently. These three modalities are capable of imaging anatomical structures in sections or slices that are viewed somewhat differently than routine diagnostic radiographs. Using computers to figuratively extract a thin slice of tissue, physicians are better able to evaluate anatomy and pathology. These sectional images can be obtained from various planes in the body, including transverse (axial), sagittal, coronal (frontal), and virtually any oblique plane *(Figure 1–5)*. To identify anatomical structures, the radiographer must know the anatomy and anatomical relationships extremely well. Anterior/posterior and medial/lateral relationships can be identified on transverse sections, and superior/inferior and medial/lateral relationships can be delineated on coronal sections. The radiographer must know the normal relationships to identify anatomical structures on sectional images. Because these modalities enable us to see muscles, vessels, and other soft tissue structures extremely well, the radiographer must know all the anatomy, not just bones and major organs!

It is often difficult for the novice to orient himself or herself to sectional images. Although it may be easier to think of sectional images as two-dimensional structures, they actually have a third dimension—depth or section thickness. The thickness of a sectional image is determined by the operator and may be established by department protocol. When viewing transverse sections, the radiographer should imagine standing at the foot of the table and looking up at the bottom of the slice; the inferior surface of the slice is being viewed. Coronal slices are viewed as if looking at the front of the patient or the anterior surface of the section. For sagittal sections, the right side of the slice is viewed.

▶ PROCEDURAL CONSIDERATIONS

Every radiology department will have established routine projections that must be included with each examination. In general, at least two projections/positions, 90° apart, are obtained for all body parts to demonstrate anatomy that may not be visible on one projection because of superimposition (eg, a lateral chest x-ray demonstrates any anatomy or pathology behind the heart). Two projections, 90° apart, are also required for localization of foreign objects and assessment of fracture alignment. To adequately demonstrate all angles and surfaces of a joint, at least three projections/positions are necessary.

To minimize patient motion, various restraint devices, such as sandbags, tape, and compression bands, can be used for immobilization *(Figure 1–6)*. In addition, clear breathing instructions can also help eliminate patient motion that contributes to blur on the image.

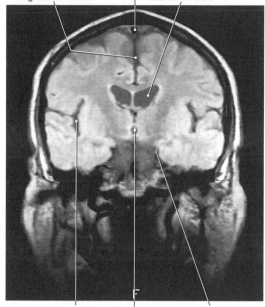

Superior sagittal sinus
Longitudinal fissure   Lateral ventricle

Lateral fissure   Internal carotid artery
3rd ventricle

C

Figure 1–5 *(continued)*.

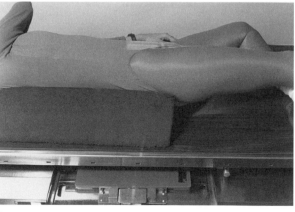

A

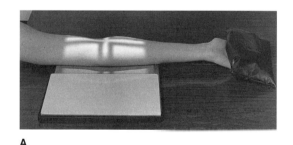

B

Figure 1–6. Sandbags **(A)** and sponges **(B)** can be used to immobilize and support the patient.

GENERAL POSITIONING TERMINOLOGY

Knowledge of specific terminology is required to understand instructions for patient positioning. Positioning terminology is used to describe anatomical planes, the direction of the central ray, movement of the body or body part, and actual patient position *(Table 1–5)*. Other terms are used to describe various projections (direction of travel of the x-ray beam). Please note that the term *lateral* can be used to describe a patient position, a projection, or the relationship between two structures.

Table 1–5. Positioning Terminology

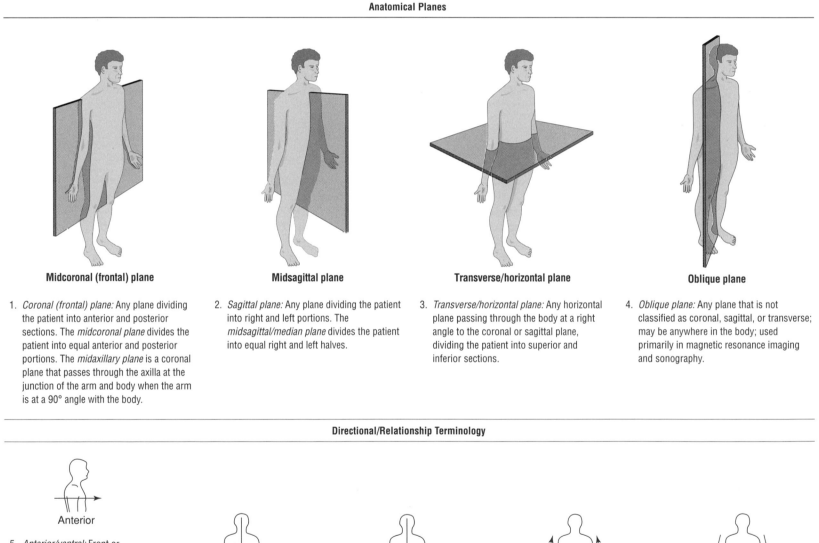

Anatomical Planes

Midcoronal (frontal) plane | **Midsagittal plane** | **Transverse/horizontal plane** | **Oblique plane**

1. *Coronal (frontal) plane:* Any plane dividing the patient into anterior and posterior sections. The *midcoronal plane* divides the patient into equal anterior and posterior portions. The *midaxillary plane* is a coronal plane that passes through the axilla at the junction of the arm and body when the arm is at a 90° angle with the body.

2. *Sagittal plane:* Any plane dividing the patient into right and left portions. The *midsagittal/median plane* divides the patient into equal right and left halves.

3. *Transverse/horizontal plane:* Any horizontal plane passing through the body at a right angle to the coronal or sagittal plane, dividing the patient into superior and inferior sections.

4. *Oblique plane:* Any plane that is not classified as coronal, sagittal, or transverse; may be anywhere in the body; used primarily in magnetic resonance imaging and sonography.

Directional/Relationship Terminology

Anterior

Posterior

Medial | Lateral | Proximal | Distal

5. *Anterior/ventral:* Front or forward aspect of the body or body part.

6. *Posterior/dorsal:* Back part of the body or body part.

7. *Medial/mesial:* Toward the median plane or middle of a part; opposite of lateral (eg, spine is medial to kidneys).

8. *Lateral:* Away from the median plane or middle of a part; opposite of medial (eg, kidneys are lateral to spine).

9. *Proximal:* Parts closest to the point of origin or attachment (eg, elbow is proximal to wrist); opposite of distal.

10. *Distal:* Parts furthest from the point of origin or attachment (eg, fingers are distal to wrist); opposite of proximal.

continued

Table 1–5. Positioning Terminology (continued)

Directional/Relationship Terminology (continued)

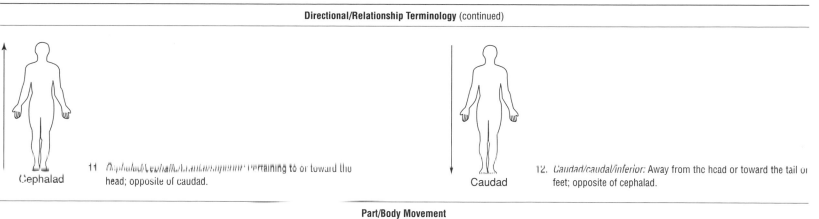

11. *Cephalad/cephalic/superior:* Pertaining to or toward the head; opposite of caudad.

12. *Caudad/caudal/inferior:* Away from the head or toward the tail or feet; opposite of cephalad.

Part/Body Movement

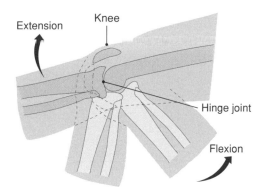

13. *Flexion:* Decrease in the angle of a joint by bending; opposite of extension. *Hyperflexion* is overflexion.
14. *Extension:* Increase in angle of a joint; straightening of a joint; opposite of flexion. *Hyperextension* is extension beyond normal limits.

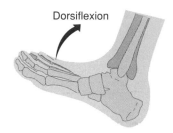

15. *Dorsiflexion:* Flexion between the lower leg and foot so the angle between the two structures is less than or equal to 90°.

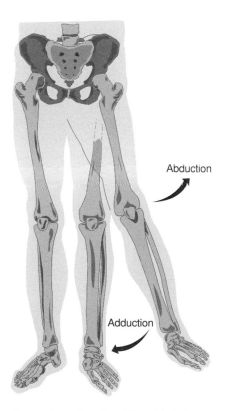

18. *Abduction:* Movement away from the midline of the body or body part; opposite of adduction.
19. *Adduction:* Movement toward the midline of the body or body part; opposite of abduction.

Eversion   **Inversion**

16. *Inversion:* Turning the foot inward at the ankle joint; opposite of eversion.
17. *Eversion:* Turning the foot outward at the ankle joint; opposite of inversion.

continued

Table 1–5. Positioning Terminology (continued)

Part/Body Movement (continued)

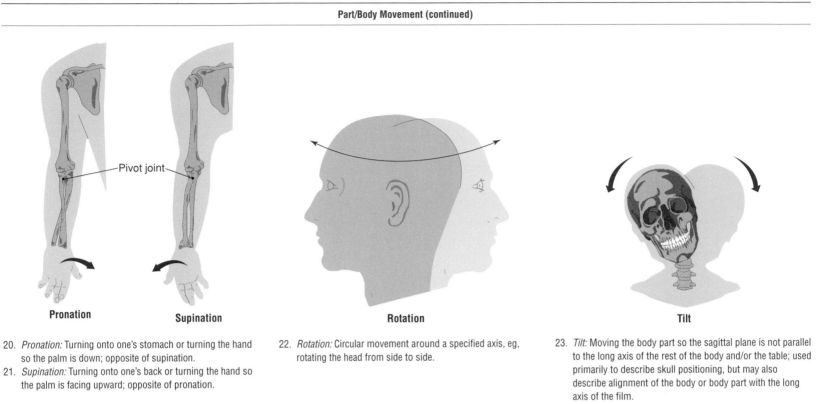

Pronation **Supination**	**Rotation**	**Tilt**

20. *Pronation:* Turning onto one's stomach or turning the hand so the palm is down; opposite of supination.
21. *Supination:* Turning onto one's back or turning the hand so the palm is facing upward; opposite of pronation.

22. *Rotation:* Circular movement around a specified axis, eg, rotating the head from side to side.

23. *Tilt:* Moving the body part so the sagittal plane is not parallel to the long axis of the rest of the body and/or the table; used primarily to describe skull positioning, but may also describe alignment of the body or body part with the long axis of the film.

Positioning Terms

24–37. *Position:* Specific body position or act of placing the patient in the desired position.
28–31. *Oblique:* Patient is rotated between lateral and prone or supine position. Amount of obliquity varies depending on the structure to be demonstrated.
32–34. *Decubitus:* Patient is recumbent. In radiography, this usually implies use of a horizontal beam. It is used to identify air–fluid levels or free air in a body cavity.

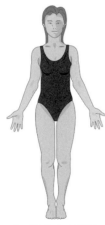

Anatomical position

24. *Anatomical:* Standing, erect position of the body with all anterior surfaces facing forward. Arms are down with palms forward.

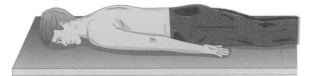

Supine (dorsal recumbent) position.

25. *Supine:* Lying flat on the back.

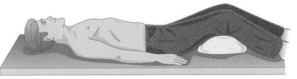

Prone (ventral recumbent) position.

26. *Prone:* Lying face down.

continued

Table 1–5. Positioning Terminology (continued)

Positioning Terms (continued)

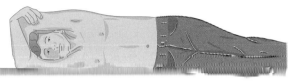

Right lateral recumbent position.

27. *Lateral:* Erect or recumbent position, 90° from true AP or PA.

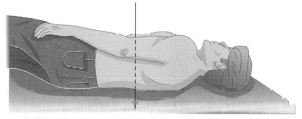

RPO (right posterior oblique) position, AP oblique projection.

28. *Right posterior oblique (RPO):* Right posterior side of the patient is nearest the film; reverse of left anterior oblique.

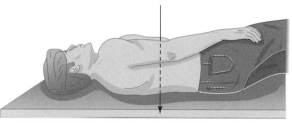

LPO (left posterior oblique) position; AP oblique projection.

29. *Left posterior oblique (LPO):* Left posterior side of the body is nearest the film; reverse of right anterior oblique.

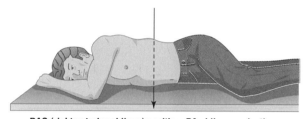

RAO (right anterior oblique) position; PA oblique projection.

30. *Right anterior oblique (RAO):* Right anterior side of the body is nearest the film; reverse of left posterior oblique.

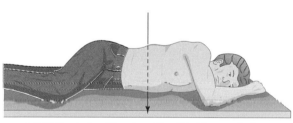

LAO (left anterior oblique) position; PA oblique projection.

31. *Left anterior oblique (LAO):* Left anterior side of the body is nearest the film; reverse of right posterior oblique.

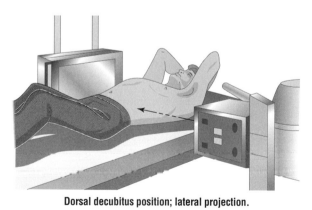

Dorsal decubitus position; lateral projection.

32. *Dorsal decubitus:* Patient is supine with central ray passing horizontally from one side to the other.

continued

Table 1–5. Positioning Terminology (continued)

Positioning Terms (continued)

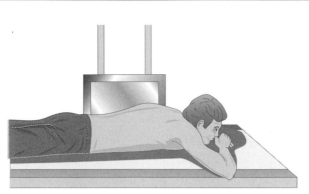

Ventral decubitus position; lateral projection.

33. *Ventral decubitus:* Patient is prone with central ray passing horizontally from one side to the other.

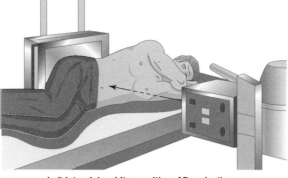

Left lateral decubitus position; AP projection.

34. *Lateral decubitus:* Patient is lying on either right or left side. Central ray travels horizontally either from front to back or back to front. When the patient is lying on left side, it is termed a *left lateral decubitus*.

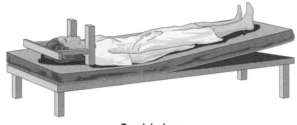

Trendelenburg

35. *Trendelenburg:* Table or bed is positioned so the patient's head is lower than the feet.

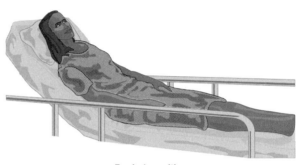

Fowler's position

36. *Fowler's:* Patient's head is elevated. Elevation of 45°–90° may be helpful for patients with respiratory distress.

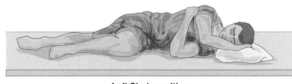

Left Sim's position

37. *Sim's:* A near lateral left anterior oblique (left Sim's) or right anterior oblique with the top leg in front of the lower leg.

Projection Terminology

38–43. *Projection:* Direction the central ray travels through the body. *Note:* The term *view* is only used when discussing a radiographic image; it is the exact opposite of projection.

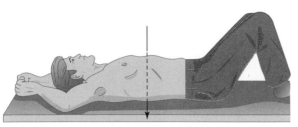

Anteroposterior (AP) projection.

38. *Anterorposterior (AP):* Central ray passes from the anterior to posterior aspect of the body.

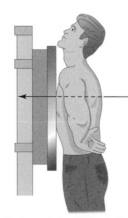

Posteroanterior (PA) projection.

39. *Posteroanterior (PA):* Central ray passes from the posterior to anterior aspect of the body.

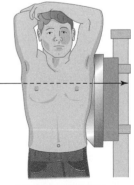

Left lateral projection.

40. *Lateral:* Central ray passes from one side to the other. For head, chest, and abdomen, it is named for the side nearest the film. For limbs, it is named for aspect of structure the central ray entered, then exited (eg, mediolateral).

continued

Table 1–5. Positioning Terminology (continued)

Projection Terminology (continued)

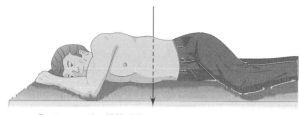

Posteroanterior (PA) oblique projection (RAO position).

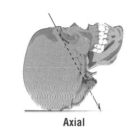

Axial

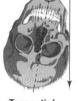

Tangential

41. *Oblique.* Central ray enters at a point between the anterior or posterior surface and the lateral aspect of the body; it exits at the exact opposite side.

42. *Axial:* Longitudinal central ray angle of 10° or more with the long axis of the body or body part.

43. *Tangential:* Central ray touches the structure at one point, skimming it and producing a profile projection.

GUIDELINES FOR USE OF LEAD MARKERS

All radiographs must include patient identification and a marker indicating the patient's right or left side *(Table 1–6)*. Patient identification may include patient name and/or x-ray number, patient age or birth date, date and time of examination, name of patient's physician, and facility name. For medicolegal reasons, patient information and right or left markers should be exposed on the film prior to processing. Other information may include time elapsed since administration of contrast, patient position (eg, upright, prone), or information related to the specific procedure (eg, scout, postevacuation, postvoid) *(Figure 1–7)*.

Table 1–6. Rules for Using Lead Markers

1. Right or left markers *must* be used on *all** films.
2. Markers should be placed on the cassette where they will be clearly seen on the radiograph, while not obscuring required anatomy.
   a. Markers should not be placed over the patient identification blocker.
   b. Markers should be placed within the collimation field.
   c. Markers should be placed away from an area where lead shielding on the patient or table may obscure the markers.
3. Markers must be placed appropriately to identify the *patient's* right or left side.
4. When the extremities and hip or shoulder girdles are being radiographed, markers should be placed on the lateral side of the body part.
5. When one film is being used for two projections of the same body part (eg, PA and oblique right hand), only one of the projections must be marked.
6. If bilateral projections (eg, right and left AP knees) are positioned on one film, both right and left markers should be used to identify the corresponding sides.
7. Auxilliary markers (eg, postevacuation, postvoid, minute markers) should be used whenever possible and positioned away from the critical anatomy.
8. When lateral decubitus projections are performed, a marker indicating the side up should be placed on the upside of the cassette, away from any anatomy of interest.
9. For lateral projections, a marker indicating the side closest to the film should be used.
10. When the spine is being radiographed in the lateral position, markers should be placed on the cassette anterior to the spine to be clearly visualized (not "burned out" or obscured by lead masking on the table behind the patient).
11. When the chest, abdomen, or spine is being radiographed in an oblique position, the side nearest the film is generally marked. For example, when an LPO projection of the lumbar spine is being obtained, a left marker would be placed on the cassette to identify the patient's left side. When both sides are on the film (eg, barium enema or oblique chest), either marker can be used.
    Note: The marker may also be used to identify the anatomical structure(s) seen on the projection. For example, when the LPO position is used to demonstrate the right sacroiliac joint, a right marker could be used. Radiographers should follow department policy when using markers.

*Exception: To prevent superimposition of the marker on critical anatomy, many hospitals have a policy restricting marker use in surgery.

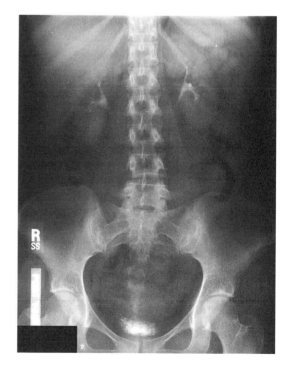

Figure 1–7. Lead *right* and *postvoid* markers were correctly positioned on the cassette prior to exposure.

Table 1–7. General Procedure Protocol

1. Assess examination request and prepare the room.
   a. Thoroughly wash hands.
   b. Collect appropriate-sized cassettes and any other equipment needed for examination (eg, immobilization devices, markers, lead shielding).
   c. Clean the radiographic table or upright unit with appropriate disinfectant.
   d. Position cassette on table or in Bucky tray for first projection.
2. Prepare the patient.
   a. Identify the patient by using a wrist band ID and/or asking the patient to state complete name, birth date, address, or any other information seen on the request form.
   b. Explain the entire procedure to the patient, offering the patient the opportunity to ask questions.
   c. Obtain a pertinent patient history and document per department policy.
   d. Determine pregnancy status (female patients of reproductive age only).
   e. Instruct the patient to remove metallic objects and clothing from the area being examined and put on a patient gown, if necessary.
   f. Assist the patient to the radiographic table, upright grid device, or stool.
   g. Explain any special breathing or procedural instructions to the patient.
   h. Measure the body part.
3. Prepare the equipment.
   Set exposure factors considering the following: Bucky versus tabletop, film-screen speed, part of interest, automatic exposure control versus manual technique, pathology.
4. Position patient and set up equipment.
   a. Accurately position patient for the projection; use appropriate restraints or immobilization devices, if necessary.
   b. Center the central ray to the grid (if Bucky is used) and body part.
   c. Center the cassette to the central ray (this step may be performed before centering the central ray when a table with a floating tabletop is used).
   d. Correctly position lead marker(s) on the cassette.
   e. Shield patient, if it will not compromise examination.
   f. Push Bucky tray in completely, if used.
   g. Recheck exposure factors prior to making exposure.
   h. Give breathing instructions or instruct the patient to hold still; make the exposure.
   i. Repeat components of item 4 for additional projections.
5. Complete postexamination procedure.
   a. Critique radiographs for technical accuracy before dismissing the patient; do not leave patient unattended without adequate safety restraints.
   b. Notify patient of end of procedure and assist patient to the dressing booth, wheelchair, stretcher, or waiting room; release patient per department policy.
   c. Clean radiographic room; change linens and disinfect table and other equipment touched by the patient.
   d. Wash hands thoroughly.

PROCEDURAL PROTOCOL

Each radiographer must establish her or his own protocol for completing a radiographic procedure efficiently. The steps may vary depending on the procedure performed and the condition of the patient. *Table 1–7* suggests how a radiographic procedure can be performed efficiently and effectively.

Although basic guidelines are provided for patient positioning and centering, every student of radiography should remember two important points:

1. There is almost always more than one way to position a patient to achieve the desired view.
2. The primary goal of patient and central ray centering is to project the part of interest into the middle of the collimated area on the film.

Finally, it is important to observe others to learn different techniques and to be creative when trying to position the less than perfect patient.

▶ TECHNICAL CONSIDERATIONS

Knowledge of correct patient positioning and equipment manipulation is not all that is required in the production of quality radiographs. There are several technical factors that the radiographer must be able to control to produce a radiograph in which the anatomical structures can be seen clearly and with good detail *(Figure 1–8)*. The radiographer must be knowledgeable of the factors that contribute to image quality and be able to vary those factors according to patient size, age, and pathologic condition.

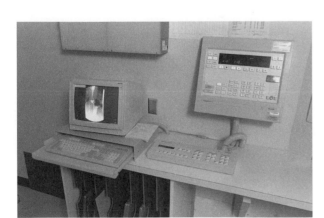

Figure 1–8. Control panel.

IMAGE CHARACTERISTICS

The qualities of a radiograph can be divided into two major categories: (1) the visibility or photographic qualities, which include density and contrast; and (2) the geometric qualities, which include definition or sharpness, magnification, and shape distortion.

Visibility Qualities

Radiographic density refers to the overall blackening of the film, and is controlled by the amount of radiation reaching the film. Three major factors affect radiographic density:

- *Milliampere seconds (mAs).* Milliamperage and exposure time control the quantity of radiation produced, thus controlling the amount reaching the film.
- *Kilovoltage peak (kVp).* Kilovoltage controls the penetration of the radiation. Radiation that is more penetrating will be more likely to pass through the patient and reach the film.
- *Source–image distance (SID).* The distance between the source of radiation and the image receptor is inversely proportional to radiographic density. As the x-ray tube is moved further from the film, the radiation diverges more, resulting in less radiation reaching all areas of the film.

   Radiographic contrast can be described as the density difference between two adjacent areas of a radiograph. A large difference is described as *high contrast, or short scale,* and would appear as a mostly black and white image. Small density differences are described as *low contrast, or long scale,* and would appear as many shades of gray. Radiographic contrast can be divided into subject contrast and film contrast.

   Subject contrast refers to differences in the intensity of areas of the x-ray beam as it exits the patient and is dependent on the following factors:

- *The patient.* The varying densities of tissues in the body will affect how the x-ray beam passes through the patient. For example, radiation penetrates easily through air, but is absorbed more by bone. Areas of anatomy with large differences in tissue densities (such as the chest with air-filled lungs, bone, and heart in the center) will result in a radiograph with high contrast. Anatomical areas with similar tissue densities (such as the abdomen with various organs of similar density) will result in a radiograph with low contrast.
- *kVp.* High kVp will produce an x-ray beam that will penetrate more anatomical structures and record those structures on the film as varying shades of gray. The resultant radiograph will have many shades of gray, or low contrast. Conversely, low kVp will produce a less penetrating beam that will penetrate and record fewer structures on the film. This type of radiograph would demonstrate few shades of gray, or high contrast. For radiography of anatomy with high subject contrast, high kVp can be used to produce a lower-contrast image. (For example, chest radiography is usually performed at 110 to 120 kVp in an effort to produce the lowest radiographic contrast possible for that anatomical area.)

   Film contrast is a characteristic of radiographic film emulsion and is dependent on the type of film used. Radiographic film can be manufactured with low-contrast characteristics, which will result in grayer images, or with high-contrast characteristics, which will result in images that are more black and white.

Geometric Qualities

Recorded detail (sharpness) refers to the ability to recognize anatomical details as being separate and distinct. A radiograph with good sharpness is clear and sharply defined, with no blurriness. The following factors affect sharpness:

- *Focal spot size.* The size of the focal spot affects sharpness. The small focal spot will produce better sharpness than the large focal spot and should be used when the technique permits it.
- *Distances.* The conditions that will produce the greatest sharpness are the longest practical source–image receptor distance (SID) and the shortest possible object–image receptor distance (OID).
- *Motion.* Anytime there is patient motion during an exposure, the radiograph demonstrates poor sharpness because of blurring. Short exposure times, correct patient communication, and use of immobilization devices can help eliminate motion.

   Magnification is a type of distortion causing the anatomical structures on the radiograph to appear larger than the actual anatomy. Magnification should be eliminated as much as possible because it results in poor sharpness. The controlling factor of magnification is the relationship between SID and OID. Any time there is space between the anatomy of interest and the film, there will be magnification; however, an increase in SID can compensate for a large OID and eliminate magnification.

   Shape distortion is the second type of distortion that can be present on a radiograph. This quality is controlled by the alignment of the x-ray beam, the part being examined, and the image receptor. To eliminate shape distortion, the part should be parallel to the film, and the beam should be perpendicular to both *(Figure 1–9).*

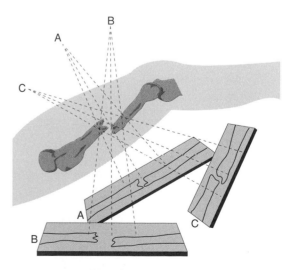

Figure 1–9. To prevent shape distortion, the central ray should be perpendicular to the part and film **(A)**. Failure to do so will result in an inaccurate representation of size and shape **(B,C)**. *(From Cullinan AM, Cullinan JE. Producing Quality Radiographs, 2nd ed. Philadelphia: JB Lippincott; 1994, with permission.)*

Table 1–8. Common Film Sizes and Their Uses

Inches	Centimeters	Example of Use
14 × 17	35 × 43	Chest, abdomen, pelvis, lumbar and thoracic spines
11 × 14	30 × 35	Stomach, pediatric chest or abdomen
10 × 12	24 × 30	Skull, cervical spine, extremities
9 × 9	24 × 24	Sinuses, facial bones, fluoro spots
8 × 10	18 × 24	Sinuses, facial bones, extremities, infants
7 × 17	18 × 43	Femur, lower leg, humerus

EQUIPMENT CONSIDERATIONS

In addition to the technical factors discussed, some equipment items affect the quality of the radiograph. The use of radiographic grids and different film/screen combinations will affect one or more of the qualities previously described.

Film/Screen Combinations

Radiographic film is available in various sizes, the most common of which are listed in *Table 1–8*. The English and metric measurements are similar, but not identical; metric film is slightly smaller than the English equivalents. Even though the film sizes are slightly different, film is often referred to by radiography professionals in terms of the English measurements, even when metric film is actually being used.

Because radiographic film is sensitive to light, it is placed in lightproof cassettes for use during exposures. Inside these cassettes are intensifying screens, which contain crystals that emit light when they are exposed to radiation. This light provides most of the exposure to the film.

The types of film and screens that are used in an imaging system affect both visibility and geometric qualities of a radiograph. The crystals in the screens can be different in terms of chemical composition, size, or layer thickness. These differences affect how much light the screen produces when it is exposed to radiation. A *fast* screen produces more light for a given exposure than a *slow* one, resulting in a radiograph with more density. A fast screen has larger crystals or a thicker layer, causing the light produced from them to be spread out over a larger area. This light spread results in a loss of sharpness. In summary, fast screens result in greater radiographic density, but less sharpness, for a given exposure than slow screens. The choice of which type to use depends on the examination being performed. Most radiology departments have two screen speeds available. In general, the slower screens are used only for nongrid radiography of the extremities, when excellent sharpness of detail is desired. The faster screens are used for all other anatomy.

Radiographic film is also composed of crystals that react to radiation and the light from the intensifying screen. To maximize the efficiency of the imaging system, radiographic film and screens must be matched so that the film is most sensitive to the type of light emitted by the screen.

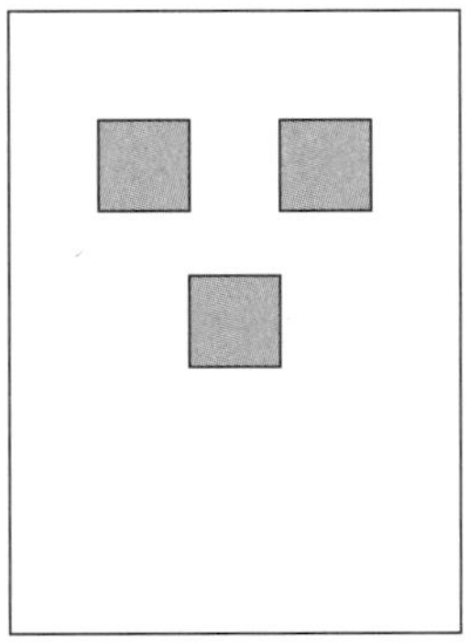

Radiographic Grids

A *radiographic grid* is a device that absorbs scatter radiation exiting the patient, thereby preventing it from reaching the image receptor. *Scatter radiation* is radiation that exits the patient at a different angle than it entered. This radiation provides no diagnostic information to the radiograph. In fact, scatter radiation serves only to add a layer of density (fog) to the image, resulting in a grayer image. A grid is made up of lead strips that, when placed between the patient and the film, absorb this scatter. If scatter radiation is prevented from reaching the film, the resulting radiograph will have less density and higher contrast.

As scatter radiation is produced in the patient, the size of the anatomy of interest determines whether or not a grid should be used. The general rule that is followed provides for the use of a grid on anatomy that measures 10 cm or more, or when the kVp is 70 or above.

Automatic Exposure Control

Automatic exposure control (AEC) is a common method used to provide consistency in radiographic density. An AEC device measures the amount of radiation that reaches the film and automatically ends the exposure when the correct amount is measured. AEC eliminates the need for the radiographer to set a specific exposure time for the examination. There are, however, still several factors that the radiographer must control, including kVp, mA, and photocell selection. The photocells are the actual devices that measure the radiation, and are located and configured in the table as indicated in *Figure 1–10*. The radiographer must make sure to select the photocell(s) that corresponds to the centering of the anatomy of interest, or the ex-

Figure 1–10. Typical configuration of photocells in a general radiographic unit.

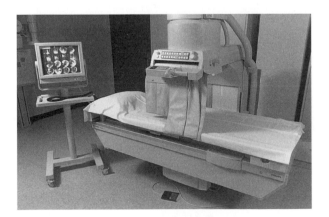

Figure 1–11. Fluoroscopic room.

posure may be too long or too short resulting in a radiograph with poor density; accurate patient centering is a critical factor in producing the optimum density when AEC is used. Photocell selection may be preset for various projections or it may be manually selected by the technologist. Suggestions for photocell selection will be included when appropriate in the radiographic positioning section of each chapter.

RADIOGRAPHIC EQUIPMENT

Radiographic Tables

The tables used in radiography have many features designed to facilitate the radiographic examination. All tables have a space under the tabletop where the Bucky mechanism is located. The Bucky consists of a tray to hold the cassette and a grid positioned above the cassette. This entire mechanism may move up and down the length of the table to correctly position the film. Another feature of the table is its motion capability. Some tables can be tilted from horizontal to raise the patient to a standing position or lower the patient's head during the examination. These tables are most often located in fluoroscopy rooms. Other tables, called *high–low tables,* can be raised or lowered vertically to aid in transfer of the patient onto the table.

The tabletop is an important part of the radiographic table. Because the film is located under the tabletop, it must be completely radiolucent so the radiation can pass directly through it. The tabletop should also be hard, smooth, and difficult to scratch so that body fluids and contrast media do not collect in crevices. The tabletop can also have different motion capabilities. A stationary tabletop does not move at all. For correct centering of anatomy, the patient must be physically moved on the table. Moving tabletops can move up and down the length of the table, and some may also move right or left across the table. Floating tabletops move freely in any direction with the release of a lock. Moving and floating tabletops provide much greater ease of patient positioning because the tabletop can move instead of the patient.

Upright Wall Units

Certain radiographic examinations, such as that of the chest, need to be performed with the patient in an upright position. To facilitate this requirement, some rooms may have upright wall units. These units are mounted on the wall and allow the patient to sit up or stand for the radiographs. Upright units consist of a square or rectangular surface for patient positioning and a Bucky mechanism behind this. Either the whole wall unit or just the Bucky moves up and down to allow for height adjustments.

Fluoroscopic Equipment

To observe dynamic physiologic function, fluoroscopy (fluoro) is needed. In fluoroscopy, the image receptor is a fluorescent screen that emits light when hit by x-ray photons. An image intensifier amplifies the image, converting x-ray photons into visible light so that images can be viewed on a video monitor. Static (still) images can be recorded using a spot film device or camera. Performed primarily by radiologists, fluoroscopy is used for gastrointestinal and some urinary and biliary examinations, as well as special procedures such as myelography, arthrography, and angiography. Radiographic rooms capable of both general radiography and fluoroscopy are commonly referred to as R/F rooms *(Figure 1–11).*

Tomographic Equipment

Tomography is a special type of radiography that uses motion to visualize specific sections, or layers, of anatomy. The motion is used to blur out all structures above and below the area of interest, leaving a clear image of the specified anatomy without superimposition of other structures. During tomography, the x-ray tube and image receptor rotate around a stationary fulcrum. The level of the fulcrum corresponds to the level of the anatomy that is seen on the tomograph. The anatomy at this level is visible because it is always projected to the same place on the film, while anatomy at other levels is blurred across the whole film *(Figure 1–12).* To set the correct fulcrum level, the patient must be measured to determine the depth in the body at which the anatomy of interest is located. This measurement is then used as the initial fulcrum level. Several subsequent tomographs are usually taken at different fulcrum settings to demonstrate different layers of anatomy.

Specialized equipment with the tube and Bucky tray attached to each other is required to perform tomography. This attachment of tube and Bucky is necessary so that their motion can be synchronized and in opposite directions. A conventional radiographic table and tube may be modified by the attachment of a bar connecting them when tomography is needed, or specialized systems specifically designed for tomography are available.

Examinations that use tomography may include excretory urography for visualization of contrast-filled kidneys; various skeletal examinations including those of the wrist, knee, temporomandibular joint,

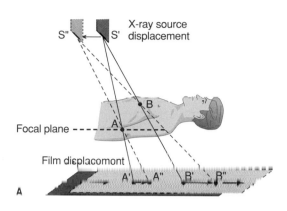

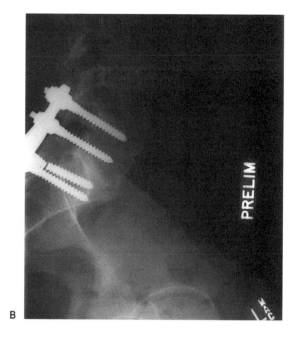

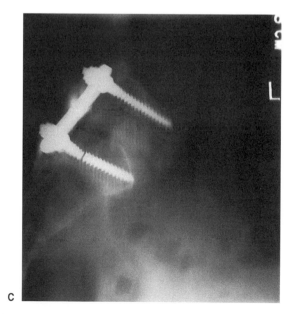

Figure 1–12. With conventional tomography, the image of objects at the level of the focal plane (fulcrum) is fairly sharp, whereas those structures above or below the level of the focal plane are blurred. When the x-ray tube moves a specified distance in one direction, the film moves the same distance in the opposite direction **(A).** Structures at the level of the focal plane stay in the same place on the film and are clearly visible; conventional radiography **(B)** and tomography **(C).** *(Drawing is from Wolbarst AB. Physics of Radiology. Norwalk, CT: Appleton & Lange; 1993, with permission.)*

and cervical spine; and chest tomography for visualization of lung masses. This type of tomography has, to some extent, been replaced by computed tomography (CT).

MOBILE EQUIPMENT

Often, radiographic procedures need to be performed on patients who are unable to come to the radiology department. For these situations, mobile radiography equipment is available. There are two basic types of mobile x-ray units. The standard radiographic unit takes only routine radiographs, such as for chest and abdominal examinations *(Figure 1–13)*. This portable machine can operate on batteries or may need to be plugged into a wall outlet. The other type of mobile unit is a portable C-arm, which is capable of fluoroscopy and radiography. This unit must be plugged into a special type of wall outlet for use. The C-arm is used most often during surgical procedures such as pacemaker insertions, open reductions of fractures, and hip pinnings.

Ancillary Equipment

There are many accessory items that can be used to make a radiographic examination easier for the radiographer to perform or more comfortable for the patient.

Measuring calipers are devices used to measure the thickness of the patient *(Figure 1–14)*. They consist of a measuring scale, a base that slides under the patient, a sliding arm that adjusts to the part thickness, and a measurement indicator. The patient is measured to determine the quantity of radiation needed for the examination.

Sandbags are bags filled with sand or small metal beads that can be used to (1) support the part of the patient that is not in the x-ray beam, (2) hold the body part in position during the x-ray exposure, and/or (3) serve as weights for some specialized examinations. The radiographer should note that sandbags are not radiolucent and should not be placed over anatomy of interest *(Figure 1–15)*.

Positioning sponges are polyurethane foam sponges that are used to cushion and support the patient during radiographic examinations. They are radiolucent and, therefore, will not show up on a radiograph.

Compression bands are wide bands of a radiolucent material that attach to both sides of the table and tighten across the patient. They are used to compress the tissue during certain examinations, to lessen superimposition of structures. They may also be used to aid in immobilization of the patient *(Figure 1–16)*.

Lead masking comes in strips or squares and is used to block x-rays from part of a cassette so that more than one exposure can be made on one cassette. It may also be used as gonadal shielding or to absorb scatter radiation *(Figure 1–17)*.

Cassette holders are designed to hold various cassette sizes for procedures that require the film to be upright with a horizontal x-ray beam, instead of in the Bucky or flat on the tabletop. Cassette holders eliminate the need for a person to hold the cassette during the exposure *(Figure 1–18)*.

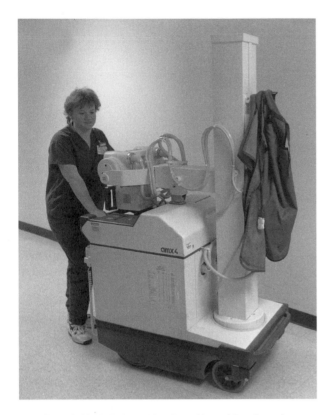

Figure 1–13. Typical portable unit used for mobile radiography.

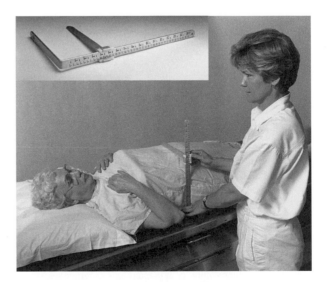

Figure 1–14. A caliper can be used to measure tissue thickness.

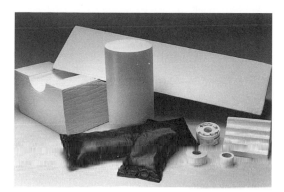

Figure 1–15. Various devices can be used for support and immobilization, including sandbags and sponges.

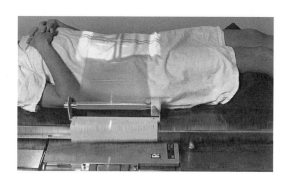

Figure 1–16. A radiolucent compression band can be used to compress abdominal tissue.

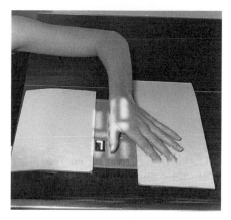

Figure 1–17. Lead masking can be used to shield part of a cassette from scatter radiation that may produce unwanted fog on the film.

► RADIATION PROTECTION

We are exposed daily to various sources of radiation. *Natural background,* or *environmental, radiation* comes from the sun (cosmic), radioactive elements in the earth (terrestrial), and naturally deposited radionuclides in the body (internal) and contributes the most to the population's exposure. On average, *human-made sources of radiation,* such as fallout from nuclear weapons, radioactive materials used in industry, consumer products, and medical/dental exposures, contribute about one-third the background exposure received by the population.

We know from observation and study that radiation can destroy or mutate cells, causing cancer, leukemia, and other pathologic conditions. Depending on which cells are affected, the effects may be *somatic,* affecting the exposed individual, or *genetic,* affecting future generations. If radiation can be damaging, then why is it used?

In radiology, ionizing radiation is used to produce a radiographic image, with the hope that the patient will benefit from the exposure and that a diagnosis can be made or a condition ruled out. Although it is important to remember that any type of radiation can be biologically harmful, we must also put risk from the procedure into perspective. We all take risks every day—crossing the street, driving a car, eating foods that are not good for our bodies. Many people smoke cigarettes, knowing that the primary cause of lung cancer is smoking. Yet, we continue to take these risks. With regard to medical uses of radiation, it is important to evaluate the benefit and risk of performing the procedure. In most cases, the risk from radiography is minimal when compared with the potential benefit of the examination; the ordering of routine chest x-rays for all hospital admissions, preemployment physicals, periodic health examinations, and mass tuberculosis screenings is not recommended.

The radiographer, as a professional who uses ionizing radiation, has two primary responsibilities with regard to radiation protection: to minimize the amount of radiation exposure to patients while producing radiographs of optimum quality and to limit radiation exposure of personnel. Although exposure levels are low, the ultimate goal of the radiographer is to keep radiation exposures *as low as reasonably achievable,* also known as the ALARA concept *(Figure 1–19).*

PATIENT PROTECTION

The radiographer can minimize the amount of radiation a patient receives in a variety of ways.

Elimination of Need for Repeat Radiographs

Anytime a repeat radiograph is required, the patient is receiving an unnecessary, excess amount of radiation. Repeat radiographs are usually attributed to poor patient communication, inaccurate patient positioning, or improper exposure factors. As stated earlier, it is important to make sure the patient understands any directions given. The radiographer must also watch for nonverbal signals that the patient may be unable to

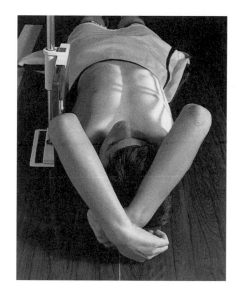

Figure 1–18. A cassette holder is helpful when performing "cross-table" images that require a horizontal beam.

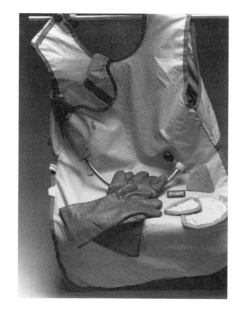

Figure 1–19. Leaded apron, gloves, shields; shadow shield; film badge monitor.

comply with the instructions and make necessary changes to ensure a good radiograph is produced. Immobilization devices should be used as necessary to eliminate voluntary motion on the finished radiograph. If the patient is difficult to position because of condition or pathology, special care must be taken to ensure the desired projection will be obtained. This may take some problem solving and some extra time. *Never* make an exposure unless you are confident that everything possible has been done to produce the desired radiograph. When radiographing very young children, it may be possible to eliminate some projections routinely performed on adults; the radiologist should be consulted prior to modifying any routine radiographic procedure.

Optimum Selection of Exposure Factors

Low kVp is associated with the photoelectric effect, an interaction between an x-ray photon and tissue that results in the absorption of the photon. When photons are absorbed into the tissue, patient dose increases. High-kVp techniques with associated lower mAs, therefore, tend to decrease patient dose. Unfortunately, high kVp also produces a longer scale of contrast (grayer film) and may be inappropriate for some examinations. To minimize patient dose without sacrificing radiographic quality, an appropriate kVp should be selected for the part to be examined. In addition to using the highest appropriate kVp for the examination, an appropriate milliamperage and exposure time (mAs) should be chosen to produce an image with the best density to avoid a repeat radiograph. Improper exposure factors may result in films that are too light or too dark. A light film that has "white" areas has areas of zero information in which pathology may go undetected; these films need repeating. Although dark films can sometimes be salvaged by using the "hot light," they also indicate the patient was overexposed.

▶ *Minimize Patient Dose By*

- *double checking patient positioning and technical factors prior to making an exposure*

- *clearly explaining the procedure to the patient*

- *using a high kVp, low mAs technique whenever doing so will not compromise the procedure*

- *using a high speed film/screen system when it is not necessary to see fine detail*

- *collimating to the area of interest*

- *using gonadal shielding when it does not compromise the examination*

Filtration

When x-rays are produced in the radiographic tube, the resulting beam contains photons of varying energies and wavelengths. The low-energy photons, unfortunately, are not very penetrating and are usually absorbed within the soft tissue of the patient, contributing to patient dose but not to the radiographic image. Radiographic tubes must contain a minimum amount of total filtration (inherent plus added filtration) based on the kVp range for the tube; radiographic and fluoroscopic tubes capable of operating above 70 kVp must have a minimum of 2.5 mm Al equivalent. This filtration removes the low-energy photons from the beam, thereby reducing patient dose.

Appropriate Selection of Image Receptors

Rare earth intensifying screens with matched photographic emulsions have varying relative speeds, up to 12 times those of a comparable calcium tungstate film/screen system. When higher-speed film/screen systems are used, exposure factors can be reduced, thus reducing patient dose. Although lower-speed systems are often used for detail examinations, such as fingers, hands, and wrists, higher-speed systems generally produce acceptable images for other parts of the body, resulting in a lower patient exposure. Although the routine for a specific body part may call for a low-speed film/screen system, follow-up studies and some pediatric examinations may be performed using higher-speed systems to reduce patient dose.

Collimation

The use of collimation can significantly reduce patient exposure, as well as improve radiographic quality. At the very least, collimation should be to film size; collimating to the part of interest further reduces patient exposure.

Protective Shielding

Because the embryo/fetus and children of any age are more susceptible to the effects of radiation, gonadal shields should routinely be used on children and adults of reproductive age. As a general rule of thumb, gonadal shielding should be used anytime the gonads are within or near (5 cm or 2 in.) the collimated field unless doing so will compromise the examination and require a repeat exposure. A shadow shield can be used to shield the breasts of young women having scoliosis series completed or as a gonadal shield when a contact shield cannot be used.

Learning a skill or set of skills is about learning good habits. Although the guidelines for shielding patients relate primarily to children and those capable of reproduction, the radiographer who provides gonadal shields for all patients on a routine basis will never have to worry about causing potentially damaging genetic effects.

Management of Potentially Pregnant Patients

During the first trimester, especially the first 2 months, the embryo is at its greatest risk for congenital abnormalities. Unfortunately, this is also a time when the mother may not know she is pregnant. Prior to exposing a female patient between the ages of 11 and 50, therefore, the radiographer must assess whether she could possibly be pregnant. Asking the patient for the date of the first day of the last menstrual period and subsequent questions regarding birth control measures, if necessary, will help determine pregnancy status. If the patient is pregnant, the patient, radiologist, and patient's physician should determine whether to proceed with the examination. When the decision is made to proceed with the study, maximum collimation, careful gonadal shielding, and high-kVp techniques should be employed; abdominal studies, such as an intravenous pyelogram (IVP), may be modified to reduce the number of radiographs obtained. Radiography should be performed on a pregnant woman only when the benefits outweigh the risks.

PERSONNEL PROTECTION

All radiation workers should follow the primary rules of radiation protection: time, distance, and shielding. The *time* the radiation worker is exposed to radiation should be kept to a minimum. The *distance* between the source of radiation and radiation worker should be maximized. Doubling the distance from the source decreases exposure to one-fourth its value at the initial distance. Increasing distance from 2 to 4 ft, therefore, can significantly reduce one's exposure. *Protective shielding* should always be positioned between the source and the radiographer. This shielding may be in the walls, built into the equipment, and/or worn as protective lead apparel, such as an apron, gloves, thyroid shield, and leaded glasses.

Unlike the case for patients, the dose that a radiation worker receives is monitored using a personnel monitor such as a film badge, thermoluminescent dosimeter (TLD), or pocket ionization chamber. Personnel monitors are worn either at the collar level outside any protective apparel or at waist level under protective apparel, depending on institutional and state guidelines. Wearing the monitor at the collar level provides a way to estimate eye and thyroid dose and effective dose equivalency. For comparison, all personnel at any one institution should wear their monitors in the same place. To prevent false readings, the monitor should also be worn so the front faces the source of the radiation. When not in use, radiation monitors should be stored in a safe place within the department, away from possible irradiation. The dose equivalent limit for the radiation worker is 5 rem per year *(Table 1–9)*.

The Pregnant Radiographer

It is the responsibility of the pregnant radiographer to inform her supervisor as soon as she suspects she is pregnant. The supervisor should review the radiographer's radiation exposure history with her. A second monitor will be worn under any protective apparel to more closely estimate the embryo/fetal dose. The dose equivalent limit for the embryo/fetus is 0.5 rem for the gestational period. In normal circumstances, the radiographer's exposure, with the film badge at the collar level outside the lead apron, is very low and the estimated embryo/fetal dose is extremely small. When possible, the radiographer should avoid fluoroscopy and mobile radiography.

▶ *Current Dose Equivalent Limits*

- *Occupational exposures* (annual)   *5 rem*
- *Public exposures (annual)*
  - *Frequent exposure*   *.1 rem*
  - *Infrequent exposure*   *.5 rem*
- *Education/training exposures*   *.1 rem* (annual)
- *Embryo/fetus exposures*   *.5 rem*

From NCRP Report No. 105, 1989.

Table 1–9. Units of Radiation Measurement

roentgen (coulomb/kg)	Describes the measurement of radiation exposure in air
rad (gray)	Describes the amount of radiation energy absorbed in a medium (tissue)
rem (seivert)	Describes occupational exposure; it is a unit of dose equivalence, taking into consideration the biological effects of various types of ionizing radiations
curie (becquerel)	Describes the amount of radioactivity emitted from a radioactive source; term used in nuclear medicine

Various terms are used to describe the quantity of radiation or radioactivity; the traditional units are italicized and the international units (SI) are in parentheses. Each is used in specific situations. Although it is not true for all types of ionizing radiation, the roentgen, rad, and rem are considered equal in diagnostic radiology.

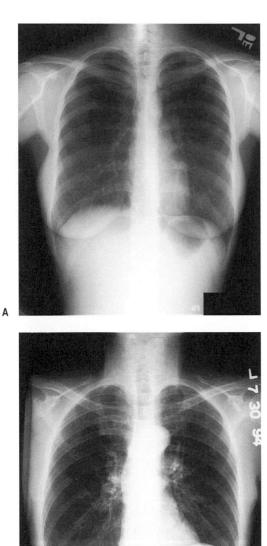

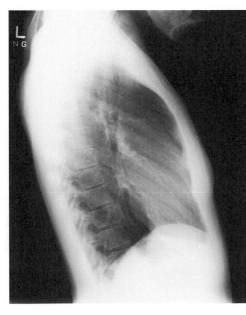

Figure 1–20. Correctly displayed PA **(A)**, AP **(B)**, and lateral **(C)** projections of the chest.

▶ IMAGE EVALUATION & FILM CRITIQUE

The ability to critique one's own radiographs for appropriate patient positioning, technique selection, and radiation protection is a required skill of any radiographer. To evaluate patient positioning, the radiographer must know what anatomy should be demonstrated on the projection. The ability to see well-defined, detailed structures is important when evaluating the selection of technical factors. Adequate collimation, appropriate exposure factors, and shielding (if appropriate) are all important components of radiation protection.

FILM DISPLAY

Before the radiographer can critique a radiographic image, however, the film must be "hung" on the viewbox. Images should be displayed as if looking at the front of the patient. The right marker on the film, therefore, should be on the radiographer's left side, regardless of how the patient was positioned. For example, both PA and AP chest radiographs are displayed so the patient's right side is on the radiographer's left side. Lateral projections are displayed as if the radiographer is looking at the patient in the actual position. For example, the radiograph of a patient positioned for a left lateral chest film is displayed so the anterior side of the patient is on the radiographer's right side *(Figure 1–20)*.

Hanging extremity radiographs is often confusing to the student radiographer. Again, the images should be displayed as if looking at the front of the standing patient. Consistently placing markers on the lateral side of the part will help. In general, any time the fingers or toes are normally demonstrated on a projection, the film is hung so the fingers or toes point upward (fingers, hand, wrist, foot, toes). Although the fingers are not necessarily seen on radiographs of the forearm, these too are usually displayed with the fingers pointing upward. Radiographs of all other extremities are displayed with the hand or foot pointing downward.

SYSTEMATIC EVALUATION

To avoid overlooking incorrect patient information, right or left marker, or other radiographic detail, a systematic method of film evaluation is a critical procedural component. Although the exact procedure can be tailor-made to the individual, it should include an assessment of correct patient and projection identification, adequate radiation protection, accurate patient positioning, centering, and tube/part/film alignment, critical anatomy demonstrated, patient preparation, and image quality.

Film Identification
- Is the correct patient identification on the film?
- Is the film correctly marked with lead markers (right/left, postvoid, etc)

Radiation Protection
- Was the maximum amount of collimation used without compromising the examination?
- Is there evidence of gonadal shielding, if appropriate?

Patient Positioning
- By looking at the radiograph, determine how the patient's body or body part was positioned. Was the actual patient positioning accurate?
- Was the central ray correctly centered to the part?
- Was the central ray correctly angled (if appropriate)?
- Was the film correctly centered to the part and central ray?

Radiographic Quality
- Do the density and contrast allow for maximum visibility of recorded detail in the radiographic image?
- Were appropriate tube/part/film alignment and SID used to minimize unwanted distortion (size or shape)?
- Are there artifacts that detract from or obscure anatomical structures?

Anatomy
- Each projection is performed to evaluate specific anatomical structures. What is the critical anatomy that should be demonstrated on the projection and is it adequately visualized (considering patient positioning, centering, collimation, and technique selection)?

► RELATED IMAGING MODALITIES

In addition to routine diagnostic radiography, several other imaging modalities can be used for diagnosis. These modalities may either supplement or replace routine radiography. The radiographer should have a basic understanding of these imaging methods and be able to respond to basic questions a patient may have.

COMPUTED TOMOGRAPHY

Computed tomography, also called *CT* or *CAT scanning,* is a special tomographic technique used to produce cross-sectional images of slices of tissue. Through use of an x-ray tube or tubes and special radiation detectors, CT produces sectional images that permit differentiation between various soft tissues and is used to image the brain, thorax, abdomen, spine, and extremities. Examinations of the brain, thorax, and abdomen are often performed following the intravenous, oral, and/or rectal administration of contrast medium *(Figure 1–21).* Because it can differentiate between fresh and old blood intracranially, CT is often used to image the brain in emergency situations, such as stroke and subdural hematoma. Although older equipment may take 20 to 60 minutes to complete a study, spiral CT scanners can complete an examination in a matter of a few minutes.

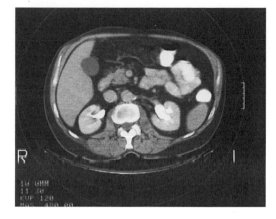

Figure 1–21. Transverse sectional CT image of the abdomen following the intravenous and oral administration of contrast medium.

MAGNETIC RESONANCE IMAGING

The newest imaging modality, magnetic resonance imaging or MRI, does not use ionizing radiation. Although it uses a computer and produces cross-sectional images similar to CT, it uses a strong magnetic field, pulsed radio waves, and the nuclei of the hydrogen atoms in the body to construct images. With MRI, very small structures can be imaged quickly and there is good contrast resolution between tissues. Muscles, vessels, organs, and other tissues, such as ligaments and tendons, can be easily visualized. Although MRI does not image bone, the bone marrow within the bone can be seen *(Figure 1–22).*

For the examination, the patient must be positioned so the part of interest is in the middle of the magnet, which generally looks like a long, narrow tunnel (some lower-strength magnets have larger openings). The examination usually lasts 45 minutes to 1 hour, but may last longer. During this time, the patient must hold still and endure a loud knocking noise. Because a strong magnet is used, not all patients are candidates for this examination. MRI is contraindicated for patients with cardiac pacemakers, aneurysm clips within the skull, or metallic foreign bodies in the eyes. In addition, patients who are claustrophobic may not be able to lie in the "tunnel" for the time required. Currently, there are no known biological hazards.

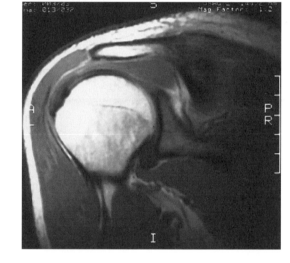

Figure 1–22. Damage to soft tissue structures within the shoulder joint is often evaluated using MRI.

DIAGNOSTIC MEDICAL SONOGRAPHY (ULTRASOUND)

Another imaging modality that is frequently used is diagnostic medical sonography, often called ultrasound. Sonography stems from the use of SONAR during World War II, when sound waves were used to locate submarines. Because of the properties of sound, sonography can differentiate between solid and fluid-filled structures (sound passes through fluid and is reflected back from solid structures). Because ultrasound does not use ionizing radiation, it is considered safe and is the modality of choice for pregnant women and children, whenever possible. It is also used to evaluate the biliary and urinary systems, other intra- and retroperitoneal structures, vessels, and the heart *(Figure 1–23).* Because air, bone, and barium act as acoustic barriers, sonography has some limitations. For example, air-filled structures of the gastrointestinal system may prohibit evaluation of structures beneath them.

NUCLEAR MEDICINE

In diagnostic radiography, x-rays are produced in a special tube and directed toward the patient. In nuclear medicine, a *radionuclide,* or radiation-emitting material, is administered to the patient either intravenously or by ingestion or inhalation. Based on the type of tracer used and the type of metabolic activity, the radioactive material localizes in specific areas. A special radiation detector, called a *gamma camera,* mea-

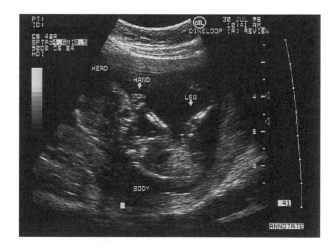

Figure 1–23. Fetal sonogram obtained approximately 15 weeks postconception. *(Courtesy of Peggy Neal (RDMS) and Stephanie Wetherell.)*

sures the amount of gamma radiation coming from the patient; the results are displayed as static images that reflect the amount of isotope activity within the organ or tissue. An unusual intensity may indicate the presence of a tumor or other pathology. Although the resolution is relatively poor when compared with other types of imaging, it can be used to assess the function of various systems and for the early detection of diseases; allergic or toxic reactions are rare. Nuclear medicine studies are done for the thyroid, bones, lungs, kidneys, liver, spleen, heart, and brain. The examinations can be fairly lengthy, often requiring delayed images *(Figure 1–24).*

$\mathcal{S}$UMMARY

- ▶ The Code of Ethics for the radiologic technologist addresses the qualities and characteristics of a professional working in radiography.

- ▶ To provide quality patient care, the radiographer must consider the psychological and emotional needs of the patient, in addition to the physical needs.

- ▶ Effective communication is important to patient care and the production of quality radiographs; it includes both verbal and unspoken messages.

- ▶ Personal attitudes may affect behavior, which may ultimately affect patient care.

- ▶ The approach the radiographer takes toward the pediatric patient can be a significant factor in the degree of cooperation received.

- ▶ One of the primary concerns when radiographing a neonate is prevention of hypothermia.

- ▶ As with children, older patients should be individually assessed and should not be stereotyped.

- ▶ Thorough handwashing and good housekeeping practices help prevent the transmission of disease.

- ▶ Health care workers should treat all patients as if they have a communicable disease, using appropriate precautions whenever there is a possibility of contact with blood or body fluids.

- ▶ When a patient is known or suspected of having a communicable disease, special precautions are followed relative to the specific disease or category of isolation.

- ▶ The term *habitus* is used to describe the shape, size, muscle tone, and position of internal organs in the body; the four general classifications are hypersthenic, sthenic, hyposthenic, and asthenic.

- ▶ Special imaging techniques, such as computed tomography, magnetic resonance imaging, and ultrasound, allow us to image sections or slices of the body in various planes (sagittal, coronal, transverse/axial, and oblique).

- ▶ For most radiographic examinations, a minimum of two projections, 90° apart, are needed to demonstrate structures that may otherwise be superimposed and not visualized; at least three projections are needed to demonstrate all angles and surfaces of joints.

- ▶ Positioning terminology is used to describe anatomical planes, direction of the central ray, anatomical relationships, part or body movement, patient position, and radiographic projections.

- ▶ A lead right or left marker should be appropriately placed on the cassette prior to exposure.

- ▶ The establishment of a procedural routine improves efficiency.

- ▶ The visible or photographic qualities of the radiograph include radiographic density and contrast.

- ▶ Recorded detail (sharpness) refers to the ability to recognize anatomical details and is affected by focal spot size, object–image distance, source–image distance, and patient motion.

- ▶ Faster screens are used when excellent sharpness of detail is not required; slower screens produce greater sharpness and are generally preferred when visibility of fine detail is needed.

- ▶ Radiographic grids, used to produce a higher radiographic contrast, are recommended whenever the part measures 10 cm or more or when 70 kVp or more is used.

- ▶ Radiographic tables may turn from the horizontal to the vertical position, may be raised and lowered in the horizontal position, and may have either a stationary, moving, or floating tabletop.

- ▶ Tomographic equipment uses motion to visualize sections of anatomy.

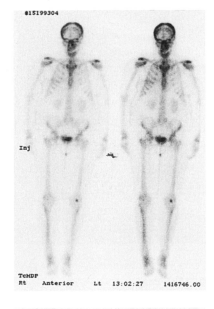
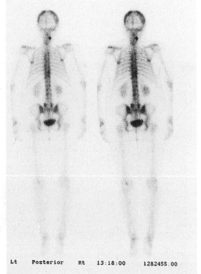

Figure 1–24. A nuclear medicine bone scan can be performed to assist in diagnosis of fractures, tumors, or other pathology of the skeletal system.

► Mobile equipment is used to image patients away from the radiology department and is capable of producing routine radiographs and/or fluoroscopy (C-arm).

► As a component of any radiation protection program, x-rays should be used only when the benefit outweighs any risk of irradiation.

► Ionizing radiation can destroy or mutate cells, affecting the exposed individual (somatic effects) or future generations (genetic effects).

► The radiographer can minimize patient dose by reducing the number of repeat radiographs, selecting optimum exposure factors, ensuring that the minimum amount of filtration is used, using high-speed film/screen systems when possible, maximizing collimation (reducing field size), and using gonadal shielding routinely.

► Radiation workers minimize occupational exposure by reducing the amount of time exposed to radiation, maximizing the distance between the source of radiation and the worker, and maximizing the amount of shielding between the radiation source and worker.

► Occupational radiation workers are monitored using a film badge, thermoluminescent or pocket dosimeter, ionization chamber; their annual dose equivalent limit is 5 rem.

► The pregnant radiographer may continue working; however, her exposure history should be reviewed and assignments may be modified to limit fluoroscopy and mobile radiography. The dose equivalent limit for the embryo/fetus is 0.5 rem for the gestational period.

► Radiographs should be displayed on the viewbox as if looking at the front of the patient; the right marker should be on the radiographer's left side.

► A systematic film evaluation should include verification of correct film identification, assessment of appropriate collimation, analysis of patient positioning and radiographic quality, and identification of critical anatomy demonstrated.

► Computed tomography, ultrasound, nuclear medicine, and magnetic resonance imaging are often used to supplement or replace routine diagnostic radiography.

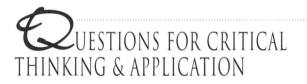

QUESTIONS FOR CRITICAL THINKING & APPLICATION

1. After observing health professionals as they care for patients, identify those behaviors that would be considered professional and those considered unprofessional. Discuss how the unprofessional behaviors should be changed.

2. You must obtain PA and lateral chest projections on a 2½-year-old child who is kicking and screaming. Discuss how you will proceed to obtain quality films.

3. A patient who is in isolation because of an infected abdominal wound must come to the department for a barium enema. Describe the procedure you will follow to minimize the risk of contaminating the equipment, other personnel, and yourself.

4. Following fluoroscopy, the radiologist requests a PA projection of the patient's entire large intestine. A quick assessment of the patient tells you that the patient is hypersthenic. Describe how you will fulfill the radiologist's request.

5. The patient is lying on her left side with a grid cassette supported vertically behind her abdomen; the central ray is directed horizontally and perpendicular to the middle of the cassette. Name the projection.

6. A PA chest radiograph was taken on an elderly male patient who had an enlarged heart (cardiomegaly). Automatic exposure control was used with a kilovoltage setting of 90 kVp. Although the density of the lungs was acceptable, the heart was underpenetrated. Describe how you would improve the radiographic quality.

7. Knee x-rays have been ordered on an unconscious patient. Identify the ancillary equipment you could use to immobilize the leg for the AP projection and describe how you would use that equipment.

8. A 1-year-old child fell down steps and injured his arm; radiographs of his entire arm have been requested. The department routine indicates that, for the adult patient, hand, wrist, forearm, elbow, and

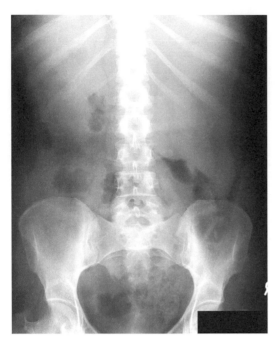

Figure 1–25.

humerus studies should be performed separately. In addition, both obliques should be obtained of each joint. You are concerned about the radiation exposure to the patient. Describe how you would proceed.

9. It is your turn to assist the radiologist in fluoroscopy. The patient is fairly agile and does not need help moving on the table. Describe the measures you would take to minimize your exposure to radiation.

10. Which of the related imaging modalities do not use ionizing radiation? What do they use instead to obtain an image?

11. What general information can a transverse (axial) CT image of the abdomen provide that would not be demonstrated on a routine AP projection?

Film Critique

Evaluate this abdominal radiograph (Figure 1–25). Is it correctly displayed?

Is the lead marker placed appropriately?

How did you determine this?

Is the part of interest in the middle of the collimation field?

How would you describe the radiographic contrast of this image?

2

RESPIRATORY SYSTEM

► OBJECTIVES.

Following the completion of this chapter the student will be able to:

- Name and identify on a drawing the structures constituting the respiratory system.

- Trace the path of oxygen and carbon dioxide through the respiratory system during inhalation and exhalation.

- Identify the skeletal landmarks associated with certain structures of the respiratory system.

- Define the terminology associated with the respiratory system, to include anatomy, procedures, and pathology.

- Describe the process for obtaining and simulate the positioning for routine and nonroutine chest radiographs.

- List and describe the type and size of film holder, central ray location, and structures best demonstrated on routine and nonroutine projections of the chest.

- Evaluate radiographs of the chest in terms of positioning, centering, image quality, and radiographic anatomy.

- Identify technical changes necessary to compensate for various pathologic conditions of the chest.

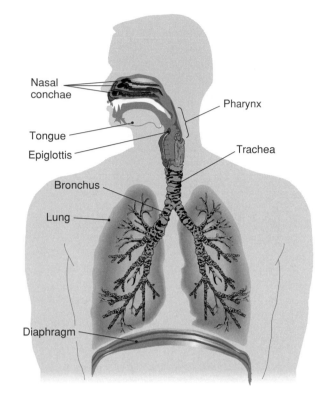

Figure 2–1. Components of the respiratory system.

Table 2–1. Progression of Air Through the Structures of the Respiratory System

Nasal and mouth cavities	Take in and warm air
Pharynx	Functions in both respiratory and digestive systems to convey air to lungs and foods fluids to esophagus
Larynx	Voicebox
Trachea	Windpipe
Bronchi	Trachea branches at T4–5 into right and left primary bronchi
Bronchioles	Smaller branches off of bronchi in lungs
Alveoli	Millions of air sacs in lungs
Lung capillaries	Small blood vessels in close contact with alveoli; function in exchange of gases

The respiratory system is responsible for performing two vital functions for the body: making oxygen available and removing carbon dioxide, a waste product. The organs or structures that are directly responsible for these functions include the nasal cavities, pharynx, larynx, trachea, bronchi, and lungs *(Figure 2–1, Table 2–1)*.

The routine examination used for evaluating the respiratory system is the chest x-ray. The chest x-ray is the most frequently performed radiographic examination and is also one that can be difficult to interpret. Accurate patient positioning and technical factor selection are integral to accurate diagnosis.

▶ ANATOMY OF THE RESPIRATORY SYSTEM

The process of respiration provides the body with oxygen needed for cell survival. Exchange of gases (air and waste products) takes place in the lungs as well as at a cellular level. The respiratory system is designed to bring oxygen-rich air into the body and at the same time rid the body of carbon dioxide. The cardiovascular system assists the respiratory system in the exchange of oxygen and carbon dioxide.

The four main structures of the respiratory system are the pharynx, trachea, bronchi, and lungs. Each plays a vital role in the function of the respiration system. These and other related structures are discussed in detail.

Initially, air is taken in through the mouth and nose. Both of these structures, and in particular the nose, warm and moisten the air before it passes into the lungs. In addition, the nasal cavities filter out dirt from the environment.

PHARYNX

The pharynx (FAR-ingks), or throat, functions in both the respiratory and digestive systems for the passage of air, fluids, and food. This passageway is approximately 3.9 in. (10 cm) long and is divided into three parts, which are named according to their location *(Figure 2–2)*.

Nasopharynx

The nasopharynx is located posteriorly to the two nasal cavities. It is also superior and posterior to the soft palate, which acts to close off the nasopharynx during the act of swallowing. This prohibits food from being regurgitated into the nasal cavities. The right and left eustachian (auditory) tubes open into the nasopharynx. These structures serve as canals between the middle ears and pharynx to equalize pressure on the eardrums. The pharyngeal tonsils (adenoids) of the lymphatic system are found in the nasopharynx. The uvula, a small piece of tissue suspended from the soft palate, has a supporting role in speech and sound production. It indicates the end of the nasopharynx and the beginning of the oropharynx.

Oropharynx

This division of the pharynx is located behind the mouth. The palatine tonsils, which are part of the lymphatic system, are found between the mouth and the oropharynx and function to protect the respiratory system by filtering out various pathogens in the environment that enter the respiratory tract. The epiglottis is a small leaf-shaped flap of cartilage found at the distal end of the oropharynx at the top of the larynx. This structure is discussed more fully with the larynx.

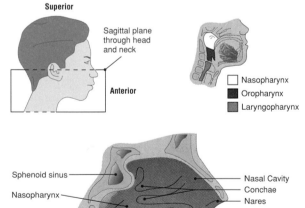

Figure 2–2. The pharynx.

Laryngopharynx

This third division of the pharynx is located inferiorly to the epiglottis. It extends from the hyoid bone to the esophagus. The hyoid bone is a small horseshoe-shaped bone located at the base of the tongue in the anterior neck. It is situated slightly above the thyroid cartilage and provides attachment for the muscles of the tongue and mouth.

LARYNX

The larynx (LAR-ingks) or voicebox is a boxlike cartilaginous structure. It is located in the anterior portion of the neck between C-3 and C-6 and is approximately 2 in. (5 cm) long. Nine cartilages compose the box or frame of the larynx. The most prominent cartilage is known as the **thyroid cartilage** or Adam's apple. It is an important positioning landmark as it is located approximately at the level of the fifth cervical vertebra. The radiographer will notice that the thyroid cartilage is more prominent in male patients than it is in female patients.

The **cricoid cartilage** is a ring of cartilage that forms the inferior margin of the larynx and attaches to the trachea by ligaments. This structure is significant, as tracheostomies are performed just below this point.

The **epiglottis** is located on the top of the larynx. This leaf-shaped flap of cartilage forms a lid over the glottis (laryngeal opening) during swallowing. When the epiglottis covers the opening, food and fluids pass into the esophagus instead of the trachea.

The **glottis** is a slitlike opening between the horizontal folds of the mucous membrane of the larynx. The upper pair of folds form the false vocal cords; the true vocal cords are formed by the lower folds. Sound is produced as air passes through the opening and vibrates the true vocal cords. Contraction of muscles of the face, mouth, lips, and pharynx changes the shape of the opening, which in turn changes the pitch of the sounds *(Figure 2–3)*.

TRACHEA

In layman's terms, the trachea (TRĀ-kē-ah) is known as the windpipe. This hollow tube is approximately 1 in. (2 to 2.5 cm) in diameter and 4 in. (10 to 11 cm) long. It is located anteriorly to the esophagus in the mediastinum and extends from the level of the sixth cervical vertebra to the fourth or fifth thoracic vertebra. The trachea is kept open by the rigid support provided by approximately 16 to 20 "C"-shaped rings of cartilage encircling the front and side walls, along with fibrous connective tissue. The open portions of the C-rings face the esophagus. When a bolus of food is swallowed, the esophagus can expand into the smooth muscular wall of the posterior tracheal wall *(Figure 2–4)*.

BRONCHI

At the approximate level of the fourth or fifth thoracic vertebra, the trachea bifurcates into the right and left primary bronchi (BRONG-kī) (singular, *bronchus*). A ridge of cartilage found at the lower end of the trachea where it branches into the bronchi is known as the **carina.** This structure is an important reference point in the placement of an endotracheal tube, which is used to assist a patient with breathing.

The primary or main-stem bronchi convey air into and out of the right and left lungs. The right primary bronchus is wider, shorter, and more vertical than the left bronchus; therefore, foreign bodies entering the airway are more likely to pass into and perhaps lodge on this side. The right bronchus branches into three smaller secondary bronchi, whereas the left bronchus branches into two secondary bronchi, corresponding respectively to the lobes in the lungs. In each lung, the secondary or lobar bronchi branch into smaller bronchi called bronchioles. This continuous branching from the trachea to the terminal bronchioles forms the bronchial tree *(Figure 2–5)*. As the bronchi branch into smaller tubes, the amount of cartilage in the structures decreases with a corresponding increase in the amount of smooth muscle. There is a complete absence of cartilage in the terminal bronchioles. The clinical significance of this is seen in asthma. This condition results in muscle spasms that can block off the air passages because there is no cartilage to support and keep them open.

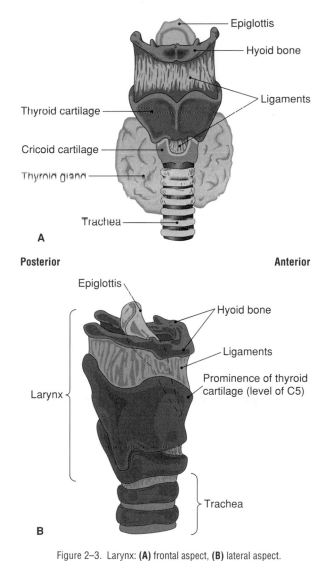

Figure 2–3. Larynx: **(A)** frontal aspect, **(B)** lateral aspect.

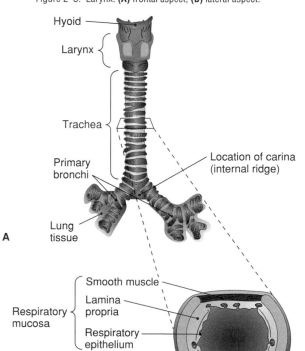

Figure 2–4. Trachea: **(A)** frontal aspect, **(B)** cross section.

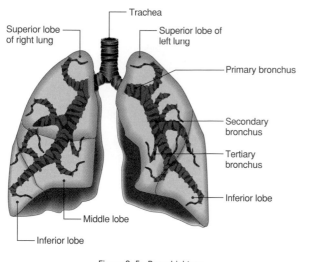

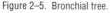

Figure 2–5. Bronchial tree.

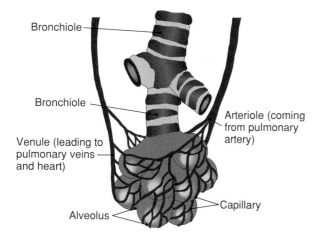

Figure 2–6. Relationship between the alveoli and capillaries.

ALVEOLI

At the termination of the branching are clusters of small air sacs called alveoli (al-VĒ-ō-lī) (singular, *alveolus*). These air sacs have very thin walls and are in close contact with the capillaries of the cardiovascular system. The alveoli are functional units within the lungs because the exchange of O_2 and CO_2 takes place between them and the surrounding capillaries. There are millions of alveoli in each lung *(Figure 2–6)*.

LUNGS

The paired lungs are located in the thoracic cavity on either side of the mediastinum. Each lung is a cone-shaped structure. The upper rounded end situated above the clavicles is called the **apex** (plural, *apices*); the broad, inferior end is called the **base.** The surface of the base is concave to rest over the convex surface of the diaphragm. The costal surface of the lungs is gently rounded and lies against the ribs. The **hilum** or **hilus** (plural, *hila* or *hili*) is a vertical depression or slit on the medial aspect of each lung where the primary bronchi, pulmonary vessels, lymphatic vessels, and nerves enter and leave the lungs. This area constitutes the lung root. Although the lungs are freely movable in the thoracic cavity, they do not move in the area of the lung roots.

The costophrenic angles are formed on the lateral lower aspects of each lung where it sits on the **diaphragm** (cost/o = rib, phren/o = diaphragm). The **cardiac notch** or angle is found on the inferior, medial aspect of the left lung. It is a concavity caused by the border of the heart resting against the lung. Because the liver pushes up on the diaphragm, the right lung is shorter and broader than the left. Horizontal and oblique fissures divide the right lung into three lobes; the left lung is divided into two lobes by the oblique fissure. These fissures are grooves that are sometimes evident on radiographs of the chest. The lobes of each lung are further divided into lobules, which include bronchioles and alveolar sacs.

The lungs and thoracic cavity are both covered with a membrane called the **pleura.** This is a double fold of serous membrane, with the inner visceral pleura lying adjacent to the lungs and the parietal pleura being closest to the ribs and lining the thoracic cavity. A small space between these two folds contains a lubricating fluid that prevents friction during the movements of respiration. The presence of air or other fluids in this space causes this space to become apparent on a radiograph.

The tissue composition of the lungs is a spongy, elastic material known as **parenchyma.** The characteristics of lung parenchyma allow for expansion and contraction during respiration *(Figure 2–7)*.

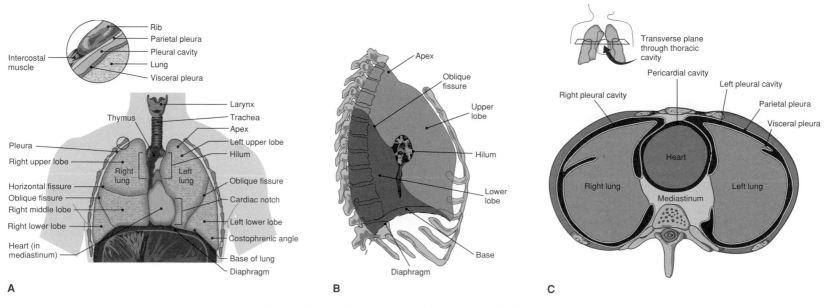

Figure 2–7. Lungs: **(A)** frontal aspect, **(B)** lateral aspect, **(C)** axial section.

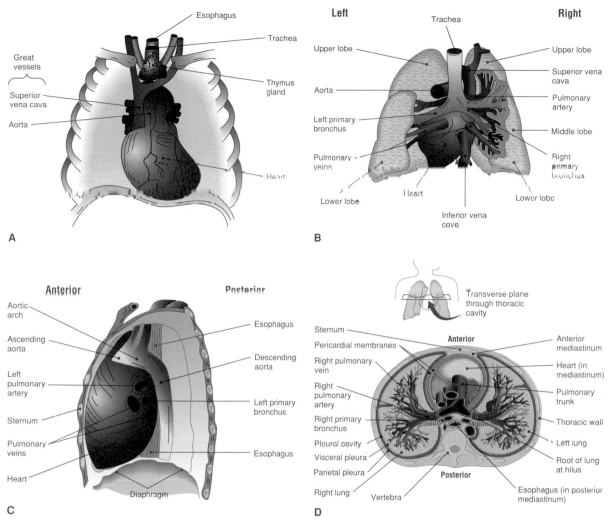

Figure 2–8. Mediastinum: **(A)** frontal aspect, **(B)** posterior aspect, **(C)** lateral aspect, **(D)** axial section.

MEDIASTINUM

The mediastinum (mē-dē-ah-STĪ-num) is located in the middle of the thoracic cavity between the two lungs. It contains all of the structures in the thorax with the exception of the lungs. This includes the heart, great vessels, thymus gland, trachea, and esophagus (*Figure 2–8*).

Heart

The heart is situated anteriorly in the thoracic cavity, just posterior to the sternum at the approximate level of the fifth through eighth thoracic vertebrae. It is positioned in an oblique plane, with most of the organ lying to the left of the midline. The size of the heart can be evaluated on routine radiographs of the chest.

Great Vessels

The aorta, superior and inferior vena cavae, pulmonary arteries, and pulmonary veins are found in the mediastinum. The aorta leaves the left ventricle of the heart to carry oxygenated blood to the body. The inferior and superior vena cavae return deoxygenated blood to the heart. The pulmonary arteries transport deoxygenated blood to the lungs, whereas the pulmonary veins return the oxygenated blood to the heart. It should be noted that the function of these vessels is the opposite of the normal function of arteries and veins. Elsewhere in the body, arteries carry oxygenated blood and veins return the deoxygenated blood to the heart. A network of capillaries that are branches of these pulmonary vessels surround the alveolar sacs in the lungs.

► Related Terminology

apnea (AP-nē-ah)—absence or cessation of respiration

aspiration (as-pi-RĀ-shun)—inhalation of a foreign material (eg, vomitus in the lungs)

asthma (AZ-mah)—condition in which spasmodic constriction of the bronchial tree causes dyspnea and wheezing; bronchial asthma may be allergic in nature

atelectasis (at-e-LEK-tah-sis)—airless portion of lung or collapsed lung, usually due to obstruction of bronchus

bifurcation (bī-fur-KĀ-shun)—branching or splitting into two divisions

bronchiectasis (brong-kē-EK-tah-sis)—chronic condition in which the bronchus or bronchi are dilated

bronchitis (brong-KĪ-tis)—chronic or acute inflammation of a bronchus or bronchi

bronchogram (BRONG-kō-gram)—radiograph obtained after iodinated contrast medium is introduced into one or both bronchi

bronchoscopy (brong-KOS-kō-pē)—examination of the bronchi in which a fiberoptic scope is passed down the trachea and into a bronchus to be visually inspected

(continued)

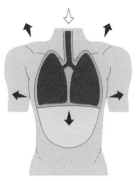 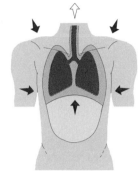

Diaphragm in inspiration **Diaphragm in expiration**

Figure 2–9. Movement of the diaphragm during breathing.

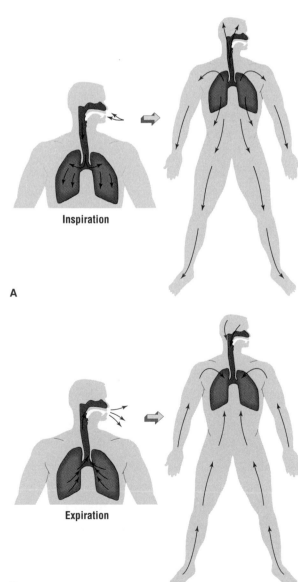

Inspiration

A

Expiration

B

Figure 2–10. Path of oxygen and carbon dioxide during inspiration **(A)** and expiration **(B)**.

Thymus Gland

This structure is part of the lymphatic system. It produces hormones as well as lymphocytes and plays a vital role in the autoimmune system of infants and children. It is located behind the upper portion of the sternum. Because the thymus gland decreases in size after puberty, it is not usually seen on chest radiographs of adults, but may be responsible for a wide mediastinum on infants.

Trachea

As discussed earlier, the trachea is located in the mediastinum. It branches into the primary bronchi in this area of the thoracic cavity.

Esophagus

The esophagus forms part of the alimentary canal. This structure branches from the pharynx and is located in the mediastinum just posterior to the trachea and anterior to the descending aorta. It passes through the diaphragm into the abdomen about the level of the tenth thoracic vertebra.

DIAPHRAGM

The diaphragm (DĪ-ah-fram) is a dome-shaped muscular structure that separates the thoracic and abdominal cavities. There are actually two domes, one under each lung, hence the term *hemidiaphragm*. The diaphragm moves up and down with respiration. The physical position of a person also affects the movement of the diaphragm. When a person is standing erect, the diaphragm can move lower. Consequently, it is at its highest point on expiration when a person is in a recumbent position, and at its lowest position on inspiration when a person is standing upright *(Figure 2–9)*.

Three openings in the diaphragm allow the aorta, inferior vena cava, and esophagus to pass between the thoracic and abdominal cavities.

MECHANICS OF RESPIRATION

During the process of breathing, otherwise known as ventilation, the respiratory system supplies oxygen to the cells of the body and rids the body of carbon dioxide, which is a waste product of metabolism *(Figure 2–10)*.

On inspiration, the diaphragm contracts and moves inferiorly, allowing the lungs to expand with air. This results in a decrease in pressure in the thoracic cavity; consequently, air is sucked into the lungs from the nose and mouth. The pulmonary veins carry the oxygenated blood to the heart, where it is then transported to the tissues of the body via the arteries. The arteries branch into smaller arteries called arterioles, which continue to branch into even smaller vessels called capillaries. The exchange of O_2 and CO_2 takes place at the capillary level. Capillaries are very small blood vessels whose thin walls allow for the transfer of gases and some fluids. As these blood vessels become bigger, they are known as venules. The venules in turn join to form veins. Veins convey deoxygenated blood to the heart, where it is then transported to the lungs. At this point, carbon dioxide is expelled during expiration and oxygen is taken in on inspiration *(Figure 2–11)*.

The average number of respirations is approximately 10 to 20 per minute. Respiration is controlled by the respiratory center of the brain located in the medulla oblongata. Although respiration patterns can be altered voluntarily by holding one's breath for a short time, breathing basically occurs automatically without conscious thought.

► PROCEDURAL CONSIDERATIONS

Although radiography of the chest may appear to be a fairly simple procedure, accurate positioning and technical factor selection are critical. Even slight errors in patient positioning and technique can affect a patient's diagnosis. Although chest x-rays are fairly routine, the technologist must provide the same attention to detail as in the most specialized of procedures.

Because the radiologist must be able to compare subsequent chest radiographs, it is important that patient positioning, exposure factors, and breathing instructions be duplicated for each examination.

PATIENT PREPARATION

After identifying and introducing yourself to the patient, it is vitally important to obtain a good, clinical, patient history *(Figure 2–12)*. A good technologist uses this information to make appropriate adjustments in patient positioning and/or exposure factors due to anatomical variants or pathology. If previous films are available, they may indicate any technical errors or adjustments made previously.

Because artifacts as innocent as emblems on T-shirts have been known to appear on chest radiographs, the patient should be instructed to remove all clothing above the waist, including bra, and put on a snapless patient gown prior to the examination. In addition, long, dangling earrings and necklaces should be removed. Hair braids or pony tails should be moved from the collimated field prior to making the exposure, as dense braids of hair, elastic bands, hair pins, and barrettes could be visualized within the lung fields *(Figure 2–13)*. In addition, oxygen tubing and monitor wires should also be moved away from the lung fields, if possible.

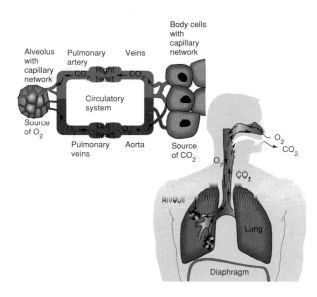

Figure 2–11. Process of respiration.

▶ **Related Terminology** *(continued)*

chronic obstructive pulmonary disease (COPD)—a condition resulting from asthma, chronic bronchitis, or pulmonary emphysema in which the person experiences shortness of breath on exertion and a chronic cough

cyanosis (si-ah-NŌ-sis)—bluish coloration of the skin resulting from deficient oxygenation

diphtheria (dif-THĒ-rē-ah)—contagious bacterial infection usually affecting children rather than adults; it affects the larynx and pharynx

dyspnea (DISP-nē-ah or disp-NĒ-ah)—difficult or painful breathing

emphysema (em-fi-ZĒ-mah)—condition in which the alveoli becomes distended, resulting in a loss of elasticity of the lung tissue and difficult breathing; the lungs appear overinflated because air is trapped in the alveoli, making respiration difficult; subcutaneous pneumothorax is a condition in which air is present in the subcutaneous tissue as the result of an infection or injury within the chest cavity *(continued)*

History Sheet: Chest Radiography

Patient Name: _____ Age: _____

Date: _____ X-ray No.: _____ Pregnant? _____

Reason for admission/complaint: _____

Symptoms (check all that apply):

_____ Chest pain: (area) _____

_____ Shortness of breath: (duration) _____

_____ Cough: (duration) _____

_____ Fever: (duration) _____

_____ Trauma: _____

_____ Other: _____

Previous history (check all that apply):

_____ Pneumonia: (when and number occurrences) _____

_____ Emphysema: (when diagnosed) _____

_____ Heart problems: (type/extent) _____

_____ Chest surgery: (reason) _____

_____ Breast surgery: (date) _____

_____ Trauma: _____

Additional comments: _____

_____

_____

Technologist: _____

Figure 2–12. Patient history form.

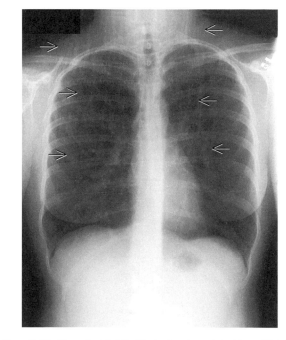

Figure 2–13. The patient in this PA chest radiograph had long, thick hair that produced vertical artifacts throughout the lungs (see arrows).

► Related Terminology *(continued)*

epiglottitis (ep-i-glot-Ī-tis)—inflammation with swelling of the epiglottis

hemothorax (hē-mō-THŌ-raks)—blood in the pleural cavity; this may be the result of a ruptured blood vessel or due to trauma

hyperventilation (hī-per-ven-ti-LĀ-shun)—excessive movement of air in and out of lungs caused by abnormally deep breathing

hypoxia (hī-POK-sē-ah)—deprivation of oxygen to the body tissues and organs

laryngitis (lar-in-JĪ-tis)—sore throat caused by inflammation of the mucous membrane of the larynx

pertussis (per-TUS-is)—whooping cough; infectious condition in which the patient makes a whooping sound on inhalation   *(continued)*

TABLE 2–2. Routine and Optional*a* Projections: Chest and Airway

Chest	Airway
PA*b*	AP
Lateral	Lateral
Supine/semierect*a*	
Obliques*a*	
Decubitus*a*	
Apical lordotic*a*	

*a*Optional projections.
*b*The single PA projection is often done without the lateral for screening purposes.

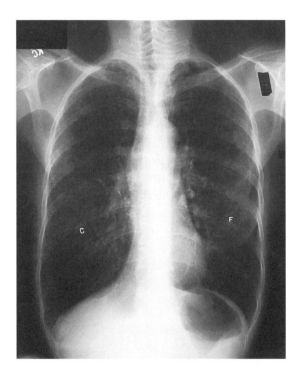

Figure 2–14. In the absence of special nipple markers, lead letters were taped over the nipples for this PA chest radiograph.

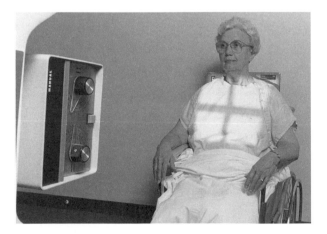

Figure 2–15. An AP chest radiograph can be obtained on wheelchair patients who are unable to stand.

POSITIONING CONSIDERATIONS

Although routines can vary, most medical facilities identify both the PA and lateral projections as the routine procedure for their department or office. Because the heart is positioned toward the left side of the thorax, the left lateral is usually performed to position the heart closer to the film and minimize magnification. Right lateral chest projections are generally obtained when the area of interest is in the right hemithorax or when the left lung has been removed *(Table 2–2)*.

When positioning a patient for a frontal projection, either PA or AP, the patient's chin should be elevated to prevent superimposition in the apices; usually there is a chin rest on the upright wall unit. With the patient's chin elevated over the top of the upright wall unit, it may be impossible to center the chest to the film. In this situation, the central ray should be centered to the part and not the film; the central ray can then be collimated to include only the lungs. To assist the diaphragm in its downward movement against the abdominal organs and to allow for visualization of fluid levels, chest x-rays should be performed with the patient in the upright position whenever possible. Patients may be standing or seated upright on a stool, stretcher, or bed. Supine and semierect projections should be obtained only on seriously ill patients who are too ill to sit erect or stand. Chest radiographs obtained by any means other than the routine upright PA projection should be clearly marked as to patient position and radiographic tube angle. Women with large breasts should be instructed to move their breasts upward and outward to provide a more uniform density of the lung tissue.

Positioning accuracy for a PA chest projection can be determined by symmetry of the sternoclavicular joints and absence of the scapulae and chin from the lung fields. The apices and costophrenic angles should be seen within the collimated area. On the lateral projection, the spinous processes and sternum should be seen in profile and the posterior margins of the lungs should be superimposed. Collimation should be used to minimize patient exposure and improve radiographic quality.

Occasionally, unusual artifacts may appear on radiographic images of the chest. These artifacts, which could mimic a disease process, may be due to lumps on the skin, prominent pectoralis muscles, skin folds, breast implants, or nipples. To assist the radiologist in diagnosis, repeat radiographs may be taken with disposable, lead nipple markers adhered to the suspected artifact(s) *(Figure 2–14)*.

ALTERNATE PROJECTIONS

Occasionally, special projections of the chest may be required. Patients with suspected fluid or free air within the thorax may require **decubitus films** to demonstrate the fluid or air. To allow the fluid to layer at the bottom of the thorax or the air to rise, the patient should be positioned in the lateral decubitus position for at least 10 minutes prior to the exposure. A horizontal beam is necessary to demonstrate air–fluid levels. If at all possible, the entire thorax should be visualized on the finished radiograph. If this is not possible because of patient size, the dependent side (side down) should be included when fluid is suspected and the independent side (side up) should be included when a pneumothorax is suspected. Although the projection is named for the dependent side (it is called a right lateral decubitus projection when the patient is on the right side), the side up is labeled on the film to ensure the marker is not in the anatomy of interest.

To better demonstrate the apices, a **lordotic projection** can be obtained. Either by leaning the patient backward or angling the central ray cephalad with the patient positioned for an AP projection, the clavicles should be projected above the thorax. This projection can prove invaluable for evaluation of the apices.

Oblique chest projections may be requested to evaluate suspicious areas seen on the PA or lateral projections or to evaluate the heart. When evaluating the heart, the patient may be instructed to drink a barium sulfate suspension. The exposure is made as the patient swallows the barium. The barium-coated esophagus should follow the contours of the heart, providing the radiologist with additional information for diagnosis. This study is commonly referred to as a *cardiac series*. Shallower obliques, 10° to 20° rotation, may be requested for further evaluation of pulmonary nodules.

AP chest projections can be performed on patients who are unable to stand. For patients seated in a wheelchair, the cassette can be positioned behind the patient with the central ray directed perpendicular to the patient's coronal plane at the level of sixth or seventh thoracic vertebra *(Figure 2–15)*. Stretcher patients who are unable to sit or stand may be radiographed semierect or while lying supine on the stretcher. Because a 72 in. (183-cm) SID is usually impossible to achieve when the patient is supine, the maximum SID should be used with an appropriate reduction in technical factors to allow for the shorter distance. To demonstrate air–fluid levels, however, at least one projection must be obtained using a horizontal beam. A dorsal decubitus, lateral chest radiograph can meet this need when the patient is supine. If the patient is semierect *(Figure 2–16)*, a horizontal beam can be used with the AP projection.

BREATHING INSTRUCTIONS

In most situations, chest radiographs are taken with the patient holding his or her breath after deep inspiration. The patient should be instructed to take in a deep breath, exhale, take in another deep breath, and hold that breath in. The second inspiration allows the lungs to expand more fully. At least 10 posterior ribs should be seen within the lung field on a good inspiration chest radiograph. Poor expansion of the lungs may cause a normal-sized heart to appear enlarged.

Occasionally, inspiration and expiration PA chest radiographs are requested to assist in diagnosing foreign bodies, pneumothorax, and function of the diaphragm *(Figure 2–17)*. Films should be clearly marked to indicate the breathing instructions used.

For AP and lateral airway projections, the patient should be instructed to take in a slow, deep breath during the exposure. This technique ensures that the airway is filled with air, allowing for a more accurate diagnosis.

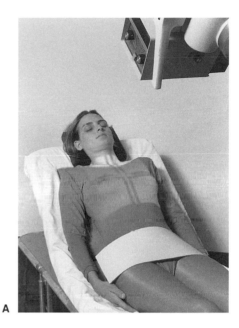

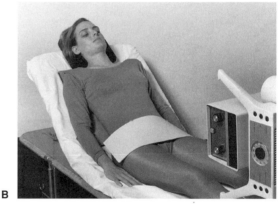

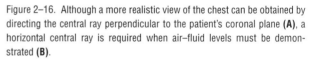

Figure 2–16. Although a more realistic view of the chest can be obtained by directing the central ray perpendicular to the patient's coronal plane **(A)**, a horizontal central ray is required when air–fluid levels must be demonstrated **(B)**.

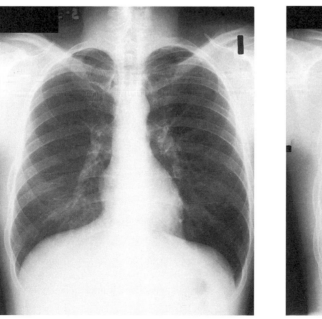

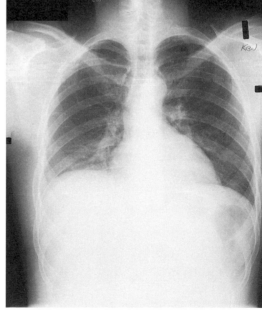

Figure 2–17. Inspiration **(A)** and expiration **(B)** chest radiographs on the same person can look very different; compare the heart size and diameter of the thorax.

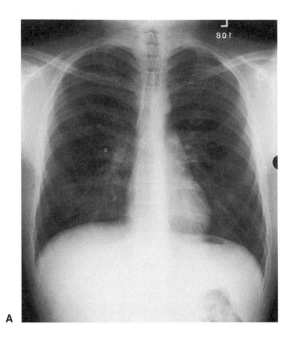

A

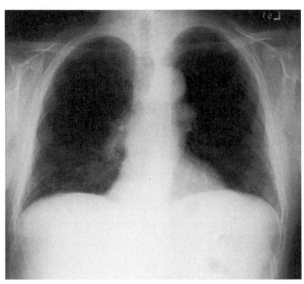

B

C

Figure 2–18. Accurate selection of technical factors is a major factor in diagnosis. **A** represents optimum density, contrast, and heart penetration. The chest in **B** was taken using 90 kVp and is underpenetrated, but overexposed (the mAs was too high). Figure **C** illustrates both underexposure and underpenetration.

EXPOSURE FACTORS

Two very important factors must be taken into consideration when selecting exposure factors. The chest is an area of high subject contrast because of the difference in tissue between the very dense heart muscle and the radiolucent lung tissue. This physical makeup will produce a finished image that appears primarily black and white, with very few shades of gray. Because the heart and mediastinum are very dense structures, the technical factors selected must be capable of penetration.

The use of low kVp enhances the bony thorax and provides higher radiographic contrast, but less penetration. Because the bony thorax can obscure vascular markings in the lung and because the chest inherently has a high subject contrast, low kVp is not desirable. High kVp is needed, however, to penetrate the heart and mediastinum and produce a scale of contrast that permits visualization of various pathologies. The outlines of the thoracic vertebral bodies and intervertebral disk spaces should be visualized through the heart shadow and mediastinum on an adequately penetrated PA chest radiograph. In addition to ensuring adequate penetration, high-kVp techniques also provide a wider exposure latitude (range of acceptable techniques) *(Figure 2–18)*.

The use of high-kVp techniques not only increases exposure latitude; it allows for adequate penetration of the heart, abnormal masses, and fluid-filled portions of the lungs. Structures or pathology within the thorax that may be more difficult to penetrate are considered additive processes and require higher kVp. Some pathologies, destructive processes, are easier than normal to penetrate and require a reduction in exposure factors *(Table 2–3)*. In this situation, a reduction in mAs is generally preferred *(Figure 2–19)*. A soft tissue technique should be used when radiographing the airway in either the AP or lateral position.

Whether or not a grid is used influences the choice in technical factors. Normally, a grid is used for any structure measuring more than 10 cm (4 in.) in thickness. Because the chest is an air-filled cavity, either a nongrid or grid technique can be used to obtain an acceptable image. Nongrid chest techniques are employed primarily for mobile radiography.

In most clinical settings, the kVp for chest radiography normally ranges between 100 and 150. Nongrid chest techniques may range from 80 to 95 kVp on an adult. Because kVp controls the penetration of the x-ray beam and also determines the contrast, all radiographers at any one facility should use the same kVp to ensure image consistency.

The mAs controls the density of the image and should be adjusted according to patient size and pathology. To minimize breathing and heart motion on the finished image, high mA and short exposure times should also be used. Generally speaking, changes in technical factors should be made by varying the mAs, not the kVp, as changing the kVp alters the contrast of the image and makes comparison of follow-up films more difficult. A correctly exposed chest radiograph allows the radiologist to visualize fine vascular markings along the outer margins of the lungs, the costophrenic angles, and bases of the lungs, while penetrating the heart adequately *(Figure 2–18)*.

As part of a routine diagnosis, the radiologist evaluates the heart size. A more accurately sized representation can be obtained when the structure of interest is positioned as close as possible to the image receptor. Objects further from the image receptor will be magnified proportional to the object–image receptor distance. Increasing the SID to 72 in. minimizes magnification of the image and also contributes to an increase in sharpness of fine lung structures.

TABLE 2–3. Pathologic Conditions

Additive Chest Pathology	Destructive Chest Pathology
Atelectasis	Emphysema
Bronchiectasis	Pneumothorax
Edema	Tuberculosis, active
Hydropneumothorax	
Malignancy	
Pleural effusion	
Pneumoconiosis	
Pneumonia	
Tuberculosis, arrested	

As with all radiographic examinations, the acquisition of a thorough patient history can be vital to appropriate selection of technical factors.

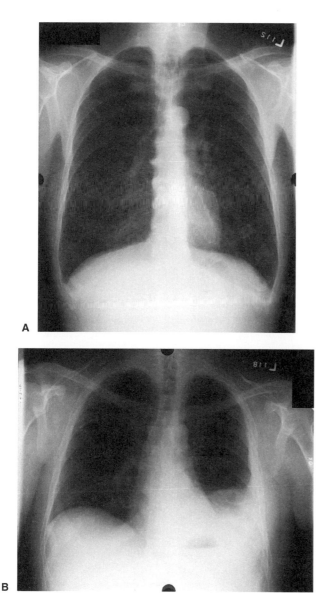

A

B

Figure 2–19. The patient in **A** has emphysema, resulting in slightly overexposed lungs. The patient in **B** has fluid in the lower lobe of the left lung.

▶ **Related Terminology** *(continued)*

pleural effusion (PLOO-ral ē-FŪ-zhun)—accumulation of excess fluid within the pleural cavity

pleurisy (PLOO-ri-sē)—inflammation of the pleura, which is the serous membranous sac enclosing the lungs and thoracic cavity; also known as pleuritis

pneumonia (nū-MŌ-nē-ah)—inflammation of the lungs with congestion; there are various types which may be caused by viruses, bacteria, protozoa, or fungi

pneumocentesis (nū-mō-sen-TĒ-sis)—surgical puncture of a lung to remove fluid

pneumothorax (nū-mō-THŌ-raks)—collapsed lung caused by the accretion of air in the pleural cavity

pulmonary edema (PUL-mō-ner-ē ed-Ē-mah)—accumulation of excess serous fluid in the lungs and alveoli

pulmonary embolism (PUL-mō-ner-ē EM-bi-lizm)—blood clot in the pulmonary artery or arterioles, resulting in obstruction of circulation

rales (rāhlz)—crackling or bubbling sounds heard in the lungs on inhalation or exhalation

respiratory distress syndrome (RDS)—condition of neonates characterized by dyspnea and cyanosis (ARDS is adult respiratory distress syndrome)

sputum (SPŪ-tum)—expectorant; mucous secretion from the lungs coughed up and expelled through the mouth

thoracentesis (thor-rah-sen-TĒ-sis)—surgical puncture of the thoracic cavity to drain fluid for therapeutic as well as diagnostic purposes

tracheostomy (tra-kē-OS-tō-mē)—artificial opening in the neck through which a tube is placed to facilitate ventilation

tuberculosis (TB) (too-ber-kū-LŌ-sis)—disease of the lungs characterized by inflamed lesions; the condition can spread to other parts of the body via the bloodstream and is an infectious disease which is reported to the health department

EQUIPMENT CONSIDERATIONS

One of the primary deterrents to high-quality radiography is scattered radiation coming from the patient. In most instances, a grid is used to stop the radiation from reaching the patient. In chest radiography, however, an air-gap technique can also accomplish the same objective in most patients. By moving the image receptor further from the patient, most scattered radiation will not reach the film. A 6-in. (15-cm) air gap is roughly equivalent to a 6:1 ratio grid. When the patient is moved further from the image receptor, however, the heart will be magnified. To overcome this increased magnification, the SID must be increased. An air gap of 10 to 12 in. (25 to 30 cm) requires an SID of 10 to 12 ft (3 to 3.7 m) *(Figure 2–20)*. This technique may not, however, provide an adequate reduction in scattered radiation for a patient with an enlarged heart or fluid-filled thorax.

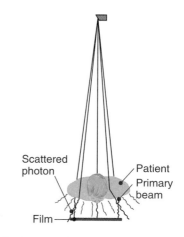

Figure 2–20. An air-gap technique can be used in place of a grid in chest radiography.

To consistently reproduce radiographic contrast and density on chest radiographs, many hospitals, imaging centers, and physicians' offices are using automatic exposure control (AEC). When using AEC, the radiographer selects the kVp, mA, focal spot size, and ionization chamber(s) (see Chapter 1). To maximize tube life, a large focal spot should be selected. Although departments may vary somewhat, the right or both right and left chambers are usually selected for a PA chest and the middle chamber for a lateral. The exposure is automatically terminated when a preselected amount of radiation is received by the ionization chambers located between the patient and the film. Most AEC devices have a density control that allows the radiographer to increase or decrease image density when an over- or underpenetrated film is desired. Accurate patient centering and appropriate AEC chamber selection are imperative for optimum density.

Dedicated chest units allow for speedier patient throughput in busy radiology departments. These units can be set up to receive either individual cassettes or a magazine of 50 to 100 films that move, one at a time, into position in front of the patient. After the exposure, the film is automatically transported to either a film receiver or an automatic film processor *(Figure 2–21)*.

Several manufacturers have developed equipment capable of producing uniform density on chest radiographs. One such model that has been successful in overcoming wide differences in chest tissue resulting from anatomy or pathology is the advance multiple-beam equalization radiography (AMBER) unit. An AMBER device, containing 21 beam modulators, is positioned in front of the radiographic tube and converts the beam into a horizontal, fanlike beam that is raised or lowered vertically. A linear detector array, positioned in front of the cassette, receives and analyzes the radiation that passes through the patient and sends a message to the corresponding modulator to provide sufficient exposure locally *(Figure 2–22)*. Studies have shown that significantly more nodules are discovered in the mediastinum and retrodiaphragmatic regions with the AMBER system *(Figure 2–23)*.

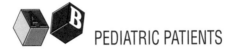

PEDIATRIC PATIENTS

Positioning for pediatric chest radiographs varies depending on the age of the patient and the department routine. Infants may be positioned upright in a device such as that in *Figure 2–24*. The patient is easily immobilized. The seat in this device rotates to facilitate positioning for the lateral projection without moving the patient. An alternative method, however, is to position the patient supine for both the AP and lateral projections, using a horizontal beam for the lateral projection to demonstrate any fluid present in the lungs.

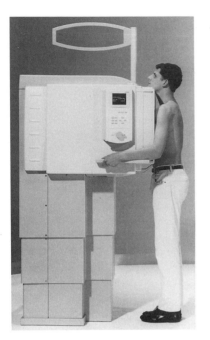

Figure 2–21. Dedicated chest unit. *(Courtesy of Philips Medical Systems.)*

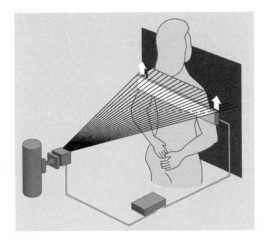

Figure 2–22. Wide tissue absorption differences can be overcome by using a scanning equalization chest unit such as the AMBER system.

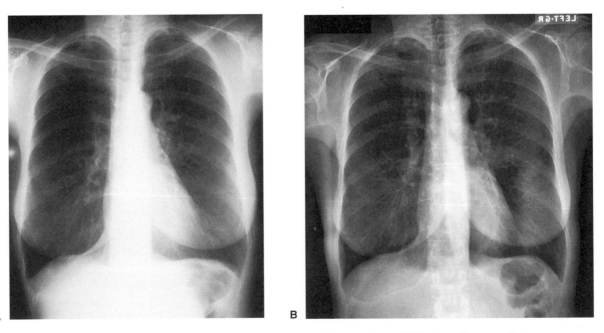

A   B

Figure 2–23. Conventional chest radiograph **(A)** versus an AMBER chest radiograph **(B)** taken on the same patient.

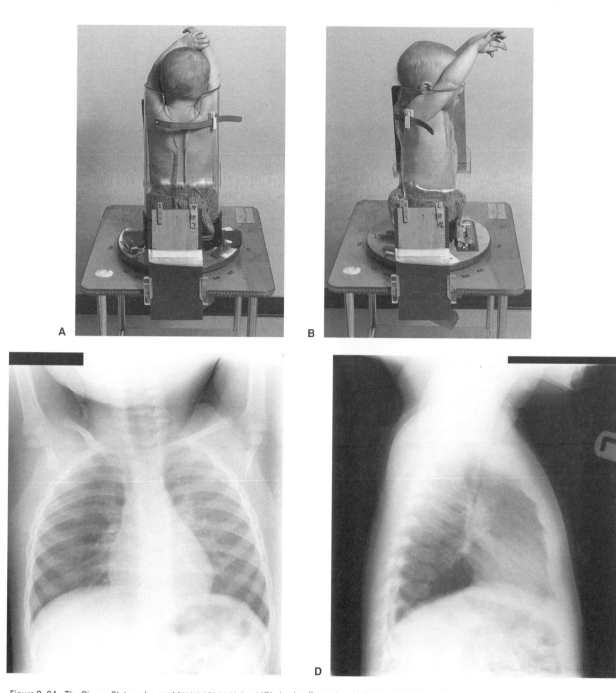

Figure 2–24. The Pigg-o-Stat can be used for PA **(A)** and lateral **(B)** chest radiography of infants and young toddlers, producing satisfactory radiographs **(C, D)**.

Toddlers can also be positioned on a chair-type device as seen in *Figure 2–25*. Both the AP and lateral projections can easily be obtained using a horizontal beam. A leaded acrylic panel provides added radiation protection for a parent or health professional who may be assisting with immobilization.

In addition to changes in patient positioning, radiographing the pediatric chest also requires an adjustment in technical factors. In most cases, both kVp and mAs will need to be decreased. Because of the increased percentage of water per body weight, which increases the production of scatter radiation, and the size of the part, kVp should be reduced 2 for each centimeter difference between the child's measurement and that of the average adult. The mAs should be reduced using a factor related to the patient's physical age *(Table 2–4)*. Generally speaking, children over age 12 do not require special compensation in technical factors.

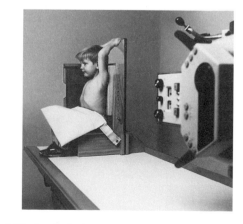

Figure 2–25. A pediatric chest chair can be used to produce AP and lateral chest radiographs on young children who are able to sit upright by themselves. *(Courtesy of Nuclear Associates.)*

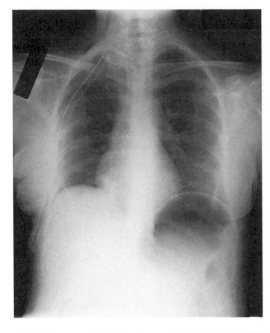

Figure 2–26. Because air–fluid levels were not anticipated, a horizontal beam was not used (note the absence of a well-defined air–fluid level in the stomach); the tip of a chest tube can be seen in the upper lobe of the right lung.

TABLE 2–4. Pediatric mAs Conversions

Using the child's physical age, multiply the adult mAs by the appropriate modification factor:

0–1 year	0.25
1–3 years	0.50
3–7 years	0.70
7–12 years	0.90

MOBILE RADIOGRAPHY

Although chest radiographs performed in a radiographic room provide the best quality, bedside, or portable, radiography is often required for patients too ill or otherwise unable to travel to the radiology department. Whenever possible, the head of the patient's bed should be moved to the upright position with the patient sitting as erect as possible. To minimize exposure to the radiographer and patient and eliminate the concern of grid lines on the finished radiograph, a nongrid cassette is used. A pillowcase can be used to cover the cassette, making it easier to slide behind the patient and maintain cleanliness. The portable unit should be situated near the foot of the bed so a 72 in. SID can be obtained. To prevent unwanted lordosis or kyphosis, the central ray should be directed perpendicular to the patient's coronal plane *(Figure 2–26)*. If the patient is unable to sit erect, a semierect or supine position must be used with the maximum obtainable SID and technique compensation for the difference in SID. To demonstrate air–fluid levels, a *horizontal beam* must be used on erect or semierect patients. For patients who must remain supine, a dorsal decubitus lateral chest projection can be performed to demonstrate air–fluid levels. The finished radiograph should be marked to indicate the conditions of the exposure: patient position, SID, and technical factors used.

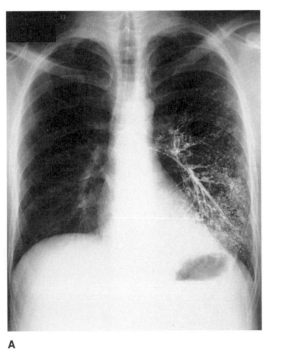

A

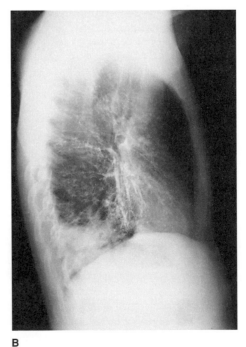

B

Figure 2–27. Bronchogram: **(A)** PA, **(B)** lateral.

ALTERNATE IMAGING PROCEDURES

Bronchography (brong-KOG-rah-fē) is the radiographic examination of the bronchial tree of the respiratory system after the introduction of radiopaque contrast medium. This examination is infrequently performed today, as bronchoscopy and computed tomography (CT) examinations have supplanted it as examinations of choice for diagnosing pulmonary pathology.

Bronchography is usually indicated in cases of bronchiectasis. It is also performed when a CT examination yields nonspecific findings. The examination is contraindicated in patients running a high fever. Other contraindications include a history of asthma, severe hypertension, and congestive heart failure. An allergic history is taken prior to the procedure. The procedure consists of introducing a catheter into the trachea and then positioning it in the main stem bronchus of the affected side under fluoroscopy. Either an oil based or aqueous iodinated contrast medium is injected into the bronchus of interest through the catheter. The patient is asked to cough lightly to distribute the agent. Spot films may be taken during the procedure. PA, lateral, and anterior oblique projections to demonstrate the side of interest are routinely taken with the patient in the erect position with a 72-in. SID. Positioning and centering are the same as for routine chest radiography. At the conclusion of the procedure, the patient is encouraged to cough and expel the contrast medium *(Figure 2–27)*.

Periodically, it is necessary to use special imaging methods to make an accurate diagnosis of pathology seen on a chest radiograph. Tomography, as described in Chapter 1, is one such method that has been used to evaluate lesions in the lung *(Figure 2–28)*. Although tomography is still used, computed tomography (CT) is often preferred and provides unobstructed sectional images of the heart and lungs *(Figure 2–29)*. Echocardiography, a specialized field of sonography, is also used in evaluation of the heart. In nuclear medicine, radiopharmaceuticals are administered to the patient to evaluate various phases of lung function. These studies may be performed when pulmonary emboli, bronchogenic carcinoma, and chronic obstructive pulmonary disease, such as bronchitis or emphysema, are suspected *(Figure 2–30)*. Although new to chest and heart examination, magnetic resonance imaging (MRI) is also used on a limited basis and has the capability of viewing the chest and heart in more than one plane *(Figure 2–31)*.

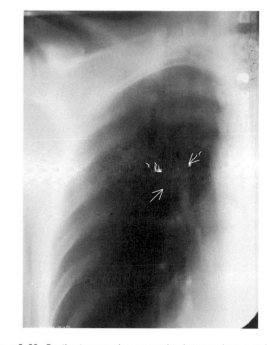

Figure 2–28. Routine tomography was used to better evaluate a nodule in the left lung.

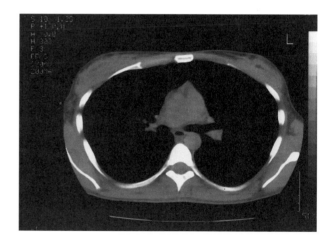

Figure 2–29. Axial computed tomography image of the chest.

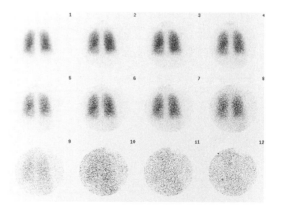

Figure 2–30. Nuclear medicine lung (ventilation) scan, posterior projections. After the patient breathed in radioactive xenon gas, these 30-second frames were obtained while the patient breathed out the gas. Areas that retain gas may indicate pathology. *(Courtesy of Linda Winkler, RT(R)(N).)*

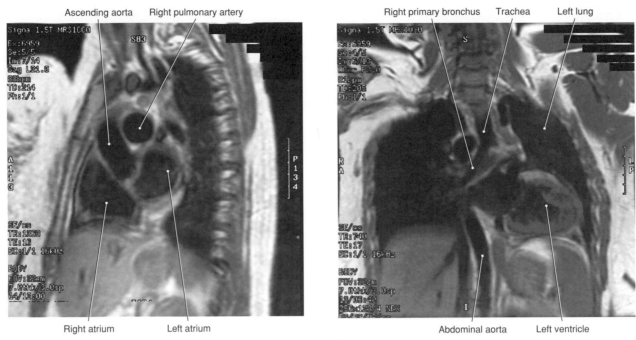

Figure 2–31. Sagittal **(A)** and coronal **(B)** magnetic resonance images of the chest.

RADIOGRAPHIC POSITIONING OF THE RESPIRATORY SYSTEM

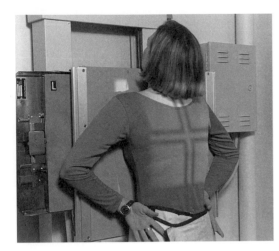

Figure 2–32. PA chest.

▶ PA CHEST

Technical Considerations

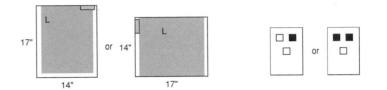

- Film size: Adult: 14 × 17 in. lengthwise on most patients, crosswise on large patients. Pediatric: size determined by patient size.
- Grid or nongrid, depending on department policy.
- 100–150 kVp, grid (adult); 80–95 kVp, nongrid (adult).
- Collimate to the rib margins crosswise and to include the apices and costophrenic angles lengthwise.

Shielding

- Use gonadal shielding on all pediatric patients and adults of reproductive age.

Patient Positioning

- Assist patient to erect position facing upright wall unit. **Note:** If patient is too ill to stand or sit on a stool or stretcher for the routine, upright PA projection, an AP projection may be obtained with patient supine on a stretcher, seated semierect on a stretcher, or seated in a wheelchair. If patient is seated semierect and fluid is suspected, a horizontal beam must be used, regardless of patient angle, to demonstrate an air–fluid level.
- Patient's feet should be separated slightly with weight equally distributed on both feet.
- Adjust the height of the wall unit so the top edge of the cassette is approximately 1.5 to 2 in. above the top of the patient's shoulders.

Part Positioning

- Center the midsagittal plane of the patient's body to the midline of the wall unit.
- Extend patient's chin upward over the top of wall unit, if possible; adjust the head so there is no rotation.
- Position backs of patient's hands on hips; depress shoulders and roll them forward so they touch wall unit. Shoulders should be relaxed and the hands should be below the area of the lung fields (Figure 2–32).

Central Ray

- Using a 72-in. SID to minimize magnification, direct the central ray horizontally to the midline of the patient at the level of T7, approximately at the level of the inferior angle of the scapula.

Breathing Instructions

- Instruct the patient to take in a breath, blow the breath out, take in another deep breath, and hold it in.

Image Evaluation

- The apices, costophrenic angles, and lateral margins of the ribs should be included in the collimated area.
- The spine should be centered crosswise on the film; the middle of collimation field should be at T7.
- The heart will be adequately penetrated; vascular markings will be clearly seen near lateral lung margins .
- The outlines of the heart and diaphragm will be sharp when there is no patient motion.
- The distance between the medial ends of the clavicles and the spine should be equal; the right and left ribs should be symmetrical.
- The scapulae should be moved lateral to the lung fields; approximately 2 in. of lung should be seen above the clavicles, demonstrating appropriate patient positioning and central ray direction.
- At least 10 posterior ribs should be demonstrated above the diaphragm on a good inspiration chest radiograph (Figure 2–33).

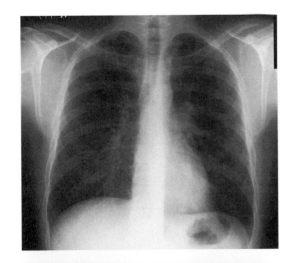

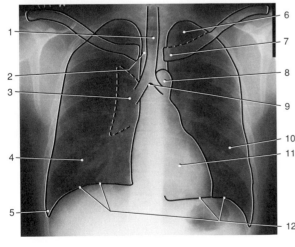

Figure 2–33. PA chest.

1. Trachea
2. Right sternoclavicular joint
3. Right hilum
4. Right lung
5. Right costophrenic angle
6. Left apex
7. Left clavicle
8. Aortic arch
9. Carina
10. Left lung
11. Heart
12. Diaphragm

► LATERAL CHEST

Technical Considerations

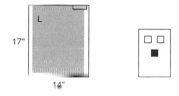

- Film size: Adult; 14 × 17 in. lengthwise. Pediatric: size determined by patient size.
- Grid or nongrid, depending on department policy.
- 100–150 kVp, grid (adult).
- 80–95 kVp, nongrid (adult).
- Collimate to include the spine and sternum crosswise and apices and diaphragm lengthwise.

Shielding

- Use gonadal shielding on all pediatric patients and adults of reproductive age.

Patient Positioning

- Assist the patient to the erect position with the side of interest nearest the upright wall unit.
- Usually a left lateral is performed; however, a right lateral may be the department routine or may be required to demonstrate the right lung.
- Patient's feet should be separated slightly with weight equally distributed on both feet.
- Adjust the height of the wall unit so the top edge of the cassette is approximately 1.5 to 2 in. above the top of the patient's shoulders.

Part Positioning

- Center the patient's midcoronal plane to the midline of the wall unit.
- Instruct patient to extend arms directly upward, flex the elbows, and grasp opposite elbows with hands. The patient should be standing straight with one shoulder touching the upright wall unit and the eyes directed straight ahead.
- Check for rotation by standing between radiographic tube and patient, placing hand on patient's back, and adjusting to true lateral position *(Figure 2–34)*.

Central Ray

- Direct the central ray horizontally to the middle of the thorax at the level of T 7, approximately the level of the inferior angle of the scapula.
- A 72-in. SID should be used to minimize magnification of the heart and vascular structures.

Breathing Instructions

- Instruct the patient to take in a breath, blow the breath out, take in another deep breath, and hold it in.

Image Evaluation

- The apices, costophrenic angles, spine, and sternum should be included within the collimated area.
- The thorax should be in the center of the collimated area.
- The heart will be adequately penetrated; vascular markings should be seen behind the sternum and heart.
- The outlines of the heart and diaphragm will be sharp when there is no patient motion.
- Posterior ribs and lung fields will be superimposed on a well-positioned lateral chest radiograph.
- Patient's arms and/or chin should not be superimposed over the upper lung fields *(Figure 2–35)*.

1. Apices, superimposed
2. Aortic arch
3. Lungs, superimposed
4. Right hemidiaphragm
5. Sternum
6. Heart
7. Left hemidiaphragm

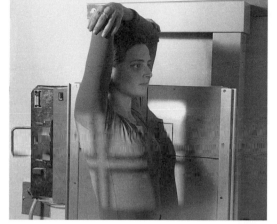

Figure 2–34. Lateral chest.

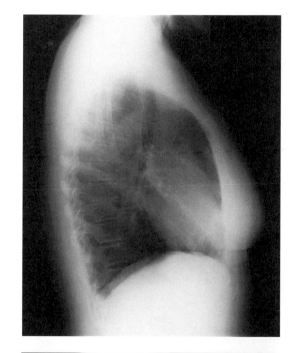

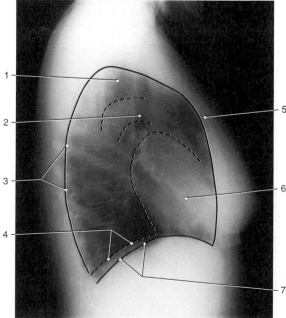

Figure 2–35. Lateral chest.

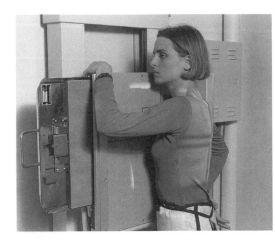

Figure 2–36. 45° RAO chest.

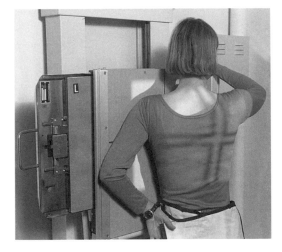

Figure 2–37. 45° LAO chest.

► PA OBLIQUE CHEST (RAO/LAO)

Technical Considerations

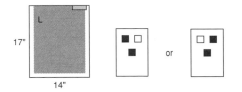

- Film size: Adult: 14 × 17 in. lengthwise on most patients, crosswise on large patients. Pediatric: size determined by patient size.
- Grid or nongrid, depending on department policy.
- 100–150 kVp, grid (adult).
- 80–95 kVp, nongrid (adult).
- Collimate to the rib margins crosswise and to include the apices and costophrenic angles lengthwise.

Shielding

- Use gonadal shielding on all pediatric patients and adults of reproductive age.

Patient Positioning

- Assist the patient to the erect position facing the upright wall unit.
- Patient's feet should be separated slightly with weight equally distributed on both feet.
- Adjust the height of the wall unit so the top edge of the cassette is approximately 1.5 to 2 in. above the top of the patient's shoulders.

Part Positioning

- Rotate the patient so the midsagittal plane is at a 45° angle with the film plane. **Note:** To demonstrate the heart, the patient should be rotated 55° to 60° in the LAO position to separate the heart and vertebral column. When oblique projections are obtained to further evaluate a pulmonary nodule, a 10° to 20° rotation may be adequate.
- Raise the arm furthest from the film and rest the hand on top of the wall unit.
- Flex the arm nearest the film and rest the back of the hand on the hip below the area of the lung.
- With the patient standing up straight, center the thorax to the upright wall unit.
- Adjust the patient's head so it is facing the same direction as the body.
- Both obliques are usually done *(Figures 2–36, 2–37).*

Central Ray

- Direct the central ray horizontally to the level of T 7, approximately the level of the inferior angle of the scapula.
- A 72-in. SID should be used to minimize magnification of the heart and vascular structures.

Breathing Instructions

- Instruct the patient to take in a breath, blow the breath out, take in another deep breath, and hold it in.

Image Evaluation

- The apices, costophrenic angles, and lateral margins of the ribs should be included within the collimated area.
- The lungs should be in the middle of the collimated area.
- The heart will be adequately penetrated without overexposure of the lungs.
- The outlines of the heart and diaphragm will be sharp when there is no patient motion.
- If the patient is correctly rotated, the width from the spine to lateral margin of thorax of the side furthest from the film will be approximately twice the width of the side nearest the film *(Figures 2–38, 2–39)*.

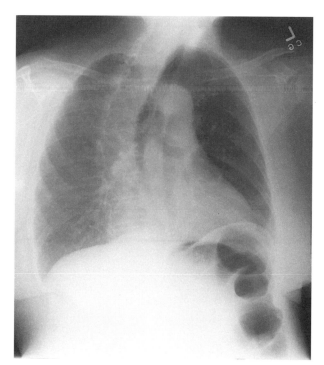
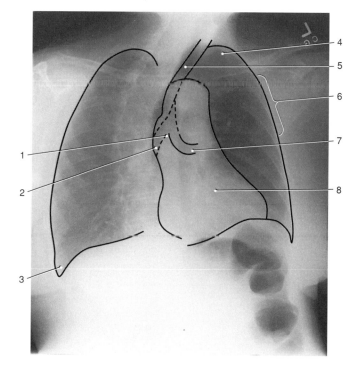

1. Carina
2. Right primary bronchus
3. Costophrenic angle
4. Apex
5. Trachea
6. Lung
7. Left primary bronchus
8. Heart

Figure 2–38. 45° RAO chest.

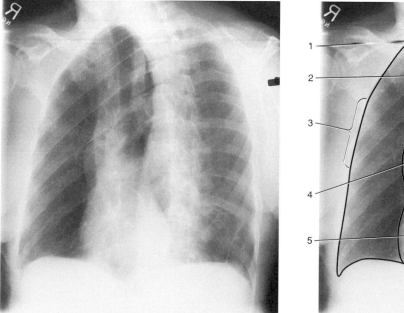
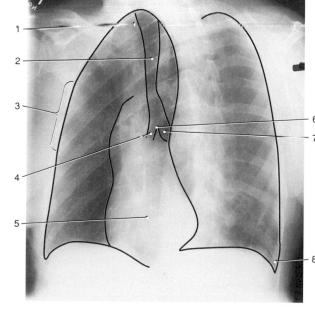

1. Apex
2. Trachea
3. Lung
4. Right primary bronchus
5. Heart
6. Carina
7. Left primary bronchus
8. Costophrenic angle

Figure 2–39. 45° LAO chest.

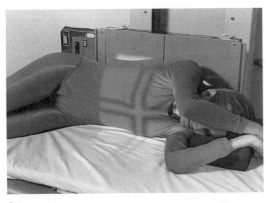

A

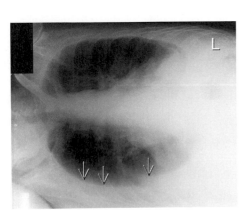

B

Figure 2–40. The decubitus chest radiograph can be obtained using a vertical grid device **(A)** or portable grid and holder **(B)**. **(A)** left lateral decubitus, **(B)** right lateral decubitus.

► LATERAL DECUBITUS CHEST

Technical Considerations

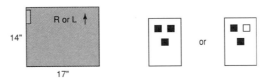

- Film size: Adult: 14 × 17 in. lengthwise with the long axis of the patient. Pediatric: size determined by patient size.
- Grid or nongrid, depending on department policy.
- 100–150 kVp, grid (adult).
- 80–95 kVp, nongrid (adult).
- Collimate to include lateral rib margins, apices, and costophrenic angles, especially of the side of interest.

Shielding

- Use gonadal shielding on all pediatric patients and adults of reproductive age.

Patient Positioning

- Position the patient in the lateral recumbent position on the radiographic table or patient stretcher.
- To demonstrate fluid levels, the patient should lie on the affected side; a pneumothorax is best demonstrated with the patient lying on the unaffected side. In either situation, the patient should be instructed to remain in the lateral position for at least 10 minutes prior to the exposure.
- When using a cassette in a portable cassette holder, the patient should be supported on radiolucent sponges or a firm support.

Part Positioning

- Extend the patient's arms above the head.
- Adjust the thorax to true lateral position. The patient's legs can be flexed for balance.
- Position either the anterior or posterior surface of the patient in front of a cassette in a cassette holder, an upright wall unit, or an upright radiographic table so the cassette extends 2 in. above the top of the shoulders.
- The long axis of the cassette should be parallel with the long axis of the patient's body *(Figure 2–40)*.

Central Ray

- Direct the central ray horizontally to the midline of the cassette at the level of T7, approximately the level of the inferior angle of the scapula; center the cassette to the central ray.
- A 72-in. SID should be used to minimize magnification of the heart and vascular structures.

Breathing Instructions

- Instruct the patient to take in a breath, blow the breath out, take in another deep breath, and hold it in.

Image Evaluation

- The apices, costophrenic angles, and lateral margins of the ribs should be included within the collimated area (especially the side of interest).
- The heart should be adequately penetrated without overexposure of the lungs.
- The outlines of the heart and diaphragm will be sharp when there is no patient motion.
- The distances between the medial ends of the clavicles and the spine should be equal; the right and left ribs should be symmetrical *(Figure 2–41)*.

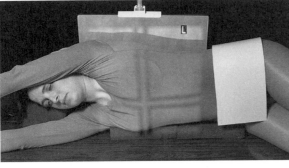

Figure 2–41. Left lateral decubitus chest; note the air–fluid levels in both lungs.

▶ LORDOTIC CHEST

Technical Considerations

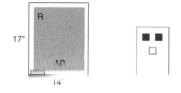

- Film size: Adult: 14 × 17 in. lengthwise or crosswise; 11 × 14 in. crosswise for apices only. Pediatric: size determined by patient size.
- Grid or nongrid, depending on department policy.
- 100–150 kVp, grid (adult); 80–95 kVp, nongrid (adult).
- Collimate to include apices and lateral margins of the thorax.

Shielding

- Use gonadal shielding on all pediatric patients and adults of reproductive age.

Patient Positioning

- Assist the patient to the erect position facing the radiographic tube and standing about 1 ft from the upright wall unit. **Note:** If the patient cannot assume the lordotic position, assist the patient into the anatomical position (seated, standing, or supine on the table) and direct the central ray 20° cephalad. Center the central ray about 2 in. below midsternum and center cassette to the central ray *(Figure 2–42)*.
- Patient's feet should be separated slightly with weight equally distributed on both feet.
- Adjust the height of the wall unit so the top edge of the cassette is just below the top of the patient's shoulders.

Part Positioning

- Center the midsagittal plane of the patient's body to the midline of the wall unit.
- Supporting the patient, lean the patient backward until the patient's shoulders are supported by the upright wall unit; the curvature of the patient's lower back will be exaggerated.
- Position the back of the patient's hands on the hips; bring shoulders and elbows forward to remove scapulae from lung fields. The shoulders should be relaxed and the hands should be below the area of the lung fields *(Figure 2–43)*.

Central Ray

- Direct the central ray horizontally to the midline of the patient at the level of the midsternum; center the cassette to the central ray.
- A 72-in. SID should be used unless the examination is completed with the patient supine.

Breathing Instructions

- Instruct the patient to take in a breath, blow the breath out, take in another deep breath, and hold it in.

Image Evaluation

- The clavicles, diaphragm, and lateral margins of the ribs should be included within the collimated area.
- The spine should be in the middle of the film crosswise.
- The vascular markings of the lungs should be clearly demonstrated, especially in the apices.
- The clavicles should be projected above the lungs; the medial ends may be slightly superimposed over the first or second ribs.
- The distances between the medial ends of the clavicles and the spine should be equal; asymmetry would indicate rotation. The clavicles and ribs will lie almost horizontally *(Figure 2–44)*.

1. Right clavicle
2. Right apex
3. Trachea
4. Right costophrenic angle
5. Left apex
6. Heart
7. Left costophrenic angle

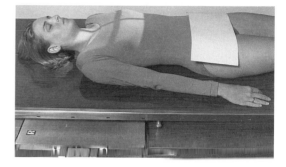

Figure 2–42. AP lordotic chest using a cephalic central ray angle.

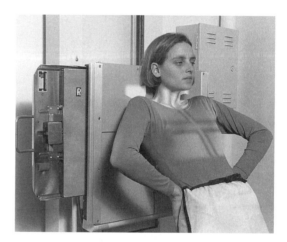

Figure 2–43. AP lordotic chest.

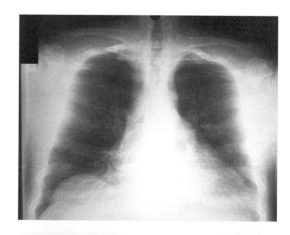

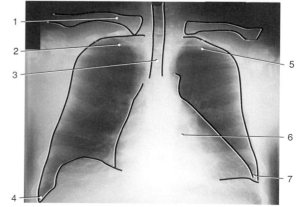

Figure 2–44. AP lordotic chest.

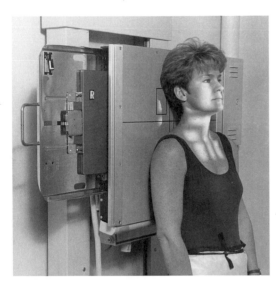

Figure 2–45. AP upper airway.

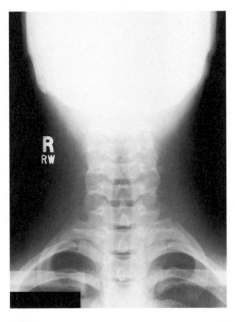

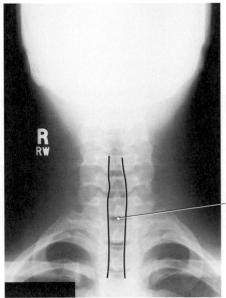

Figure 2–46. AP upper airway.

► AP UPPER AIRWAY

Technical Considerations

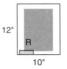

- Film size: 10 × 12 in. lengthwise.
- Grid or nongrid, depending on patient size and department policy.
- 65–75 kVp.
- Collimate to the soft tissue of the neck crosswise and include the posterior part of the mandible and the sternoclavicular joints lengthwise.

Shielding

- Use gonadal shielding on all pediatric patients and adults of reproductive age.

Patient Positioning

- Assist the patient to the erect position, standing or seated, with back against the upright wall unit. **Note:** This projection can also be obtained with the patient supine on the table. In addition, some department routines specify centering to the level of the suprasternal notch to include the upper mediastinum.
- Patient's feet should be separated slightly with weight equally distributed on both feet.
- Adjust the height of the wall unit so the top edge of the cassette is approximately at the level of the mouth.

Part Positioning

- Center the median plane of the patient's body to the midline of the wall unit.
- Extend the patient's chin upward slightly and adjust the head so there is no rotation.
- The patient's shoulders should be in the same transverse plane with no rotation (*Figure 2–45*).

Central Ray

- Using a 40-in. SID, direct the central ray perpendicular to the film at the level of the thyroid cartilage.
- Center the cassette to the central ray.

Breathing Instructions

- Instruct the patient to inhale slowly and deeply and make the exposure during slow inhalation to ensure an air-filled trachea.

Image Evaluation

- The region from C3 to T3 should be visualized on the radiograph.
- Technical factors should allow visualization of air in the pharynx, larynx, and trachea.
- The mandible should be superimposed over the base of the skull.
- The sternoclavicular joints should be equidistant from the spine.
- The airway should be in the middle of the film (*Figure 2–46*).

1. Trachea

► LATERAL UPPER AIRWAY

Technical Considerations

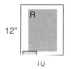

12"

10

- Film size: 10 × 12 in. lengthwise.
- Grid or nongrid depending on patient size and department policy.
- 65–75 kVp.
- Collimate to the soft tissue of the neck crosswise and include the inferior margin of the mandible and the sternoclavicular joints lengthwise.

Shielding

- Use gonadal shielding on all pediatric patients and adults of reproductive age.

Patient Positioning

- Assist the patient to the upright lateral position, standing or seated, against the wall unit.
- Patient's feet should be separated slightly with weight equally distributed on both feet.
- Adjust the height of the wall unit so the top edge of the cassette is approximately at the level of the gonions.

Part Positioning

- Center the coronal plane that passes through the gonions to the midline of the upright wall unit.
- Extend the patient's chin slightly and adjust the patient's head so it is aligned with the body and there is no rotation.
- The patient's arms should be positioned at sides with shoulders back *(Figure 2–47)*.

Central Ray

- Direct the central ray perpendicular to the film at a point 1 to 2 in. superior to the level of the suprasternal notch. **Note:** Some department routines may specify centering to the level of the suprasternal notch to include the upper mediastinum.
- A 72-in. SID should be used to minimize the magnification caused by the increased OID.

Breathing Instructions

- Instruct the patient to inhale slowly and deeply and make the exposure during inhalation to ensure an air-filled trachea.

Image Evaluation

- The region from C1 to T3 should be visualized on the radiograph.
- Technical factors should allow visualization of air in the pharynx, larynx, and trachea.
- The mandible should be elevated slightly to prevent superimposition over the anterior vertebral bodies.
- There should be no rotation of the vertebrae and the mandibular bodies should be superimposed.
- The airway should be in the middle of the film *(Figure 2–48)*.

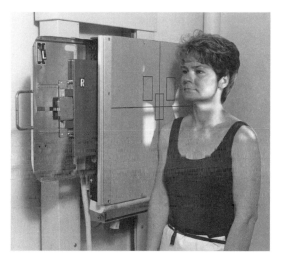

Figure 2–47. Lateral upper airway.

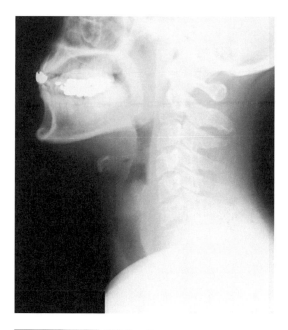

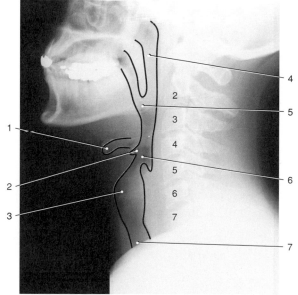

1. Hyoid bone	4. Nasopharynx	6. Laryngopharynx
2. Epiglottis	5. Oropharynx	7. Trachea
3. Larynx		

Figure 2–48. Lateral upper airway.

$\mathcal{S}$UMMARY

► The primary functions of the respiratory system are to provide oxygen to the circulatory system and to eliminate carbon dioxide from the body.

► The principal structures of the respiratory system are the pharynx, trachea, bronchi, and lungs.

► Oxygen and carbon dioxide are exchanged in the alveoli of the lungs.

► Routine chest examinations usually include both the PA and lateral projections.

► Chest radiography is generally performed with a grid or air-gap technique employing 100 to 150 kVp.

► To ensure consistency, automatic exposure control is frequently used in chest radiography.

► The apices, the cone-shaped lung regions above the clavicles, and the costophrenic angles, formed by the lower, lateral margins of the ribs and diaphragm, must be included on chest radiographs.

► When checking positioning accuracy on a PA chest radiograph, the sternoclavicular joints should be equidistant from the spine and the scapulae should be out of the lung field.

► On a lateral chest radiograph, the posterior ribs should be superimposed and the arms should be elevated to prevent superimposition over the lungs.

► Oblique projections can be used to evaluate the heart or pulmonary nodules, whereas lordotic projections are used to better visualize the apices.

► Lateral decubitus projections are used to demonstrate the presence of free air or fluid in the thoracic cavity; the side of interest will be up when looking for free air and down when looking for fluid.

► Consistent patient positioning and technique selection are critical to accurate diagnosis.

► Bronchography, tomography, CT, echocardiography, MRI, and nuclear medicine are specialized imaging procedures that can be used to further evaluate the lungs and/or heart.

$\mathcal{Q}$UESTIONS FOR CRITICAL THINKING & APPLICATION

1. A patient has been brought to the radiology department on a stretcher for a chest radiograph. Because she was unable to sit or stand, you obtained an AP chest radiograph with the patient supine. After looking at the radiograph, the radiologist requested a film to demonstrate air–fluid levels in the lungs. What projection(s) can you obtain to achieve this goal?

2. Describe the location of the trachea with reference to the esophagus and vertebral column.

3. Why might the nasal cavities be referred to as "air conditioners"?

4. Your patient had an upper respiratory infection for the past week and is now complaining of pain in her right ear. Explain the connection between these two conditions.

5. You have an order to take a soft tissue neck examination on a 6-month-old infant for possible epiglottitis. How could this condition impede respiration?

6. Young children often insert small objects up their nostrils. You receive an order from the ER for a chest radiograph on a 4-year-old patient who is experiencing respiratory difficulties after inserting a little metal bolt up her nose. If the child's mother has given you this history, where would you expect to see a foreign body on the exposed radiograph? Why?

7. Diagram the path of O_2 as it enters the mouth and nasal cavities on inhalation, is transported to the body, and is expelled as CO_2 on exhalation.

8. Why is a 72-in. or greater SID preferred for chest radiography?

9. Describe the possible methods that could best be used to demonstrate the apices on both agile patients and immobile patients.

10. Why is it important to make the exposure during slow, deep inhalation when imaging the upper airway?

11. Why is high kilovoltage preferred when radiographing the chest?

12. Which is the best projection to demonstrate fluid in the right lung?

FILM CRITIQUE

What structures should you look at to evaluate positioning on this PA chest radiograph *(Figure 2–49)*?

Was this patient correctly positioned?

How can you tell?

Was there adequate inhalation for this projection?

How is this determined?

These PA *(Figure 2–50A)* and lateral *(Figure 2–50B)* chest radiographs were taken to locate a foreign body. Can you identify the foreign body?

Although it is not well demonstrated, a straight pin was inhaled.

Where is it located?

Why did the foreign body position itself where it did?

Describe the route of travel of the foreign object.

What effect might this foreign body have on the lung(s)?

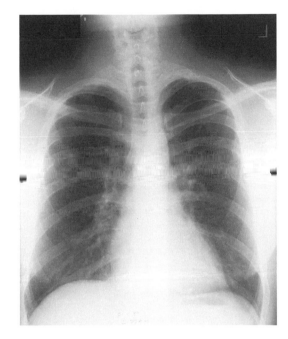

Figure 2–49.

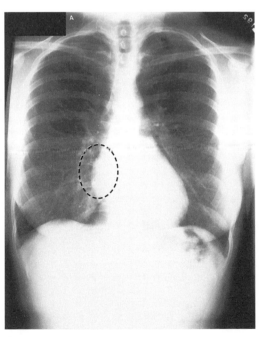

A

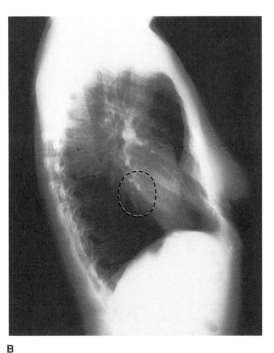

B

Figure 2–50.

3

THE ABDOMEN

► OBJECTIVES

Following the completion of this chapter the student will be able to:

- Name and identify those structures contained within the abdominopelvic cavity, to include the digestive system, urinary system, adrenal glands, hepatobiliary system, spleen, and pancreas.

- Differentiate between the four quadrant and nine-region methods of localization of structures within the abdominopelvic cavity and identify structures normally located in each quadrant and/or region.

- Define the terminology associated with the abdomen, to include anatomy, procedures, and pathology.

- Describe the procedure for obtaining supine, prone, upright, and decubitus projections of the abdomen to include patient positioning, centering, and technical considerations.

- Discuss the technical considerations needed for producing optimum radiographs of the abdomen and how these technical considerations must be changed to accommodate the pediatric patient.

- Evaluate radiographs of the abdomen in terms of positioning, centering, image quality, and radiographic anatomy.

- Differentiate between radiographs of the abdomen taken in the supine, prone, upright, and decubitus positions.

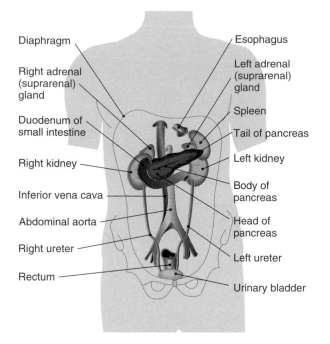

Figure 3–1. The abdomen.

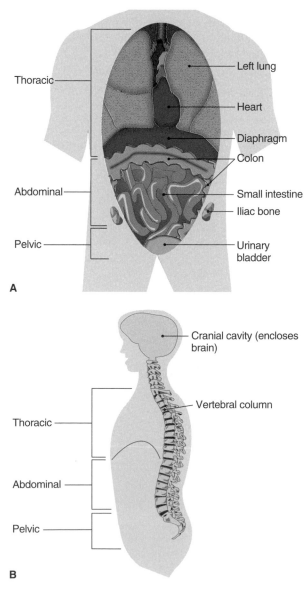

Figure 3–2. Abdominal cavity: **(A)** frontal view, **(B)** lateral view.

Radiography of the abdomen may be done simply to evaluate the abdominal contents, check tube placements, or as a preliminary step prior to the administration of contrast medium. The abdomen contains organs vital to digestion, metabolism, reproduction, and waste removal. Many of these organs can be visualized radiographically following the administration of contrast medium.

Plain, noncontrast films of the abdomen are usually obtained prior to administration of contrast medium to rule out residual contrast from earlier examinations and to identify any pathology that may be obscured following the administration of contrast medium. Plain films may also be obtained to rule out free air in the abdomen, identify radiopaque stones in the kidneys or gallbladder, or localize foreign objects.

▶ ANATOMY OF THE ABDOMEN

The abdominopelvic cavity *(Figure 3–1)* is separated from the thoracic cavity by the muscular diaphragm. It can be arbitrarily divided into abdominal and pelvic cavities as follows. The abdominal cavity is located above an imaginary plane at the level of the iliac crests and houses the stomach, small intestine, most of the large intestine, liver, gallbladder, spleen, pancreas, kidneys, and ureters. The lower portion of the abdomen, or pelvic cavity, is located below this plane. The sigmoid colon, rectum, urinary bladder, and some of the reproductive organs are contained within this area *(Figure 3–2)*.

The abdominopelvic cavity is lined with a double-walled membrane known as the **peritoneum** (per-i-tō-NĒ-um). The visceral portion of the peritoneum encloses the organs in the abdomen, whereas the parietal peritoneum lines the walls of the abdominal cavity. The peritoneum secretes a serous fluid which acts as a lubricant for the movable abdominal organs. Double layers of peritoneum called mesentery and omentum are extensions of the parietal peritoneum. These tissues stretch from the abdominal walls to the abdominal organs, thereby supporting them and holding them in place. A condition known as peritonitis occurs if the potential space between the two walls of the peritoneum, referred to as the peritoneal cavity, becomes infected through contamination (eg, perforated ulcer, ruptured appendix, or stab wound to abdomen) *(Figure 3–3)*.

Many bony, soft tissue, and vascular structures are contained within the abdominopelvic cavity. It would be impossible to discuss radiography of the abdomen without acquiring a rudimentary knowledge of these structures *(Table 3–1)*, which accounts for their inclusion in this chapter; however, most of the structures are discussed in much greater detail in other chapters dealing with the related body systems.

Although many of the structures in the abdomen cannot be adequately visualized without the aid of a contrast medium, they can still be identified by the radiographer. Knowledge of the structures and their general location and shape is critical for radiographic positioning and technical evaluation of abdominal radiographs.

METHODS OF DESCRIBING LOCATIONS OF STRUCTURES

Medical personnel must use a method of describing the exact location of internal structures or pathology within the abdominopelvic cavity. Two methods are commonly used.

Nine-Region Method

To divide the abdominopelvic cavity into nine regions, an imaginary grid (like Tic–Tac–Toe) is used. The upper horizontal plane is situated near the lower margin of the ribs, and the lower horizontal plane is located slightly inferior to the iliac crests. The right and left vertical planes are parallel to the midsagittal plane and are located slightly medial to each nipple *(Figure 3–4)*.

The regions can be described as follows:
- *Right (1) and left hypochondriac (3).* Hypochondriac means "under or below the cartilage" and refers to the upper, lateral portions of the abdomen under the ribs.
- *Epigastric (2).* This region is in the upper central part of the grid and is located over the stomach.
- *Right (4) and left lumbar (6).* These middle regions of the grid are located lateral to the umbilicus. They may also be called the right and left lateral regions.
- *Umbilical (5).* The umbilical is the central region of the grid which is located around the navel.
- *Right (7) and left iliac (9).* These lower side regions of the grid correspond to the ilia of the pelvis, but are also referred to as the inguinal regions as they are located near the groin.
- *Hypogastric (8).* Located below the umbilicus, the hypogastric region is the lower middle region. *Hypogastric* means "below the stomach."

Table 3–1. Summary of the Abdomen

Bony Structures
Vertebral column
  Thoracic spine
  Lumbar spine
  Sacrum
  Coccyx
Pelvis
  Ilium
  Ischium
  Pubis

Muscles
Diaphragm
Right and left psoas major muscles

Digestive System
Stomach
  Cardiac orifice
  Fundus
  Body
  Pyloric portion
  Pyloric orifice
Small intestine
  Duodenum
  Jejunum
  Ileum
Large intestine
  Cecum
  Ascending colon
  Right colic (hepatic) flexure
  Transverse colon
  Left colic (splenic) flexure
  Descending colon
  Sigmoid colon
  Rectum
  Anus

Biliary System
Liver
Gallbladder
Biliary ducts

Urinary System
Right and left kidneys
Right and left ureters
Urinary bladder

Reproductive System
Female
  Right and left ovaries
  Right and left uterine tubes
  Uterus
  Vagina
Male
  Testes
  Duct system
  Accessory glands
  Scrotum
  Penis
  Prostate gland

Miscellaneous Soft Tissue Structures
Pancreas
Spleen
Adrenal glands

Vascular Structures
Aorta
Inferior vena cava

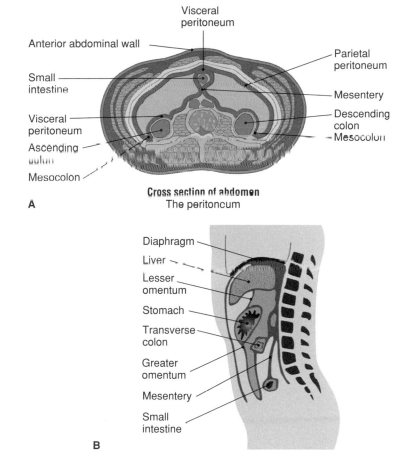

Cross section of abdomen
The peritoneum

A

B

Figure 3–3. Peritoneum: **(A)** axial section of abdomen, **(B)** sagittal view.

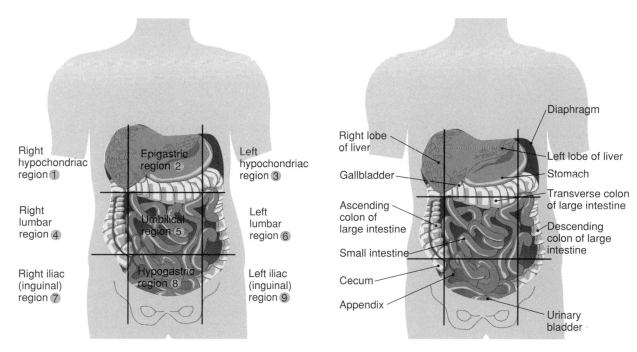

Figure 3–4. Nine-region method.

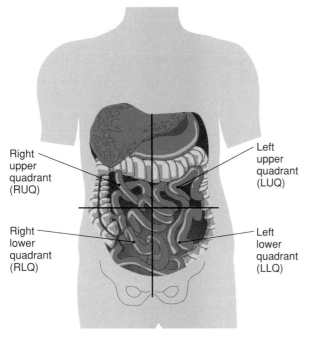

Right upper quadrant (RUQ)

Left upper quadrant (LUQ)

Right lower quadrant (RLQ)

Left lower quadrant (LLQ)

Figure 3–5. Quadrant method.

Quadrant Method

The abdominopelvic cavity can also be divided into four compartments or quadrants by drawing an imaginary line vertically down the midsagittal plane and horizontally through the umbilicus. The resulting divisions are known as right upper (RUQ), left upper (LUQ), right lower (RLQ), and left lower (LLQ) quadrants *(Figure 3–5)*.

Although the nine-region method is more precise, the quadrant method is usually considered sufficient for use by radiographers in the localization of abdominal structures and pathology. For example, when taking a patient's history prior to examination, the radiographer might indicate that "the patient complained of pain in the right lower quadrant."

BODY HABITUS

As discussed in Chapter 1, body habitus affects the size, shape, and relative position of internal organs. Those organs in the abdominopelvic cavity most affected by body habitus are the stomach and gallbladder. The dimensions of the abdomen are subject to wide variation depending on body type. This affects centering and film orientation. For example, a hypersthenic patient may require two radiographs to adequately demonstrate the upper and lower abdomen.

BONY STRUCTURES

The bony structures that can be visualized on an abdominal radiograph include the lower vertebral column and pelvis. The proximal femurs are sometimes demonstrated depending on the size of the patient, but are included in this discussion mainly because they are important positioning landmarks.

The lower vertebral column is located posteriorly in the abdominopelvic cavity. The sections that are relevant to this discussion of the abdomen are the thoracic spine, lumbar spine, sacrum, and coccyx *(Figure 3–6)*.

Thoracic Spine

There are 12 thoracic (tho-RĀS-ik) vertebrae, most of which are above the level of the diaphragm in the thoracic cavity. The position of the diaphragm is variable depending on bodily habitus, patient position (upright versus supine), and respiration, but usually only the lower two or three thoracic vertebrae are considered to be in the abdominopelvic cavity.

Lumbar Spine

There are five lumbar (LUM-bar) vertebrae. This portion of the vertebral column is just inferior to the thoracic spine and is visible on an abdominal radiograph. Each lumbar body is large and boxlike. Right and left transverse processes project laterally to either side of the body. The spinous process of each vertebra can be visualized on end through the body and appears in the shape of a teardrop. These processes are blunt and can usually be palpated on the patient's back. The space between adjacent vertebral bodies is known as the intervertebral joint or disk space.

Sacrum

The sacrum (SĀ-krum) is inferior to the lumbar spine. This structure is shaped like a shovel and formed by five fused vertebrae. The upper sides of the sacrum articulate with the ilia of the pelvis to make the sacroiliac joints.

Coccyx

The coccyx (KOK-siks) is a small structure made up of three to five fused vertebrae. In layman's terms, it is known as the tailbone and can be easily palpated at the inferior end of the vertebral column *(Figure 3–7)*.

Ilia

The right and left ilia (IL-ē-ah) (singular, ilium) of the pelvis are located to either side of the sacrum. The upper flared portion of each ilium is called the *ala* or *wing*. The superior border is known as the crest of the ilium or iliac crest and is situated approximately at the level of the disk space between the 4th and 5th lumbar vertebrae. It can be palpated just below the patient's waistline. Located at the anterior edge of the iliac

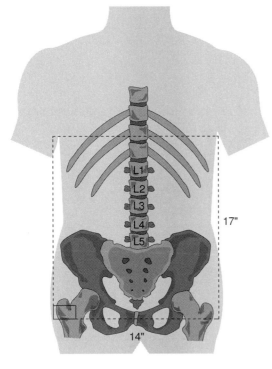

L1
L2
L3
L4
L5

17"

14"

Figure 3–6. The dashed lines indicate the parameters of a 14 × 17-in. (35 × 43-cm) cassette and illustrate the area that would be included on an abdominal radiograph.

crest, the anterior superior iliac spine (ASIS) is a prominent bony projection, which can also be palpated. The iliac crest and ASIS are commonly used positioning landmarks. The lower portion of the each ilium forms part of the acetabulum (as-e-TAB-ū-lum), or socket, of the hip joint *(Figure 3–8)*.

Pubic Bones

The lateral portions of the right and left pubic (PŪ-bik) bones also assist in the formation of each acetabulum. The pubic bones meet medially to form the symphysis pubis. The upper margin of the symphysis (SIM-fi-sis) pubis can be palpated and is an important landmark for locating the urinary bladder.

Ischia

Along with the ilia and pubic bones, the right and left ischia (ISH-ē-ah) (singular, ischium) form a portion of the acetabulum. The ischia are located inferior and posteriorly to the pubic bones. The rounded process on the posterior aspect of each ischium is called the ischial tuberosity. It can be palpated just below the gluteal folds (cheeks of the buttocks) and lateral to the anus. When a person is sitting, most of his or her body weight will be borne by the ischial tuberosities. These structures can be used as positioning landmarks for a PA projection of the abdomen, as the ischial tuberosities lie approximately 1.5 in. below the level of the symphysis pubis. The large opening found between each ischium and pubic bone is called the obturator (ob-tū-RĀ-tor) foramen. These foramina will not usually be demonstrated on a correctly centered radiograph of the abdomen.

Femur

The proximal portion of each femur may be partially demonstrated on an abdominal radiograph if the patient is small to average in size. Although they are not considered to be critical anatomy, certain structures on the femur can be identified on the radiograph. The head of the femur is rounded and fits in the acetabulum to form the hip joint. The constricted neck is inferior to the head. The greater trochanter is a large bump or prominence located on the lateral margin of the upper femur at the junction of the neck and shaft. It can be palpated on the upper lateral aspect of the thigh and may be used as a centering landmark as it lies approximately 1.5 in. (almost 4 cm) above the level of the symphysis pubis.

MUSCLES

Diaphragm

The diaphragm (DĪ-ah-fram) is a dome-shaped muscular structure. It serves as the roof of the abdominal cavity, as well as the floor of the thoracic cavity. If breathing is not suspended during abdominal radiography, blurring will occur as a result of movement of the diaphragm. The movement of the diaphragm during respiration affects the physical location of some organs in the abdomen. For example, the diaphragm moves inferiorly on inhalation, displacing the kidneys downward approximately 1 in. (2.5 cm).

Psoas Major Muscles

The right and left psoas (SŌ-as) major muscles are located in the posterior abdomen and help to form the posterior wall of the abdominopelvic cavity. These muscles are situated lateral to the lumbar spine. The origin of the muscles is the bodies and transverse processes of the 12th thoracic through 5th lumbar vertebrae, whereas the insertion is the lesser trochanter of the femurs. These muscles help to flex the trunk and also flex and rotate the thighs medially. As they are particularly dense soft tissue structures, they will be visible on a properly exposed radiograph of the abdomen *(Figure 3–9)*.

DIGESTIVE SYSTEM

The digestive system is a continuous hollow tube known as the alimentary canal. The alimentary canal extends from the mouth through the pharynx, esophagus, stomach, small intestine, and large intestine, terminating at the anus. A characteristic shared by all of the structures in the alimentary canal is the presence of a mucosal membrane that forms the lining of this hollow tube.

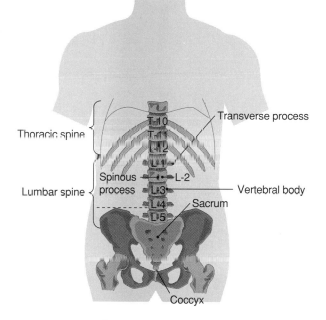

Figure 3–7. Vertebral column.

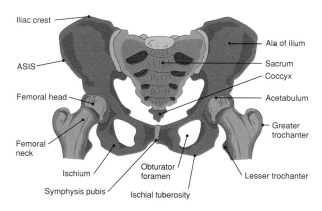

Figure 3–8. Bony landmarks of the pelvis.

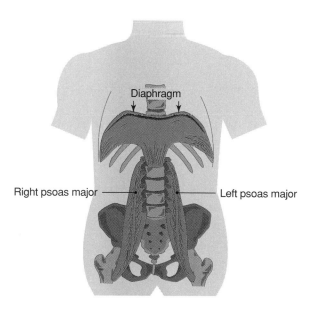

Figure 3–9. Location of the diaphragm and psoas major muscles within abdomen.

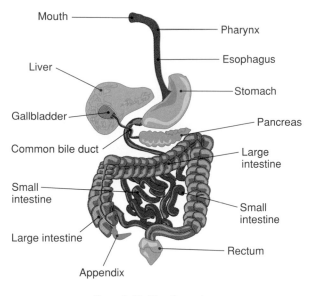

Figure 3–10. Digestive system.

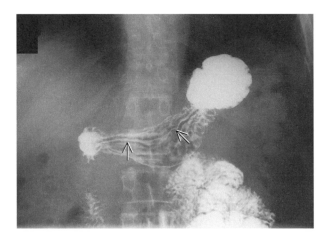

Figure 3–11. Rugae in the body of the stomach demonstrated on an AP projection.

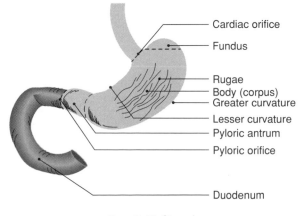

Figure 3–12. Stomach.

Most of the alimentary canal is located within the abdominopelvic cavity; however, the mouth and pharynx are not found in this region and as such are not discussed at this time *(Figure 3–10)*.

Esophagus

The esophagus (e-SOF-ah-gus) is a hollow, muscular tube that is contained primarily in the thoracic cavity. It does, however, pass through the diaphragm into the abdomen approximately at the level of the 10th thoracic vertebra. The abdominal esophagus is usually only 1 to 2 cm long, and may be referred to as the cardiac antrum. It terminates at the cardiac orifice to the stomach.

Stomach

The stomach (STUM-ak) is located predominately in the left upper quadrant of the abdomen, or more specifically in the epigastric, umbilical, and left hypochondriac regions. It extends from the esophagus to the small intestine. The stomach will characteristically collapse when empty, but has the ability to expand greatly. In the sthenic patient, the stomach assumes a "J" shape. As the shape is affected by bodily habitus, the radiographer will notice that the stomach is higher and more transverse in the hypersthenic patient but situated lower and closer to the spine in the asthenic patient. When the stomach is empty, the mucosal lining falls into longitudinal folds called *rugae* (ROO-gee or ROO-guy). Rugae are visible on a radiograph of the stomach when contrast medium is employed, and might also be demonstrated on plain films as gas-filled rugae *(Figure 3–11)*.

The stomach has two openings or orifices on it. The entrance or opening where the esophagus empties into the stomach is known as the cardiac orifice. The stomach ends at the pyloric orifice, where it connects with the duodenum of the small intestine. Located at both the proximal and distal orifices of the stomach are sphincters (SFINGK-ters), which are round muscles designed to regulate the movement of food substances into and out of the stomach.

The three main portions of the stomach are the fundus (FUN-dus), body (corpus), and pylorus or pyloric (pī-LOR-ik) antrum. The fundus is the rounded upper portion of the stomach. It is located above and to the left of the cardiac orifice and just inferior to the left hemidiaphragm. Gas in the fundus can usually be visualized on a PA upright projection of the chest, as well as on an erect projection of the abdomen. The body is the large central area of the stomach, and the pyloric antrum is the inferior portion. The pyloric antrum terminates at the pyloric orifice *(Figure 3–12)*.

Small Intestine

Although widely variable in length, the small intestine averages 20 ft (6 m). Without the use of contrast medium, it is generally not well visualized on plain radiography of the abdomen. Large amounts of gas are not usually seen in the small intestine unless an obstruction exists. Generally, small air pockets in the small intestine are visible on a plain radiograph of the abdomen. If an ileus, or bowel obstruction, is present, gas will distend the small intestine, causing it to take on the appearance of stacked coins.

The duodenum (dū-ō-DĒ-num) is the first of three segments of the small intestine. Approximately 10 in. (25 cm) long, the duodenum is usually C-shaped. It crosses from the right side of the upper abdomen to the left, where it meets the second segment, the jejunum (je-JOO-num). Measuring approximately 8 ft or 2.5 m, the jejunum is located mainly in the left upper and lower quadrants. It merges with the ileum (IL-ē-um), which forms the last part of the small intestine. Situated primarily in the middle and right regions of the abdomen, the ileum measures in as the longest segment at approximately 11 ft (3.3 m). The terminal portion of the ileum connects to the large intestine at the ileocecal valve, which is generally located in the right lower quadrant of the abdomen. A muscular sphincter at the ileocecal valve prevents backflow from the large intestine into the ileum *(Figure 3–13)*.

Large Intestine

Extending from the ileum of the small intestine to the anus, the large intestine is approximately 5 ft (1.5 m) long. It is larger in diameter than the small intestine. In the average body build, the large intestine spans all four quadrants as it is located around the periphery of the abdomen. Divided into three primary regions, it begins in the right lower quadrant at the ileocecal valve.
A. The **cecum** (SĒ-kum) is a rounded sac or pouch located inferior to the ileocecal valve. The appendix, or vermiform process, projects from the posteromedial surface of the cecum.
B. The **colon** (KO-lon) is a long tube that continues from the cecum to the rectum. It can be divided into four portions:
1. The ascending colon is directed superiorly from the cecum to right upper quadrant, where it bends medially and anteriorly. This bend is known as the right colic (hepatic) flexure as it is located under the liver.
2. The transverse colon crosses the upper anterior abdomen from the right to left sides, where it bends inferiorly and posteriorly under the spleen to form the left colic (splenic) flexure.

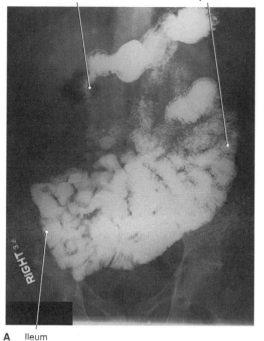

Duodenum　　　Jejunum

RIGHT

A　　Ileum

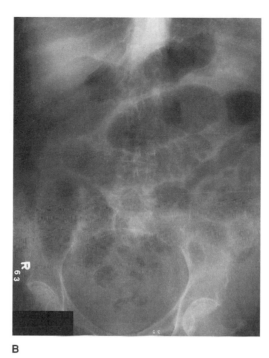

B

Figure 3–13. Small intestine: **(A)** AP projection of contrast filled small intestine, **(B)** KUB demonstrating a small bowel obstruction.

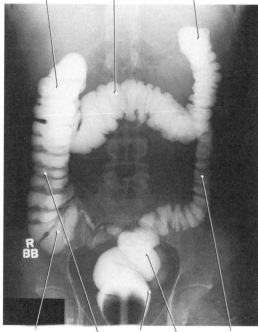

Right colic (hepatic) flexure　Transverse colon　Left colic (splenic) flexure

R BB

A　Cecum　　　　　Rectum　　　　Descending colon

Ascending colon　　　Sigmoid colon

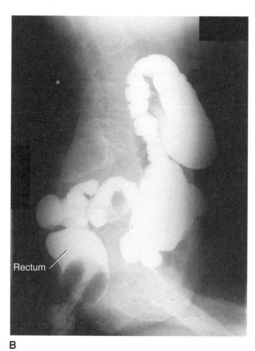

Rectum

B

Figure 3–14. Large intestine: **(A)** AP projection, **(B)** lateral projection.

3. The descending colon is located on the left side of the abdomen and extends inferiorly from the left colic (splenic) flexure into the pelvis, where it becomes the sigmoid colon.

4. The sigmoid colon is an "S"-shaped segment of the colon. It extends approximately from the level of the iliac crest inferiorly to the third segment of the sacrum (S3), where it connects to the rectum.

C. The rectum (REK-tum) is approximately 6 in. (15 cm) long and is the last section of the large intestine. It begins about the level of S3 and is situated just anterior to the sacrum. The inferior or terminal portion is known as the anal canal and constitutes the last 1 in. (2–3 cm) of the rectum. The external opening of the large intestine is the anus.

A barium enema is the radiographic examination usually performed to evaluate the large intestine *(Figure 3–14)*; however, a plain radiograph of the abdomen will demonstrate gas and the presence of fecal material. The radiographer can determine that gas is in the large intestine not only by its location, but also by the characteristic shape. Bands of muscle fibers running the length of the large intestine produce a puckering effect. Sacs or pouches called *haustra* (HAUS-tra) (singular, haustrum) are formed. Gas accumulates in the haustra and is demonstrated radiographically.

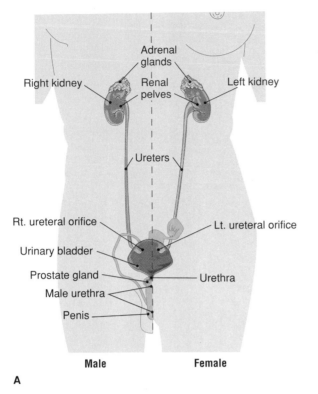

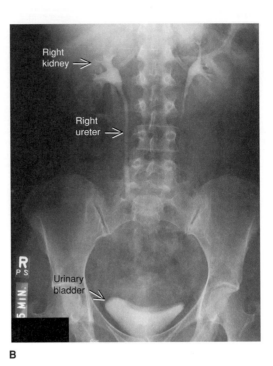

Figure 3–15. Urinary system: **(A)** frontal aspect, **(B)** intravenous pyelogram.

► Related Terminology

anastomosis (ah-nās-tō-MŌ-sis)—joining or connection between two tubular structures which may be abnormal in nature or due to surgery (eg, ileorectal)

anorexia (an-ō-REK-sē-ah)—lack of appetite

appendicitis (ah-pen-di-SĪ-tis)—condition in which the vermiform appendix is inflamed and infected, generally requiring surgical removal

ascites (ah-SĪ-tēz)—abnormal accumulation of fluid in the abdominal (peritoneal) cavity

atresia (ah-TRĒ-zē-ah)—occlusion or absence of a normal opening to a tubular structure of the body (eg, esophageal atresia)

calculus (KAL-kū-lus)—formation of a stone (concretion) in body tissues as the result of an accumulation of mineral salts (eg, a renal calculus is a kidney stone)

cirrhosis (si-RŌ-sis)—degenerative disease of the liver in which the liver cells are progressively destroyed

colostomy (kō-LOS-tō-mē)—creation of an artificial opening in the large intestine from the abdominal wall

constipation (kon-sti-PĀ-shun)—difficulty in eliminating fecal material

cryptorchidism (krip-TOR-ki-dizm)—condition in males in which one or both of the testes remain in the abdomen and fail to descend to the scrotum

diarrhea (dī-ah-RĒ-ah)—frequent and abnormally liquid bowel movements resulting from accelerated passage of fecal material through the intestine

dyspepsia (dis-PEP-sē-ah)—discomfort after eating (indigestion)

emesis (EM-e-sis)—vomiting

fistula (FIS-tū-lah)—abnormal tubelike opening between two internal organs or between an internal organ and the body surface (eg, tracheoesophageal fistula)

(continued)

URINARY SYSTEM

The urinary system is located in the abdomen and functions to remove waste and excess water from the body. It consists of the two kidneys, two ureters, one urinary bladder, and one urethra. To adequately study the functional ability of the urinary system, either ionic or nonionic iodinated contrast medium must be used *(Figure 3–15)*. The kidneys and urinary bladder, however, may be identified by the radiographer on a plain radiograph of the abdomen.

Kidneys

The kidneys (KID-nez) are paired, bean-shaped organs that are situated in the posterior abdomen above the waist. They function to remove liquid waste products from the blood. They are located bilaterally to the lumbar spine, with the right kidney in a slightly lower position than the left because of the large mass of the liver in the right upper quadrant. The kidneys are considered to be retroperitoneal structures as they are located behind the peritoneum. The kidneys may be localized on a plain radiograph of the abdomen because of the presence of fat, which surrounds each one. This fat is known as the adipose capsule.

Ureters

Urine produced in the kidneys drains to the urinary bladder via the right and left ureters (UR-e-ters or ū-RĒ-ters). These hollow tubes are approximately 10 to 12 in. (25–30 cm) long and are also located behind the peritoneum.

Urinary Bladder

The urinary bladder is an expandable sac that serves as a temporary reservoir for urine before it is excreted. It is located behind the symphysis pubis and under the peritoneum (infraperitoneal). To adequately study the urinary bladder, it must be filled with iodinated contrast medium; however, the shadow or outline of the bladder may be visualized on a radiograph of the abdomen if it is distended with urine.

Urethra

The urethra (ū-RĒ-thrah) serves as the passageway for urine as it is excreted from the body. It is a narrow canal that extends from the urinary bladder to the outside of the body. Although it is not possible to demonstrate the urethra on a plain radiograph of the abdomen, it can be evaluated during an examination called a voiding cystourethrogram.

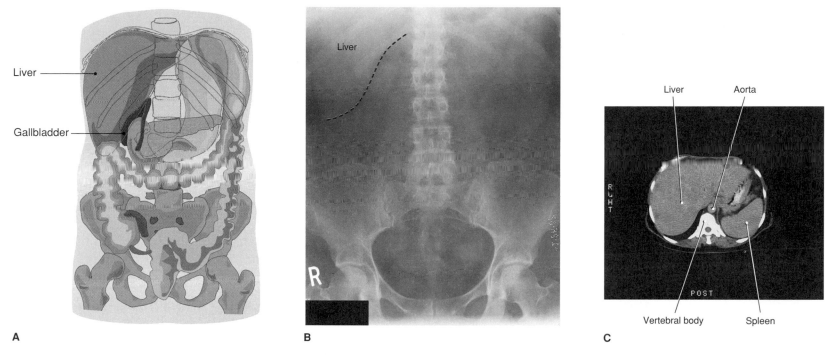

Figure 3–16. Liver: **(A)** frontal aspect, **(B)** KUB with lower margin of liver outlined, **(C)** axial CT image.

Adrenal Glands

The adrenal (ah-DRĒ-nal) glands are also known as the suprarenal glands because of their location. These structures are part of the endocrine system, but are included in this discussion because of their proximity to the kidneys. The adrenal glands are paired and are situated superiorly and medially to each kidney. Although not usually visualized on a radiograph of the abdomen, they might be seen if they are calcified or enlarged. A CT image of the abdomen may demonstrate the adrenal glands.

BILIARY SYSTEM

The structures of the biliary system are the liver, gallbladder, and duct system. These structures are located in the upper right quadrant of the abdomen.

Liver

The liver (LIV-er) is a large, solid organ found just inferior to the right hemidiaphragm. On a plain radiograph of the abdomen, an area of decreased radiographic density can be seen in the right upper quadrant because of its presence. The liver performs a multitude of functions, including the formation of bile, which aids in digestion by breaking down fats in the small intestine *(Figure 3–16)*.

Gallbladder

The gallbladder is a pear-shaped sac located on the inferior aspect of the liver. Once bile is produced by the liver, it is stored in the gallbladder. It is here that the bile is concentrated. When the gallbladder contracts, the bile is released. It is then conveyed to the small intestine to assist in digestion, specifically in the breakdown of fats. The gallbladder is not readily visible on a plain radiograph of the abdomen. It can be examined radiographically after the oral administration of an iodinated contrast medium. Alternative methods of examination include CT and ultrasonography.

► Related Terminology (*continued*)

gastroenteritis (gas-trō-en-te-RĪ-tis)—inflammation of the stomach and the small intestine, specifically the lining of these structures

hemoperitoneum (he-mō-per-i-tō-NĒ-um)—abnormal presence (effusion) of blood in the peritoneal cavity

hiatal hernia (hī-A-tal HER-nē-ah)—protrusion of part of the stomach up through the esophageal opening of the diaphragm

hysterectomy (his-te-RECK-tō-mē)—surgical removal of the uterus

ileus (IL-ē-us)—obstruction of the intestines caused by lack of forward movement of the bowel contents

incontinence (in-KON-ti-nens)—inability to control urination; may also refer to the inability to control defecation

inguinal hernia (ING-gwi-nal HER-nē-ah)—protrusion of the intestine through the abdominal wall; in the case of a male, the intestine may protrude into the scrotal sac

jaundice (JAWN-dis)—condition in which an increase in bilirubin and bile pigments in the blood causes a yellow discoloration of the skin; usually due to a disorder of the gallbladder or liver

laparoscopy (lap-ah-ROS-kō-pē)—examination of the abdomen in which an endoscope is inserted through a small incision in the abdominal wall; may be performed on a woman to evaluate the ovaries and also for a tubal ligation procedure

megacolon (meg-ah-KŌ-lon)—condition in which the colon is dilated

nausea (NAW-zē-ah)—sick feeling or sensation that may result in vomiting

(continued)

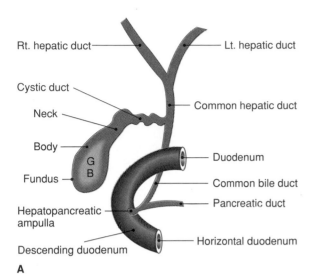

A

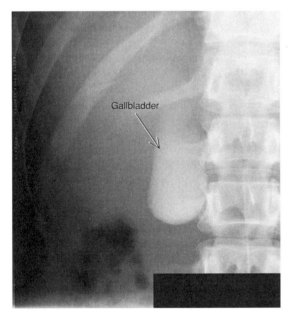

B

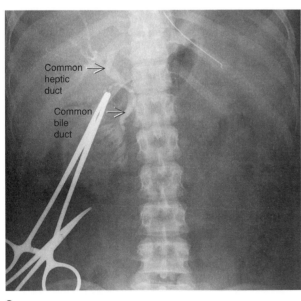

C

Figure 3–17. Biliary system: **(A)** frontal aspect of the ducts and gallbladder, **(B)** PA cholecystogram demonstrating the gallbladder, **(C)** OR cholangiogram demonstrating the ducts.

Biliary Ducts

A series of ducts serve to convey the bile from the liver to the gallbladder and then on to the small intestine. Bile leaves the liver via the right and left hepatic (he-PAT-ik) ducts. These ducts merge to form the common hepatic duct. Bile enters and leaves the gallbladder through the cystic duct. This duct unites with the common hepatic duct to form the common bile duct. The common bile duct empties into the duodenum *(Figure 3–17)*.

REPRODUCTIVE SYSTEM

The female reproductive organs are located in the abdominopelvic cavity. Although they are not visualized on a plain radiograph of the abdomen, they are discussed briefly in this chapter because of their presence in the abdomen.

The female reproductive anatomy includes left and right ovaries, left and right uterine tubes, uterus, vagina, and external genitalia. As the external genitalia are situated inferiorly to the symphysis pubis, this anatomy is not included in this discussion. The location of the reproductive anatomy makes it difficult, if not impossible, for the radiographer to shield the female patient during abdominal radiography *(Figure 3–18)*.

Ovaries

The paired almond-shaped ovaries (Ō-var-ēz) are located in the pelvic cavity to each side of the uterus and are held in place by ligaments. As the female gonads, the ovaries produce eggs (ova), as well as secrete sexual hormones.

Uterine Tubes

The uterine (Ū-ter-in) tubes are also known as oviducts or fallopian tubes. These hollow tubes are approximately 5 in. (13 cm) long and serve to transport the ova from the ovaries to the uterus. The medial end of each tube connects to the upper angles of the uterus; the other end opens into the peritoneal cavity. This end lies very close to the adjacent ovary but is not actually attached to it.

Uterus

The uterus (Ū-ter-us) is a pear-shaped hollow organ. It is situated anterior to the rectum and posterosuperior to the urinary bladder. The uterus is the structure that nourishes and protects the developing embryo after conception. The lower end of the uterus is constricted and is known as the cervix.

Vagina

The vagina (vah-JĪ-nah) is a tubelike canal that serves as a passageway between the cervix and the outside of the body. It is situated behind the urinary bladder and urethra and anterior to the anal canal.

The female reproductive anatomy is most commonly visualized during an ultrasound examination. A more detailed radiographic examination of the uterus and uterine tubes is known as a *hysterosalpingogram*. This examination can be performed to determine causes of infertility (eg, blocked uterine tubes).

Testes

The male reproductive anatomy is situated primarily below the symphysis pubis and therefore is not included on an abdominal radiograph. It is important for the radiographer to know the location of the male reproductive anatomy to properly apply the lead shielding during radiography of the abdomen. For this reason, certain structures of the male reproductive system are discussed in this chapter *(Figure 3–19)*.

The male reproductive organs or gonads are known as the testes (TES-tēz). The two testes are responsible for producing spermatozoa and male sex hormones. They are enclosed by the scrotum (SKRŌ-tum), which is a sac suspended below the symphysis pubis and anterior to the anus.

Accessory Structures

Accessory structures in the male reproductive system are involved with the secretion of semen. Besides the scrotum, other accessory structures include the duct system, glands, and penis. As the mature sperm are conveyed along a series of ducts, they mix with fluids secreted by accessory glands to form semen. The duct system is composed of the epididymis (ep-i-DID-i-mis), ductus (vas) deferens (DUK-tus DEF-erens), and urethra. The semen is discharged from the penile urethra during ejaculation.

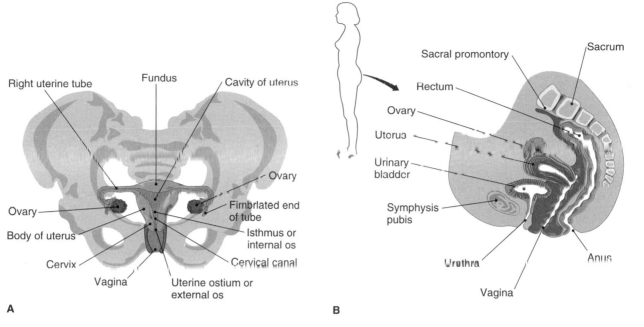

A

B

Figure 3–18. Female reproductive anatomy: **(A)** frontal aspect, **(B)** lateral aspect.

One of the accessory glands of the male reproductive system is the prostate (PROS-tāt) gland. It is situated just inferior to the urinary bladder and encircles the proximal portion of the urethra. The prostate gland can harden and enlarge in the elderly male, causing difficulty in urination.

The radiographer should attempt to shield the male gonads as long as the radiographic anatomy will not be compromised. During radiography of the abdomen, a gonadal shield can be placed below the symphysis pubis to adequately protect the gonads.

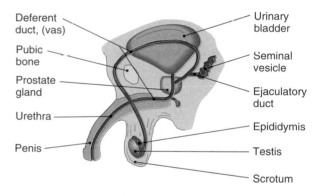

Figure 3–19. Lateral aspect of male reproductive anatomy.

MISCELLANEOUS STRUCTURES

Several other structures are found in the abdomen that should be mentioned in this chapter. Although they may not be visualized on a radiograph of the abdomen without employing contrast media, it is important to know of their location relative to other abdominal structures.

Pancreas

The pancreas is a gland that has both endocrine and exocrine functions. It secretes hormones, including insulin and glucagon, which regulate the concentration of glucose (sugar) in the blood. In addition, the pancreas serves as an accessory to digestion by producing enzymes necessary for the breakdown of proteins, carbohydrates, and fats. Pancreatic juices which contain these enzymes are excreted into the duodenum via the pancreatic duct. Approximately 8 to 10 in. (2–25 cm) long, the pancreas spans the right and left upper quadrants of the abdomen. The large head is situated in the C-loop or curve of the duodenum, whereas the body and tail taper toward the spleen.

Spleen

The spleen is an organ of the lymphatic system. It plays an important role in the formation and storage of blood cells. Located in the left upper quadrant under the diaphragm, the spleen is situated between the stomach and the left kidney *(Figure 3–20)*.

Aorta and Inferior Vena Cava

Blood from the circulatory system supplies oxygen necessary to the well-being of organs and tissues in the abdomen. Although there is a large network of blood vessels present in the abdomen, only the two main vessels are mentioned in this chapter.

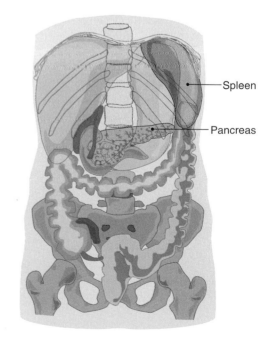

Figure 3–20. Location of spleen and pancreas in relationship to other abdominal structures.

The aorta is the largest artery in the body. In the abdomen, the aorta is positioned just anterior to the lumbar spine. Branches off of the aorta supply blood to various organs and structures in the abdomen and lower extremities.

The inferior vena cava (IVC) is the largest vein in the body. Deoxygenated blood from structures below the diaphragm is returned to the heart by way of the IVC. This structure is also located posteriorly in the abdomen and to the right of the aorta. Both the aorta and the IVC are retroperitoneal structures *(Figure 3–21)*.

► PROCEDURAL CONSIDERATIONS

Noncontrast radiography of the abdomen is very common in most radiology departments. Plain films are usually obtained prior to the administration of contrast medium for an upper gastrointestinal (UGI) study, small bowel examination, barium enema (colon or large intestinal study), or excretory urogram, also called an intravenous urogram or intravenous pyelogram (IVP). Films obtained for this purpose can be used to identify stones or calcifications in the kidneys or gallbladder, check for residual barium from a previous contrast study, evaluate bowel gas patterns, assess the size and location of abdominal organs, rule out congenital disorders and gross abnormalities, or identify foreign bodies or pathology which may be evident on plain films of the abdomen. Plain abdominal projections include the AP (supine), PA (prone), upright, and lateral or dorsal decubitus.

PATIENT PREPARATION

Unless the patient is scheduled for a contrast examination of the abdomen or other procedure requiring cathartics or fasting, there is no advance preparation. After the patient is correctly identified, an outpatient should be instructed to remove long necklaces and all clothing except shoes and socks. Although most undergarments do not contain metal, the elastic may cause unwanted artifacts on the radiograph and inconsistent density in the area of the elastic. Patients should be checked for radiopaque objects that might obscure abdominal anatomy on the radiograph. The radiographer should then obtain a pertinent patient history. This history can be used to assist the radiologist in diagnosis and may help determine whether exposure factors need to be adjusted due to pathology *(Figure 3–22)*.

Patients scheduled for an upright or decubitus abdominal projection must remain in that position for a minimum of 10 minutes to allow air in the abdomen to rise and fluid to settle. A patient who has been sitting in a wheelchair or outpatient waiting area should have the upright projection performed first to expedite completion of the procedure. Likewise, a patient traveling to the department on a stretcher can be positioned on the left side prior to transport and will be ready for the left lateral decubitus projection upon arrival in the radiology department.

POSITIONING CONSIDERATIONS

Preliminary or scout films of the abdomen are taken with the patient lying supine or prone on the table. These films, called KUBs, include the kidneys, ureters, and urinary bladder. To ensure inclusion of the bladder on the radiograph, the symphysis pubis must be included on the film.

When positioning a patient for abdominal radiography, the radiographer should check for patient rotation and alignment. The anterior superior iliac spines, as well as the shoulders, should be equidistant from the table. Very thin, asthenic patients may need small radiolucent supports positioned under the buttocks for comfort and to prevent rotation. A pillow may be placed under the patient's head and a small support may be positioned under the patient's knees to relieve stress on the back. Alignment can be checked by standing at the head or foot of the table and ensuring that the patient is straight and parallel with the long axis of the table.

The cassette is generally centered to the iliac crest. Based on patient size or build, this centering may need slight adjustment to ensure inclusion of the symphysis pubis on the radiograph. The frontal projection may also be obtained with the patient prone. When done prone, palpation of the greater trochanters or ischial tuberosities can be used to identify the level of the symphysis pubis. Normally, a 14 × 17-in. (35 × 43-cm) cassette is positioned lengthwise in the Bucky tray. Large patients, however, may require the use of two 14 × 17-in. cassettes positioned crosswise, the first to include the symphysis pubis and the second centered higher to include the upper abdomen with at least 2- to 3-in. overlap of the first film.

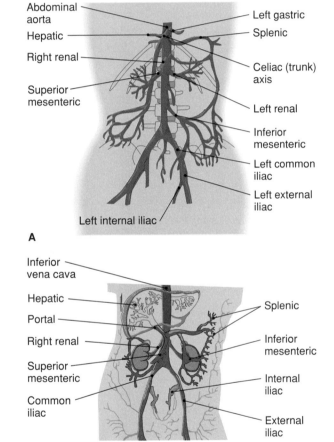

Figure 3–21. Major blood vessels of the abdomen: **(A)** arteries, **(B)** veins.

History Sheet: Abdominal Radiography

Patient Name: _____   Age: _____

Date: _____   X-ray No.: _____   Pregnant? _____   LMP: _____

Reason for admission/complaint: _____

Symptoms (check all that apply):

_____ Nausea	_____ Fever
_____ Vomiting	_____ Back pain
_____ Diarrhea	_____ Abdominal pain
_____ Constipation	_____ Blood in stool/urine
_____ Unexplained weight gain	_____ History of stones
_____ Unexplained weight loss	_____ Trauma
_____ General weakness or tiredness	

Duration of symptoms: _____

Abdominal surgical history: _____

Previous abdominal problems: _____

Additional comments: _____

_____

_____

Technologist: _____

Figure 3–22. Patient history form.

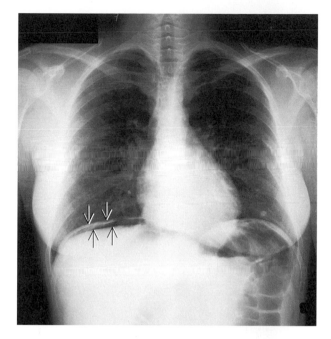

Figure 3–23. A PA chest radiograph may be a part of an acute abdominal series; note the presence of free air under the right hemidiaphragm.

Although most noncontrast abdominal radiographs are taken with the patient in the supine or prone position, upright and decubitus films are sometimes obtained to evaluate air–fluid levels and the presence of free air in the abdominal cavity. Free air can be a result of recent abdominal surgery, abdominal infection, or a perforation in the stomach or bowel. An acute abdominal series may include an upright PA projection of the chest and supine or prone, upright, and/or decubitus radiographs of the abdomen, depending on the department routine and patient condition *(Figure 3–23)*. An acute abdominal series is sometimes called a three-way or two-way abdomen, depending on the number of abdominal projections included in the departmental routine *(Table 3–2)*.

Table 3–2. Acute Abdominal Series

Two-way Abdomen	Three-way Abdomen
AP or PA abdomen	AP or PA abdomen
Upright or decubitus abdomen	Upright abdomen
	Decubitus abdomen
PA chest[a]	PA chest[a]

[a]Optional.

► Related Terminology *(continued)*

peristalsis (per-i-STAL-sis)—wavelike movement or process by which contents of the alimentary canal move forward

pneumoperitoneum (nū-mō-per-i-tō-ÑE-um)—condition in which air or gas is present in the peritoneal cavity; may be caused by trauma or surgically induced (also referred to as "free air")

pylorospasm (pī-l OR-ō-spazm)—spasm or contraction of the pyloric portion of the stomach or the pyloric sphincter

stenosis (ste-NŌ-sis)—constriction or narrowing of a body opening or passage (eg, pyloric stenosis)

tubal ligation (TOO-bal lī-GĀ-shun)—surgical procedure in which the uterine tubes are cut or tied off to prevent pregnancy

transposition (trans-pō-ZISH-un)—normal positions of the organs are reversed; in the abdomen; those organs normally found on the right side may lie on the left side (also called *situs inversus*)

ulcer (UL-ser)—hollow or craterlike lesion on the surface of an organ or tissue resulting from necrosis of inflamed tissue

umbilicus (um-BIL-i-kus)—navel; scar at the site of connection of the umbilical cord in the fetus

vasectomy (vah-SEK-tō-mē)—surgical procedure in which a portion of the ductus (vas) deferens is excised to result in sterility of the male

volvulus (VOL-vū-lus)—twisting of the intestine that results in obstruction

vomiting (VOM-it-ing)—forcible expulsion of the contents of the stomach through the mouth

Table 3–3. Evaluation Criteria for the Recumbent Abdomen Radiograph

- Spine is straight as possible and centered on the film.
- Symphysis pubis is included on the film.
- Ilia are symmetrical.
- Renal shadows, psoas major muscles, inferior margin of the liver, and transverse processes of lumbar spine are visualized.
- Gas shadows and other structures are relatively sharp.

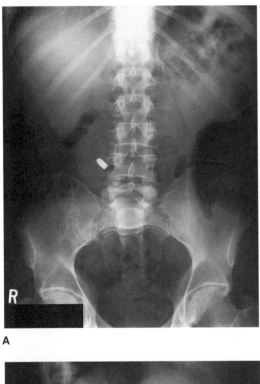

A

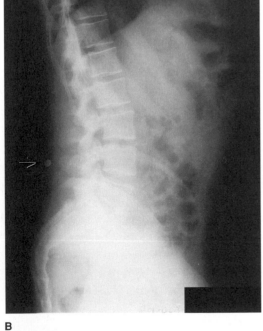

B

Figure 3–24. By looking at this AP projection of the abdomen **(A)**, it is impossible to determine anterior/posterior location of the bullet. The lateral projection **(B)**, however, can be used to demonstrate its location in the soft tissue behind the spine.

The upright abdominal projection is obtained with the patient standing with the back against an upright grid device. The arms should be relaxed at the patient's side, but not in the collimated area. If a patient is unable to stand, this projection may also be obtained with the patient seated on a stool or stretcher in front of the upright grid device. It should, however, be noted that the patient's legs will obscure the lower part of the abdomen. The cassette height should be adjusted to include the entire diaphragm. Although the cassette is usually positioned lengthwise with the body, very large patients may require a crosswise orientation.

If a patient is unable to sit or stand, the left lateral decubitus projection can be obtained to evaluate gas patterns or the presence of free air in the abdomen. For this projection, the patient lies on the left side, allowing any free air to accumulate along the smooth surface of the liver. In this position, the liver will drop slightly, creating a space between it and the diaphragm, referred to as the subphrenic space. Any free air in the abdomen should then be visualized under the right hemidiaphragm along the lateral aspect of the liver in the subphrenic space.

When positioning a patient for the left lateral decubitus projection, care must be taken to ensure there is no patient rotation. Lines passing between the right and left shoulders and between the right and left hips should be perpendicular to the table or stretcher. In addition, the right leg should be directly over the left leg and the arms should be raised with the elbows near the head. The cassette can be either behind (AP projection) or in front of (PA projection) the patient, with the central ray directed perpendicular to the cassette. The central ray should pass through the transverse plane 2 to 3 in. superior to the iliac crests on the average patient; adjustments may need to be made, however, to ensure the diaphragm is included on the film. Upright and decubitus projections should be obtained only after the patient has been in that position for at least 10 minutes, to allow any free air to rise.

Positioning accuracy for these projections can be evaluated by symmetric appearance of the right and left ilia, ischial spines, and ribs (Table 3–3). The diaphragm should be included on the upright and decubitus projections and the symphysis pubis should be visualized on the supine or prone projection. Crosswise collimation should be adjusted to the lateral margins of the thorax to minimize patient dose and improve radiographic quality.

Because the aorta is sometimes calcified and visualized radiographically in older patients, AP supine and dorsal decubitus projections are sometimes obtained to evaluate the presence of abdominal aortic aneurysms. The dorsal decubitus projection is performed with the patient supine on the table and the central ray directed horizontally and perpendicular to the film. A grid cassette or Bucky can be on either the patient's right or left side with the x-ray tube directed about 2 in. above the level of the iliac crests. This projection may also be used to evaluate abdominal masses and air–fluid levels.

Occasionally, abdominal radiographs are obtained to determine the presence and location of foreign bodies. Although a single projection can demonstrate presence of a foreign object, a second projection is required to demonstrate exact location of the object. In this situation, AP supine and lateral abdominal radiographs are usually ordered (Figure 3–24).

BREATHING INSTRUCTIONS

A significant problem relevant to abdominal radiography is motion. Involuntary motion, such as peristalsis in the alimentary canal, or voluntary motion, such as breathing, can cause unsharpness or poor definition of the abdominal structures. Although a short exposure time will help prevent involuntary motion on the finished radiograph, appropriate breathing instructions prevent voluntary motion. To move the diaphragm upward and avoid compression of the abdominal organs, the exposure should be made during suspended expiration. The patient should be instructed to "take in a breath . . . , blow it all out . . . , and hold the breath out." Suspended expiration also reduces tissue thickness, thereby requiring less radiation to produce a diagnostic film.

EXPOSURE FACTORS

The abdomen is an area of low subject contrast. Various organ tissue densities and the presence of radiolucent fat in the abdomen help to demonstrate specific abdominal structures. Because of the low subject contrast, a moderate kilovoltage, 70–80, is usually employed to enhance the subject contrast, demonstrate soft tissue, and penetrate the abdomen. The use of 70 kVp will penetrate even the most fatty of abdomens. Very muscular patients may require 80 kVp. Higher kilovoltages, 100–120, are used following the administration of barium sulfate contrast medium. A grid is used to improve radiographic contrast and quality. The milliampere-seconds, mAs, is adjusted according to patient size, equipment, and film/screen system speed and will vary from department to department or from room to room. A fast exposure time, 0.5 second or less, should be used to minimize breathing and peristaltic motion. A correctly exposed radiograph will clearly demonstrate the transverse processes of the vertebrae, the inferior margin of the liver, the kidneys, and the psoas major muscles.

Physical evaluation of the patient's abdomen prior to exposure may be important in the selection of technical factors. An air-distended bowel increases the thickness of the abdomen but does not require an increase in the amount of radiation needed to produce a diagnostic image. Increasing the kilovoltage in this situation will produce a dark, gray film. On the other hand, a fluid (ascites)- or blood-filled (hemoperitoneum) abdomen will be harder to penetrate and may require an increase in exposure factors. Generally speaking, an abdomen with an air-distended bowel will feel taut, whereas a fluid-filled abdomen may be hard or soft, depending on the amount of fluid present.

Most urinary tract and some gallbladder calculi contain calcium, allowing them to be visualized on plain radiographs of the abdomen. Demonstration of flecks of calcium, which may also be seen in arteries or veins, requires the use of moderate kilovoltage.

Many departments use an automatic exposure device (AED/AEC) for all or some of the Bucky procedures performed in the department. When used for plain films of the abdomen, both side cells are usually used for the supine films and all three cells are used for the upright and lateral decubitus films. This can vary, however, depending on the calibration of the equipment and radiologist preference.

EQUIPMENT CONSIDERATIONS

Supine or prone radiography can be performed on any radiographic table or with a mobile unit at the patient's bedside or stretcher using a grid cassette. To perform upright abdominal radiography, a wall unit with a grid or a radiographic table capable of being turned 90° upright is preferred. A grid cassette can also be positioned behind a patient seated on a bed, if necessary. The x-ray tube must be directed horizontally to demonstrate air–fluid levels within the abdomen.

For the left lateral decubitus projection of the abdomen, the patient must be lying on her or his left side on a radiographic table, stretcher, or bed with x-ray tube directed horizontally. If the patient is on a stretcher, the stretcher can be easily positioned in front of an upright wall unit or erect radiographic table. In this situation, the cassette holder can be raised or lowered and appropriately centered to the abdomen. The projection may be AP or PA; however, the AP projection with the patient's back nearest the cassette holder is usually easier to perform and generally reduces object–image receptor distance (OID).

If the patient is on the radiographic table or bed, a grid cassette must be positioned vertically either in front or behind the patient (PA or AP projection). A special cassette holder or sandbags and tape will be needed to hold the cassette in the vertical position. Sponges or other radiolucent supports should be used to elevate the patient to center the abdomen in the middle of the film. Compression bands may also be used to immobilize the patient.

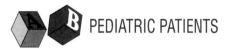

PEDIATRIC PATIENTS

Depending on age and level of cooperation, the pediatric patient can pose additional challenges for the radiographer. Special immobilization devices have been developed to restrain children of various ages. The approach to the child, as well as various immobilization techniques, is more fully discussed in Chapter 1. Because children are more sensitive to the effects of radiation than adults, accurate collimation and gonadal shielding, if possible, are critical (*Figure 3–25*).

As with all abdominal radiography, a fast exposure time is important when radiographing children. Exposure factors also need to be modified. Because children have a higher percentage of water per body weight that adults, a lower kVp should be used to reduce scatter and improve radiographic contrast. Gen-

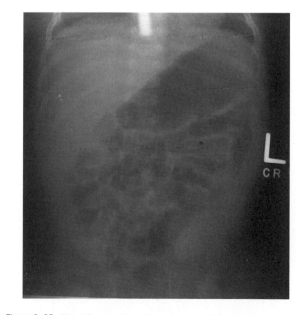

Figure 3–25. This AP projection of a newborn was taken in the nursery using a portable unit.

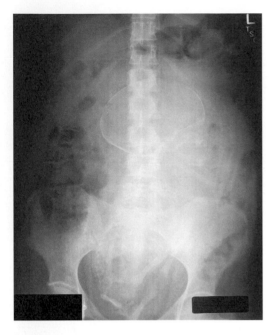

Figure 3–26. This AP projection of the abdomen was taken with the mobile unit in the Labor & Delivery Department. Note the position of the fetus on the radiograph.

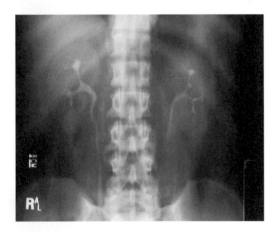

Figure 3–27. Tomogram of the kidneys taken as part of an intravenous pyelogram.

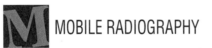

Liver   Aorta   Transverse colon

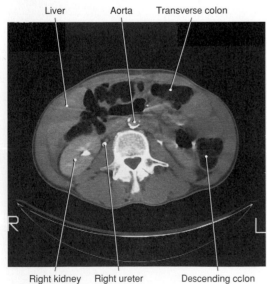

Right kidney   Right ureter   Descending colon

Figure 3–28. Axial CT image of the abdomen.

Table 3–4. Technique Selection for the Pediatric Patient

- Select appropriate adult kVp; reduce 2 kVp/cm difference.
- Using the child's physical age, multiply the adult mAs by the appropriate modification factor:

0 to 1 year	0.25
1–3 years	0.50
3–7 years	0.70
7–12 years	0.90

erally speaking, the kVp should be reduced 2 kVp for each centimeter of difference between the child and the adult technique for the same procedure.

A reduction in mAs is also necessary to compensate for the reduced tissue thickness. Patient age is usually used as a guide for mAs selection. An mAs modification factor is assigned to specific age groups to assist the radiographer in technique selection. Children 13 years of age and older can usually be radiographed using adult techniques appropriate for their size. Children younger than 13 are separated into categories. Because children may be small or large for their age, patient size—not chronological age—should determine the age bracket used for technique selection *(Table 3–4)*.

MOBILE RADIOGRAPHY

At times it is necessary to perform abdominal radiography on patients who are too ill to travel to the department. A mobile, or portable, unit and grid cassette will be required for the examination. When performing portable radiography, the technologist must consider the potential problems. Positioning the cassette so it is level in the bed under the patient can be challenging. To prevent grid cutoff, the central ray must be perpendicular to and centered to the grid. In addition, the source–image receptor distance (SID) used must be within the range of the grid. A low grid ratio, 8:1 or less, is usually recommended. When a low grid ratio is used, 80 to 85 kVp or less is recommended to minimize radiation fog on the film *(Figure 3–26)*.

ALTERNATE IMAGING PROCEDURES

Because of overlying bowel gas or other structures, it is sometimes necessary to use other methods of imaging to demonstrate specific anatomy or pathology. Tomography, as discussed in Chapter 1, is frequently performed as part of the excretory urogram and can play an important role in the identification of renal stones and masses or cysts *(Figure 3–27)*.

Computed tomography now plays a significant role in the diagnosis of abdominal disorders. CT produces a sectional image with excellent visualization of bony and soft tissue structures comparable to that seen in *Figure 3–28*. Contrast medium can be administered intravenously, orally, and rectally to better delineate abdominal structures.

Ultrasound is the primary imaging modality for the biliary system and plays an integral role in the diagnosis of gallstones *(Figure 3–29)*. It is also used to diagnose other abnormalities of the abdomen and pelvis. Magnetic resonance imaging (MRI) is also used in some facilities to screen for hepatic metastases and evaluate pelvic abdominal structures and pathology *(Figure 3–30)*. Nuclear medicine plays a role in the diagnosis of pathology of the liver, spleen, and kidneys, including liver function, cirrhosis, splenomegaly, renal hypertension, cysts, and tumors *(Figure 3–31)*.

SPECIAL RADIOGRAPHIC PROCEDURES

Hysterosalpingography (HSG) (his-ter-ō-sal-ping-GOG-rah-fē) is the radiographic examination of the uterus and uterine (fallopian) tubes of the female reproductive system after the injection of contrast medium. This procedure may be performed for both diagnostic and therapeutic purposes. It is used to make diagnoses in cases of abnormal uterine bleeding (amenorrhea or dysmenorrhea), infertility, chronic spontaneous abortions, pelvic masses, endometrial polyps, and fistulas. In some cases, an HSG also acts therapeutically to reverse infertility by dilating and restoring patency to blocked or tortuous uterine tubes.

An HSG is contraindicated in cases of pregnancy, active uterine bleeding, or pelvic inflammatory disease (PID). The examination is usually scheduled for the 10th day following the start of menstruation to avoid the possibility of pregnancy.

Preparation of the intestinal tract is necessary to allow for adequate visualization of structures. The patient should take a non-gas-forming laxative on the evening prior to the examination and use a cleansing enema on the day of the examination. The meal prior to the examination is usually withheld. If the patient's history reveals a sensitivity to iodinated contrast medium, the physician can premedicate her with steroids and/or antihistamines. Premedication with glucagon can be used to reduce pain and spasms during the procedure. Immediately preceding the examination, the patient irrigates the vagina, cleans the perineal area, and urinates to empty her bladder.

A HSG is generally performed in a radiographic/fluoroscopic room. If possible, gynecologic leg stirrups should be attached to the table. A sterile tray consists of the cannulation equipment, vaginal speculum, antiseptic solution, lubricating jelly, swabs, syringes, towels, and drapes.

Either an oily or water-soluble iodinated contrast medium may be used. There are advantages and disadvantages to each, although the water-soluble medium is used more frequently today. The oily contrast medium is well tolerated by the patient with little or no reactions and provides high visibility of structures; however, it is absorbed so slowly that it remains in body cavities for a long period. Its use also presents the danger of intravasation, resulting in a pulmonary embolism. Although the water-soluble contrast medium provides satisfactory visibility and rapid absorption by the body, it often causes pain on instillation. Carbon dioxide, a negative contrast medium, may also be introduced to outline the reproductive structures in the peritoneal cavity.

For the procedure, the patient is placed supine on the table in the lithotomy position with her legs in the stirrups, if available. The table is then tilted to a slight Trendelenburg position to aid in the flow of the contrast medium. The physician introduces the cannulation device through the cervix and into the uterus. The cervical os is occluded, usually by a balloon on the catheter, to prevent retrograde spillage of the contrast medium. Sterile technique is used by the physician performing the examination and the assisting radiographer. Complications resulting from an HSG might include hemorrhage, peritonitis, and oil embolism (if oily contrast medium is used).

Radiographs may be taken using either a fluoroscopic or overhead method. If fluoroscopy is used, spot films are taken as the contrast medium is injected. An overhead AP projection is usually taken on a 10 × 12-in. (25 × 30-cm) cassette; however, RPO and LPO projections may also be necessary to demonstrate the anatomy. The central ray and film are centered to the point 2 in. superior to the symphysis pubis. The radiographs should demonstrate the cannula in the cervix, the uterus (body and horns), and uterine tubes. If the tubes are patent, spillage of the contrast medium will be seen in the peritoneal cavity (*Figure 3–32*).

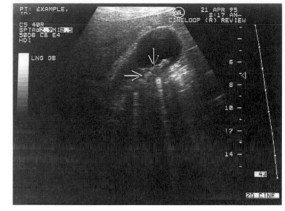

Figure 3–29. Ultrasound image of the gallbladder; note the presence of stones.

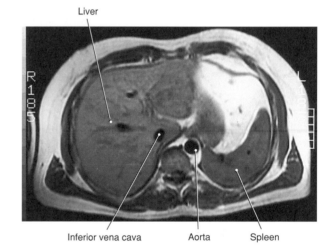

Liver

Inferior vena cava　　Aorta　　Spleen

Figure 3–30. MRI can be used effectively to evaluate the liver.

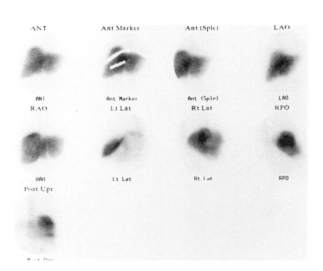

Figure 3–31. Nuclear medicine scan of the liver. This patient has had a splenectomy. Lead markers are used to measure and to note anatomical landmarks.

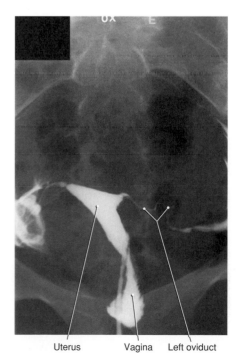

Uterus　　Vagina　　Left oviduct

Figure 3–32. Normal hysterosalpingogram.

RADIOGRAPHIC POSITIONING OF THE ABDOMEN

- ► AP ABDOMEN

- ► UPRIGHT AP ABDOMEN

- ► LEFT LATERAL DECUBITUS ABDOMEN

- ► DORSAL DECUBITUS ABDOMEN

► AP ABDOMEN

Technical Considerations

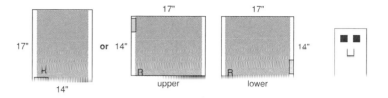

- Film size: Adult: 14 × 17 in. lengthwise on most patients, two cassettes crosswise on large patients. Pediatric: size determined by patient size.
- Grid required.
- 70–80 kVp, adult.
- Collimate to the abdominal walls laterally and to film size lengthwise.

Shielding

- Male patients can be shielded according to department policy.

Patient Positioning

- Assist the patient to the supine position on the radiographic table. **Note:** A comparable radiograph can be obtained with the patient prone.
- Place a pillow under the patient's head and position a small support under the patient's knees for comfort.
- Adjust the long axis of the patient parallel with the long axis of the table; pull gently on patient's legs or under patient's arms to move and straighten the patient.

Part Positioning

- Center the median plane of the patient's body to the midline of the table.
- Check for rotation of the pelvis by palpating the anterior superior iliac spines and ensuring they are equidistant from the table; use sponges for support and immobilization, if necessary *(Figure 3–33)*.

Central Ray

- Direct the central ray perpendicular to the level of the iliac crests.
- Center the cassette to the central ray. **Note:** Make any needed adjustment in cassette centering to ensure the symphysis pubis is included on the film (palpate the symphysis pubis directly or palpate the greater trochanter to determine the level of the symphysis pubis).

Breathing Instructions

- Instruct the patient to take in a deep breath, blow it out, and hold it out during the exposure.

Image Evaluation

- The symphysis pubis and lateral margins of the abdomen should be included within the collimated area.
- The renal shadows, psoas major muscles, transverse processes of the lumbar spine, and inferior margin of the liver should be clearly visualized on a properly exposed abdominal radiograph.
- Asymmetry of the iliac crests and ischial spines indicates rotation of the pelvis; the narrower ilium would have been elevated.
- Unless pathology is present, the spine should be straight and centered to the film *(Figure 3–34)*.

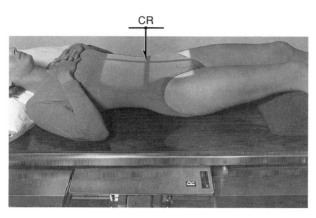

Figure 3–33. AP abdomen (KUB).

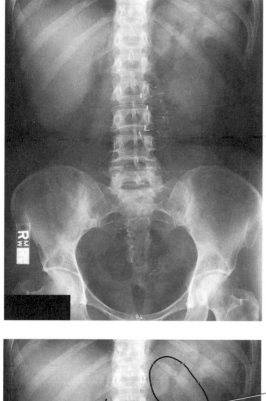

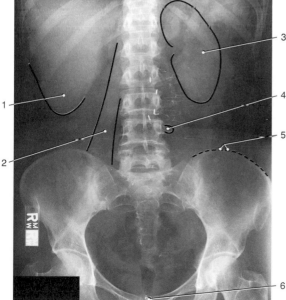

1. Liver
2. Psoas major muscle
3. Kidney
4. Transverse process
5. Iliac crest
6. Symphysis pubis

Figure 3–34. AP abdomen (KUB).

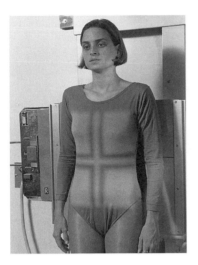

Figure 3–35. Upright abdomen.

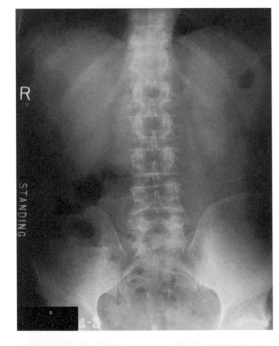

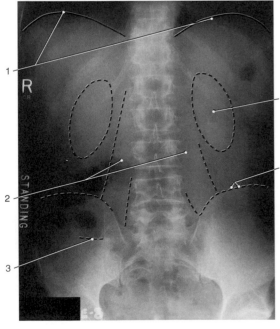

Figure 3–36. Upright abdomen; note the air–fluid levels.

► UPRIGHT AP ABDOMEN

Technical Considerations

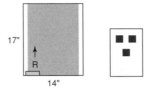

- Film size: Adult: 14 × 17 in. lengthwise on most patients; two cassettes crosswise on large patients. Pediatric: size determined by patient size.
- Grid required.
- 70–80 kVp, adult.
- Collimate to the abdominal walls laterally and to film size lengthwise.

Shielding

- A shadow shield or drape can be used to shield male patients whenever possible according to department policy.

Patient Positioning

- Assist the patient to the erect position with the back to an upright table or wall unit; the patient may also be seated on a stool, stretcher, or bed with a grid device or grid cassette behind the patient.
- Position the patient's arms comfortably at the patient's sides and out of the collimated area.

Part Positioning

- Center the midsagittal plane of the patient to the midline of the upright grid device or grid cassette.
- When an upright grid device is used, a compression band may be used to immobilize the patient.
- Check for rotation of the pelvis by palpating the anterior superior iliac spines and ensuring they are equidistant from the table; use sponges for support and immobilization, if necessary *(Figure 3–35).*

Central Ray

- Direct the central ray to a point approximately 2 to 3 in. above the level of the iliac crests.
- Center the cassette to the central ray; the top edge of the cassette should be at the level of the axilla. **Note:** Adjust the height of the central ray and cassette to compensate for patients who are shorter or taller than average.

Breathing Instructions

- Instruct the patient to take in a breath, blow it out, and hold it out during the exposure.

Image Evaluation

- The diaphragm and lateral margins of the abdomen should be included within the collimated area.
- Air–fluid levels should be adequately exposed and demonstrated.
- Asymmetry of the iliac crests indicates rotation of the pelvis; the narrower ilium would have been elevated.
- Unless pathology is present, the spine should be straight and centered to the film *(Figure 3–36).*

1. Diaphragm
2. Psoas major muscles
3. Air-fluid levels
4. Kidneys
5. Iliac crests

► LEFT LATERAL DECUBITUS ABDOMEN

Technical Considerations:

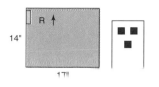

- Film size: Adult: 14 × 17 in. lengthwise with the patient's body. Pediatric size determined by patient size.
- Grid required.
- 70–80 kVp, adult.
- Collimate to the abdominal walls laterally and to film size lengthwise.

Shielding:

- Although shielding can be difficult for decubitus projections, a shadow shield or lead drape can be used to shield male patients.

Patient Positioning

- Assist the patient to the left lateral decubitus position on the table or stretcher; the right leg should be directly over the left leg and the right arm should be directly over the left.
- Extend the arms upward so the elbows are near the face.

Part Positioning

- Adjust the thorax and pelvis to a true lateral position; check for rotation by standing at the head or foot of the patient and making sure the shoulders and hips are superimposed.
- The patient should be positioned so the plane passing 2 to 3 in. superior to the iliac crests is centered to the midline of the upright table, wall unit, or vertically positioned grid cassette.
- The midsagittal plane of the patient should also be aligned to the midline of the film.
- If a grid cassette is used, sponges should be used to elevate the patient, if necessary, to center the midsagittal plane of the patient to the grid *(Figure 3–37)*.

Central Ray

- Direct the central ray horizontally to the midline of the grid device.
- Adjust the patient and/or cassette so the top edge of the cassette is at the level of the axilla.

Breathing Instructions

- Instruct the patient to take in a breath, blow it out, and hold it out during the exposure.

Image Evaluation

- The diaphragm, renal shadows, and air–fluid patterns should be illustrated on the radiograph.
- Air–fluid levels should be adequately exposed and demonstrated.
- Asymmetry of the iliac crests or ribs indicates rotation of the pelvis or shoulders, respectively.
- Unless pathology is present, the spine should be fairly straight and centered to the film *(Figure 3–38)*.

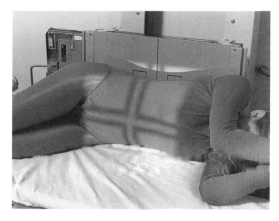

Figure 3–37. Left lateral decubitus abdomen.

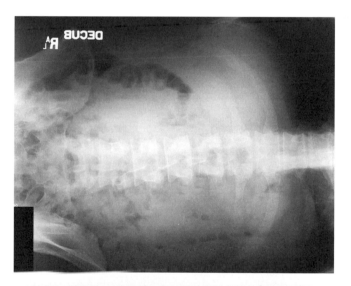

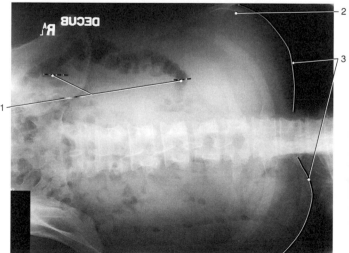

Figure 3–38. Left lateral decubitus abdomen.

1. Air-fluid levels	2. Subphrenic space	3. Diaphragm

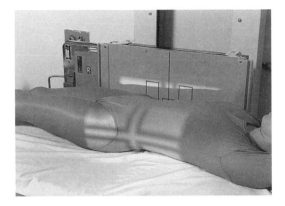

Figure 3–39. Dorsal decubitus abdomen.

▶ DORSAL DECUBITUS ABDOMEN

Technical Considerations

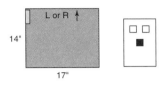

- Film size: Adult: 14 × 17 in. lengthwise with the patient's body. Pediatric: size determined by patient size.
- Grid required.
- 80–90 kVp, adult.
- Collimate to the abdominal walls anteriorly and posteriorly and to film size lengthwise.

Shielding

- Gonadal shields should be used on all male patients or according to department policy.

Patient Positioning

- Assist the patient to the supine position on the radiographic table or stretcher; place a pillow under the patient's head and raise the arms above the head.
- Adjust the long axis of the patient parallel with the long axis of the table or stretcher.

Part Positioning

- Center the plane 2 in. superior to the iliac crests to the midline of the upright table, wall unit, or vertically positioned grid cassette.
- The plane 2 in. anterior to the midaxillary plane of the patient should also be aligned to the midline of the film.
- If a grid cassette is used, sponges should be used to elevate the patient, if necessary, to center this plane to the grid (Figure 3–39).

Central Ray

- Direct the central ray horizontally to the midline of the grid.
- Adjust the patient and/or cassette so the top edge of the cassette is at the level of the axilla.

Breathing Instructions

- Instruct the patient to take in a breath, blow it out, and hold it out during the exposure.

Image Evaluation

- The diaphragm, spine, and anterior margin of the abdomen should be included within the collimated area.
- Air–fluid levels should be adequately exposed and demonstrated on the radiograph.
- Superimposition of the ribs and ilia indicates a true lateral position (Figure 3–40).

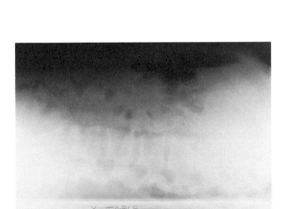

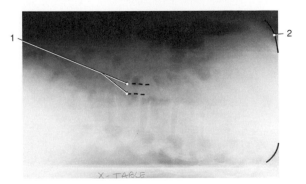

Figure 3–40. Dorsal decubitus abdomen.   1. Air-fluid levels   2. Diaphragm

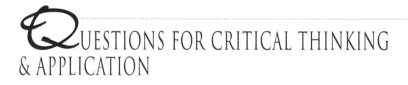

SUMMARY

▶ Radiography of the abdomen may be done to evaluate abdominal contents, check tube placements, or as a preliminary step prior to the administration of contrast medium.

▶ The abdomen contains organs vital to digestion, metabolism, reproduction, and waste removal.

▶ Plain films of the abdomen may be obtained to rule out free air in the abdomen, identify radiopaque stones in the kidneys or gallbladder, or localize foreign objects.

▶ Although contrast medium is required to adequately demonstrate many of the abdominal organs, plain noncontrast films of the abdomen are usually obtained prior to administration of contrast medium to rule out residual contrast from previous examinations and identify any pathology that may be obscured by contrast medium.

▶ Precontrast examinations of the abdomen generally consist of an AP or PA projection (KUB), whereas an acute abdominal series usually includes the supine, upright, and/or decubitus projections.

▶ Plain abdominal radiography is performed with a grid, a kilovoltage of approximately 70 to 80, and a short exposure time.

▶ To minimize tissue thickness and elevate the diaphragm, exposures should be made during suspended expiration.

▶ A properly exposed abdominal radiograph should demonstrate the kidney shadows, inferior margin of the liver, psoas major muscles, and transverse processes of the lumbar vertebrae.

▶ When evaluating positioning accuracy on an AP or PA projection of the abdomen, the iliac crests and ischial spines should be symmetrical and the spine should be straight on the film.

▶ While the supine projections of the abdomen should include the symphysis pubis, upright and decubitus projections should include the diaphragm.

▶ When radiographing pediatric patients, kVp and mAs are reduced according to the patient's age and size.

▶ Some pathologies of the abdomen require an adjustment in technical factors: the air-distended bowel may require a decrease in exposure factors, whereas a fluid-filled abdomen necessitates an increase.

QUESTIONS FOR CRITICAL THINKING & APPLICATION

1. Using the nine-region method of localization, describe the location of the pancreas.

2. Discuss why a patient with a history of a gunshot wound to the abdomen is likely to develop peritonitis.

3. You just completed an acute abdominal series on a patient who was stabbed in the right lower quadrant of his abdomen. On evaluation of the radiographs, the ER physician noted the presence of "free air." Discuss what is meant by the term "free air" in this case to include the following: where it is demonstrated on the radiographs, what structures might be involved, and possible implications for the patient.

4. An AP supine projection of the abdomen demonstrates a considerable amount of gas. How can you distinguish if the gas is in the small or the large intestine?

5. In the course of taking a supine abdominal radiograph, the patient, who is female, asks you to please shield her. How will you respond to her?

6. In abdominal radiography, why must the patient be given specific breathing instructions prior to making the exposure? Discuss the effect inhalation and exhalation have on the diaphragm and abdominal organs.

7. List possible reasons for obtaining noncontrast radiographs of the abdomen.

8. Your patient is a victim of a motor vehicle accident (MVA) and has an obviously fractured lower leg. The patient's physician is concerned about abdominal injuries and requests an abdominal series to rule out free air in the abdomen. Describe possible methods and projections you might follow in obtaining the requested films.

9. Why are abdominal radiographs taken during suspended expiration?

10. How should technical factors for the abdomen be adjusted for very obese patients? Consider both manually set technique and AEC.

11. How can the radiographer ensure that the urinary bladder is included on an AP radiograph of the abdomen?

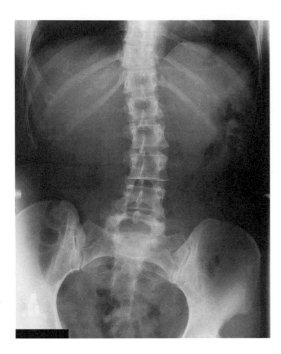

Figure 3–41.

FILM CRITIQUE

Evaluate the abdominal radiograph *(Figure 3–41)*. Describe how the patient was positioned. Was the patient accurately positioned and centered?

What criteria were used to determine positioning accuracy or error?

Was the film adequately exposed?

How is appropriate exposure determined in abdominal radiography?

4

MUSCULOSKELETAL SYSTEM

► OBJECTIVES

Following the completion of this chapter the student will be able to:

- Define terminology of the musculoskeletal system, to include anatomy, procedures, and pathology related to bones, joints, and muscles.

- Describe the basic anatomic structure of bone and discuss the process of bone development and growth.

- Describe the fracture process, to include physical signs of fracture and the healing process.

- Discuss the technical and equipment considerations involved in producing optimum radiographs of the skeletal system and how these must be modified to accommodate pediatric and geriatric patients.

- Explain the rationale for taking a minimum of two projections at 90° from each other when radiographing the skeletal system and the need for an additional (oblique) projection when radiographing a joint.

- Describe the procedural and technical modifications to be considered when performing a radiographic examination of an extremity in a cast or splint.

► ANATOMY OF THE MUSCULOSKELETAL SYSTEM

SKELETAL SYSTEM

The scientific study of bones is known as *osteology* (os-tē-OL-ō-jē). This is an especially relevant subject for radiographers as much of diagnostic radiography focuses on the skeletal system *(Table 4–1)*.

There are approximately 206 bones in the average adult skeleton *(Figure 4–1)*. Together they form and shape the body and perform the following important functions:

- *Support*. The bones form a structural frame to which the soft tissues of the body can attach. Without this support, a person would not be able to stand upright.
- *Protection*. The hard frame of the skeleton protects delicate organs and tissues. For example, the brain is protectively enclosed by the skull. The ribs, sternum, and thoracic spine form a bony cage around the heart, great vessels, and lungs.
- *Movement*. The bones of the skeleton serve as levers for the attachment of muscles. Movement takes place when the muscles contract. The type of movement depends on which levers, or bones, are being affected.
- *Storage*. Important minerals, such as calcium and phosphorus, are stored in the tissue of bones. The bones act as a reservoir for these minerals, storing them until they are needed by the body. Fat is also stored in the form of yellow bone marrow in the inner cavity of adult long bones.
- *Hematopoiesis* (hem-ah-tō-poi-Ē-sis). This term refers to the process of blood cell formation. Red and white blood cells are continually produced in the red marrow of bones.

With the exception of the enamel on teeth, bones are the strongest structures in the human body. They are so durable that radiographs of mummies have demonstrated that their skeletons were still intact after many years; it is interesting to note that the word *skeleton* has a Greek origin which means "mummy." As sturdy and enduring as bones seem to be, it may be surprising to learn that bones are relatively lightweight and constitute only about 20% of the body's mass.

Osseous tissue, or bone, is a very hard substance primarily because of the presence of mineral salts such as calcium carbonate and calcium phosphate. Collagen fibers serve to reinforce the osseous tissue and also provide some flexibility to the bone. The two basic types of osseous tissue are **compact** and **cancellous** (KAN-cell-us) **bone** *(Figure 4–2)*.

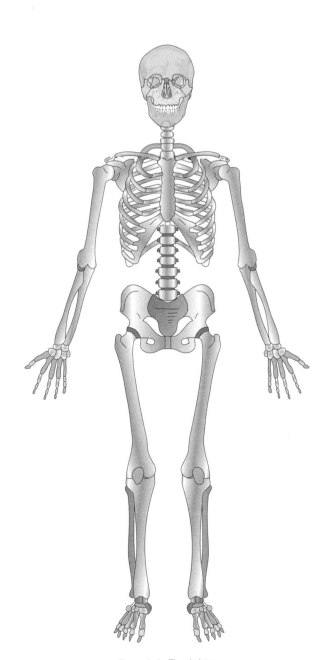

Figure 4–1. The skeleton.

Table 4–1. Summary of the Musculoskeletal System

Functions of the Skeleton	Bone Structure
Support	Periosteum
Protection	Diaphysis
Movement	Epiphysis
Storage	Medullary cavity
Hematopoiesis	Endosteum
	Nutrient foramen
Divisions of Skeleton	Bone marrow
Axial	
Appendicular	*Joints*
	Synarthrodial
Classification of Bones	Fibrous
Long	
Short	Amphiarthrodial
Flat	Fibrous
Irregular	Cartilaginous
Sesamoid	
Wormian	Diarthrodial
	Cartilaginous
Osteogenesis	
Intramembranous ossification	*Musculature*
Endochondral ossification	Muscles
	Movement
Bone Cells	Form
Osteocyte	Heat
Osteoblast	
Osteoclast	Tendons
	Attach muscles to bone
Bone Tissue	Ligaments
Compact	Hold bones together
Cancellous	

Compact bone tissue appears smooth and solid like the ivory tusks of an elephant. **Haversian canals** (osteon systems) form the structure of compact bone. In these systems, bone cells are arranged in a ringlike fashion around a canal to form columns or pillars. The canals contain blood vessels, lymphatic vessels, and nerves. Because it is so dense, compact bone is strong. It is also referred to as cortical bone because it surrounds each bone, forming the cortex or outer shell. The shell is particularly dense in areas of stress, such as the shafts of the femurs, which bear the weight of the body when a person is standing.

Cancellous bone is also known as spongy bone. Although it is not actually soft and spongy to the touch, it has the physical appearance of a sponge. A network or honeycomb effect called **trabeculae** (trah-BEK-ū-lē) is formed by fine bony spikes. The spaces within the network are filled with red bone marrow *(Figure 4–3)*.

The outer covering of a bone is known as **periosteum** (per-ē-OS-tē-um). This structure actually consists of two layers: a white outer layer, which is dense, fibrous, and vascular, and an inner cellular layer, which is composed of bone-forming cells. Periosteum plays a vital role in the growth, repair, and nutrition of bones. It contains blood vessels, lymphatic vessels, and nerve fibers. It also serves as an attachment site for tendons and ligaments. In the area of joints, periosteum is continuous with hyaline (articular) cartilage.

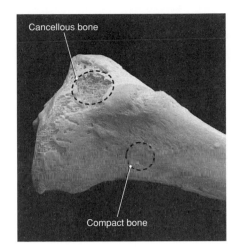

Figure 4–2. Compact and cancellous bone identified on a long bone (tibia).

Classification

There are a variety of shapes and sizes among the bones of the adult skeleton. Basically, the shape of the bone is determined by the particular role or job it performs. For example, the flat sternum forms a shield to protect the heart, whereas the femurs of the legs are long with a large amount of compact bone for strength. Bones are generally described as belonging to one of the following six classes:

1. *Long.* These bones are found primarily in the extremities. They consist of a shaft and two articular ends. Their length is much greater than their width and they are slightly curved for increased strength. The cylindrical shaft of a long bone is known as the diaphysis (dī-AF-i-sis). It is composed primarily of compact bone. A cavity extends longitudinally through the center of the shaft. It is called the medullary or marrow cavity. This cavity is occupied by red bone marrow in children. As a person ages, the red bone marrow is gradually replaced by yellow or fatty bone marrow. The medullary cavity is lined with endosteum. This inner lining contains bone-forming and bone-breaking cells which are necessary for bone repair. The nutrient foramen is a small opening located approximately midshaft. It provides a passageway for blood vessels, lymphatic vessels, and nerves into the medullary cavity. Each expanded, articular end of a long bone is called an epiphysis (ē-PIF-i-sis). The epiphyses are formed predominately of cancellous bone and contain red bone marrow. Although still classified as long bones, the metacarpals and phalanges of the hands, as well as the metatarsals and phalanges of the feet, are often referred to as "mini-long bones" because of their shorter length; however, they have all of the same characteristic features of long bones *(Figure 4–3)*.

2. *Short.* These cube- or box-shaped bones are composed primarily of cancellous bone covered by compact bone. The carpals of the wrist and tarsals of the foot are examples of short bones.

3. *Flat.* These bones are thin and flat, although they may have a slightly curved surface, such as the bones forming skull cap and the ilia of the pelvis. Flat bones are best described as cancellous bone sandwiched between two parallel plates of compact bone. In the skull, the cancellous layer is known as *diploe,* and the two plates of compact bone are referred to as the *inner and outer tables.* In addition to providing protection, such as in the cases of the sternum and the skull, flat bones allow for the production of red blood cells and also the attachment of muscles.

4. *Irregular.* These complex-shaped bones do not fit into any of the previously discussed categories. Their composition is similar to that of short bones in that they are formed primarily from cancellous bone covered by compact bone. Examples of irregular bones include vertebrae and the bones forming the base of the skull (eg, temporal bone).

5. *Sesamoid.* These bones are usually short, rounded, and somewhat flat. They develop near joints in areas of stress and are usually embedded within a tendon. Although the number of sesamoid bones varies among individuals, everyone has at least two in the form of patellas (kneecaps).

6. *Wormian.* These bones are also referred to as sutural bones as they develop between the joints or sutures of the bones forming the roof of the skull. Not only are these bones oddly shaped, they vary in number and actual position from person to person *(Figure 4–4)*.

The skeleton can be divided into two distinct categories: axial and appendicular. The skeleton basically consists of a central axis that runs along the center of gravity with other bones attached to it. Therefore, the bones that lie on and around this axis are referred to as the axial skeleton, and the bones that attach or append to the axial skeleton are known as the appendicular skeleton. Eighty bones constitute the axial skeleton. These include the cranium, face, hyoid, ossicles of the ears, and vertebral column. The appendicular skeleton comprises the bones of the upper and lower extremities, shoulder girdle, and pelvic girdle. There are a total of 126 bones in this division of the skeleton *(Table 4–2)*.

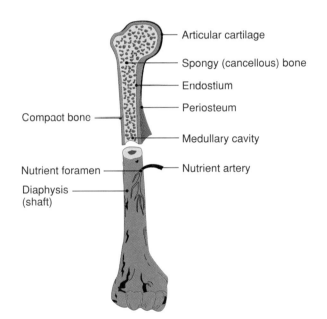

Figure 4–3. Characteristics of a long bone.

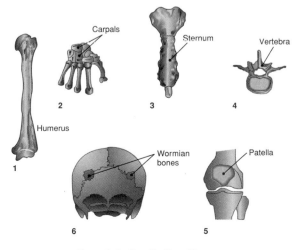

Figure 4–4. Classification of bones.

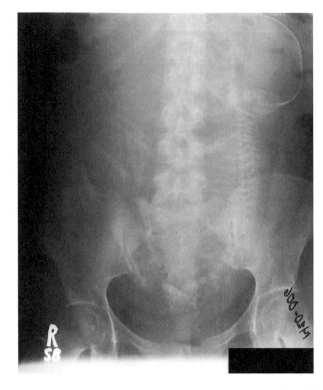

Figure 4–5. The fetal skeleton is demonstrated on an abdominal radiograph of a term pregnancy.

Table 4–2. The Skeleton

Axial (80)	Appendicular (126)
1. Skull (22)	1. Upper extremities (60)
a. Cranium (8)	a. Humerus (2)
b. Face (14)	b. Radius (2)
2. Hyoid (1)	c. Ulna (2)
3. Ossicles (6)	d. Carpals (16)
a. Malleus (2)	e. Metacarpals (10)
b. Incus (2)	f. Phalanges (28)
c. Stapes (2)	2. Lower extremities (60)
4. Vertebral column (26)	a. Femur (2)
a. Cervical (7)	b. Tibia (2)
b. Thoracic (12)	c. Fibula (2)
c. Lumbar (5)	d. Patella (2)
d. Sacrum (1)	e. Tarsals (14)
e. Coccyx (1)	f. Metatarsals (10)
5. Thorax (25)	g. Phalanges (28)
a. Ribs (24)	3. Shoulder girdle (4)
b. Sternum (1)	a. Clavicle (2)
	b. Scapula (2)
	4. Pelvic girdle (2)
	a. Hip bones (os coxae) (2)

Bone Growth & Development

Within 6 weeks of conception, a fetus has developed a skeleton. At this point, however, the "bones" are actually composed of hyaline (HĪ-ah-lin) cartilage. This connecting tissue, or gristle as it is also called, is clear and glassy in appearance. The process of bone formation is known as **ossification** or **osteogenesis** and begins at this stage of fetal development. The soft cartilaginous bones are gradually replaced by osseous tissue. Mature bone cells are known as osteocytes; osteoblasts are the cells responsible for the formation of bone. Bone formation occurs in two manners. In intramembranous ossification, bones form from the fibrous membrane that is already present. Endochondral ossification results in the replacement of cartilage by osseous tissue *(Figure 4–5)*.

Intramembranous Ossification. Intramembranous ossification is a rapid form of bone growth which takes place primarily in flat bones such as the calvarium, or skull cap, although the mandible and clavicles also form in this manner. Initially, cells in the fibrous membrane or connective tissue of the structure differentiate into **osteoblasts.** This occurs in the center of ossification. The bone-forming osteoblasts begin to secrete osteoid, an intercellular substance which becomes calcified. A trabecular network covered with a layer of compact bone is formed through this process. Thus, cancellous bone is the resulting product; however, the bone can undergo a remodeling process through which it then produces primarily compact bone.

Endochondral Ossification. Prior to birth, a group of osteoblasts found in the center of a bone divide repeatedly. New bone tissue is formed to replace the cartilage that previously composed the bodies or shafts of these bones. This primary center of ossification becomes known as the **diaphysis** (dī-AF-i-sis).

Secondary ossification centers known as **epiphyses** (ē-PIF-i-sēz) (singular, epiphysis) appear in bones around the time of birth. Depending on the specific bone, this may be shortly before birth or up to several years later. Clusters of bone cells in the end of a long bone or in bony processes divide repeatedly and eventually replace the cartilage in that area of the bone. There may be more than one secondary center of ossification on a bone. For example, the femur has an epiphysis at each end of its length and also at the site of its processes, the greater and lesser trochanters *(Figure 4–6)*.

A long bone increases in length at the ends of the diaphysis adjacent to the epiphysis. This area of growth is known as the **metaphysis** (me-TAF-i-sis). During a person's growing years, the diaphysis and epiphysis of a bone are separated by cartilage at the metaphysis known as the **epiphyseal** (ep-i-FIZ-ē-al) **plate.** This cartilage allows the bone to grow in length as it is gradually replaced by bony tissue on the side of the diaphysis *(Figure 4–7)*. On a radiograph, the epiphyseal plate would be visualized as a dark line as

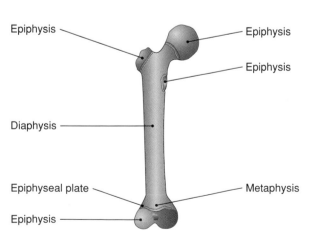

Epiphysis — Epiphysis

Epiphysis

Diaphysis

Epiphyseal plate — Metaphysis

Epiphysis

Figure 4–6. Ossification centers of a long bone (femur).

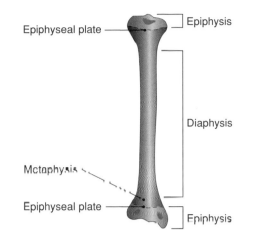

Figure 4–7. Diaphysis, epiphysis, and metaphysis identified on a long bone (tibia).

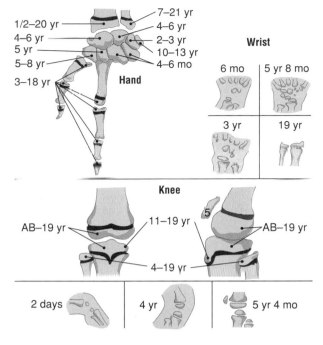

Figure 4–8. Bone ages. *(Adapted with permission from Camp JD, Cilley El. American Journal of Roentgenology. 1931; 26–905.)*

no calcium is present. As a person matures, the production of cartilage diminishes, then halts as the production of bone increases. The cartilaginous plates at the metaphysis become progressively thinner and then cease to exist. The diaphysis and epiphysis fuse completely. This point of fusion is known as the epiphyseal line. A faint linear image at the fusion sight may be visualized radiographically. Radiographs of a child's knee at various stages of growth would demonstrate the epiphyseal plates becoming progressively thinner. Tables have been constructed demonstrating the normal ages at which epiphyseal fusion takes place. These charts depict what is referred to as "bone age" *(Figure 4–8)*. It is possible to determine whether a child's growth is accelerated or delayed for his or her chronologic age by radiographing his or her extremities and comparing the films with the standard ages represented on the chart.

Throughout the process of ossification, the circumference of a bone also increases at a corresponding rate. Ossification is generally complete in females by age 18 and in males by age 21.

Bone Physiology

Recall that bones serve as storehouses for minerals. Throughout life, calcium salts and other mineral components are continually being removed and replaced. Bones are dynamic structures in the sense that they are constantly undergoing change. Old, worn-out bone tissue is replaced by new bone tissue. Bone resorption occurs as **osteoclasts** (bone-destroying cells) break down and demineralize old bone tissue. In a healthy individual, homeostasis exists as the skeleton achieves a sort of status quo; that is, the amount of bone removed equals the amount replaced. This process of bone remodeling continues throughout a person's lifetime. For example, the distal femur undergoes a remodeling process that results in complete replacement of itself every 4 months. Approximately one fifth of the skeleton is replaced each year through normal bone remodeling.

The remodeling process of bones lends itself to the ability to self-repair. In the case of a fracture or break in the bone, the bone begins to repair itself in stages. In the first step, a hematoma occurs at the site of the fracture because of injured blood vessels. Second, a capillary network forms in the hematoma site and bone cells within the bone begin to divide rapidly to develop an internal **callus** (KAL-us) or network of bone. An external callus also forms a thickened ring around the bone at the injury site. The repair process continues in step 3 as osteoblasts replace the callus with bone cells, forming spongy bone. This is demonstrated radiographically as a white haziness around the fracture. Remodeling of the bone in step 4 continues with replacement of the spongy bone by compact bone. The remodeling process results in enlargement of the bone at the injury site because of new bone growth; however, through normal homeostatic functions, the bone gradually returns to nearly normal size *(Figure 4–9)*.

Bone Markings

Bones are rarely smooth structures. On their external surfaces, they have bumps, processes, depressions, and holes. Each of these surface markings has a specific function which is usually evident by its appearance. Processes grow outward or project from the bone. They are prominent and roughened in appearance and often serve as attachment sites for muscles, tendons, and ligaments. They also assist in the formation of joints. Included among this group are heads, tubercles, tuberosities, trochanters, spines, and condyles. Depressions and openings usually allow for the passage of blood vessels and nerves. Some depressed areas receive the rounded processes of other bones in the formation of joints. Sinuses, fossae, meati, and foramina are examples of this group. *Table 4–3* summarizes the different surface markings of bones.

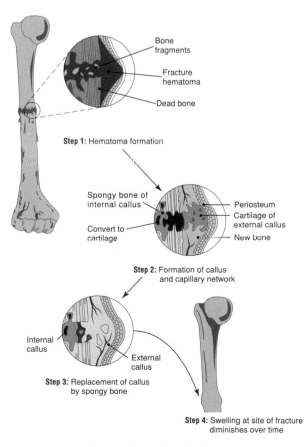

Figure 4–9. Repair of a fracture.

Table 4–3. Surface Markings of Bones

Name	Description	Example
Processes That Help Form Articulations		
Condyle	Rounded, knucklelike process	Lateral condyle of femur
Facet	Small, flat articular surface	Articular facets on sternum for ribs
Head	Rounded, ball-like structure above a constricted neck	Head of the humerus
Ramus	Armlike extension of bone	Ramus of the pubis in the pelvis
Processes That Act as Attachment Sites for Muscles, etc		
Crest	Prominent ridge or border	Crest of the ilium
Epicondyle	Prominence or raised area above or on a condyle	Medial epicondyle of the humerus
Line	Ridge of bone more narrow and less prominent than a crest	Intertrochanteric line on anterior surface of proximal femur
Spine	Slender, pointed process (spinous process)	Ischial spines in the pelvis
Styloid process	Sharp, slender process	Styloid process of ulna
Trochanter	Blunt, large projections found only on each femur	Greater and lesser trochanters of femur
Tubercle	Small, rounded, knoblike process	Greater tubercle of humerus
Tuberosity	Large, rounded process; may be roughened	Ischial tuberosity
Openings, Grooves, and Depressions		
Fissure	Narrow slit or cleftlike opening	Superior and inferior orbital fissures
Foramen	Round opening for passage of blood vessels and nerves	Mental foramina in mandible
Fossa	Shallow depression or hollow area on a bone for articulation	Olecranon fossa on humerus
Fovea	Small depression or pit	Fovea capitis on head of femur
Groove	Linear depression or furrow (also called a sulcus)	Intertubercular (bicipital) groove on humerus
Meatus	Canal-like opening or passage in a bone	Internal auditory meatus of temporal bone
Sinus	Hollow cavity or recess in a bone (also called an antrum)	Maxillary sinuses in maxillary bones of face

Bony Pathologies

Various skeletal disorders can occur if the homeostatic process of bone is disturbed. Each of the following conditions can interrupt normal homeostasis: congenital defects, hormone imbalance, malnutrition, degenerative and inflammatory diseases, and injuries.

Talipes equinovarus (TAL-i-pēz ē-kwī-nō-VĀ-rus) is a congenital deformity of the foot commonly referred to as "clubfoot." It may be seen in approximately 1 of every 1000 births. The defect occurs in the 9th or 10th week of fetal development and causes the affected foot to turn downward and inward.

Osteopenia (os-tē-ō-PĒ-nē-ah) is a condition that results from insufficient ossification. To some extent, every adult suffers from this condition. Between the ages of 30 and 40, the mass of both compact and spongy bone decreases because bone resorption exceeds new bone formation. Although osteoclasts continue to break down old bone at a fairly constant rate, osteoblastic activity decreases. Absorption and deposition of minerals are also diminished. The outcome is thinner, more fragile bones. As spongy bone is more affected by this process than compact bone, a person may become shorter as the vertebral bodies lose mass.

If more than the expected amount of bone mass is lost, **osteoporosis** (os-tē-ō-pō-RŌ-sis) occurs. Women over the age of 50 seem to be more susceptible to this condition than any other group, as it is strongly related to the lack of estrogen secretion after menopause.

Osteomalacia (os-tē-ō-mah-LĀ-shē-ah) results from a deficiency of vitamin D. This condition causes the bones to soften as a result of insufficient calcium and phosphorus deposition. The childhood form of the disease is known as *rickets.*

In **Paget's disease,** for some unknown reason (possibly a virus), the normal bone-forming and bone-destroying processes become unbalanced. This results in abnormal thickening and softening of the bones. The condition is usually localized to the skull, pelvis, and extremities. It is seldom seen in individuals under the age of 50 and it strikes both sexes with equal frequency.

Inflammatory and infectious diseases of bone are known as **osteomyelitis** (os-tē-ō-mī-LĪ-tis). The microorganism most often responsible for this condition is *Staphylococcus aureus,* otherwise known as "staph." It reaches and infects the bone through many different modes, such as fractures and abscesses or through the bloodstream from another infected body structure. This condition is generally treatable by antibiotics.

Lesions occurring in bones, whether benign or malignant, are classified as either **osteoblastic** (bone-forming) or **osteolytic** (bone-destroying). Although bones can be the sight of primary or secondary cancer,

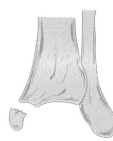
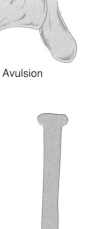
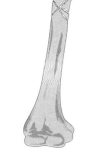
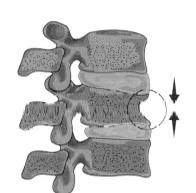
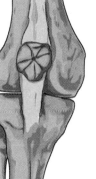

Avulsion—Chip fractures which occur from pulling or tearing of the ligaments or muscle attachments at joint articulations.

Comminuted—The bone is broken into small fragments; often a compound fracture.

Compression—Usually seen in the vertebral column; the anterior aspect of the vertebral body compresses together as force results in compaction of the cancellous bone.

Epiphyseal—Fracture extends through the ununited epiphysis of a growing bone; can result in arrested growth if not treated promptly.

Avulsion   Comminuted   Compression   Epiphyseal plate fracture

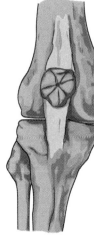

Greenstick—Type of incomplete fracture in which one side of the cortex is fractured and the other side of the bone is bent; seen in children.

Impacted—Fractured ends of bone are forced or compacted together.

Spiral—Fracture spirals through the shaft of a bone as a result of a twisting type of injury.

Stellate—Star-shaped fracture.

Greenstick fracture   Impacted   Spiral   Stellate

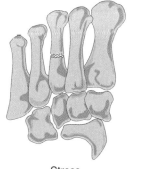

Stress/march—Occurs at sites of stress, such as metatarsals of foot.

Torus—Bulging fractures in which the cortex of the bone buckles; often occur in children.

Transverse—Fracture extends transversely across the bones.

Stress   Torus   Transverse

Figure 4–10. Types of fractures.

the most common malignancy of bone is metastatic cancer. Multiple myeloma and osteosarcoma are the two most frequently seen types of bone cancer; however, only about 1% of all malignancies are attributed to bone cancer.

Bones are remarkably strong and resilient structures, yet they are susceptible to breaking as the result of traumatic injury or a disease process. Any break in the cortex of a bone is termed a **fracture** (FRAK-chur). Fractures are the most common ailment affecting bones. There are many different types of fractures. The criteria for naming or classifying them are as follows:

1. Outward appearance (eg, open versus closed)
2. Mechanics of the injury (eg, spiral fracture)
3. Site/location (eg, Colles fracture of the radius)

The following descriptive terms may be used to characterize fractures: A *closed* fracture is a break in a bone with no interruption of the skin; also called a simple fracture. A *complete* fracture extends completely through the cross section of bone. A *compound* fractured bone breaks through the skin; also known as an open fracture. In a *displaced* fractured bone, fragments are separated and are not in normal alignment. In an *incomplete* fracture, only the cortex on one side of the bone is fractured; in a *nondisplaced* fracture, the bone fragments lie in the normal alignment. A *pathologic* fracture occurs in a weak, diseased bone upon normal activity.

Usually more than one criterion applies to the fracture. *Figure 4–10* identifies some of the more common classifications of fractures. A fracture may be evident even before a radiograph is taken for a definitive diagnosis. The signs a radiographer can be aware of when evaluating a patient prior to filming include the following:

1. Abnormal movement or motion of the body part
2. Differences in shape and length of corresponding bones on the two sides of the patient's body
3. Obvious deformities, such as a large bump over the injury or a misalignment of articulating bones
4. An open wound over the bone
5. Swelling of the soft tissue around the injury
6. Discoloration (blanching or bruising) of the skin at the site of the injury
7. Pain or tenderness in response to gentle pressure at the site of the injury

Arthrology

The rigidity of bones prevents them from bending for normal movements of the body. The skeleton would be a very unyielding structure incapable of movement if all of its 206 bones were affixed to one another. Fortunately, many of the bones are attached to one another by connective tissue, which allows for varying degrees of movement. A **joint** or **articulation** is formed by the juncture of two or more bones. Any movement of the skeleton occurs at its joints. Almost every bone in the body articulates with at least one other bone to form a joint. The exceptions are the hyoid bone in the neck and sesamoid bones. Some joints are extremely flexible and permit a wide range of movement, whereas other joints permit only slight movement or no movement at all. There are three classifications of joints based on the type and degree of movement permitted: synarthrosis (sin-ar-THRŌ-sis), amphiarthrosis (am-fi-ar-THRŌ-sis), and diarthrosis (dī-ar-THRŌ-sis). In addition to being classified according to function (movement), joints are classified according to their structure. *Table 4–4* summarizes the classifications of joints.

► *Classification of Joints According to Movement*

• *Synarthrosis—no movement*

• *Amphiarthrosis—limited movement*

• *Diarthrosis—movable*

Synarthroses

Synarthrodial joints are immovable. Structurally, they have no joint cavity. The articulating bones are joined together and held in place by fibrous connective tissue. The four types of fibrous synarthrodial joints are sutures, synchondroses, synostoses, and gomphoses.

A **suture** (SOO-cher) is a joint between bones of the skull. The bones have irregular edges that interlock like the pieces of a jigsaw puzzle. Fibrous tissue between the bones holds them tightly in place.

Recall that an epiphyseal plate is cartilage located between the shaft and epiphysis of a bone. Because the two elements of bone are held together by rigid cartilage, initially this joint is classified as **synchondrosis** (sin-kon-DRŌ-sis). It is a temporary joint, however, because the diaphysis and epiphysis eventually fuse together. Once this fusion has taken place, the joint is classified as a **synostosis** (sin-os-TŌ-sis) and is completely immovable.

A **gomphosis** (gom-FŌ-sis) is a joint found in the mouth. The cone-shaped roots of the teeth fit into the bony socket of the maxillae and the mandible bones. Fibrous ligaments aid in holding the teeth in place *(Figure 4–11)*.

Table 4–4. Summary of Joint Classifications

Functional Category	Structural Type	Description	Example
Synarthrosis	Fibrous	No movement permitted	
	Suture	Bones interlock with each other	Between the bones of the skull
	Synchondrosis	Rigid cartilaginous connection	Epiphyseal plates (temporary joint that eventually fuses completely)
	Synostosis	Complete fusion of two bones	Epiphyseal plate in adult
	Gomphosis	Articulation of a cone-shaped structure in a bony socket	Between the teeth and alveolar process of the jaw
Amphiarthrosis	Cartilaginous	Slight movement permitted	
	Symphysis	Bones separated by pad or disk of cartilage	Between the vertebral bodies in the spinal column, symphysis pubis
	Fibrous	Slight movement permitted	
	Syndesmosis	Bones connected by fibrous tissue	Articulation between distal tibia and fibula
Diarthrosis	Synovial	Joint capsule containing synovial fluid; permits movement in varying degrees	
	Ball and socket	Ball-shaped head of one bone fits in cup-shaped socket of another bone; freely movable	Shoulder and hip joints
	Condyloid	Gently rounded surface of one bone articulates with slight cavity of another bone; movement in four directions at right angles to each other	Wrist joint (radiocarpal joint); 2nd–5th metacarpophalangeal joints
	Saddle	Articular surfaces are saddle-shaped; considerable movement	Carpometacarpal joint of thumbs
	Hinge	Articular surface of one bone is convex, while surface of other bone is concave; flexion and extension movement	Elbow, knee, and ankle joints
	Pivot	Rounded surface of bone rotates in concave surface of another bone; twisting movement	Axis and atlas of vertebral column; proximal radioulnar joint
	Gliding	Surface of bones is flat or slightly curved, allowing bones to slide or glide against one another; slight movement	Intercarpal, acromioclavicular, and costovertebral joints

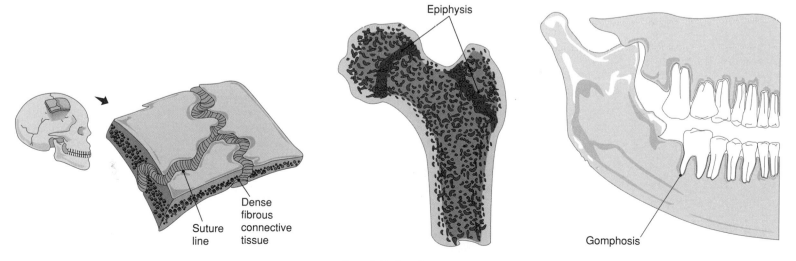

Figure 4–11. Synarthroses.

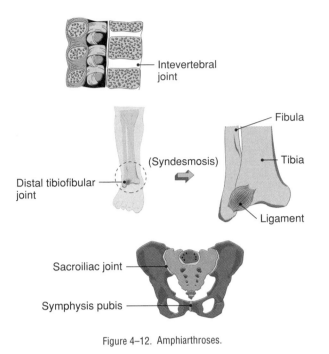

Figure 4–12. Amphiarthroses.

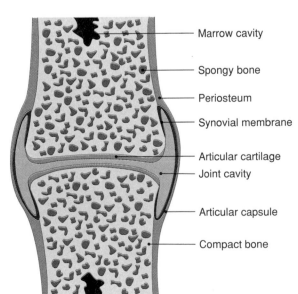

Figure 4–13. General structure of a synovial (diarthrodial) joint.

Amphiarthrosis

Joints that are slightly movable are termed amphiarthrodial. They can be either cartilaginous or fibrous in structure and, like synarthrodial joints, they do not possess a joint cavity.

In cartilaginous joints, the bones are held closely together and are connected by cartilage. A **symphysis** (SIM-fi-sis) is a cartilaginous joint in which the bones of the joint are separated by a pad or disk of cartilage. This type of articulation is found between the bodies of the vertebral column and also between the right and left pubic bones in the pelvis.

A **syndesmosis** (sin-des-MŌ-sis) is a fibrous joint in which the bones are connected by dense fibrous tissues known as ligaments. The bones are a little further apart than in a fibrous synarthrodial joint and the ligaments do allow for slight movement. The distal articulation between the tibia and fibula of the lower leg is a good example of a syndesmosis *(Figure 4–12)*.

Diarthrosis

Diarthrodial joints allow for varying degrees of motion. Structurally they are significantly different from either synarthrodial or amphiarthrodial joints. The articular surfaces of the bones involved are covered with hyaline, or articular, cartilage. An articular capsule encloses the joint, forming a cavity. The capsule is fibrous in nature and is continuous with the periosteum of the bones. Strong ligaments form the outer layer, whereas a smooth **synovial** (si-NŌ-vē-al) **membrane** lines the inside of the capsule. The synovial membrane secretes a slippery fluid called synovial fluid, which provides nourishment to the articular cartilage. It also functions to lubricate the articular cartilage to reduce friction during movement. For this reason, diarthrodial joints are also known as synovial joints. In most diarthrodial joints, muscle tendons cross the joint to stabilize it and provide support during movement *(Figure 4–13)*.

Many diarthrodial joints also contain one or more **bursae** (BER-sē) (singular, bursa). A bursa is a sac of synovial fluid that is positioned between tissues around a joint. It may be located between the skin and bone, muscle and bone, or tendon and bone. Synovial fluid is secreted from the bursa to reduce friction when the parts come in contact with one another.

Some diarthrodial joints contain either fat pads or articular disks made of fibrocartilage. These structures act as shock absorbers during movement of the articulating bones. For example, the knee has articular disks called **menisci** (me-NIS-kī) to help absorb shock in the joint when a person is walking, running, or jumping.

Diarthrodial joints are subdivided into six categories according to movement type. The range of motion of a particular joint is determined by several factors:
1. Shape of the articular surfaces of the bones involved in the joint
2. Action of the muscle and its attachment point on the bone
3. Tension of the ligaments forming the articular capsule around the joint

Ball-and-socket joints permit more movement than any other diarthrodial joint subtype. They are characterized by a rounded, ball-shaped head of one bone that fits into a cup-shaped depression or socket of another bone. Movement occurs in almost any direction through rotation, flexion, extension, abduction, and adduction. The shoulder and hip joints are ball-and-socket joints.

Condyloid joints are characterized by an elliptical-shaped or knucklelike structure on one bone that articulates with a corresponding concave surface on another bone. Movement in two planes is permitted: flexion/extension and abduction/adduction. The wrist joint, which is formed by the articulation of the radius and carpal bones, is a good example of this type of joint.

In a **saddle joint,** the articular surfaces of the two bones are saddle-shaped. That is, one bone is concave and the other is convex, with these surfaces fitting together like a cowboy sitting in the saddle. This joint is similar to a condyloid joint but allows for slightly more movement. Saddle joints are capable of circumduction in addition to flexion, extension, abduction, and adduction. The best example is the carpometacarpal joint of each thumb.

A **pivot joint** consists of a conical, rounded, or pointed surface of bone articulating with a ringlike structure on another bone. Rotation is the only movement permitted. The ulna and head of the radius form a pivot joint. As the name suggests, the radius pivots around the ulna. Another example is the axis and atlas, which are the first and second cervical vertebrae. Turning one's head from side to side is possible because of this pivot joint.

In a **hinge joint,** a convex surface or cylindrical structure on one bone fits into a concave surface on another bone. Movement occurs in a single plane in the form of flexion and extension. The elbow and knee joints are both hinge joints.

In a **gliding joint,** the articular surfaces of the bones are basically flat or minimally curved, allowing the bones to slide or glide against one another in a back-and-forth movement. The intercarpal joints of the wrist and the costotransverse joints of the spine (formed by the articulation of a rib with the transverse process of the thoracic vertebra) are gliding joints *(Figure 4–14)*.

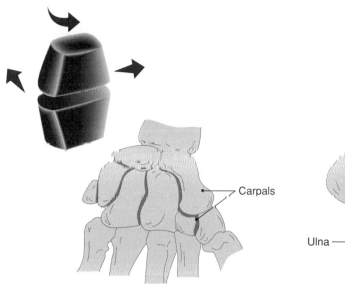

Gliding

Carpals

Humerus

Ulna

Hinge

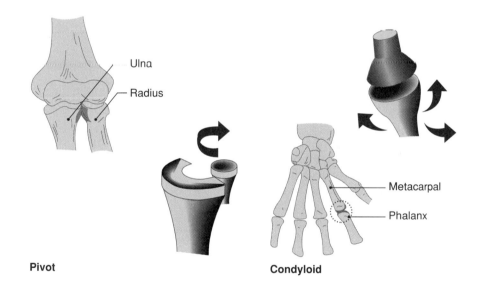

Ulna

Radius

Pivot

Metacarpal

Phalanx

Condyloid

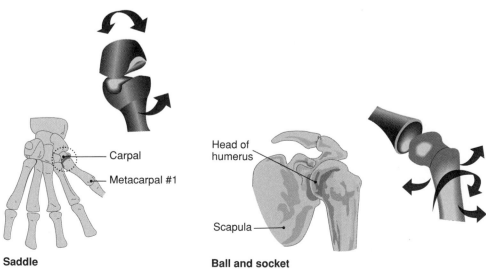

Carpal

Metacarpal #1

Saddle

Head of
humerus

Scapula

Ball and socket

Figure 4–14. Diarthroses.

► Related Terminology

ankylosis (ang-ki-LŌ-sis) — fusion or fixation of a joint usually resulting from an inflammatory disease or injury, but may be achieved artificially through a surgical procedure

arthralgia (ar-THRAL-jē-ah) — pain in a joint

arthrectomy (ar-THREK-tō-mē) — surgical excision of a joint

arthritis (ar-THRĪ-tis) — condition of the joints of the musculoskeletal system characterized by inflammation, redness, heat, pain, stiffness, and swelling; can cause degenerative changes in the connective tissue; two primary varieties are osteoarthritis and rheumatoid arthritis

arthrocentesis (ar-thrō-sen-TĒ-sis) — surgical puncture of a joint with a hollow needle to withdraw synovial fluid for microscopic examination

arthrogram (AR-thrō-gram) — radiograph taken of a joint after the introduction of contrast medium

arthroscopy (ar-THROS-kō-pē) — examination of the interior of a joint by means of an arthroscope, which is an endoscope designed specifically for examination of a joint

atrophy (AT-rō-fē) — shrinking or wasting away of tissue, specifically muscle, as a result of disuse or a disease process

bursitis (ber-SĪ-tis) — inflammation of a bursa, usually because of overuse of the joint

calcification (kal-si-fi-KĀ-shun) — deposition of calcium salts in the tissues of the body

chondritis (kon-DRĪ-tis) — inflammation of cartilage

chondromalacia (kon-dro-mah-LĀ-shē-ah) — condition of abnormal softening of cartilage

(continued)

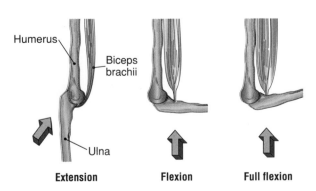

Extension   **Flexion**   **Full flexion**

Figure 4–15. Movement and the forces acting at an articulation.

MUSCULAR SYSTEM

Myology (mī-OL-ō-jē) refers to the study of muscles. There are more than 700 muscles in the body. If the skeleton provides the structural framework of the body, then the muscles are the moving force behind it. They have the ability to contract, stretch, return to normal length, respond to stimuli, and conduct impulses from nerves. Approximately one half of a person's body weight and mass are attributed to the presence of muscles. Because muscles are a soft tissue, they are generally not demonstrated on a radiograph; however, very dense muscles such as the psoas major muscles are moderately visible on films of the abdomen or lumbar spine. Some injuries to muscles and their associated structures can be determined radiographically. For example, stress projections of the ankle will demonstrate ligament damage because of the abnormal movement of the bones forming the joint.

Classification

Muscles are classified according to location, function, and structure. The three types of muscles are skeletal, visceral, and cardiac.

Skeletal muscles are usually attached to bones. They make up the red meat of the body. They are voluntary muscles because they can be controlled on command. The contractions of the skeletal muscles result in movement of the joints of the skeleton.

Viscus or *visceral* (VIS-er-al) refers to an organ. Therefore, **visceral muscles** are smooth muscles found in the walls of some organs, such as the stomach and intestines. These muscles are involuntary as they function without a conscious command to do so.

Cardiac muscle is actually the myocardium or muscle of the heart. It is also an involuntary muscle as it beats rhythmically and automatically.

Function

Muscles work hard and perform vital functions for the body. The four most notable functions are:

1. *Movement.* The skeletal muscles contract, pulling on the bones to produce movement. Involuntary muscles contract to move food through the alimentary canal or blood through the vessels of the circulatory system.
2. *Posture.* The muscles work synchronously to maintain a person's posture, such as holding the head up and standing or sitting upright.
3. *Support.* The muscles provide support and stability to the joints of the skeleton. They also help to support soft tissue structures, such as the abdominal and pelvic organs.
4. *Heat.* Heat generated as energy is expended through muscle contractions. This heat is necessary to maintain the body's relatively constant internal temperature.

In addition, ringlike muscles called **sphincters** (SFINK-terz) are found throughout the body. Situated at an orifice, or opening, each sphincter constricts the opening to regulate the flow of fluids or other materials and also to prevent backflow.

Attachment

Each skeletal muscle has at least two points of attachment on the skeleton. The immovable or more fixed attachment is known as the **origin** and is usually located at the proximal end of the muscle. The **insertion** is the more movable attachment situated at the distal end of the muscle. The bones that serve as attachment points also act as levers. When a muscle contracts, the movable bone is pulled toward the immovable bone; thus, movement occurs *(Figure 4–15)*.

Associated Structures

A **tendon** is a band of white fibrous connective tissue that connects a muscle to bone. Tendons are very strong but do not have the ability to contract or stretch. A **ligament** is also a band of fibrous connective tissue, but it connects one bone to another. Ligaments usually extend across joints to hold the articulating structures together and provide support.

Naming System

With so many muscles in the body, it could be quite difficult to remember all of their names. Actually, muscles tend to be named according to their functional and structural characteristics. There are seven criteria by which muscles are named:

1. *Shape.* Muscles come in a variety of shapes. The deltoid muscle is triangular (*deltoid* = "triangle") and the rhomboid is a diamond-shaped muscle (*rhombo* = "diamond").

2. *Size.* Terms to indicate the length or size of muscles are often used, such as the longissimus, which is a long group of muscles extending from the lumbar spine to the skull. The pectoralis minor refers to the smaller of the chest muscles.

3. *Sections.* Muscles may have more than one section or part. The quadriceps muscle has four heads (*quad* = "four," *cep* = "head"). The digastric muscle has two bellies or bodies (*di* = "two," *gastro* = "belly" or "stomach").

4. *Location.* Muscles may be named according to their location. The subscapularis muscle forms part of the posterior wall of the axilla and is located under the scapula (*sub* = "under," *scapularis* = "scapula"). The tibialis anterior is a muscle located on the anterior side of the tibia.

5. *Direction of fibers.* The name of a muscle may indicate the direction in which the muscle fibers run in relationship to the body part on which they are located. The transversus abdominis muscle extends horizontally across the abdomen (*trans* = "across"), whereas the rectus abdominis extends straight up from the pubis to the rib cage (*rectus* = "straight").

6. *Action.* The terms *supinator, pronator, extensor, flexor, abductor, adductor, levator,* and *depressor* refer to specific actions performed by the muscle. For example, rotation of the arm from pronation to supination is possible because of the action of the supinator muscle and the pronator quadratus muscle in the arm.

7. *Origin/insertion.* Muscles may be named for their points of attachment, with the origin always named first. The origin of the coracobrachialis muscle is the coracoid process of the scapula; the insertion is the humerus (*coraco* = "coracoid process," *brachial* = "arm"). The sternothyroid muscle originates on the posterior aspect of the sternum and inserts on the thyroid cartilage.

► PROCEDURAL CONSIDERATIONS

Musculoskeletal trauma contributes significantly to the workload in most radiology departments. Although departments generally have routines identified that indicate the normal projections for each body part, these routines may be altered by the physician.

PATIENT PREPARATION

Following identification of the patient, a thorough patient history should be obtained and recorded for the radiologist. An example of a history sheet that might be used to convey this information to the radiologist is illustrated in *Figure 4–16*. It is not only important to know what kind of problem the patient is having, but exactly how long the patient has been having the problem, how the injury occurred (in trauma cases), and exactly where the pain is located. Because some pathologies look very similar to normal variants in anatomy, a pertinent patient history may make the difference between a normal and abnormal diagnosis.

All radiopaque objects should be removed from the area to be included within the collimation field, if possible. Radiopaque objects may obscure the anatomy of interest and can be distracting to the radiologist interpreting the images. Patients frequently arrive in the radiology department with immobilization splints in place. Although these devices can affect the quality of the finished images, it is sometimes necessary to initially radiograph the part with the immobilization device in place. A physician should approve the removal of splints, braces, or other orthopedic immobilization devices. When an immobilization device is removed from a long bone, the joints proximal and distal to the injury should be supported to prevent additional injury from displacement of fracture fragments.

POSITIONING CONSIDERATIONS

To adequately demonstrate long bones of the body such as the femur or humerus, at least two projections 90° from each other must be obtained. When evaluating joints, at least one oblique projection should be obtained to demonstrate all the surfaces of the joint. For example, the routine projections for a wrist might include the PA, PA oblique, and lateral projections. Many institutions require that both oblique projections be obtained when radiographing any joint. Using the previous example, the AP oblique wrist projection would also be obtained.

Because body parts move only in certain directions, it is important to know the normal joint movements and learn to position patients without causing unnecessary pain or discomfort. Elderly patients may not be able to move as quickly or easily as younger patients. Care must be taken to prevent new injuries or

► Related Terminology *(continued)*

electromyography (ē-lek-trō-mī-OG-rah-fē) — examination in which the skeletal muscles are electrically stimulated; changes in the muscles are recorded and provide feedback about the nerves supplying them

exostosis (ek-sos-TŌ-sis) — development of abnormal bony projections

ganglion (GANG-glē-on) — cystlike tumor or mass on a tendon, usually seen in the wrist

gout (gowt) — form of arthritis in which there is an excessive amount of uric acid in the bloodstream; affects the cartilage in the joint and causes inflammation, pain, and swelling, particularly in the big toe; long-term effects include renal impairment

luxation (luk-SĀ-shun) — dislocation, specifically of a bone from a joint

muscular dystrophy (mus-KŪ-lar DIS-trō-fē) — degenerative, crippling disease of the muscles that results in progressive weakening and atrophy

myopathy (mī-OP-ah-thē) — disease of the muscles (eg, cardiac myopathy refers to disease of the heart muscle)

orthopedics (or-thō-PĒ-dix) — branch of medicine that deals with the function, correction, and prevention of abnormalities of the musculoskeletal system; the surgeon who specializes in this branch of medicine is known as an orthopedist

osteitis (os-tē-Ī-tis) — inflammation of bone tissue

osteolysis (os-tē-OL-ī-sis) — loss of calcium resulting in dissolution of bony tissue

osteomalacia (os-tē-ō-mah-LĀ-shē-ah) — condition of demineralization of bony tissue, resulting in abnormal softening

osteosclerosis (os-tē-ō-skle-RŌ-sis) — condition of abnormal hardness or density of a bone

rheumatism (ROO-mah-tizm) — inflammatory condition affecting connective tissue of the joints and their associated structures; can cause limitation of movement, pain, and degenerative changes

sprain (SPRĀN) — twisting injury to a joint that involves damage to the tendons, ligaments, or muscles, resulting in swelling, pain, and discoloration of the joint

strain (STRĀN) — minor injury to muscle tissue that usually results from overstretching; not as serious as a sprain

synovitis (sin-ō-VĪ-tis) — inflammation of the synovial membrane in a joint cavity

tendinitis (ten-di-NĪ-tis) — inflammation of the tendons, which may result from straining them

---

History Sheet: Skeletal Radiography

Patient Name: _____   **Age:** _____

Reason for complaint:

_____   Non-injury (make additional comments below)

 _____   Pain: _____

 _____   Follow-up: _____

 _____   Other: _____

_____   Injury

 How injury occurred (e.g. fall, car accident, sports): _____

 _____

 Type of injury (e.g. impact, twist, etc.): _____

 _____

 Location of tenderness (be specific): _____

 _____

 Date of injury: _____

Additional comments: _____

_____

_____

Technologist: _____   **Date:** _____

Figure 4–16 Patient history form.

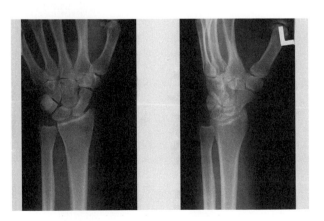

Figure 4–17. When more than one projection is included on one film, the parts should be positioned so comparable joints will be at the same level on the radiograph.

aggravate current injuries. Performing cross-table projections or angling the radiographic tube may be necessary to obtain the required views. Whenever modifying a patient position or a projection, tube–part–film alignment is critical. The central ray must be directed perpendicular to the structure of interest to prevent distortion, which could obscure pathology or lead to misinterpretation of fracture alignment (see Chapter 1).

When centering the patient for any procedure, the primary objective is to position the part of interest in the middle of the film and/or collimated area. The cassette should be oriented according to the part. In other words, the long axis of the film should be parallel to the long axis of the bone. The cassette, therefore, is usually oriented lengthwise for long bones. In most situations where two projections of a joint are included on the film, the cassette is usually masked crosswise, with the parts centered to one half of the film and centered to each other; associated joints or bones should be level with each other when the radiograph is displayed on the viewbox *(Figure 4–17)*.

To help prevent blurring of the recorded image and assist the patient in maintaining the desired position, immobilization devices or restraints may be needed. Depending on the situation, sponges, sandbags, tape, compression bands, or plexiglass "paddles" can be used to immobilize the patient. Infants can also be "mummy wrapped" in a sheet for some procedures (see Chapter 1).

Table 4–5. Recommended kVp Ranges

Small extremities	50–60 kVp
Large extremities	65–75 kVp
Ribs	60–70 kVp
Vertebral column (AP)	70–80 kVp
Vertebral column (lateral)	80–90 kVp
Skull	70–90 kVp

BREATHING INSTRUCTIONS

Although suspended respiration is not usually required for radiography of the extremities, the patient should be instructed to hold very still. Patients who are shaking because of nervousness, anxiety, pain, or room temperature may hold more still if they are instructed to suspend respiration during the exposure.

Special breathing instructions may be used for specific body parts. A patient may be instructed to breathe quietly during the exposure for a lateral thoracic spine or an RAO projection of the sternum *(Figure 4–18)*. While suspending respiration following inspiration or expiration may not be important in some situations, certain projections require specific instructions to better visualize anatomical structures. For example, the patient should be instructed to suspend respiration following deep inspiration for the AP upper rib projection to move the diaphragm inferiorly, whereas suspended expiration should be used to move the diaphragm superiorly for the AP lower rib projection.

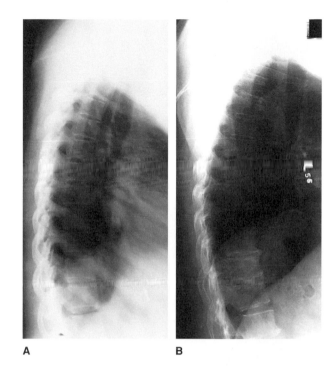

A **B**

Figure 4–18. The lateral thoracic spine projection is often obtained using a long exposure time while the patient breathes quietly **(A)**. In this instance, the rib and lung detail are blurred, allowing for better visualization of the thoracic vertebrae than when the patient suspends respiration **(B)**.

EXPOSURE FACTORS

Proper exposure factors are necessary for accurate diagnosis. Both soft tissue and bony structures must be demonstrated. Soft tissue areas may show muscle atrophy, soft tissue swelling, calcifications, opaque foreign bodies, or presence of air, which could indicate a pathologic process.

The relationship between cortical bone and soft tissue must also be clearly demonstrated for evaluation of new bone formation or erosion of the cortex, which could indicate a response to trauma or arthritis, respectively *(Figure 4–19)*. Internal bony structures (trabeculae) must be visualized to determine abnormally altered texture, alterations in the amount of mineralization, or areas of destruction.

Exposure factors must produce an optimal level of radiographic contrast and density for visualization of bony and soft tissue detail. Kilovoltage may range from 50 kVp for a finger to 70 kVp for a hip or shoulder to 85 kVp for a lateral projection of the lumbar spine. Generally, 70 to 90 kVp is used for the various projections of the spine and skull *(Table 4–5)*. Although lower kVp will produce a higher-contrast radiograph, it will require higher mAs and, therefore, increased patient dose. An appropriate kVp should be used to minimize patient dose while not sacrificing radiographic quality.

For most skeletal radiography, short exposure times should be used to minimize the blurring on the film caused by motion and to improve the visibility of radiographic detail. In several specific situations, however, a long exposure time is used to produce blurring, as described earlier.

Some pathologic conditions of the skeletal system require a change in routine technical factors. These conditions may be additive, such as Paget's disease and osteoma, and require an increase in kVp or mAs; others may be destructive conditions, such as osteoporosis and carcinoma, and require a decrease in exposure factors. *Table 4–6* lists some of the more common pathologic conditions that require compensation of technical factors. How much the technique is adjusted depends on the stage or severity of the patient's disease. A thorough patient history and examination of previous films, if available, assist the radiographer in making this determination.

EQUIPMENT CONSIDERATIONS

Most radiology departments today use slow-speed intensifying screens and/or radiographic film when radiographing the extremities to produce better recorded detail. When converting technical factors from the regular department film/screen combination, the kVp remains the same, whereas the mAs is increased according to the difference in system speeds. In addition to slower-speed film/screen systems, a small focal spot should be used when radiographing small skeletal structures to improve visualization of detail.

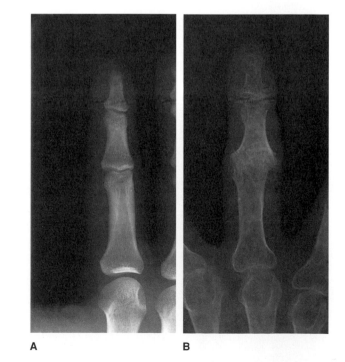

A **B**

Figure 4–19. Cortical bone and trabeculae must be demonstrated to evaluate pathology **(A)**. Destruction of the trabeculae is indicative of demineralization **(B)**.

Table 4–6. Pathologic Conditions

Additive Skeletal Pathology	Destructive Skeletal Pathology
Acromegaly	Active osteomyelitis
Callus	Aseptic necrosis
Exostosis	Atrophy
Hydrocephalus	Carcinoma
Osteoma	Degenerative arthritis
Osteopetrosis	Ewing's tumor (children)
Paget's disease	Gout
Sclerosis	Hodgkin's disease
	Neuroblastoma
	Osteoporosis

► *The Following Skeletal Exams Usually Require a Grid:*

- *Skull*

- *Spine*

- *Ribs*

- *Pelvis*

- *Shoulder*

- *Femur*

- *Humerus[a]*

- *Knee[a]*

[a]May also be performed without a grid

In general, a grid should be used for all body parts measuring 10 cm or greater. When changing from a nongrid to a grid technique, or vice versa, the kilovoltage usually remains unchanged. A nongrid technique can be converted to a grid technique by using the conversion factors in *Table 4–7* to change the mAs. For example, if 5 mAs was used without a grid and an 8:1 ratio grid was added to improve radiographic contrast, the grid technique would be 5 mAs × 4, or 20 mAs. The conversion factors can also be used to change a grid technique to a nongrid technique, as might be necessary in mobile radiography. For example, a grid technique might be used to radiograph a knee in the department, but to perform the same examination at the patient's bedside, a nongrid technique is used.

Occasionally, special techniques such as magnification radiography and tomography are employed to evaluate subtle fractures or other pathology. If the magnification technique is used or if very fine detail is needed, a small focal spot, 0.3 mm or less, must be used.

ORTHOPEDIC CAST RADIOGRAPHY

Following diagnosis of a fracture, a physician may need to reduce the fracture by manipulating the part to align the bone fragments. The radiographer may then be asked to perform *post-reduction* radiographs to assess alignment and position of the bones. These radiographs are often taken after the fracture has been immobilized in an orthopedic cast. When performing cast radiography, the routine procedure is often modified to include just AP/PA and lateral projections to demonstrate alignment of the bones.

Orthopedic casts are made of either plaster of Paris or fiberglass and may be either wet or dry at the time of the examination. To produce an acceptable film, the technical factors need to be adjusted depending on the type of casting material, the thickness of the cast, and the amount of moisture in the cast. Although authorities differ on whether kVp or mAs should be adjusted, *Table 4–8* provides some general guidelines for adjusting technique. Because fine detail is not necessary or desired in cast radiography (the detail in the cast detracts from the bony anatomy), regular or fast-speed screens are preferred over detail or slow-speed screens. The use of faster-speed film/screen systems also minimizes patient dose, an important feature considering the potential number of follow-up examinations the patient may need.

Table 4–7. Grid Conversion Factors When Converting From Nongrid to Grid Technique

Grid Ratio	Conversion Factor
5:1	2 × mAs
6:1	3 × mAs
8:1	4 × mAs
12:1	5 × mAs
16:1	6 × mAs

Table 4–8. Cast Conversions

Small to medium dry plaster cast	Increase 5–7 kVp
Large or wet plaster cast	Increase 8–10 kVp or double mAs
Wet fiberglass cast	Increase 0–4 kVp
Dry fiberglass cast	Usually no change

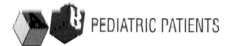

PEDIATRIC PATIENTS

Patient restraint and radiation protection are important considerations in pediatric radiography. Because children may be frightened or may not understand instructions, patient restraint is critical to producing quality films without motion. In addition to restraints, fast exposure times should also be used to minimize blurring from motion. Because young children are highly radiosensitive, high-speed film/screen systems and modification of procedures (radiologist elimination of views not necessary for diagnosis) should be employed whenever possible to minimize patient dose. Although gonadal shields should be used for all patients, when possible, their use is especially important when radiographing children, providing they do not interfere with the procedure. Because children have a higher percentage of water per body weight than adults, the kilovoltage used should be lower than that used for adults to reduce the amount of scatter that could detract from the quality of the finished image. Technique charts for children should be available in the radiology department to minimize the possibility of repeat films.

GERIATRIC PATIENTS

Because of physical or mental limitations that some elderly patients might have, a fast exposure time should be used to minimize motion. Due to atrophy of the skin, restraints should be used carefully to avoid abrasion and possible bleeding. The lack of muscle tone in the older patient often contributes to overpenetrated, overexposed radiographs. When radiographing an elderly patient, kVp should be reduced to produce optimum radiographic contrast. The mAs may also need to be decreased depending on patient condition and any pathology present. For example, a technique for a lumbar spine on an elderly woman with osteoporosis should be reduced 5 to 6 kVp and 25 to 30% in mAs to compensate for her age and condition. Evaluating the first film prior to completing the procedure will help prevent unnecessary repeat radiographs.

SPECIAL SKELETAL PROCEDURES

Radiographic evaluation of the skeletal system may be performed for reasons other than the identification of fractures. A **metastatic bone survey,** sometimes called a **skeletal survey,** may be obtained to determine whether a patient's cancer has spread, or metastasized, to the bone. Because they are highly vascular, bones that contain red bone marrow are the primary sites for metastatic lesions. Although routines vary, the examination usually includes a PA chest, AP and lateral projections of the skull and spine, and an AP projection of the pelvis. A nuclear medicine bone scan is often preferred over this plain film study because a significant amount of demineralization must occur before changes are noted radiographically.

Individuals with chronic renal disease are at risk of developing hyperparathyroidism, a disruption of the serum calcium and phosphate ratio caused by an excess of parathyroid hormone (PTH). The elevated levels of PTH overstimulate the osteoclasts responsible for removal of bone and cause bone destruction. Radiographic evaluation would demonstrate subperiosteal bone resorption, especially in the diaphyses of the phalanges, the distal clavicles, and the medial side of the proximal third of the tibias *(Figure 4–20)*. Patients on renal dialysis because of chronic renal failure are particularly prone to this condition. A **dialysis survey** may be obtained to evaluate the demineralization of the bones as a result of this process. Lateral spine, AP pelvis, PA hand, AP clavicle, lateral skull, and AP knee projections might be included in a skeletal survey done for this purpose, according to department routine or radiologist preference.

Bone age studies are performed to determine skeletal bone maturation in young children. A PA projection of the left hand and wrist, and occasionally additional projections, is obtained and compared with an atlas of standard radiographs for each age and sex. The presence or absence of ossification centers, their configuration, and the fusion of epiphyses at various sites are used to determine bone age.

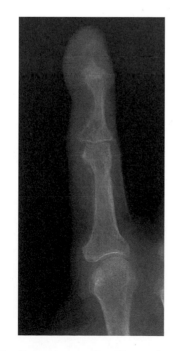

Figure 4–20. The effects of hyperparathyroidism can be seen on this radiograph of the finger.

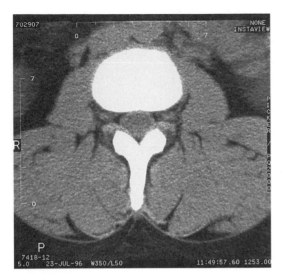

Figure 4–21. CT image of the lumbar spine. *(Courtesy of Terri Gosney, RT(R)(CT)).*

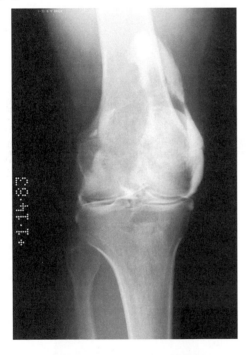

Figure 4–22. Contrast arthrogram of the knee.

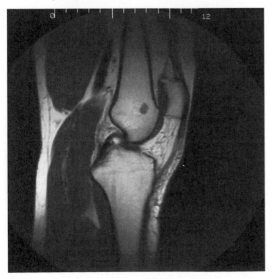

Figure 4–23. Magnetic resonance image of the knee.

Radiography of the skeletal system is also used to help diagnose child abuse. Sometimes referred to as a "Silverman series," this skeletal survey often includes AP/PA and lateral projections of both upper and lower limbs, the chest for ribs, pelvis, spine, and skull. Multiple fractures, especially those that are unusual for the location, child's age, or type of trauma, may be indicative of child abuse; a history of excessive radiography, even when normal, may also indicate possible child abuse. Although child abuse may be suspected prior to radiography, the radiographer should be aware of bruises, burns, abrasions, bite marks, and joint pain exhibited by pain on movement. Concerns about child abuse should be directed to the radiologist.

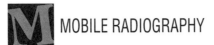 MOBILE RADIOGRAPHY

Mobile radiographic units are frequently used to perform follow-up examinations of fractures at the patient's bedside or assist the surgeon during surgery. Patients in traction in an orthopedic bed are usually unable to travel to the radiology department for progress examinations. Manipulating the mobile unit around the orthopedic bed provides a significant challenge to the radiographer. Because the patient may be in great pain, it is important to avoid bumping the bed or traction weights in this process. Frequently, a shorter or longer SID must be used, requiring a decrease or increase in exposure factors, respectively. To accurately represent the alignment of the fracture, the central ray must be perpendicular to the part of interest, as described in Chapter 1. Although most portable examinations of the extremities can be performed using non-grid cassettes, grid cassettes are usually required for the pelvis, spine, and skull. Close collimation is required for control of scatter radiation that could detract from radiographic quality. Recording the conditions of the exposure (kVp, mAs, and SID) on the radiographs assists technologists required to obtain subsequent radiographs.

ALTERNATE IMAGING PROCEDURES

Although plain-film radiography is the primary means for evaluation of the musculoskeletal system, other methods are also used. **Tomography** is used to evaluate fractures (their presence and the healing process), the mandible, and lesions. Tomographic examination of the mandible, often referred to as a "Panorex" or "Panolipse" after the manufacturer's name for the equipment, is described in Chapter 12. In addition to conventional tomography, **computed tomography** is frequently used to image the lumbar spine, skull, facial bones, and limbs *(Figure 4–21).*

Arthrography is performed to evaluate the soft tissue structures of the joints (ligaments, menisci, bursae, and articular cartilage). Although an arthrogram can be performed on any encapsulated joint, the knee is the most frequently examined joint; the shoulder, hip, wrist, and temporomandibular joints are also common sites for this procedure. Using aseptic techniques, the area of interest is carefully cleansed prior to administration of a local anesthetic. After aspiration of any effusion, a water-soluble iodine and/or air or gas contrast medium is injected into the joint of interest; when both are used for one examination, it is referred to as a **double-contrast study.** Once the contrast is in the joint, the joint must be exercised to distribute the contrast medium throughout the joint space. Fluoroscopy is used to assess the joint and obtain spot films; traditional overhead films may be requested by the radiologist *(Figure 4–22).* Because it is a noninvasive procedure, **magnetic resonance imaging** is frequently substituted for arthrography *(Figure 4–23).*

Another modality used to evaluate the skeletal system is **nuclear medicine.** The nuclear medicine bone scan can be used to evaluate injuries (fractures), metastases, tumor, arthritis, osteomyelitis, or Paget's disease. A calcium-seeking compound that is labeled with a radioactive isotope is injected intravenously into the patient. Areas of increased concentration, often called "hot spots," would indicate a problem related to the patient's medical history *(Figure 4–24).*

Myelography and **discography** are two additional procedures related to the musculoskeletal system and are described in Chapter 10.

SUMMARY

▶ The skeleton forms the bony framework of the body and serves to support and protect many vital organs; through the attachment of muscles, it permits movement.

▶ Understanding the bony anatomy and how the body moves is integral to providing the best patient care and producing quality radiographs of the skeletal system.

▶ A pertinent patient history that includes the reason for the complaint and the exact site of the pain/injury can be critical to accurate diagnosis.

▶ When radiographing long bones, at least two projections 90° from each other must be obtained; when evaluating joints, at least one oblique projection should be obtained.

▶ To prevent distortion, the central ray should be directed perpendicular to the structure of interest and the part-to-film distance (OID) should be minimized.

▶ In general, the part of interest should be centered to the film and collimated area.

▶ Patient immobilization and a fast exposure time should be used to minimize motion on the finished radiograph.

▶ Gonadal shielding, appropriately high-kVp and low-mAs techniques, and proper film/screen combination for the examination should be used to minimize patient dose.

▶ Additive and destructive skeletal pathologies may require adjustment in technical factors.

▶ Although a grid is recommended for structures measuring 10 cm or more, a nongrid technique may be preferred in some mobile radiography to minimize patient and technologist exposure.

▶ Technical compensation for casts depends on the type of casting material, the thickness of the cast, and the amount of moisture in the cast.

▶ Geriatric and pediatric patients may have special patient care needs and may require adjustment in technical factors.

▶ Metastatic bone surveys, dialysis surveys, and bone age studies are special examinations that may include radiographs of various parts of the skeletal system to evaluate specific conditions.

▶ Tomography, computed tomography, magnetic resonance imaging, arthrography, nuclear medicine, myelography, and discography are alternate methods for evaluating the musculoskeletal system.

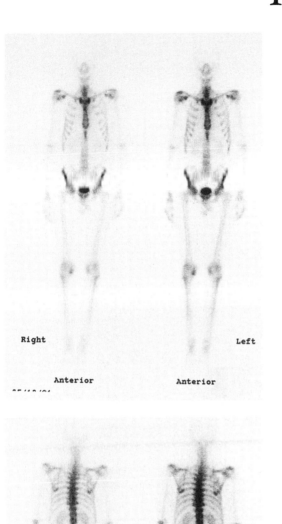
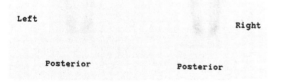

Figure 4–24. Nuclear medicine bone scan.

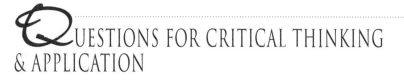

QUESTIONS FOR CRITICAL THINKING & APPLICATION

1. A 4-year-old child fell out of a tree, fracturing her right tibia. The injury was located at the proximal end of the bone and consequently damaged the epiphyseal plate. Explain the implications this injury might have on the future growth of the leg.

2. Discuss the process of bone remodeling as it relates to the healing of a fracture.

3. Why do geriatric patients usually seem small and frail? How does aging affect the skeletal system?

4. A weight lifter may be able to press more than 500 pounds over his head, thus placing an extreme amount of stress on the bones of the arms. Discuss how the construction of the bones in the arms prevents them from bending or breaking during this activity.

5. Mr. Jones stubbed his big toe against a chair leg causing the toe to swell and bruise. He did not seek treatment initially after the injury, but contacted his doctor approximately 2 weeks later when he was still experiencing pain. His physician ordered a radiographic examination of the toe which indicated that it had been fractured but was now healing satisfactorily. How can this be determined from the radiographs?

6. A patient has been involved in a car accident and has multiple injuries of the head and leg. List the questions you would ask when obtaining a pertinent patient history on this patient.

7. A patient arrives in the radiology department with an immobilization splint on her arm. Keeping patient care in mind, discuss the procedure that should be followed when radiographing her forearm.

8. A patient was admitted through the emergency room with multiple injuries. Lower leg radiographs must be obtained; however, the patient is unable to extend the knee or turn onto either side. Describe how the AP and lateral projections should be obtained.

9. A knee was radiographed using 65 kVp and 5 mAs without a grid. To produce a higher scale of contrast, a follow-up film was taken using an 8:1 grid. If the kVp remains the same, what mAs will be needed to produce a radiograph with density comparable to that of the first?

10. Preliminary films of the forearm were taken using a 50-speed film/screen combination, 55 kVp, 10 mAs. Describe the conditions under which the post-reduction radiographs should be obtained following the application of a plaster of Paris cast.

FILM CRITIQUE

Identify compact bone.

Identify cancellous bone. What is the term used to describe the honeycomb appearance?

How would the bones demonstrated on this radiograph be classified?

Approximately what kVp should be used to radiograph the wrist?

What scale of contrast is exhibited on this radiograph?

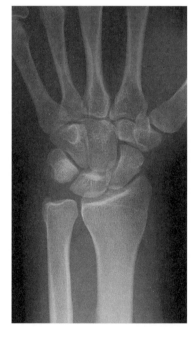

Figure 4–25. PA wrist.

5

UPPER LIMB (EXTREMITY)

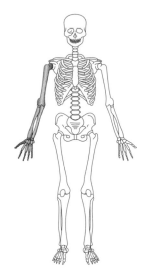

Figure 5–1. The upper limb (extremity).

► ANATOMY OF THE UPPER LIMB (EXTREMITY)

The upper limb consists of the bones of the hand, wrist, forearm, and humerus, as well as the shoulder girdle *(Figure 5–1, Table 5–1)*. Discounting the shoulder girdle, which will be discussed in the next chapter, there are a total of 30 bones on each upper limb *(Figure 5–2)*.

HAND AND WRIST

The bony structures constituting the hand and wrist are demonstrated in *Figure 5–3*. Both anterior and posterior aspects are illustrated.

Phalanges

The fingers of each hand are known as digits. They are numbered 1 through 5 beginning on the lateral side with the thumb. The bones of the digits are the phalanges (fah-LAN-jēz) (singular, *phalanx*). There are 14 of these miniature long bones in each hand. They are arranged in three rows: distal, middle, and proximal. Each of the second through fifth digits has a distal, middle, and proximal phalanx, whereas the first digit has only a distal and proximal phalanx. The thumb or first digit may also be referred to as the *pollex* (POL-eks).

Structurally, each phalanx has a head, shaft, and base. The rounded head is located distally; the more flattened base is found at the proximal end of the bone. The roughened clump of bony tissue seen at the anterior distal end of each digit on the distal phalanx is the **ungulate** (UNG-ū-lāt) **process** or **tuft.** The ungulate process acts as a support for the fingernail.

Metacarpals

The five bones forming the palm of the hand are the metacarpals (met-ah-KAR-palz). *Meta-* means "beyond" and *carpus* refers to "wrist"; thus, the metacarpus is the area beyond the wrist. Like the phalanges, the metacarpals are also numbered 1 through 5 beginning on the lateral side. These bones are also classi-

Table 5–1. Summary of Bones of the Upper Limb

Bones of Each Upper Limb	Description
Phalanges (14)	• Fingers or digits • Distal, middle, proximal • Mini-long bones • Articulate with metacarpals
Metacarpals (5)	• Palm of hand • Mini-long bones • Articulate with phalanges and carpals
Carpals (8) 　• Scaphoid 　• Lunate 　• Triquetrum 　• Pisiform 　• Trapezium 　• Trapezoid 　• Capitate 　• Hamate	• Wrist • Short bones • Arranged in two rows—distal and proximal • Articulate with metacarpals and radius
Radius (1)	• Lateral bone of forearm • Long bone • Primarily helps form wrist joint • Articulates with carpals and capitulum of humerus
Ulna (1)	• Medial bone of forearm • Long bone • Primarily helps form elbow joint • Articulates with trochlea of humerus
Humerus (1)	• Upper arm • Long bone • Assists in formation of shoulder and elbow joints • Articulates with radius and ulna at elbow joint and glenoid cavity of scapula at shoulder joint

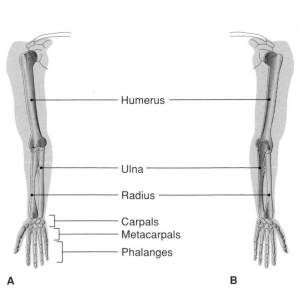

Humerus

Ulna

Radius

Carpals
Metacarpals
Phalanges

A　　　　　　　　　　**B**

Figure 5–2. The bones of the upper limb are illustrated on **(A)** anterior and **(B)** posterior views.

Table 5–2. Carpal Bones Identified by Row

Proximal Row	Distal Row
Scaphoid	Trapezium
Lunate	Trapezoid
Triquetrum	Capitate
Pisiform	Hamate

fied as miniature long bones. Each metacarpal has a head, shaft, and base. When a person clenches his or her hand to make a fist, prominent knuckles are seen. These are formed by the heads of the metacarpals. It is common to have one or two small sesamoid bones on the anterior surface of the head of the first metacarpal. The metacarpals articulate distally with the phalanges and proximally with the carpals.

Carpals

Eight bones make up the carpus (KAR-pus) or wrist. They are situated between the metacarpals of the hand and the bones of the forearm. In fact, a wristwatch is misnamed as it is actually worn on the distal forearm and not on the wrist. The carpal bones are short bones tightly arranged in two transverse rows of four bones *(Table 5–2)*. They are held securely in this formation by ligaments. When naming the carpal bones, the radiographer should begin on the lateral side with the proximal row, followed by the distal row on the lateral side.

With the exception of the pisiform, the carpal bones have alternate names. As both names may be commonly used, it is necessary for the radiographer to be familiar with them.

- *Scaphoid* (SKAF-oid). The scaphoid is also called the *navicular* (nah-VIK-u-lar). It is a boat-shaped bone situated on the lateral side of the wrist. It is the most commonly fractured carpal bone.
- *Lunate* (LŪ-nāt). The lunate, or *semilunar,* bone is crescent-shaped. As the name implies, it resembles a half-moon.
- *Triquetrum* (trī-KĒ-trum). The triquetrum is also called the *triangular* or *triquetral* bone. This triangular-shaped bone is located on the medial side of the wrist.
- *Pisiform* (PĒ-sē-form). The pisiform is the smallest carpal bone. It is a pea-shaped bone located anterior to the triquetral bone. It can be palpated on the anteromedial side of the wrist.
- *Trapezium* (trah-PĒ-zē-um). The trapezium is a four-sided bone which is also called the *greater multangular.* It articulates directly with the first metacarpal.
- *Trapezoid* (TRAP-i-zoid). The trapezoid bone is similar in shape to the trapezium, except it is smaller. Hence, it is also known as the *lesser multangular.*
- *Capitate* (KAP-i-tāt). The capitate is the largest bone of the wrist. It has a rounded area shaped like a head (*capito-* = "head"). It is also called the *os magnum.*
- *Hamate* (HAM-āt). The hamate is located on the medial side of the distal row. It is also known as the *unciform* (UN-si-form), which means "hook-shaped." The hamular process is a hooklike process that projects from the anterior aspect of the hamate bone. It can be palpated on the palmar surface of the wrist.

A mnemonic is often used to remember the names and arrangement of the carpal bones. An example of such a memory device is the following statement: "*Steve Left The Party To Take Carol Home.*" *Table 5–3* relates the mnemonic with the carpal bones.

Table 5–3. Mnemonic for Learning the Arrangement of the Carpal Bones

Mnemonic	Carpal Bones
*St*eve	*S*caphoid
*L*eft	*L*unate
*T*he	*T*riquetrum
*P*arty	*P*isiform
*T*o	*T*rapezium
*T*ake	*T*rapezoid
*C*arol	*C*apitate
*H*ome	*H*amate

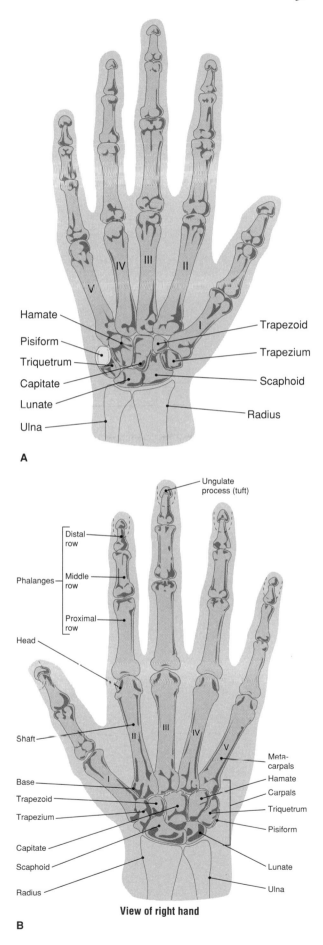

View of right hand

Figure 5–3. The hand and wrist. The position and relationship of the bones of the hand and wrist are demonstrated on **(A)** anterior and **(B)** posterior views.

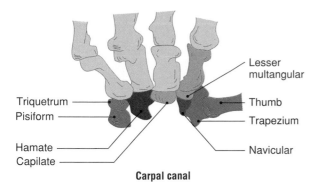

Figure 5–4. Carpal canal. The carpal bones are demonstrated in an arch arrangement.

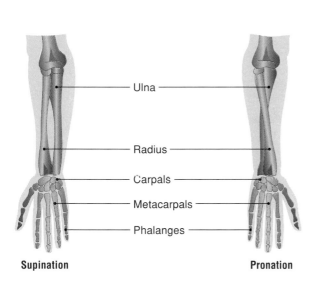

Figure 5–5. Supination versus pronation. Notice that the radius crosses the ulna when the hand is pronated.

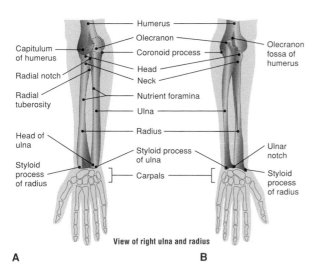

Figure 5–6. The forearm. The bones of the forearm are seen on **(A)** anterior and **(B)** posterior views.

The anterior surface of the carpus is curved. The **carpal tunnel** or canal is formed by the transverse carpal ligament, which extends transversely from the trapezium and scaphoid to the hamate and pisiform. Blood vessels, nerves, and tendons pass through the carpal tunnel. The condition known as carpal tunnel syndrome (CTS) occurs when the median nerve is pinched by the ligament, resulting in a loss of sensation in the fourth and fifth digits of the hand. When the wrist is hyperextended, an arch arrangement of the carpal bones can be demonstrated radiographically. This projection may be useful in the diagnosis of CTS *(Figure 5–4)*.

FOREARM

The forearm or lower arm comprises two long bones, the radius (RĀ-dē-us) and ulna (UL-nah), which extend from the wrist to the elbow. In the true anatomic position, these bones are parallel to one another and are connected by an interosseous membrane. If the hand is rotated to a pronated or palm-down position, the radius crosses over the ulna. As this position could possibly obscure anatomy and pathology, the radiographer should remember to keep the hand supinated for a true AP projection of the forearm *(Figure 5–5)*.

Radius

The radius is situated on the lateral side of the forearm and is the shortest of the two bones. The base of the radius is located at its distal end and is the broadest part of the bone. The concave surface of the base articulates with the proximal row of carpal bones, specifically the scaphoid and lunate. A pointed or conical projection of bone on the lateral aspect of the base is known as the **styloid** (STĪ-loid) **process.** This bony projection can be palpated on the thumb side of the distal forearm. The **ulnar notch** is located on the medial side of the base. The head of the ulna fits in this depressed area. The long central body of the radius is the **shaft** or **diaphysis.** The head of the radius is at its proximal end and is disk-shaped to fit into the radial notch on the proximal ulna. The superior aspect of the radial head is concave where it articulates with the capitulum of the humerus. The neck of the radius is the constricted area just distal to the head. A rough projection of bone on the anteromedial aspect of the radius just distal to the neck is called the **radial tuberosity.** The biceps muscle of the arm inserts at this point.

Ulna

The ulna is located medially to the radius. Whereas the radius primarily forms the wrist joint, the ulna plays a major role in the elbow joint.

Situated at the bone's distal end, the head of the ulna articulates with the ulnar notch of the radius. A fibrocartilaginous pad located on the inferior end of the ulna prevents it from directly articulating with the carpal bones. Like the radius, the ulna also has a styloid process. This pointed projection is on the medial side of the ulnar head, or on the side of the fifth digit. The shaft or diaphysis of the ulna gradually expands so that the proximal end is significantly larger than the distal end. The proximal end is hook-shaped with two processes and two notches. The **olecranon** (ō-LEK-rah-non) **process** is the very prominent, pointed tip of the elbow. It is located on the posterior and superior aspect of the ulna and can be palpated, especially when the arm is flexed. When the arm is extended, the olecranon process of the ulna fits into the olecranon fossa of the humerus. The **coronoid** (KOR-ō-noid) **process** is smaller than the olecranon process. It is a beak-shaped process located anteriorly and inferiorly to the olecranon process. The medial aspect of the coronoid process is called the **coronoid tubercle.** The **radial notch** is a smooth shallow depression located on the lateral aspect of the proximal ulna just to the lateral side of the coronoid process. The head of the radius articulates with the ulna at the radial notch. The large concave depression on the anterior side of the olecranon process is called the **trochlear** (TRŌ-K-lē-ar) **notch** or **semilunar notch.** The trochlea of the humerus sits in the trochlear notch to form the major component of the elbow joint *(Figure 5–6)*.

UPPER ARM

Humerus

The single bone forming each upper arm is known as the humerus *(Figure 5–7)*. It is a long bone that extends from the elbow to the shoulder and assists in the formation of both joints. The broadened distal end of the humerus is called the **condyle** (KON-dīl). It is divided into two distinct regions for articulation with the radius and ulna. The **capitulum** (ka-PIT-ū-lum) is a rounded process found on the anterior and inferior condylar surface of the humerus and is also known as the capitellum. It articulates with the head of the radius. The **trochlea** (TRŌ-K-lē-ah) is located on the medial inferior condylar aspect of the humerus. It is shaped like a pulley or a spool of thread to fit into the trochlear notch of the ulna. The central area of the trochlea is more constricted than its rimlike ends and is known as the **trochlear sulcus.** On a lateral radiograph of the distal humerus, the trochlear sulcus will have a cylindrical appearance.

Three depressions are found on the distal end of the humerus. The **olecranon fossa** is a large, deep depression located on the posterior surface. When the forearm is extended, the olecranon process of the ulna latches into this fossa and prevents hyperextension of the arm. The **coronoid fossa** is on the anterior surface just above the trochlea. It is a more shallow depression which accommodates the coronoid process of the ulna when the elbow joint is flexed. The third depression is the **radial fossa,** which is found on the anterior surface slightly above the capitulum. It receives the head of the radius when the arm is flexed.

There are two rough bony prominences on the distal humerus situated along the same plane as the depressions. They are known as the **epicondyles** (*epi* = "on") and are palpable on the distal humerus. The prominent medial epicondyle is situated above the trochlea. In layman's terms, the medial epicondyle is referred to as either the "funny bone" or "crazy bone." When this structure is accidentally bumped, a painful or tingling sensation is felt in the arm because of the presence of the ulnar nerve on its posterior side. The smaller lateral epicondyle is found above the capitulum.

The shaft or body of the humerus is long and cylindrical. It is also known as the diaphysis. It is more narrow than either the proximal or distal end of the bone. Approximately midway down the shaft on the lateral surface is a rough prominence known as the **deltoid** (DEL-toid) **tuberosity.** This area serves as the attachment site for the deltoid muscle.

The expanded proximal end of the humerus is the head. This smooth hemispherical structure articulates with the glenoid cavity of the scapula to form the shoulder joint. Just below the head is a slightly constricted area known as the anatomical neck. There are two bony prominences located slightly inferior to the anatomical neck. The **greater tubercle (tuberosity)** is large and lies near the head on the lateral border of the humerus. The **lesser tubercle (tuberosity)** is smaller and is situated on the anteromedial surface. Both tubercles serve as attachment sites for muscles. The greater and lesser tubercles are separated from each other by the **intertubercular,** or **bicipital, groove.** This furrow runs longitudinally on the proximal humerus and houses the tendon of the biceps muscle. The **surgical neck** is the constricted area at the junction between the proximal humerus and the shaft. It is located just inferior to the tubercles. Although the anatomical neck is seldom injured, the surgical neck is often the site of fractures. Surgical intervention is usually necessary to repair and stabilize the fractures.

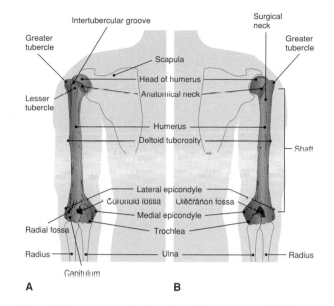

Figure 5–7. The humerus. The single bone of the upper arm is illustrated on **(A)** anterior and **(B)** posterior views.

ARTHROLOGY

The bones of the upper limb form many articulations or joints *(Figure 5–8).* The joints can be classified as synovial joints with varying degrees of movement. Each joint or group of joints is summarized below.

Interphalangeal (in-ter-fah-LAN-jē-al) **joints** are formed by the articulation of two phalanges. In each upper limb, there are a total of nine interphalangeal joints which are named according to their location. The distal interphalangeal (DIP) joints are found between the bases of the distal phalanges and the heads of the middle phalanges. The proximal interphalangeal (PIP) joints are located between the bases of the middle phalanges and the heads of the proximal phalanges. As the thumb has only two phalanges, it has a single interphalangeal joint. Interphalangeal joints are hinge joints with flexion and extension movements.

The **metacarpophalangeal** (met-ah-KAR-pō-fah-LAN-jē-al) (MCP) **joints** are formed by the bases of the phalanges and the heads of the metacarpals. The first metacarpophalangeal joint is a saddle joint, which allows circumduction in addition to flexion, extension, adduction, and abduction. The second through the fifth metacarpophalangeal joints are condylar joints, which permit flexion, extension, adduction, and abduction.

The **carpometacarpal** (KAR-pō-met-ah-kar-pal) **joints** are found between the distal row of carpal bones and the bases of the metacarpal bones. Like the first metacarpophalangeal joint, the first carpometacarpal joint is a saddle joint. The second through the fifth carpometacarpal joints are gliding joints.

The **intercarpal** (in-ter-KAR-pal) **joints** are formed by the articulation of the carpal bones with one another. The flat or slightly curved surfaces of the bones allow gliding movement to take place within the joint capsule.

The **radiocarpal** (rā-dē-ō-KAR-pal) **joint** is actually the joint typically referred to as the wrist joint. It is formed by the articulation of the carpal bones and the radius. The carpal bones specifically involved in this joint are the scaphoid, lunate, and triquetrum, although only the scaphoid and lunate articulate directly with the radius. This is a condylar joint permitting movement in four directions: flexion, extension, adduction, and abduction.

The **distal radioulnar joint** is formed by the head of the ulna articulating with the ulnar notch on the distal radius. The **proximal radioulnar joint** is found between the head of the radius and the radial notch

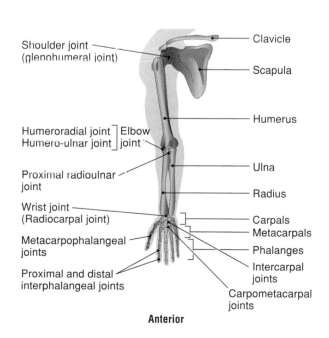

Figure 5–8. Joints of the upper limb. The articulations formed by the bones of the upper limb are illustrated on an anterior view.

Table 5–4. Summary of the Joints of the Upper Limb

Name of Joint	Classification	Structure	Movement
Interphalangeal	Diarthrodial	Synovial	Hinge
Metacarpophalangeal	Diarthrodial	Synovial	
1st			Saddle
2nd to 5th			Condylar
Carpometacarpal	Diarthrodial	Synovial	
1st			Saddle
2nd to 5th			Gliding
Intercarpal	Diarthrodial	Synovial	Gliding
Radiocarpal	Diarthrodial	Synovial	Condylar
Radioulnar	Diarthrodial	Synovial	
Distal			Pivot
Proximal			Pivot
Elbow	Diarthrodial	Synovial	Hinge
Humeroradial			
Humeroulnar			
Shoulder	Diarthrodial	Synovial	Ball and socket
Glenohumeral			

on the proximal ulna. Both radioulnar joints are pivot joints that allow for rotational movement. Together, these joints permit supination and pronation movements of the hand.

The **elbow joint** is actually formed by two articulations of the humerus: the **humeroradial joint** and the **humeroulnar joint.** The humeroradial joint is found between the capitulum of the humerus and the head of the radius. The humeroulnar joint is formed by the articulation of the trochlea of the humerus with the trochlear notch of the ulna. The elbow joint is a hinge joint that enables flexion and extension movements.

The anatomic name for the shoulder joint is the **glenohumeral joint.** It is a ball-and-socket joint formed by the glenoid cavity of the scapula (socket) and the ball-like head of the humerus. It is discussed more completely in Chapter 6.

Table 5–4 summarizes the joints of the upper limb and their movement type.

► PROCEDURAL CONSIDERATIONS

Because the upper limb includes many small bones and structures, accurate patient positioning, immobilization, and selection of appropriate technical factors and equipment are critical to producing optimum radiographs. The radiographer must understand all the procedural variables and be able to make decisions relative to alternate positioning, adjustments in technical factors, and equipment selection based on the patient's age and condition.

PATIENT PREPARATION

After proper identification, the patient should be instructed to remove jewelry, watches, and clothing from the area of interest. For radiographic examination of the humerus, women should be asked to remove all clothing above the waist and wear a patient gown. Immobilization devices, such as ACE bandages and splints, should be removed only with a physician's permission.

POSITIONING CONSIDERATIONS

For most radiographic examinations of the upper limb *(Table 5–5)*, the patient is seated at the end of the table with the side of interest nearest the table *(Figure 5–9)*. To assist in immobilization and patient comfort, the elbow and forearm should be resting on the tabletop; the patient's head should be turned away from the central ray during exposure. This general positioning maximizes the distance between the pa-

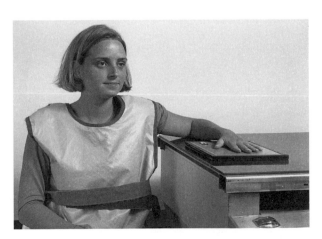

Figure 5–9. Patient correctly prepared for radiography of upper limb.

Table 5–5. Routine and Optional Projections: Upper Limb

Fingers (2nd to 5th)	*Forearm*
PA	AP
Oblique	Lateral
Lateral	*Elbow*
Thumb	AP
AP	Medial (internal) oblique[a]
Oblique	External (lateral) oblique[a]
Lateral	Lateral
Hand	Radial head (axial)[a]
PA	Trauma AP[a]
Oblique	
Lateral	*Humerus*
	AP
Wrist	Lateral
PA	AP neutral position[a]
PA oblique	Transthoracic lateral[a]
AP oblique[a]	
Lateral	
Ulnar/radial flexion[a]	
Carpal canal[a]	

While routine procedures can vary widely from one department to another, this table identifies some of the more common routine and optional projections.

[a]Optional projections; may be routine in some departments.

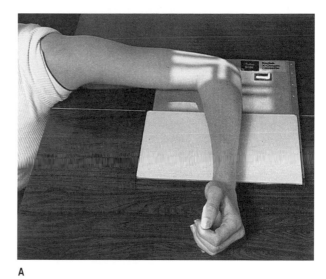

A

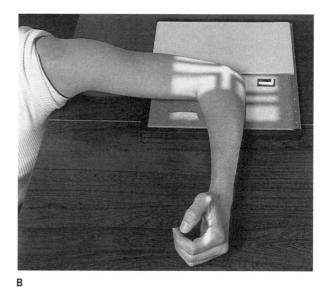

B

tient's head/neck and the central ray, minimizing the dose to the eyes and thyroid. As a habit, gonadal shielding should be used on all patients. Collimation should be seen on all four sides of the film, if permitted by patient and/or structure size. In general, the smallest film size possible should be used for each projection. This makes lengthwise collimation on long bones, other than to film size, often impossible.

Whenever more than one projection is obtained on one film, lead masking should be used to shield the unexposed side of the film from scatter radiation that could detract from the image. The use of lead masking also aids in accurate part centering. When the forearm or elbow is radiographed, two projections are generally taken on one film. Care must be taken to avoid having the patient lean over the unexposed side of the cassette; the part should be positioned so the forearm does not cross over the unexposed part of the cassette *(Figure 5–10)*. The easiest way to avoid this problem is to obtain the lateral projection first, then slide the cassette over for the AP projection. The humerus on each projection will be parallel to the other, and the forearm on the lateral projection will be directed away from the AP projection.

For radiographs of the forearm and elbow, it is important to position the shoulder and elbow on the same plane, perpendicular to the central ray. Normally, this is accomplished by moving the patient's hips forward in the chair and instructing the patient to "slouch" down. This can, however, be very difficult for tall patients. Tall patients may be seated on a footstool that has been covered with a towel. An alternative is to elevate the cassette and arm on a firm level support, adjusting the tube to maintain a 40-in. SID.

Trauma patients may need to be radiographed while in the recumbent position on the table or a stretcher. While patient positioning might be modified, *it is important to obtain two projections 90° apart* for accurate evaluation of potential fractures. It is sometimes easier to use one film per projection, especially when obtaining lateral forearm and elbow projections. Sandbags, sponges, tape, or other radiolucent immobilization devices may be used to prevent movement. Additional projections may be required to adequately demonstrate the anatomic structures. For example, two AP projections of the elbow are required when the patient is unable to extend the elbow completely, as described later in this chapter.

EXPOSURE FACTORS

The kilovoltage used for projections of the upper extremities ranges from 45 to 70 kVp. The appropriate mAs depends on the type of equipment generator, film/screen speed, pathology, and presence or absence of a splint or cast, as discussed in Chapter 4.

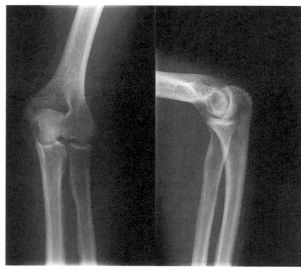

C

Figure 5–10. When positioning the cassette for lateral projections of the elbow and forearm, the arm should be placed on one half of the cassette without crossing over the other half. **(A)** Incorrect positioning. **(B)** Correct positioning. **(C)** Incorrect orientation of the projections.

EQUIPMENT CONSIDERATIONS

When using low kVp, it is possible that tape from lead markers or the plastic covering on some positioning sponges may show up on the finished radiograph. Care should be taken to position the tape on markers away from soft tissue structures and to use appropriate radiolucent supports, when available. The general guidelines for appropriate placement of lead markers can be found in Chapter 1. Radiolucent supports and sandbags should be used for immobilization as long as they do not interfere with anatomy of interest.

The cassette size is determined by part size, number of projections included on one film, department protocol, and availability. Normally, the smallest film that will include all required anatomy is used to minimize costs. Detail, or slow-speed, film/screen combinations are often used for radiographs of small anatomic parts for which the Bucky is not used. Many departments have "detail" cassettes with slower-speed screens in the smaller sizes. Larger parts, such as the lower leg, humerus, and sometimes forearm, are generally radiographed using the department's regular-speed cassettes.

RADIOGRAPHIC POSITIONING OF THE UPPER LIMB (EXTREMITY)

- ▶ PA FINGERS (2ND–5TH DIGITS)

- ▶ OBLIQUE FINGERS (2ND–5TH DIGITS)

- ▶ LATERAL FINGERS (2ND–5TH DIGITS)

- ▶ AP THUMB (1ST DIGIT)

- ▶ OBLIQUE THUMB (1ST DIGIT)

- ▶ LATERAL THUMB (1ST DIGIT)

- ▶ PA HAND

- ▶ PA OBLIQUE HAND

- ▶ LATERAL HAND IN EXTENSION

- ▶ PA WRIST

- ▶ PA OBLIQUE WRIST (SEMIPRONATION)

- ▶ AP OBLIQUE WRIST (SEMISUPINATION)

- ▶ LATERAL WRIST

- ▶ PA WRIST IN ULNAR FLEXION (RADIAL DEVIATION)

- ▶ PA WRIST IN RADIAL FLEXION (ULNAR DEVIATION)

- ▶ TANGENTIAL CARPAL CANAL

- ▶ AP FOREARM

- ▶ LATERAL FOREARM

- ▶ AP ELBOW

- ▶ AP ELBOW IN PARTIAL FLEXION: TWO PROJECTIONS REQUIRED

- ▶ MEDIAL (INTERNAL) OBLIQUE ELBOW

- ▶ LATERAL (EXTERNAL) OBLIQUE ELBOW

- ▶ LATERAL ELBOW

- ▶ AXIAL LATERAL ELBOW

- ▶ AP HUMERUS

- ▶ LATERAL HUMERUS

- ▶ TRANSTHORACIC LATERAL HUMERUS: NEUTRAL POSITION (TRAUMA)

- ▶ AP HUMERUS: NEUTRAL POSITION (TRAUMA)

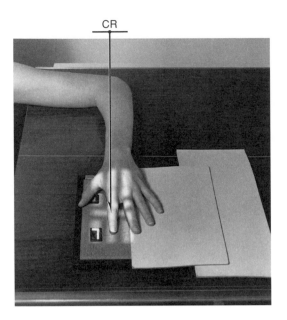

Figure 5–11. PA 2nd digit.

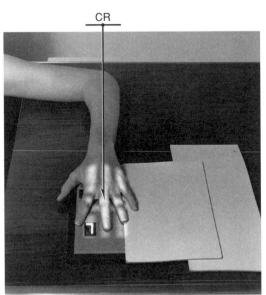

Figure 5–12. PA 3rd digit.

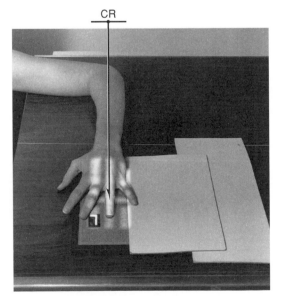

Figure 5–13. PA 4th digit.

▶ PA FINGERS (2ND-5TH DIGITS)

Technical Considerations

- Film size: 8 × 10 in. crosswise or 9 × 9 in. masked in thirds.
- Nongrid, detail cassette if available.
- 45–50 kVp.
- Collimate to soft tissue crosswise and include one third of distal metacarpal.

Shielding

- Gonadal shielding should be used on all patients, especially children and adults of reproductive age.

Patient Positioning

- Assist the patient to a seated position at the end of the radiographic table.
- The patient's side of interest should be nearest the table; the arm should rest comfortably on the table.

Part Positioning

- Pronate the hand and separate the fingers slightly.
- Center the proximal interphalangeal joint of the affected finger to the unmasked third of the cassette with the finger parallel to the long axis of the unmasked portion of the cassette *(Figures 5–11 to 5–14)*.

Central Ray

- Direct the central ray perpendicular to the proximal interphalangeal joint.

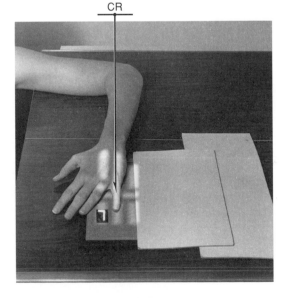

Figure 5–14. PA 5th digit.

Image Evaluation

- Soft tissue structures and one third of the metacarpal should be included in the collimated area.
- The cortex and trabeculae should be visualized and sharp.
- The long axis of the finger should be parallel to the long axis of the unmasked portion of the cassette.
- The interphalangeal and metacarpophalangeal joints should be open and well demonstrated.
- The proximal and middle phalanges should exhibit symmetrical curvatures on the medial and lateral sides (*Figures 5–15 to 5–19*).

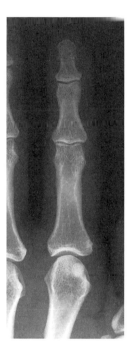

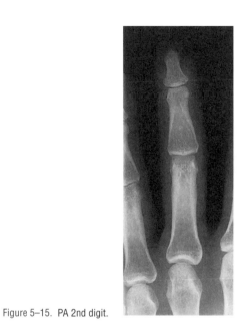

Figure 5–15. PA 2nd digit.

Figure 5–16. PA 3rd digit.

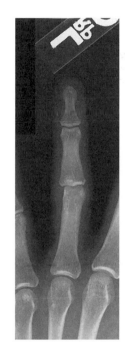

Figure 5–17. PA 4th digit. Note the subluxation at the proximal interphalangeal joint.

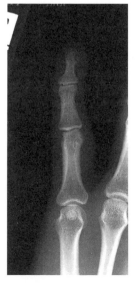

Figure 5–18. PA 5th digit.

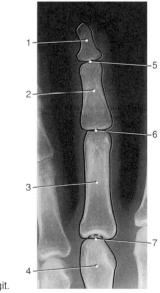

Figure 5–19. PA 3rd digit.

1. Distal phalanx
2. Middle phalanx
3. Proximal phalanx
4. Metacarpal, distal
5. Distal interphalangeal joint
6. Proximal interphalangeal joint
7. Metacarpophalangeal joint

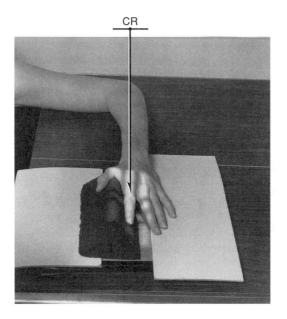

Figure 5–20. Oblique 2nd digit.

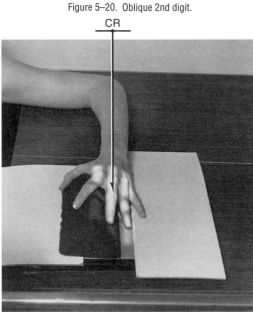

Figure 5–21. Oblique 3rd digit.

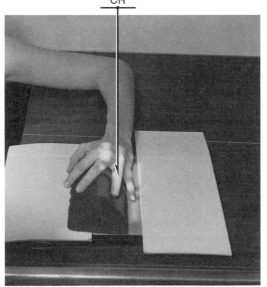

Figure 5–22. Oblique 4th digit.

▶ OBLIQUE FINGERS (2ND-5TH DIGITS)

Technical Considerations

- Film size: 8 × 10 in. crosswise or 9 × 9 in., masked in thirds.
- Nongrid, detail cassette if available.
- 45–50 kVp.
- Collimate to soft tissue crosswise and include one third of distal metacarpal.

Shielding

- Gonadal shielding should be used on all patients, especially children and adults of reproductive age.

Patient Positioning

- Assist the patient to a seated position at the end of the radiographic table.
- The patient's side of interest should be nearest the table; the arm should rest comfortably on the table.

Part Positioning

- Rotate the finger to a 45° angle with the film plane. To demonstrate joint spaces and prevent foreshortening, the finger must be parallel to the film; radiolucent supports can be used to assist with positioning and immobilization *(Figures 5–20 to 5–23)*.
- Center the proximal interphalangeal joint of the affected finger to the unmasked third of the cassette with the finger parallel to the long axis of the unmasked portion of the cassette.

Central Ray

- Direct the central ray perpendicular to the proximal interphalangeal joint.

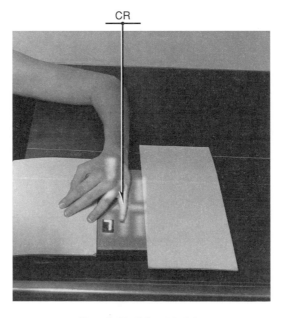

Figure 5–23. Oblique 5th digit.

Image Evaluation

- Soft tissue structures and one third of the metacarpal should be included in the collimated area.
- The cortex and trabeculae should be visualized and sharp.
- The long axis of the finger should be parallel to the long axis of the unmasked portion of the cassette.
- The interphalangeal and metacarpophalangeal joints should be open and well demonstrated.
- The proximal and middle phalanges should be curved on one side and relatively straight on the other side *(Figures 5–24 to 5–28)*.

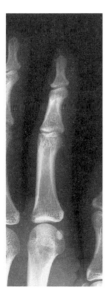

Figure 5–24. Oblique 2nd digit.

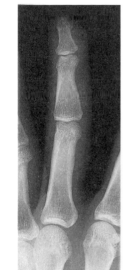

Figure 5–25. Oblique 3rd digit.

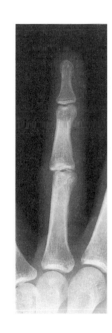

Figure 5–26. Oblique 4th digit. Note the subluxation at the proximal interphalangeal joint. This is the same patient imaged in Figure 5–17.

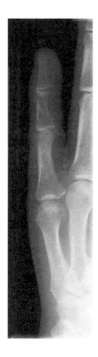

Figure 5–27. Oblique 5th digit.

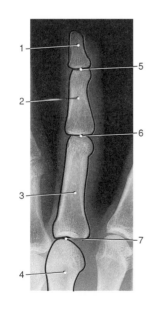

Figure 5–28. Oblique 3rd digit.

1. Distal phalanx
2. Middle phalanx
3. Proximal phalanx
4. Metacarpal, distal
5. Distal interphalangeal joint
6. Proximal (interphalangeal) joint
7. Metacarpophalangeal joint

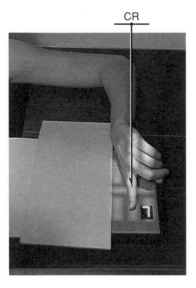

Figure 5–29. Lateral 2nd digit.

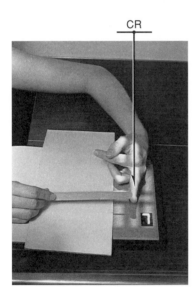

Figure 5–30. Lateral 3rd digit.

► LATERAL FINGERS (2ND–5TH DIGITS)

Technical Considerations

- Film size: 8 × 10 in. crosswise or 9 × 9 in., masked in thirds.
- Nongrid, detail cassette if available.
- 45–50 kVp.
- Collimate to soft tissue crosswise and include one third of distal metacarpal.

Shielding

- Gonadal shielding should be used on all patients, especially children and adults of reproductive age.

Patient Positioning

- Assist the patient to a seated position at the end of the radiographic table.
- The patient's side of interest should be nearest the table; the arm should rest comfortably on the table.

Part Positioning

- Rotate the hand to the lateral position with the affected finger extended and the other fingers flexed or extended out of the way (the thumb can be used to hold unaffected fingers away from the interested finger); to minimize OID while minimizing patient discomfort, the hand should be internally rotated for the 2nd digit and externally rotated for the 3rd through 5th digits (Figures 5–29 to 5–32).
- Center the proximal interphalangeal joint of the affected finger to the unmasked third of the cassette with the finger parallel to the long axis of the unmasked portion of the cassette.

Central Ray

- Direct the central ray perpendicular to the proximal interphalangeal joint.

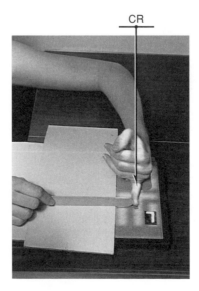

Figure 5–31. Lateral 4th digit.

Figure 5–32. Lateral 5th digit.

Image Evaluation

- Soft tissue structures and one third of the metacarpal should be included in the collimated area.
- The cortex and trabeculae should be visualized and sharp.
- The long axis of the finger should be parallel to the long axis of the unmasked portion of the cassette.
- The interphalangeal joints should be open and well demonstrated.
- The "minicondyles" at the heads and bases of the proximal and middle phalanges should be superimposed; the joint spaces should be open and well delineated.
- The posterior aspect of the phalanges will be straight while the anterior aspect will be slightly concave (*Figures 5–33 to 5–37*).

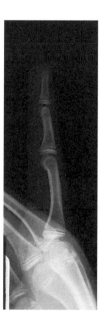

Figure 5–33. Lateral 2nd digit.

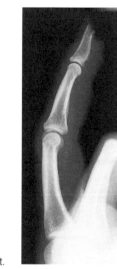

Figure 5–34. Lateral 3rd digit. Note the avulsion of soft tissue and part of the tuft of the distal phalanx.

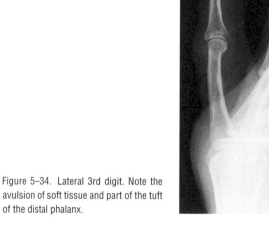

Figure 5–35. Lateral 4th digit. There appears to be a small avulsion (chip) fracture on the posterior aspect of the distal interphalangeal joint.

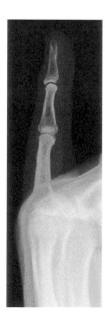

Figure 5–36. Lateral 5th digit.

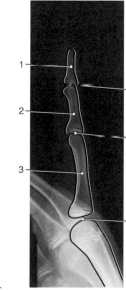

Figure 5–37. Lateral 2nd digit.

1. Distal phalanx
2. Middle phalanx
3. Proximal phalanx
4. Distal interphalangeal joint
5. Proximal interphalangeal joint
6. Metacarpophalangeal joint

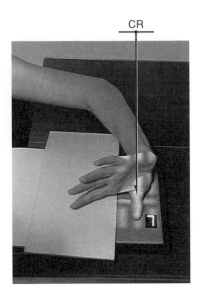

Figure 5–38. AP 1st digit.

► AP THUMB (1ST DIGIT)

Technical Considerations

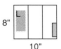

- Film size: 8 × 10 in. crosswise or 9 × 9 in., masked in thirds
- Nongrid, detail cassette if available.
- 45–50 kVp.
- Collimate to soft tissue crosswise and include the trapezium.

Shielding

- Gonadal shielding should be used on all patients, especially children and adults of reproductive age.

Patient Positioning

- Assist the patient to a seated position at the end of the radiographic table.
- The patient's side of interest should be nearest the table; the arm should rest comfortably on the table.

Part Positioning

- Internally rotate the hand and wrist to place the dorsal surface of the thumb on the unmasked third of the cassette; the forearm and elbow will be elevated and the hand will be in somewhat of a reverse lateral position. Care should be taken to ensure that the hand is not superimposed over the thumb.
- Center the metacarpophalangeal joint to the unmasked third of the cassette with the thumb parallel to the long axis of the unmasked portion of the cassette *(Figure 5–38)*.

Central Ray

- Direct the central ray perpendicular to the metacarpophalangeal joint.

Image Evaluation

- Soft tissue structures and the trapezium should be included in the collimated area.
- The cortex and trabeculae should be visualized and sharp.
- The long axis of the thumb should be parallel to the long axis of the unmasked portion of the cassette and the collimation field.
- The interphalangeal and metacarpophalangeal joints should be open and well demonstrated.
- The proximal phalanx should exhibit symmetrical curvatures on the medial and lateral sides *(Figure 5–39)*.

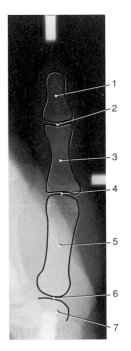

1. Distal phalanx
2. Interphalangeal joint
3. Proximal phalanx
4. Metacarpophalangeal joint
5. Metacarpal
6. 1st carpometacarpal joint
7. Trapezium

Figure 5–39. AP 1st digit.

► OBLIQUE THUMB (1ST DIGIT)

Technical Considerations

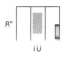

- Film size: 8 × 10 in. crosswise or 9 × 9 in., masked in thirds.
- Nongrid, detail cassette if available.
- 45–50 kVp.
- Collimate to soft tissue crosswise and include the trapezium.

Shielding

- Gonadal shielding should be used on all patients, especially children and adults of reproductive age.

Patient Positioning

- Assist the patient to a seated position at the end of the radiographic table.
- The patient's side of interest should be nearest the table; the arm should rest comfortably on the table.

Part Positioning

- Pronate the hand and separate the thumb from the fingers; the thumb is naturally obliqued when the hand is in a PA position.
- Center the 1st metacarpophalangeal joint to the unmasked third of the cassette with the thumb parallel to the long axis of the unmasked portion of the cassette (Figure 5–40).

Central Ray

- Direct the central ray perpendicular to the 1st metacarpophalangeal joint.

Image Evaluation

- Soft tissue structures and the trapezium should be included in the collimated area.
- The cortex and trabeculae should be visualized and sharp.
- The long axis of the thumb should be parallel to the long axis of the unmasked portion of the cassette and the collimation field.
- The interphalangeal and metacarpophalangeal joints should be open and well demonstrated.
- The medial aspect of the proximal phalanx should be curved while the lateral side should be relatively straight (Figure 5–41).

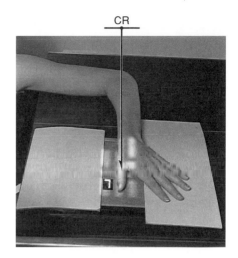

Figure 5–40. Oblique 1st digit.

1. Distal phalanx
2. Interphalangeal joint
3. Proximal phalanx
4. Metacarpophalangeal joint
5. 1st metacarpal
6. 1st carpometacarpal joint
7. Trapezium

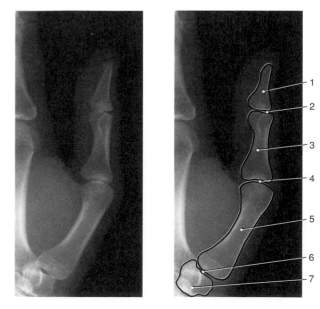

Figure 5–41. Oblique 1st digit.

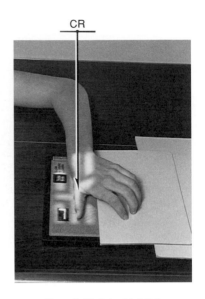

Figure 5–42. Lateral 1st digit.

▶ LATERAL THUMB (1ST DIGIT)

Technical Considerations

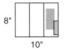

- Film size: 8 × 10 in. crosswise or 9 × 9 in., masked in thirds.
- Nongrid, detail cassette if available.
- 45–50 kVp.
- Collimate to soft tissue crosswise and include the trapezium.

Shielding

- Gonadal shielding should be used on all patients, especially children and adults of reproductive age.

Patient Positioning

- Assist the patient to a seated position at the end of the radiographic table.
- The patient's side of interest should be nearest the table; the arm should rest comfortably on the table.

Part Positioning

- Arch the fingers, placing the fingertips on the cassette; adjust the thumb so it is in a true lateral position. Make sure the hand will not be superimposed over the thumb; instructing the patient to position the hand as if "hitchhiking" often facilitates positioning.
- Center the 1st metacarpophalangeal joint to the unmasked third of the cassette with the thumb parallel to the long axis of the unmasked portion of the cassette *(Figure 5–42)*.

Central Ray

- Direct the central ray perpendicular to the 1st metacarpophalangeal joint.

Image Evaluation

- Soft tissue structures and the trapezium should be included in the collimated area.
- The cortex and trabeculae should be visualized and sharp.
- The long axis of the thumb should be parallel to the long axis of the unmasked portion of the cassette and the collimation field.
- The interphalangeal and metacarpophalangeal joints should be open and well demonstrated.
- The "minicondyles" at the head and base of the proximal phalanx should be superimposed; the joint spaces should be open and well delineated.
- The posterior aspect of the proximal phalanx should be straight, while the anterior side will be concave *(Figure 5–43)*.

Figure 5–43. Lateral 1st digit.

1. Sesamoid bone
2. Distal phalanx
3. Interphalangeal joint
4. Proximal phalanx
5. Metacarpophalangeal joint
6. 1st metacarpal
7. Trapezium

► PA HAND

Technical Considerations

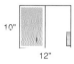

- Film size: 10 × 12 in., masked in half crosswise or 8 × 10 in. lengthwise.
- Nongrid, detail cassette if available.
- 50–55 kVp.
- Collimate to include soft tissue and at least 1 in. of distal radius and ulna; the right/left marker can be included on opposite projection.

Shielding

- Gonadal shielding should be used on all patients, especially children and adults of reproductive age.

Patient Positioning

- Assist the patient to a seated position at the end of the radiographic table.
- The patient's side of interest should be nearest the table; the arm should rest comfortably on the table with the elbow flexed approximately 90°.

Part Positioning

- Pronate the hand and separate the fingers slightly.
- Center the 3rd metacarpophalangeal joint to the unmasked half of the cassette with the hand and distal forearm parallel to the long axis of the unmasked portion of the cassette (Figure 5–44).

Central Ray

- Direct the central ray perpendicular to the 3rd metacarpophalangeal joint.

Image Evaluation

- Soft tissue structures and at least 1 in. of the distal radius and ulna should be included in the collimated area.
- The cortex and trabeculae should be visualized and sharp.
- The long axis of the hand should be parallel to the long axis of the unmasked portion of the cassette.
- The interphalangeal and metacarpophalangeal joints should be open and well demonstrated.
- The metacarpals and phalanges of the 2nd through 5th digits should exhibit symmetrical curvatures on the medial and lateral sides; the thumb will be in the oblique position (Figure 5–45).

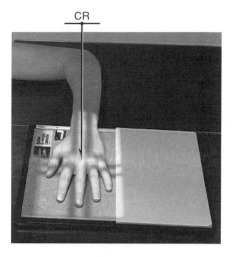

Figure 5–44. PA hand

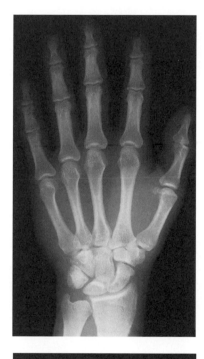

1. Distal phalanx (digits 1–5)
2. Middle phalanx (digits 1–5)
3. Proximal phalanx (digits 1–5)
4. Metacarpal (1–5)
5. Capitate
6. Hamate
7. Triangular
8. Lunate
9. Ulnar styloid process
10. Ulnar head
11. Distal interphalangeal joint (digits 2–5)
12. Proximal interphalangeal joint (digits 2–5)
13. Interphalangeal joint, 1st digit
14. Metacarpophalangeal joint (1–5)
15. Trapezium
16. Trapezoid
17. Scaphoid
18. Radial styloid process
19. Radius

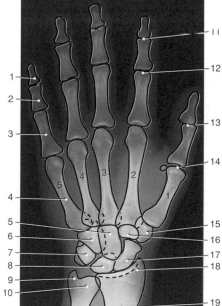

Figure 5–45. PA hand.

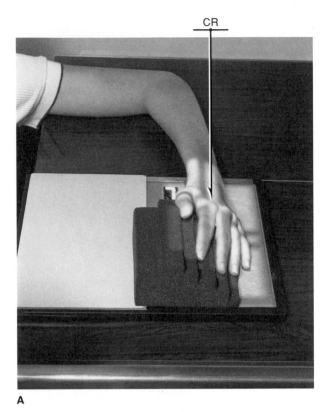

A

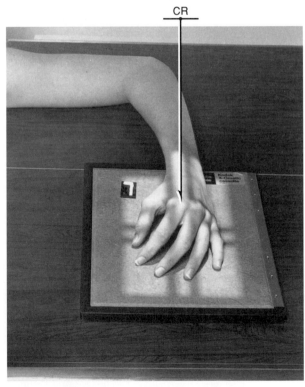

B

Figure 5–46. **(A)** PA oblique hand with fingers parallel with the film plane. **(B)** PA oblique hand with fingers curved and fingertips touching the cassette.

▶ PA OBLIQUE HAND

Technical Considerations

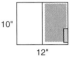

- Film size: 10 × 12 in., masked in half crosswise or 8 × 10 in. lengthwise.
- Nongrid, detail cassette if available.
- 50–60 kVp.
- Collimate to include soft tissue and at least 1 in. of distal radius and ulna.

Shielding

- Gonadal shielding should be used on all patients, especially children and adults of reproductive age.

Patient Positioning

- Assist the patient to a seated position at the end of the radiographic table.
- The patient's side of interest should be nearest the table; the arm should rest comfortably on the table with the elbow flexed approximately 90°.

Part Positioning

- From a pronated position, rotate the hand approximately 45°, elevating the lateral side of the hand (1st, 2nd, and 3rd digits); to prevent foreshortening of the distal phalanges and closure of the interphalangeal joints, the fingers must be parallel to the film plane—a radiolucent support may be used to assist with patient comfort and immobilization *(Figure 5–46A)*. **Note:** If the primary interest is the metacarpals, it may not be necessary to ensure that the fingers are parallel with the film; department protocol should be followed *(Figure 5–46B)*.
- Center the lateral aspect of the 3rd metacarpophalangeal joint to the unmasked half of the cassette with the hand and distal forearm parallel to the long axis of the unmasked portion of the cassette.

Central Ray

- Direct the central ray perpendicular to the lateral aspect of the 3rd metacarpophalangeal joint.

Image Evaluation

- Soft tissue structures and at least 1 in. of the distal radius and ulna should be included in the collimated area.
- The cortex and trabeculae should be visualized and sharp.
- The long axis of the hand should be parallel to the long axis of the unmasked portion of the cassette.
- The interphalangeal and metacarpophalangeal joints should be open and well demonstrated.
- The metacarpals and phalanges of the 2nd through 5th digits should be curved on the lateral aspect and relatively straight on the medial side.
- The heads of the 3rd, 4th, and 5th metacarpals should be slightly superimposed with space between the shafts of these three bones.
- A small space should be seen between the heads of the 2nd and 3rd metacarpals *(Figures 5–47 and 5–48)*.

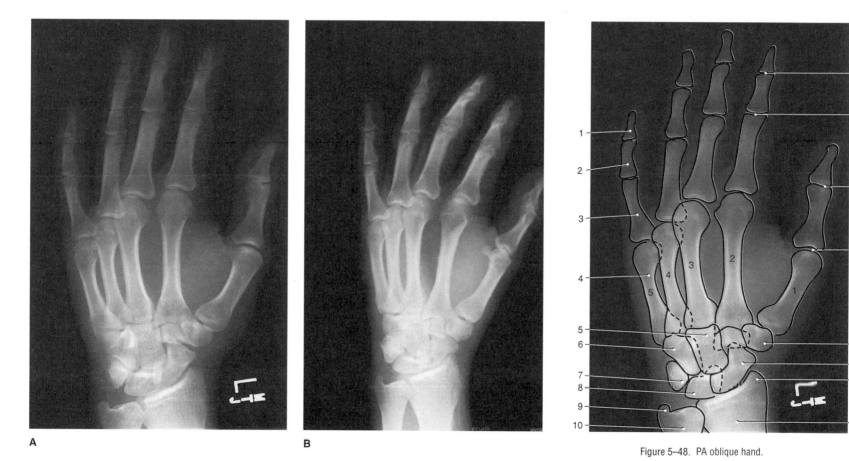

A

B

Figure 5–47. **(A)** PA oblique hand with interphalangeal joints demonstrated. **(B)** PA oblique hand demonstrating foreshortening of phalanges and closure of interphalangeal joints due to curvature of fingers during positioning.

Figure 5–48. PA oblique hand.

1. Distal phalanx (digits 1–5)
2. Middle phalanx (digits 2–5)
3. Proximal phalanx (digits 1–5)
4. Metacarpal (1–5)
5. Capitate
6. Hamate
7. Triquetrum
8. Lunate
9. Ulnar styloid process
10. Ulnar head
11. Distal interphalangeal joint (digits 2–5)
12. Proximal interphalangeal joint (digits 2–5)
13. Interphalangeal joint, 1st digit
14. Metacarpophalangeal joint (1–5)
15. Trapezium
16. Scaphoid
17. Radial styloid process
18. Radius

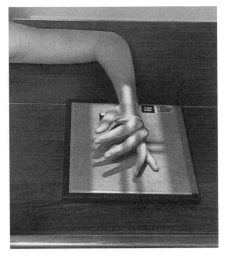

Figure 5–49. Fan lateral hand.

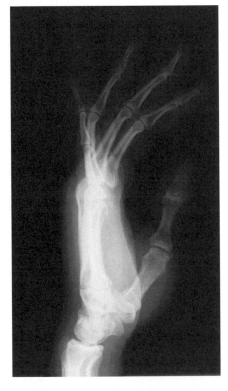

Figure 5–50. Fan lateral hand.

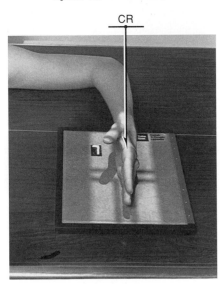

Figure 5–51. Lateral hand in extension.

► LATERAL HAND IN EXTENSION

Technical Considerations

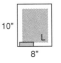

- Film size: 10 × 12 in., masked in half crosswise; 8 × 10 in. lengthwise or 9 × 9 in.
- Nongrid, detail cassette if available.
- 55–60 kVp.
- Collimate to include soft tissue and at least 1 in. of distal radius and ulna.

Shielding

- Gonadal shielding should be used on all patients, especially children and adults of reproductive age.

Patient Positioning

- Assist the patient to a seated position at the end of the radiographic table.
- The patient's side of interest should be nearest the table; the arm should rest comfortably on the table with the elbow flexed 90°.

Part Positioning

- Rotate the hand to a true lateral position with the 5th digit resting on the cassette; the hand should be in line with the forearm and the fingers should be extended. **Note:** The fan lateral hand projection may also be obtained with the fingers separated with the 1st, 2nd, 3rd, and 4th digits slightly flexed and lateral to the film plane; a radiolucent support may be used for immobilization *(Figure 5–49)*. A lateral projection of each digit will be demonstrated while the metacarpals will be superimposed *(Figure 5–50)*.
- The thumb should be positioned anterior to the metacarpals and will be in a PA position; to assist with patient comfort and immobilization, a radiolucent support may be used.
- Center the metacarpophalangeal joints to the cassette, keeping the hand and distal forearm parallel to the long axis of the cassette *(Figure 5–51)*.

Central Ray

- Direct the central ray perpendicular to the metacarpophalangeal joints.

Image Evaluation

- Soft tissue structures and at least 1 in. of the distal radius and ulna should be included in the collimated area.
- The cortex and trabeculae should be visualized and clear.
- The long axis of the hand should be parallel to the long axis of the unmasked portion of the cassette.
- The metacarpals should be superimposed.
- Fingers should be superimposed and straight *(Figure 5–52)*.
- Demonstrates anterior or posterior localization of foreign bodies or displacement of fractured bone.

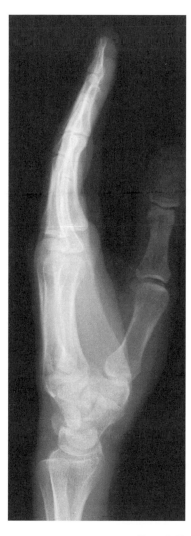
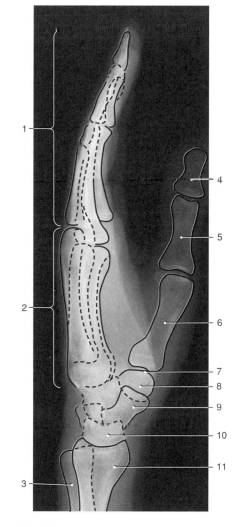

Figure 5–52. Lateral hand in extension.

1. Phalanges, superimposed digits 2–5	4. Distal phalanx, 1st digit	8. Trapezium
	5. Proximal phalanx, 1st digit	9. Scaphoid
2. Metacarpals, superimposed 2–5	6. 1st metacarpal	10. Lunate
3. Ulna	7. 1st metacarpophalangeal joint	11. Radius

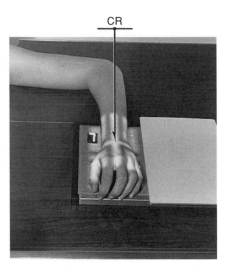

Figure 5–53. PA wrist.

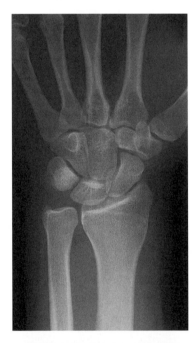

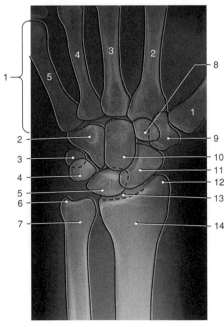

Figure 5–54. PA wrist.

► PA WRIST

Technical Considerations

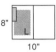

- Film size: 8 × 10 in., masked in half crosswise, or 8 × 10 in. lengthwise; 10 × 12 in., masked in thirds crosswise, or 9 × 9 in.
- Nongrid, detail cassette if available.
- 50–55 kVp.
- Collimate to include soft tissue and at least 2 in. of distal radius and ulna; the right/left marker can be included on the opposite projection.

Shielding

- Gonadal shielding should be used on all patients, especially children and adults of reproductive age.

Patient Positioning

- Assist the patient to a seated position at the end of the radiographic table.
- The patient's side of interest should be nearest the table.
- Rest the patient's arm comfortably on the table with the elbow flexed approximately 90°.

Part Positioning

- Pronate the hand.
- Center the midcarpal region to an unmasked section of the cassette with the forearm parallel to the long axis of the unmasked section of the cassette.
- Arch the hand by resting the fingertips on the cassette; cupping the hand in this manner minimizes OID and distortion of the carpals (Figure 5–53).

Central Ray

- Direct the central ray perpendicular to the midcarpal region.

Image Evaluation

- Soft tissue structures, the metacarpals, and at least 2 in. of the distal radius and ulna should be included in the collimated area.
- The cortex and trabeculae should be visualized and clear.
- The long axis of the forearm should be parallel to the long axis of the unmasked portion of the cassette.
- The capitate, proximal scaphoid, lunate, hamate, and radioulnar joint should be well demonstrated.
- The pisiform will be partially to completely under the triquetrum and the trapezoid will be partially superimposed over the trapezium (Figure 5–54).

1. Metacarpals
2. Hamate
3. Pisiform
4. Triquetrum
5. Lunate
6. Ulnar styloid process
7. Ulna
8. Trapezoid
9. Trapezium
10. Capitate
11. Scaphoid
12. Radial styloid process
13. Radiocarpal joint
14. Radius

► PA OBLIQUE WRIST (SEMIPRONATION)

Technical Considerations

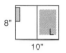

- Film size: 8 × 10 in., masked in half crosswise, or 8 × 10 in. lengthwise; 10 × 12 in., masked in thirds crosswise, or 9 × 9 in.
- Nongrid, detail cassette if available.
- 50–55 kVp.
- Collimate to include soft tissue and at least 2 in. of distal radius and ulna.

Shielding

- Gonadal shielding should be used on all patients, especially children and adults of reproductive age.

Patient Positioning

- Assist the patient to a seated position at the end of the radiographic table.
- The patient's side of interest should be nearest the table.
- Rest the patient's arm comfortably on the table with the elbow flexed approximately 90°.

Part Positioning

- From a pronated position, rotate the hand and wrist approximately 45°, elevating the lateral side of the hand; a small radiolucent support can be positioned under the hand for immobilization.
- Center the midcarpal region, approximately 0.5 in. distal to the radiocarpal joint, to an unmasked section of the cassette with the forearm parallel to the long axis of the unmasked section of the cassette (Figure 5–55).

Central Ray

- Direct the central ray perpendicular through the midcarpal area, approximately 0.5 in. distal to the radioulnar joint.

Image Evaluation

- Soft tissue structures, the metacarpals, and at least 2 in. of the distal radius and ulna should be included in the collimated area.
- The cortex and trabeculae should be visualized and clear.
- The long axis of the forearm should be parallel to the long axis of the unmasked portion of the cassette.
- The trapezoid and trapezium should be separated from each other; the lunate, distal scaphoid, and radiocarpal joint should be well demonstrated (Figure 5–56).

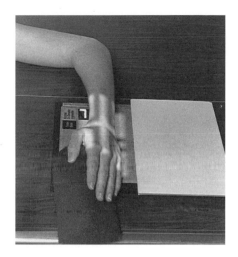

Figure 5–55. PA oblique wrist.

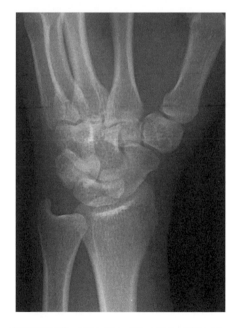

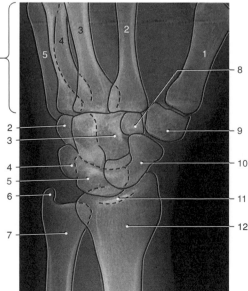

Figure 5–56. PA oblique wrist.

1. Metacarpals	5. Lunate	9. Trapezium
2. Hamate	6. Ulnar styloid process	10. Scaphoid
3. Capitate	7. Ulna	11. Radiocarpal joint
4. Triquetrum	8. Trapezoid	12. Radius

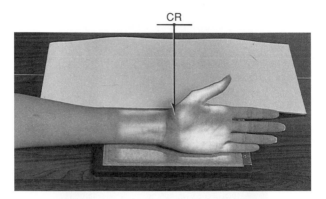

Figure 5–57. AP oblique wrist.

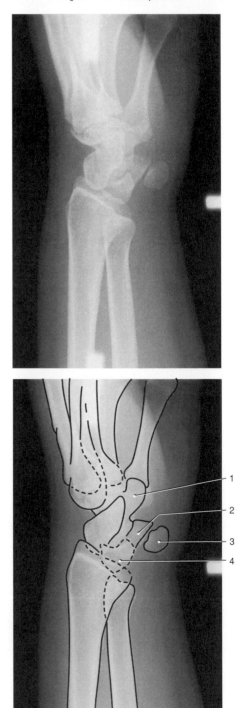

▶ AP OBLIQUE WRIST (SEMISUPINATION)

Technical Considerations

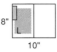

- Film size: 8 × 10 in., masked in half crosswise, or 8 × 10 in. lengthwise; 10 × 12 in., masked in thirds crosswise, or 9 × 9 in.
- Nongrid, detail cassette if available.
- 50–55 kVp.
- Collimate to include soft tissue and at least 2 in. of distal radius and ulna.

Shielding

- Gonadal shielding should be used on all patients, especially children and adults of reproductive age.

Patient Positioning

- Assist the patient to a seated position at the end of the radiographic table.
- The patient's side of interest should be nearest the table.
- Extend the patient's arm, resting it comfortably on the table.

Part Positioning

- From a supinated position, rotate the hand and wrist approximately 45° medially, elevating the lateral side of the hand; a small radiolucent support can be positioned under the hand for immobilization.
- Center the midcarpal region to an unmasked section of the cassette with the forearm parallel to the long axis of the unmasked section of the cassette (Figure 5–57).

Central Ray

- Direct the central ray perpendicular to the midcarpal region.

Image Evaluation

- Soft tissue structures, the metacarpals, and at least 2 in. of the distal radius and ulna should be included in the collimated area.
- The cortex and trabeculae should be visualized and clear.
- The long axis of the forearm should be parallel to the long axis of the unmasked portion of the cassette.
- The pisiform should be separated from the triquetrum (Figure 5–58).

1. Hamate
2. Triquetrum
3. Pisiform
4. Lunate

Figure 5–58. AP oblique wrist.

► LATERAL WRIST

Technical Considerations

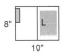

- Film size: 10 × 12 in., masked in half crosswise, 8 × 10 in. lengthwise, or 9 × 9 in.
- Nongrid, detail cassette if available.
- 55–60 kVp.
- Collimate to include soft tissue and at least 2 in. of distal radius and ulna.

Shielding

- Gonadal shielding should be used on all patients, especially children and adults of reproductive age.

Patient Positioning

- Assist the patient to a seated position at the end of the radiographic table.
- The patient's side of interest should be nearest the table; the arm should rest comfortably on the table with the elbow flexed 90°.

Part Positioning

- Rotate the hand to a true lateral position with the 5th digit resting on the cassette; the hand should be in line with the forearm.
- Center the midcarpal region to the cassette, keeping the forearm parallel to the long axis of the cassette *(Figure 5–59)*.

Central Ray

- Direct the central ray perpendicular to the midcarpal region.

Image Evaluation

- Soft tissue structures, the metacarpals, and at least 2 in. of the distal radius and ulna should be included in the collimated area.
- The cortex and trabeculae should be visualized and clear.
- The head of the ulna will be superimposed over the distal radius, while complete superimposition of the radius and ulna decreases proximally.
- The long axis of the forearm should be parallel to the long axis of the unmasked portion of the cassette.
- The carpals and metacarpals should be superimposed *(Figure 5–60)*.

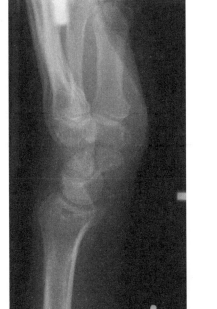

Figure 5–59. Lateral wrist.

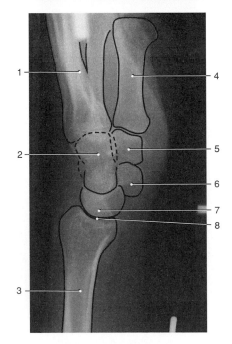

Figure 5–60. Lateral wrist.

1. Metacarpals, superimposed	4. 1st metacarpal	7. Lunate
2. Capitate	5. Trapezium	8. Radiocarpal joint
3. Radius/ulna, superimposed	6. Scaphoid	

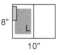
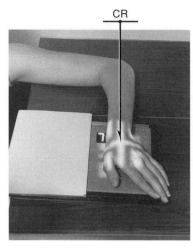

Figure 5–61. PA wrist in ulnar flexion.

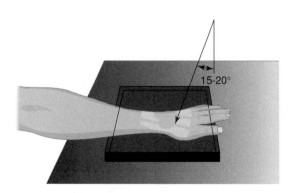

Figure 5–62. PA wrist in ulnar flexion with central ray angulation.

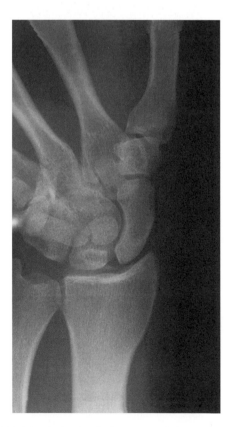

Figure 5–63. PA wrist in ulnar flexion with angulation of the central ray; notice the elongation of the scaphoid bone.

► PA WRIST IN ULNAR FLEXION (RADIAL DEVIATION)

Technical Considerations

- Film size: 8 × 10 in., masked in half crosswise, or 8 × 10 in. lengthwise, or 9 × 9 in.
- Nongrid, detail cassette if available
- 50–55 kVp.
- Collimate to include soft tissue and at least 1 in. of proximal metacarpals and 1 in. of distal radius and ulna.

Shielding

- Gonadal shielding should be used on all patients, especially children and adults of reproductive age.

Patient Positioning

- Assist the patient to a seated position at the end of the radiographic table.
- The patient's side of interest should be nearest the table.
- Rest the patient's arm comfortably on the table with the elbow flexed approximately 90°.

Part Positioning

- Pronate the hand.
- Center the midcarpal region to an unmasked section of the cassette with the forearm parallel to the long axis of the unmasked section of the cassette.
- Keeping the hand pronated, deviate the hand outward in extreme ulnar flexion (Figure 5–61).

Central Ray

- Direct the central ray perpendicular through the scaphoid. **Note:** This projection can also be performed with the central ray directed 15° to 20° toward the forearm; elongation of scaphoid often provides better visualization of fractures (Figures 5–62, 5–63).

Image Evaluation

- Soft tissue structures, the proximal metacarpals, and at least 1 in. of the distal radius and ulna should be included in the collimated area.
- The cortex and trabeculae should be visualized and clear.
- The long axis of the forearm should be parallel to the long axis of the unmasked portion of the cassette.
- The hand should be flexed toward the ulnar side of the forearm *(Figure 5–64)*.
- The carpal bones on the lateral aspect of the wrist, particularly the scaphoid, should be well demonstrated.

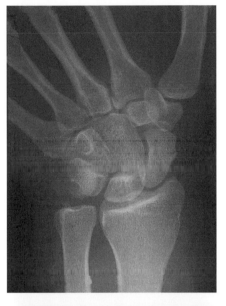

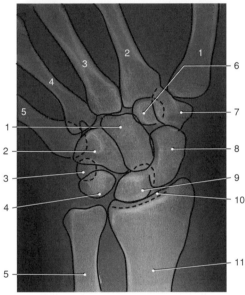

Figure 5–64. PA wrist in ulnar flexion.

1. Capitate	5. Ulna	9. Lunate
2. Hamate	6. Trapezoid	10. Radiocarpal joint
3. Pisiform	7. Trapezium	11. Radius
4. Triquetrum	8. Scaphoid	

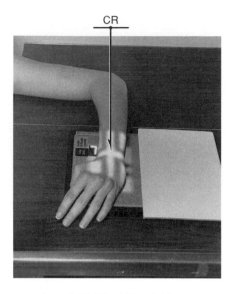

Figure 5–65. PA wrist in radial flexion.

▶ PA WRIST IN RADIAL FLEXION (ULNAR DEVIATION)

Technical Considerations

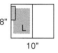

- Film size: 8 × 10 in., masked in half crosswise, or 8 × 10 in. lengthwise, or 9 × 9 in.
- Nongrid, detail cassette if available.
- 50–55 kVp.
- Collimate to include soft tissue and at least 1 in. of proximal metacarpals and 1 in. of distal radius and ulna.

Shielding

- Gonadal shielding should be used on all patients, especially children and adults of reproductive age.

Patient Positioning

- Assist the patient to a seated position at the end of the radiographic table.
- The patient's side of interest should be nearest the table.
- Rest the patient's arm comfortably on the table with the elbow flexed approximately 90°.

Part Positioning

- Pronate the hand.
- Center the midcarpal region to an unmasked section of the cassette with the forearm parallel to the long axis of the unmasked section of the cassette.
- Keeping the hand pronated, deviate the hand inward to extreme radial flexion *(Figure 5–65)*.

Central Ray

- Direct the central ray perpendicular through the midcarpal region.

Image Evaluation

- Soft tissue structures, the proximal metacarpals, and at least 1 in. of the distal radius and ulna should be included in the collimated area.
- The cortex and trabeculae should be visualized and clear.
- The long axis of the forearm should be parallel to the long axis of the unmasked portion of the cassette.
- The hand should be flexed toward the radial side of the forearm *(Figure 5–66)*.
- The carpals on the medial side of the wrist should be well demonstrated.

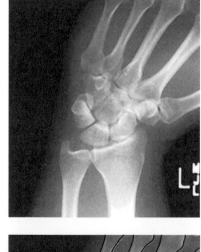

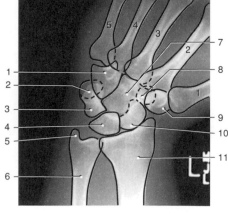

Figure 5–66. PA wrist in radial flexion.

1. Hamate	5. Ulnar styloid process	9. Trapezium
2. Pisiform	6. Ulna	10. Scaphoid
3. Triquetrum	7. Capitate	11. Radius
4. Lunate	8. Trapezoid	

► TANGENTIAL CARPAL CANAL

Technical Considerations

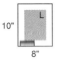

- Film size: 10 × 12 in., masked in half crosswise, 8 × 10 in. lengthwise, or 9 × 9 in.
- Nongrid, detail cassette if available.
- 60–65 kVp.
- Collimate to include soft tissue.

Shielding

- Gonadal shielding should be used on all patients, especially children and adults of reproductive age.

Patient Positioning

- Assist the patient to a seated position at the end of the radiographic table.
- Extend affected arm, resting it on the table.

Part Positioning

- Position the affected arm so it is parallel with the radiographic table.
- Hyperextend the hand and wrist of the affected side; the distal forearm should remain in contact with the cassette. **Note:** This position will be uncomfortable. Set the technical factors and center the cassette and central ray before hyperextending the hand and wrist to minimize the discomfort.
- Using the opposite hand, or a small immobilization band, immobilize the affected hand *(Figure 5–67)*.

Central Ray

- Direct the central ray 25° to 30° toward the long axis of the hand to a point 1 in. distal to the base of the 3rd metacarpal; a greater angle is required when the patient cannot adequately hyperextend the hand and wrist.

Image Evaluation

- Soft tissue structures and anterior aspect of carpal bones should be included in the collimated area.
- The carpal bones will be demonstrated in an arch arrangement *(Figure 5–68)*.

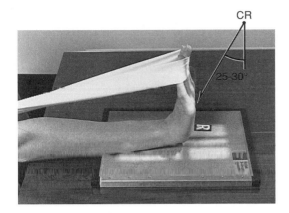

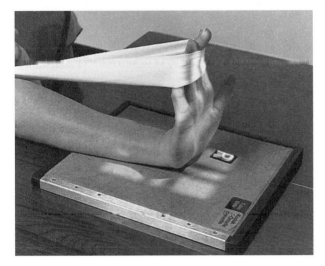

Figure 5–67. Tangential carpal canal.

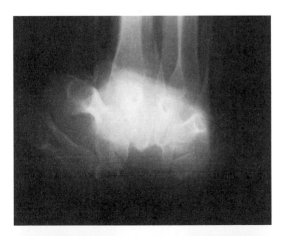

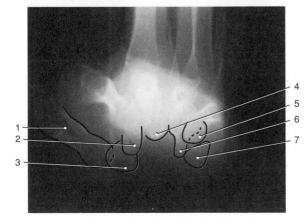

Figure 5–68. Tangential carpal canal.

1. 1st metacarpal	4. Capitate	6. Hamate (hamulus)
2. Scaphoid	5. Triquetrum	7. Pisiform
3. Trapezium		

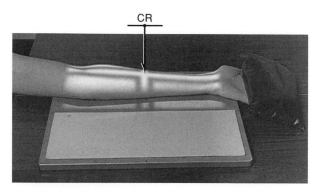

Figure 5–69. AP forearm.

► AP FOREARM

Technical Considerations

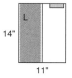

- Film size: 11 × 14 in. or 10 × 12 in., masked in half lengthwise.
- Nongrid, detail cassette if available.
- 60–65 kVp.
- Collimate to include soft tissue, proximal metacarpals, and at least 2 in. of distal humerus.

Shielding

- Gonadal shielding should be used on all patients, especially children and adults of reproductive age.

Patient Positioning

- Assist the patient to a seated position at the end of the radiographic table.
- Extend affected arm, resting it on the table.
- Adjust the patient's position to place the patient's elbow and shoulder on the same plane.

Part Positioning

- Supinate the hand; immobilize by placing a small sandbag over the hand, if necessary.
- Center the midforearm to the unmasked half of the cassette with the arm parallel to the long axis of the cassette *(Figure 5–69)*.

Central Ray

- Direct the central ray perpendicular to the middle of the forearm, midway between the wrist and elbow joints; both joints should be included.

Image Evaluation

- Soft tissue structures, the carpals, proximal metacarpals, and at least 2 in. of the distal humerus should be included in the collimated area.
- The cortex and trabeculae should be visualized and clear.
- The long axis of the forearm should be parallel to the long axis of the cassette.
- The radial tuberosity will be slightly superimposed over the ulna; the shafts of the radius and ulna should be separated.
- The proximal metacarpals should have an equal distance between them.
- The wrist and elbow joints should be well defined without unnecessary superimposition of adjacent bones; space should be seen between the radial head and capitulum.
- No foreshortening or elongation of the radius and ulna should be evident *(Figure 5–70)*.

Figure 5–70. AP forearm.

1. Radial styloid process
2. Radial body (shaft)
3. Radial tuberosity
4. Radial neck
5. Radial head
6. Lateral epicondyle, humerus
7. Distal radioulnar joint
8. Ulnar head
9. Ulnar body (shaft)
10. Olecranon process, ulna
11. Medial epicondyle, humerus

► LATERAL FOREARM

Technical Considerations

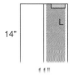

- Film size: 11 × 14 in. or 10 × 12 in. masked in half lengthwise.
- Nongrid, detail cassette if available.
- 60–65 kVp.
- Collimate to include soft tissue, proximal metacarpals, and at least 2 in. of distal humerus.

Shielding

- Gonadal shielding should be used on all patients, especially children and adults of reproductive age.

Patient Positioning

- Assist the patient to a seated position at the end of the radiographic table.
- Extend affected arm, resting it on the table.
- Adjust the patient's position to place the patient's elbow and shoulder on the same plane.

Part Positioning

- Flex the patient's elbow to a 90° angle.
- Adjust the patient's hand to a true lateral position; place a small sandbag anterior to the fingers if necessary for immobilization.
- Center the midforearm to the unmasked half of the cassette with the arm parallel to the long axis of the cassette (Figure 5–71).

Central Ray

- Direct the central ray perpendicular to a point midway between the humeral epicondyles and the radiocarpal joint; adjust the part to film centering, if necessary.

Image Evaluation

- Soft tissue structures, the carpals, proximal metacarpals, and at least 2 in. of the distal humerus should be included in the collimated area.
- The cortex and trabeculae should be visualized and clear.
- The long axis of the forearm should be parallel to the long axis of the cassette.
- The proximal and distal radius and ulna will be somewhat superimposed; the shafts of the radius and ulna will be slightly separated.
- The elbow should be flexed 90° with the humeral epicondyles superimposed; the trochlear notch should be well demonstrated.
- The proximal metacarpals should be superimposed.
- The radial tuberosity should be directed anteriorly.
- No foreshortening or elongation of the radius and ulna should be evident (Figure 5–72).

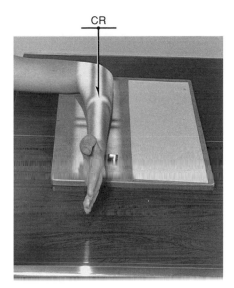

Figure 5–71. Lateral forearm.

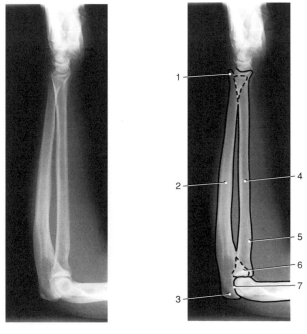

1. Ulnar styloid process
2. Ulnar body (shaft)
3. Olecranon process, ulna
4. Radial body (shaft)
5. Radial tuberosity
6. Radial head
7. Trochlear notch

Figure 5–72. Lateral forearm.

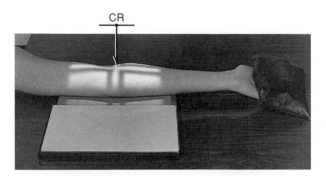

Figure 5–73. AP elbow.

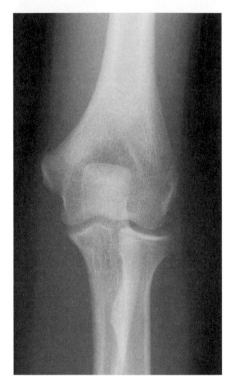

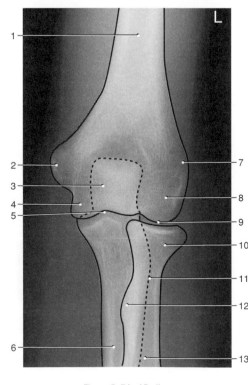

Figure 5–74. AP elbow.

► AP ELBOW

Technical Considerations

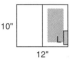

- Film size: 10 × 12 in., masked in half crosswise, or 8 × 10 in. lengthwise.
- Nongrid, detail cassette may be used.
- 60–65 kVp.
- Collimate to include soft tissue, distal humerus, and proximal radius and ulna.

Shielding

- Gonadal shielding should be used on all patients, especially children and adults of reproductive age.

Patient Positioning

- Assist the patient to a seated position at the end of the radiographic table.
- Extend affected arm, resting it on the table.
- Adjust the patient's position to place the patient's elbow and shoulder on the same plane, parallel with the plane of the film.

Part Positioning

- Supinate the hand; immobilize by placing a small sandbag over the hand, if necessary.
- Center the elbow joint to the unmasked half of the cassette with the arm parallel to the long axis of the cassette *(Figure 5–73)*.

Central Ray

- Direct the central ray perpendicular to the elbow joint, found at the crease seen on the antecubital surface.

Image Evaluation

- Soft tissue structures and at least one third of the distal humerus and proximal radius/ulna should be included in the collimated area.
- The cortex and trabeculae should be visualized and clear.
- The long axis of the arm should be parallel to the long axis of the unmasked portion of the cassette.
- The radial tuberosity will be slightly superimposed over the ulna; the olecranon process should extend into the shadow of the olecranon fossa of the distal humerus; the shadow of the olecranon fossa should be symmetrical.
- Space should be seen between the radial head and capitulum.
- No foreshortening of the forearm or humerus should be evident *(Figure 5–74)*.

1. Humerus
2. Medial epicondyle, humerus
3. Olecranon process (ulna) in olecranon fossa (humerus)
4. Medial condyle, humerus
5. Trochlea, humerus
6. Ulna
7. Lateral epicondyle, humerus
8. Lateral condyle, humerus
9. Capitulum, humerus
10. Radial head
11. Radial neck
12. Radial tuberosity
13. Radius

► AP ELBOW IN PARTIAL FLEXION: TWO PROJECTIONS REQUIRED

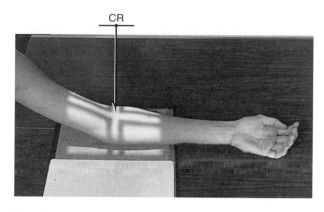

Figure 5–76. AP elbow in partial flexion, demonstrating proximal forearm.

Technical Considerations

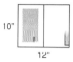

- Film size: 10 × 12 in., masked in half crosswise, or 8 × 10 in. lengthwise.
- Nongrid, detail cassette may be used.
- 60–65 kVp.
- Collimate to include soft tissue, distal humerus, and proximal radius and ulna.

Shielding

- Gonadal shielding should be used on all patients, especially children and adults of reproductive age.

Patient Positioning

- Assist the patient to a seated position at the end of the radiographic table.
- Extend affected arm as much as possible, resting it on the table.
- Adjust the patient's position so the patient's elbow and shoulder are on the same plane.

Part Positioning

Projection 1
- Supinate the hand and support on sandbags.
- Center elbow joint to unmasked half of cassette with humerus parallel to the long axis of the cassette *(Figure 5–75)*.

Projection 2
- Elevate shoulder until forearm is parallel to and resting on cassette; the hand should be supinated.
- Center elbow joint to unmasked half of cassette with the arm parallel to long axis of the cassette *(Figure 5–76)*.

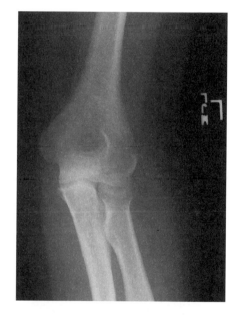

Figure 5–77. AP elbow in partial flexion, demonstrating distal humerus. Note the superimposition of the radial head over the capitulum and the fore-shortening of the olecranon.

Central Ray

- Direct the central ray perpendicular to the elbow joint, found at the crease seen on the antecubital surface.

Image Evaluation

- Soft tissue structures and at least 3 in. of the distal humerus (projection 1) and proximal radius/ulna (projection 2) should be included in the collimated area.
- The cortex and trabeculae should be visualized and clear.
- The long axis of the arm should be parallel to the long axis of the unmasked portion of the cassette.
- The elevated anatomic structures will be foreshortened and not well visualized *(Figures 5–77, 5–78)*.

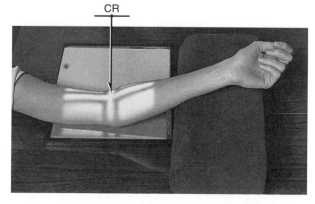

Figure 5–75. AP elbow in partial flexion, demonstrating distal humerus.

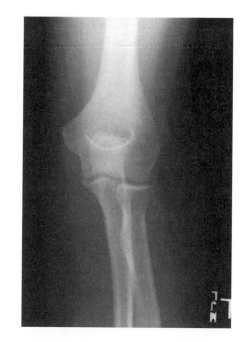

Figure 5–78. AP elbow in partial flexion, demonstrating proximal radius and ulna. Note the distorted appearance of the olecranon fossa.

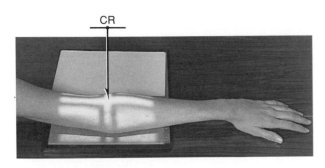
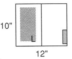

Figure 5–79. Medial oblique elbow.

► MEDIAL (INTERNAL) OBLIQUE ELBOW

Technical Considerations

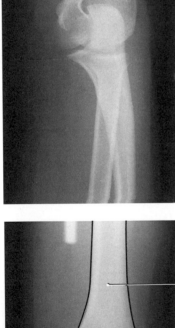

- Film size: 10 × 12 in., masked in half crosswise, or 8 × 10 in. lengthwise.
- Nongrid, detail cassette may be used.
- 60–65 kVp.
- Collimate to include soft tissue, distal humerus, and proximal radius and ulna.

Shielding

- Gonadal shielding should be used on all patients, especially children and adults of reproductive age.

Patient Positioning

- Assist the patient to a seated position at the end of the radiographic table.
- Extend affected arm, resting it on the table.
- Adjust the patient's position so the patient's elbow and shoulder are on the same plane, parallel with the plane of the film.

Part Positioning

- With the arm extended in anatomical position, internally rotate the entire arm 45°; the hand may be pronated to immobilize the arm.
- Check to be sure a line passing between the humeral epicondyles is at a 45° angle with the film plane.
- Center the elbow joint to the unmasked half of the cassette with the arm parallel to the long axis of the cassette *(Figure 5–79)*.

Central Ray

- Direct the central ray perpendicular to the elbow joint, found at the crease on the antecubital surface.

Image Evaluation

- Soft tissue structures and at least one third of the distal humerus and proximal radius/ulna should be included in the collimated area.
- The cortex and trabeculae should be visualized and clear.
- The long axis of the arm should be parallel to the long axis of the unmasked portion of the cassette.
- The coronoid process should be projected free of superimposition and demonstrated in profile *(Figure 5–80)*.

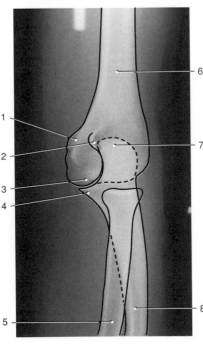

Figure 5–80. Medial oblique elbow.

1. Medial epicondyle, humerus
2. Olecranon fossa, humerus
3. Trochlea, ulna
4. Coronoid process, ulna
5. Radius
6. Humerus
7. Olecranon process, ulna
8. Ulna

► LATERAL (EXTERNAL) OBLIQUE ELBOW

Technical Considerations

- Film size: 10 × 12 in., masked in half crosswise, or 8 × 10 in. lengthwise.
- Nongrid, detail cassette if available.
- 60–65 kVp.
- Collimate to include soft tissue, proximal humerus, and distal radius and ulna.

Shielding

- Gonadal shielding should be used on all patients, especially children and adults of reproductive age.

Patient Positioning

- Assist the patient to a seated position at the end of the radiographic table.
- Extend affected arm, resting it on the table.
- Adjust the patient's position so the patient's elbow and shoulder are on the same plane, parallel with the plane of the film.

Part Positioning

- With the arm extended in anatomic position, externally rotate the entire arm 45°; the patient may have to lean laterally, moving the shoulder and body to achieve this position without undue pain; a sandbag can be used behind the hand to immobilize the arm.
- Check to be sure a line passing between the humeral epicondyles is at a 45° angle with the film plane.
- Center the elbow joint to the unmasked half of the cassette with the arm parallel to the long axis of the cassette *(Figure 5–81)*.

Central Ray

- Direct the central ray perpendicular to the elbow joint, found at the crease seen on the antecubital surface.

Image Evaluation

- Soft tissue structures and at least one third of the distal humerus and proximal radius/ulna should be included in the collimated area.
- The cortex and trabeculae should be visualized and clear.
- The long axis of the arm should be parallel to the long axis of the unmasked portion of the cassette.
- The proximal radioulnar joint should be well demonstrated; the radius and ulna will be completely separated *(Figure 5–82)*.

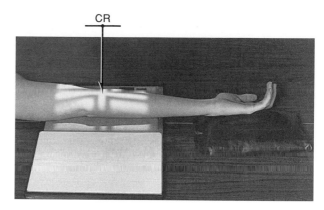

Figure 5–81. Lateral oblique elbow.

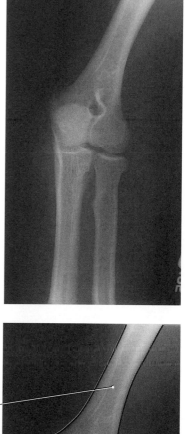

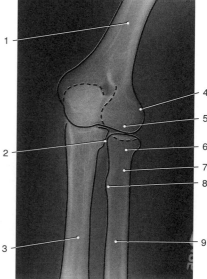

Figure 5–82. Lateral oblique elbow.

1. Humerus	4. Lateral epicondyle, humerus	7. Radial neck
2. Proximal radioulnar joint	5. Capitulum, humerus	8. Radial tuberosity
3. Ulna	6. Radial head	9. Radius

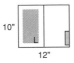

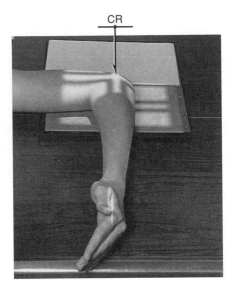

Figure 5–83. Lateral elbow.

► LATERAL ELBOW

Technical Considerations

- Film size: 10 × 12 in., masked in half crosswise, or 8 × 10 in. lengthwise.
- Nongrid, detail cassette if available.
- 60–65 kVp.
- Collimate to include soft tissue, proximal humerus, and distal radius and ulna.

Shielding

- Gonadal shielding should be used on all patients, especially children and adults of reproductive age.

Patient Positioning

- Assist the patient to a seated position at the end of the radiographic table.
- Extend affected arm, resting it on the table.
- Adjust the patient's position so the patient's elbow and shoulder are on the same plane, parallel with the plane of the film.

Part Positioning

- Flex the patient's elbow to a 90° angle.
- Adjust the patient's hand to a true lateral position; place a small sandbag anterior to the hand if necessary for immobilization.
- Center the humeral epicondyles to the unmasked half of the cassette with the humerus parallel to the long axis of the cassette (Figure 5–83).

Central Ray

- Direct the central ray perpendicular to humeral condyles which are located at the elbow joint.

Image Evaluation

- Soft tissue structures and at least one third of the distal humerus and proximal radius/ulna should be included in the collimated area.
- The cortex and trabeculae should be visualized and clear.
- The long axis of the humerus should be parallel to the long axis of the cassette.
- The epicondyles should be superimposed, with the trochlear notch and olecranon process demonstrated free of superimposition.
- The radial head will be mostly superimposed over the coronoid process of the ulna.
- The radial tuberosity will be directed anteriorly (toward the antecubital region), indicating that the hand was in a lateral position (Figure 5–84).

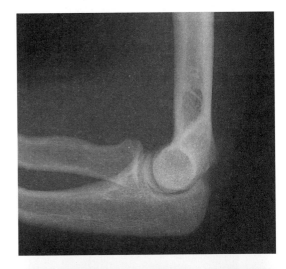

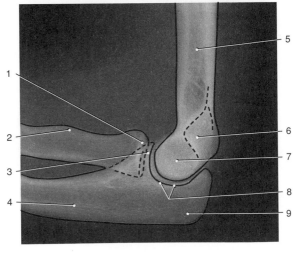

Figure 5–84. Lateral elbow.

1. Radial head
2. Radial tuberosity
3. Coronoid process
4. Ulna

5. Humerus
6. Humeral epicondyles, superimposed

7. Humeral condyles, superimposed
8. Trochlear notch, ulna
9. Olecranon process, ulna

► AXIAL LATERAL ELBOW

Technical Considerations

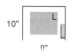

- Film size: 8 × 10 in. lengthwise or 9 × 9 in.
- Nongrid, detail cassette if available.
- 60–65 kVp.
- Collimate to include soft tissue, proximal humerus, and distal radius and ulna.

Shielding

- Gonadal shielding should be used on all patients, especially children and adults of reproductive age.

Patient Positioning

- Assist the patient to a seated position at the end of the radiographic table.
- Extend affected arm, resting it on the table.
- Adjust the patient's position so the patient's elbow and shoulder are on the same plane, parallel with the plane of the film.

Part Positioning

- Flex the patient's elbow to a 90° angle.
- Adjust the patient's hand to a true lateral position; place a small sandbag anterior to the hand if necessary for immobilization.
- Center the humeral epicondyles to the bottom half of the cassette with the humerus parallel to the long axis of the cassette *(Figure 5–85)*.

Central Ray

- Direct the central ray at a 45° angle toward the shoulder through the humeral epicondyles.
- Adjust the centering of the cassette to correspond with the central ray.

Image Evaluation

- Soft tissue structures, the distal humerus, and the proximal radius/ulna should be included in the collimated area.
- The cortex and trabeculae should be visualized and clear.
- The long axis of the humerus should be parallel to the long axis of an 8 × 10-in. cassette.
- The elbow joint should be well demonstrated.
- The radial head and capitulum will be somewhat elongated *(Figure 5–86)*.

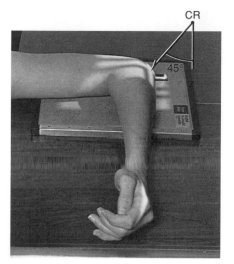

Figure 5–85. Axial lateral elbow.

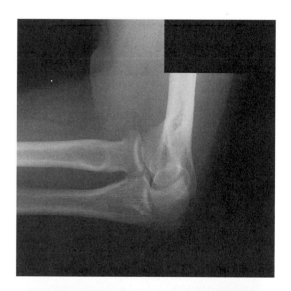

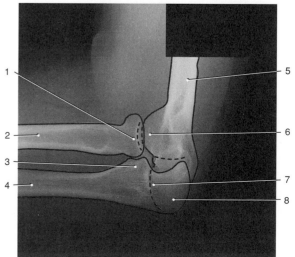

1. Radial head
2. Radius
3. Coronoid process, ulna
4. Ulna
5. Humerus
6. Capitulum, humerus
7. Trochlea, humerus
8. Olecranon process, ulna

Figure 5–86. Axial lateral elbow.

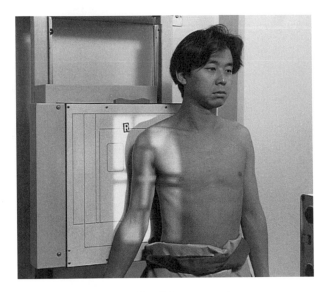

Figure 5–87. AP humerus, erect.

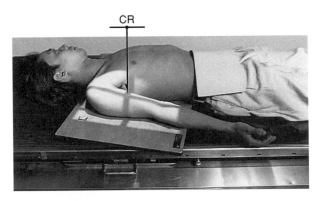

Figure 5–88. AP humerus, recumbent.

▶ AP HUMERUS

Technical Considerations

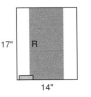

- Film size: 14 × 17 in. or 7 × 17 in. lengthwise.
- Grid recommended; nongrid acceptable for very small adults, children, and mobile radiography.
- 65–70 kVp.
- Collimate to include soft tissue, acromion, glenoid cavity, and 1 in. of proximal forearm.

CAUTION: The arm should not be externally rotated when a fracture is suspected; perform a single projection with the arm in neutral position to rule out fracture, if necessary.

Shielding

- Gonadal shielding should be used on all patients, especially children and adults of reproductive age.

Patient Positioning

- Assist the patient to the supine position on the radiographic table. **Note:** This projection may also be obtained with the patient seated or standing in front of an upright grid device *(Figure 5–87). If a fracture is suspected,* the neutral AP and transthoracic lateral projections should be obtained.
- Extend affected arm as much as possible, resting it on the table.
- Elevate the unaffected side slightly to place the affected arm in contact with the table; a sponge or sandbag may be used to support the patient.
- Adjust the patient's position so the affected arm is parallel with the long axis of the table.

Part Positioning

- Center the arm of interest to the cassette.
- Supinate the hand and adjust the rotation of the arm so the humeral epicondyles lie in the same plane parallel to the film; immobilize with a small sandbag, if necessary; large-breasted women may need to hold the breast out of the way with the opposite hand.
- Without rotating the patient's body, turn the patient's head away from the side of interest *(Figure 5–88).*

Central Ray

- Direct the central ray perpendicular to the midhumerus.
- Center the cassette to the central ray.

Image Evaluation

- Soft tissue structures, the acromion, the glenoid cavity, and at least 1 in. of the proximal forearm should be included in the collimated area.
- The cortex and trabeculae should be visualized and clear.
- The long axis of the arm should be parallel to the long axis of the cassette.
- The greater tubercle (tuberosity) and epicondyles should be seen in profile.
- The head of the humerus will be slightly superimposed over the glenoid cavity (*Figure 5–89*).

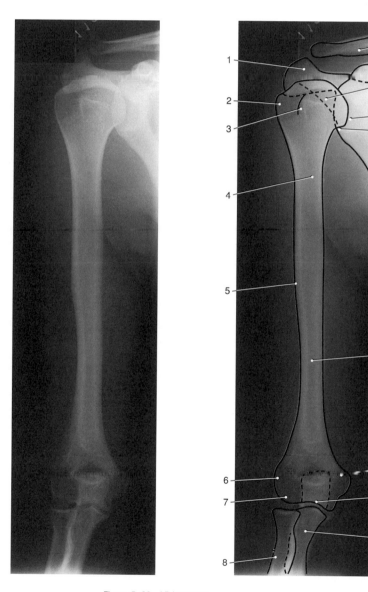

Figure 5–89. AP humerus.

1. Acromion, scapula
2. Greater tubercle
3. Intertubercular groove
4. Surgical neck
5. Deltoid tubercle
6. Lateral epicondyle

7. Capitulum
8. Radius
9. Clavicle
10. Humeral head
11. Glenoid cavity, scapula

12. Anatomical neck
13. Humeral body (shaft)
14. Medial epicondyle
15. Trochlea
16. Ulna

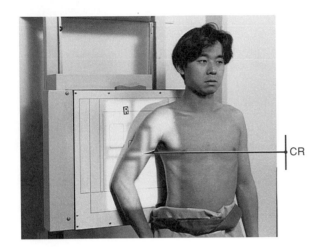

Figure 5–90. Lateral humerus, erect.

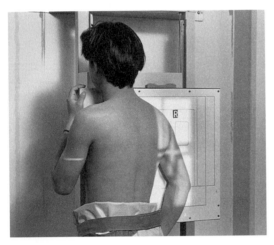

Figure 5–91. Lateral humerus, PA projection.

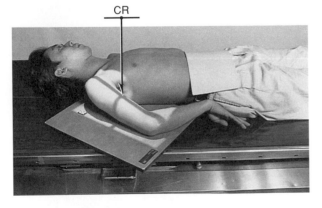

Figure 5–92. Lateral humerus, recumbent.

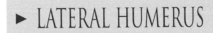

► LATERAL HUMERUS

Technical Considerations

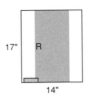

- Film size: 14 × 17 in. or 7 × 17 in. lengthwise.
- Grid recommended; nongrid acceptable for very small adults, children, and mobile radiography.
- 65–70 kVp.
- Collimate to include soft tissue, acromion, glenoid cavity, and 1 in. of proximal forearm.

CAUTION: The arm should not be internally rotated when a fracture is suspected; perform a single projection with the arm in neutral position to rule out fracture, if necessary.

Shielding

- Gonadal shielding should be used on all patients, especially children and adults of reproductive age.

Patient Positioning

- Assist the patient to the supine position on the radiographic table. **Note:** This projection may also be obtained with the patient seated or standing in front of an upright grid device *(Figure 5–90).* A PA lateral projection may also be obtained with the patient facing the upright grid device, minimizing OID *(Figure 5–91). If a fracture is suspected,* the neutral AP and transthoracic lateral projections should be performed.
- Extend affected arm as much as possible, resting it on the table.
- Elevate the unaffected side slightly to place the affected arm in contact with the table; a sponge or sandbag may be used to support the patient.
- Adjust the patient's position so the patient's arm is parallel with the long axis of the table.

Part Positioning

- Center the arm of interest to the table.
- Internally rotate the arm so the dorsal surface of the hand is resting against the patient's side; the elbow may be flexed slightly for comfort.
- Immobilize the hand with a small sandbag; large-breasted women may need to hold the breast out of the way with the opposite hand.
- Without rotating the patient's body, turn the patient's head away from the side of interest *(Figure 5–92).*

Central Ray

- Direct the central ray perpendicular to the midhumerus.
- Center the cassette to the central ray.

Image Evaluation

- Soft tissue structures, the acromion, the glenoid cavity, and at least 1 in. of the proximal forearm should be included in the collimated area.
- The cortex and trabeculae should be visualized and clear.
- The long axis of the arm should be near parallel to the long axis of the cassette.
- The lesser tubercle (tuberosity) should be seen in profile near the glenoid cavity.
- The epicondyles should be almost superimposed with only slight lack of superior–inferior superimposition due to the diverging rays.
- The head of the humerus will be slightly superimposed over the glenoid cavity *(Figure 5–93)*.

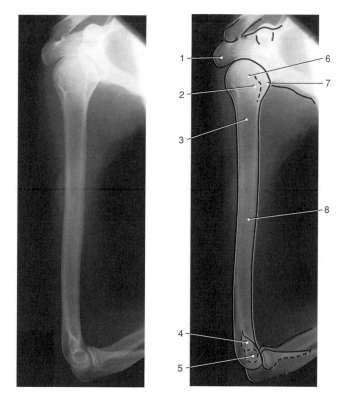

Figure 5–93. Lateral humerus.

1. Acromion, scapula
2. Greater tubercle
3. Surgical neck

4. Epicondyles, superimposed
5. Condyles, superimposed
6. Humeral head

7. Lesser tubercle
8. Humeral body (shaft)

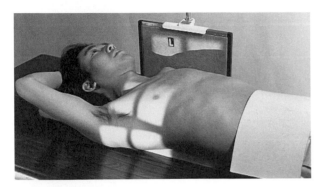

Figure 5–94. Transthoracic lateral humerus with patient supine, using horizontal beam.

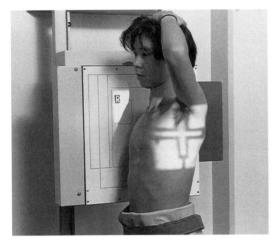

Figure 5–95. Transthoracic lateral humerus, arm in neutral position.

▶ TRANSTHORACIC LATERAL HUMERUS: NEUTRAL POSITION (TRAUMA)

Technical Considerations

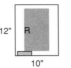

- Film size: 10 × 12 in. or 11 × 14 in. lengthwise.
- Grid recommended; nongrid acceptable for very small adults, children, and mobile radiography.
- 70–80 kVp.
- Collimate to include acromion, glenoid cavity, and elbow joint.

Shielding

- Gonadal shielding should be used on all patients, especially children and adults of reproductive age.

Patient Positioning

- Assist the patient to the standing or seated position with the side of interest nearest the upright grid device. **Note:** This projection may also be obtained with the patient supine on the radiographic table by using a horizontal beam *(Figure 5–94)*. Shoulder and arm injuries may be extremely painful. When possible, the upright position permits the weight of the arm to act as traction, generally providing more comfort to the patient when a fracture is present.
- If standing, the patient's feet should be separated slightly with weight equally distributed on both feet.
- Center the affected arm to the midline of the upright grid device.

Part Positioning

- Suspend the affected arm at the patient's side; for comfort, the elbow may be flexed with the forearm supported by a sling.
- Elevate the patient's unaffected arm and rest the forearm on the patient's head; the affected shoulder should be depressed slightly to assist in separating the shoulders.
- Adjust the rotation of the patient's body to place the humerus midway between the spine and the sternum *(Figure 5–95)*.

Central Ray

- Direct the central ray perpendicular to the surgical neck of the humerus.
- Center the cassette to the central ray; the top of the cassette should be 1.5 to 2 in. above the top of the affected shoulder.

Breathing Instructions

- Instruct the patient to breathe normally or take slow, deep breaths; using a long exposure time of 2 to 5 seconds helps blur lung detail, providing a better view of the humerus.
- Or instruct the patient to take in a deep breath and hold the breath in; suspended deep inspiration enhances the contrast between the lung and bone.

Image Evaluation

- Head and neck of the humerus, the acromion process, the glenoid cavity, and proximal two thirds of the humeral shaft should be included in the collimated area.
- The cortex should be clearly visualized.
- The long axis of the arm should be parallel to the long axis of the cassette.
- The humerus should be demonstrated between the spine and sternum without superimposition.
- This projection should be 90° rotation from the neutral AP projection *(Figure 5–96)*.

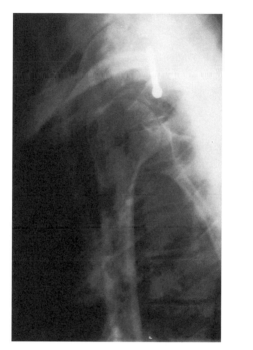 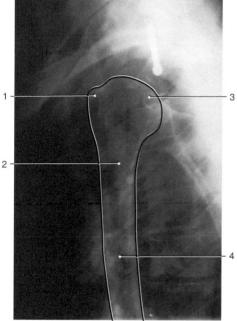

Figure 5–96. Transthoracic lateral humerus, arm in neutral position.

1. Greater tubercle
2. Surgical neck

3. Humeral head

4. Humeral body (shaft), proximal

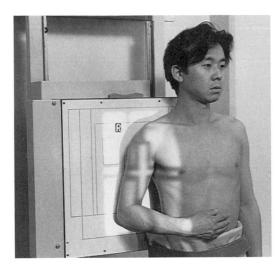

Figure 5–97. AP humerus, arm in neutral position.

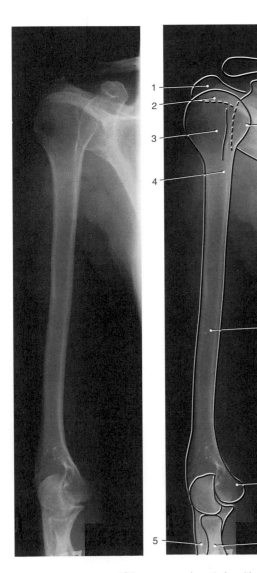

Figure 5–98. AP humerus, arm in neutral position.

▶ AP HUMERUS: NEUTRAL POSITION (TRAUMA)

Technical Considerations

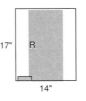

- Film size: 14 × 17 in. or 7 × 17 in. lengthwise.
- Grid recommended; nongrid acceptable for very small adults, children, and mobile radiography.
- 65–70 kVp.
- Collimate to include soft tissue, acromion, glenoid cavity, and elbow joint.

Shielding

- Gonadal shielding should be used on all patients, especially children and adults of reproductive age.

Patient Positioning

- Assist the patient to the seated or standing position in front of an upright grid device. **Note:** This projection may also be obtained with the patient supine on the radiographic table. Shoulder and arm injuries may be extremely painful. The upright position permits the weight of the arm to act as traction, generally providing more comfort to the patient when a fracture is present.
- Rotate the patient slightly toward the side of interest to bring the affected arm in contact with the upright grid device.
- Center the affected arm to the midline of the upright grid device.

Part Positioning

- Suspend the affected arm at the patient's side; for comfort, the elbow may be flexed with the forearm supported by the opposite hand or a sling.
- Without rotating the patient's body, turn the patient's head away from the side of interest (*Figure 5–97*).

Central Ray

- Direct the central ray perpendicular to the midhumerus.
- Center the cassette to the central ray.

Image Evaluation

- Soft tissue structures, the acromion, the glenoid cavity, and at least 1 in. of the proximal forearm should be included in the collimated area.
- The cortex and trabeculae should be visualized and clear.
- The long axis of the arm should be parallel to the long axis of the cassette.
- The greater tubercle will be superimposed over the head of the humerus (*Figure 5–98*).

1. Acromion, scapula
2. Humeral head
3. Greater tubercle
4. Surgical neck

5. Ulna
6. Coracoid process, scapula
7. Lesser tubercle

8. Humeral body (shaft)
9. Medial epicondyle
10. Radius

SUMMARY

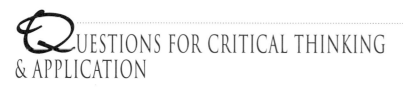

▸ For lateral projections of the forearm and elbow, the patient's shoulder and elbow must be on the same horizontal plane.

▸ In all radiographic examinations of the upper limb, at least two projections must be taken, 90° apart from each other.

▸ Radiographic examinations of the joints generally require a minimum of three projections: AP/PA, lateral, and at least one oblique.

▸ Kilovoltages for imaging of the upper limb range from 45 to 70 kVp.

▸ Detail, or slow-speed, film/screen combinations are preferred for small, bony structures.

▸ To prevent foreshortening or elongation, the central ray should be directed perpendicular to long bones.

▸ Anatomic structures should be aligned parallel to the long axis of the cassette.

▸ When radiographing long bones, both joints should be included in the collimation field.

▸ Rotation of the arm is contraindicated when a humeral fracture or shoulder dislocation is suspected.

▸ The use of a breathing technique when obtaining a transthoracic lateral projection blurs the lung detail, allowing for better visualization of the cortex of the humerus.

QUESTIONS FOR CRITICAL THINKING & APPLICATION

1. Describe the growth process of bones as it relates to the radius and ulna. In your discussion, describe the location of the epiphyses, metaphyses, and diaphysis of each bone.

2. In the narrative, the surgical neck of the humerus was described as an area susceptible to fractures. Why do you suppose this is a weak area of the bone? What is the strongest part of this bone? Relate your reasons to the anatomic structure of the humerus.

3. Your patient is a 25-year-old man who had been involved in a fight. He states that his right arm has been twisted and he is not unable to straighten his elbow completely. He has a big "bump" on the anterior surface of his elbow. What type of injury or pathology has the patient sustained? What projection(s) of the elbow best demonstrates this problem? What bones and/or structures are involved in the injury?

4. Develop a chart that summarizes the surface markings of the bones of the upper limb.

5. A young man came to the radiology department for an examination of his hand. According to his history, he was cleaning his BB gun when it accidentally discharged in his hand. Identify and describe the projections you would use to localize a foreign object in the hand. What do you expect the foreign object to look like? What projection will demonstrate anterior or posterior localization of the foreign object?

6. A 40-year-old man fell from a ladder injuring his elbow. He is in extreme pain, unable to fully extend his elbow, and is somewhat uncooperative. Describe the procedure you would follow to complete the radiographic examination to include necessary projections, methods of obtaining patient compliance to obtain the projections needed, the film/screen combination to be used, immobilization techniques, and optimum technical factors.

7. A patient was admitted to the emergency room with a fractured wrist. Following reduction of the fracture, the physician requests postreduction films. Which projections would you take? What type of film/screen combination would you select?

8. Following radiographic examination of the wrist, the radiologist suspects a scaphoid fracture. Describe the projection(s) you could obtain to adequately demonstrate a possible fracture of the scaphoid.

9. A patient has come to the department for radiographic examination of the humerus. When you identify the patient, you discover the patient's arm is in a sling. Describe the patient preparation and projections you would obtain for this examination.

10. Describe the two breathing techniques that can be used for a transthoracic lateral humerus and identify the one you feel will produce a better-quality radiograph. Justify your answer.

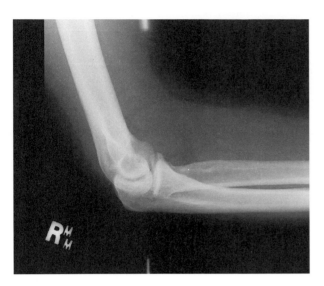

Figure 5–99.

FILM CRITIQUE

Describe the positioning and centering accuracy of the lateral elbow projection shown *(Figure 5–99)*. Is the part correctly positioned?

What criteria did you use to evaluate positioning accuracy?

Was the part correctly centered to the film?

Was the central ray correctly centered to the part and film?

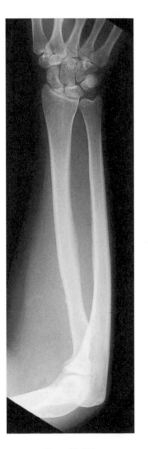

Figure 5–100.

Name this projection *(Figure 5–100)*. How was the patient positioned?

Was patient positioning accurate?

What criteria did you use to determine positioning accuracy or error?

6

SHOULDER GIRDLE

▶ OBJECTIVES

Following the completion of this chapter the student will be able to:

- Given diagrams, radiographs, or dry bones, name and describe the bones of the shoulder girdle, to include the scapula, clavicle, and proximal humerus.

- Describe the relationship of the structures on the shoulder girdle (ie, the coracoid process is anterior and medial to the glenoid cavity).

- Classify the articulations of the shoulder girdle and identify their type of movement.

- Describe patient positioning, equipment considerations, and exposure factors relative to radiography of the shoulder girdle.

- Describe procedural modifications for patients suspected of having a humeral fracture.

- Evaluate radiographs of the shoulder girdle in terms of positioning, accuracy, centering, image quality, radiographic anatomy, and pathology.

- Define terminology associated with the shoulder girdle, to include anatomy, procedures, and pathology.

- Identify the reason(s) for radiographing the acromioclavicular joints in the erect position and taking radiographs with and without weights.

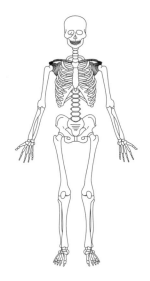

Figure 6–1. The shoulder girdle.

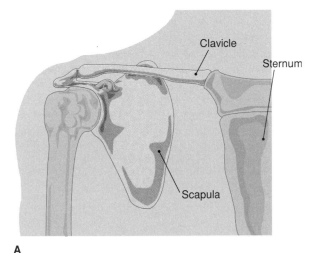

A

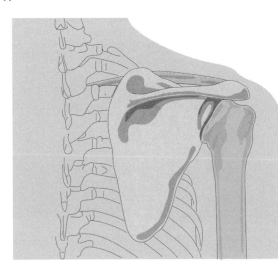

B

Figure 6–2. Bones of the shoulder girdle: **(A)** anterior view, **(B)** posterior view.

► ANATOMY OF THE SHOULDER GIRDLE

Each of the two shoulder girdles is formed by a clavicle and scapula *(Figure 6–1, Table 6–1)*. Together, these bones function to attach the upper limb to the axial skeleton. The term *girdle* is somewhat misleading, however, as it implies that the bones wrap completely around and provide support. As the only direct articulations between the shoulder girdles and the axial skeleton occur at the sternoclavicular joints, the shoulder girdles are somewhat weak. They rely on muscles for support and stability *(Figure 6–2)*.

CLAVICLE

The clavicle (KLAV-i-kal) or collarbone is situated over the anterior aspect of the upper trunk and can be seen and felt just below the skin. It is a slender, long bone which is so classified because it has a shaft and two articular ends. The **sternal** (STER-nal) **end** or **extremity** is found at the medial end of the bone. This area is roughly triangular in shape and articulates with the manubrium of the sternum to form the sternoclavicular joint. The lateral end of the clavicle is the **acromial** (ah-KRŌ-mē-al) **end** or **extremity.** It is broad, flat, and larger than the sternal end. It articulates with the acromion of the scapula to form the acromioclavicular joint.

The **shaft** or body of the clavicle is the central portion of the bone, or that area between the sternal and acromial extremities. It has a double curvature on it as it extends laterally and posteriorly from the sternal to the acromial end. The medial two thirds of the clavicle is convex forward, whereas the lateral third of the bone is concave forward.

A prominence located on the posterior aspect of the inferior surface of the clavicle is known as the **conoid** (KO-noid) **tubercle.** It projects over the coracoid process of the scapula and serves as an attachment site for the coracoclavicular ligament *(Figure 6–3)*.

The radiographer may notice a slight difference in shape between the clavicles of male and female patients. On males, the clavicles are usually longer and more curved. This is because the clavicles act as braces for the shoulders. The more muscular a person is, the more curved the clavicles become to render them stronger. The position of the each clavicle limits movement of the shoulder girdle, which aids in preventing a dislocation of the shoulder. Because the clavicle is located rather superficially, it is susceptible to fractures, particularly as the result of falls or contact sports.

SCAPULA

The scapula (SKAP-ū-lah) is a triangular bone commonly known as the shoulder blade. It lies against the rib cage, but does not directly articulate with the axial skeleton. Instead, it is fairly mobile because of the presence of many muscles in the shoulder girdle. There are two scapulae (SKAP-ū-lē), which are situated on either side of the posterior bony thorax between the second and the seventh ribs.

Each scapula has three borders, three angles, and two surfaces. The lateral border is adjacent to the patient's axilla or armpit, and is sometimes referred to as the axillary border. The medial or vertebral border is the margin of the scapula closest to and parallel with the vertebral column. It is vertical and lies approximately 2 to 3 in. lateral to the spine. The superior border is the short, upper margin of the scapula. The area between the borders is the body or ala (wing) of the scapula *(Figure 6–4)*.

Table 6–1. Summary of the Bones of the Shoulder Girdle

Bones for Each Shoulder Girdle	Description
Clavicle	• Collarbone • Long bone • Sternal and acromial articular ends • Double curvature • Conoid tubercle
Scapula	• Shoulder blade • Triangular • Flat bone • 3 borders, 3 angles, and 2 surfaces • Acromion, coronoid process, and glenoid cavity

The angles of the scapula are corners formed by the junctions of the borders. The inferior angle is the most inferior point or tip of the scapula. It is a sharp angle where the lateral and medial borders meet. The superior angle is formed by the junction of the superior and medial borders. The superior and lateral borders join to form the lateral angle. This is the thickest part of the scapula and is also referred to as the head. Although the heads of bones are typically rounded, this area on the scapula is blunt and concave. The shallow, oval concavity on the head is referred to as the glenoid cavity or fossa. It articulates with the head of the humerus to form the glenohumeral (shoulder) joint. Just medial to the head of the scapula is a slight constriction known as the neck *(Figure 6–5)*.

The two surfaces of the scapula are the ventral and dorsal surfaces. The ventral or anterior surface of the scapula is also known as the costal surface because it is adjacent to the rib cage *(Figure 6–6)*. This surface is slightly concave to add strength to the scapula.

The spine of the scapula is a sharp ridge of bone that projects from the dorsal or posterior surface of the scapula. Beginning on the medial border approximately one third of the way down, the spine passes transversely to the lateral border. At this point, it becomes larger and flatter to extend off of the scapula. This extension or process is called the **acromion** (ah-KRO-mē-on). As a continuation of the spine, it projects laterally to extend over the shoulder joint. It articulates with the lateral end of the clavicle to form the acromioclavicular joint.

There are three depressions on the body of the scapula which are named according to their location. A concavity in the middle of the body on the ventral surface is called the **subscapular** (sub-SKAP-ū-lar) **fossa.** On the dorsal surface, there are two shallow depressions situated above and below the spine. They are known respectively as the **supraspinous** (soo-prah-SPĪ-nus) and **infraspinous** (in-frah-SPĪ-nus) **fossae.** These fossae are the sites of muscle attachments.

The **coracoid process** is a fingerlike or beaklike projection that arises from the superior border of the scapula. Located just medial to the glenoid cavity, it projects anteriorly and can be palpated beneath the clavicle. The coracoclavicular ligament attaches the coracoid process of the scapula to the conoid tubercle of the clavicle. The **scapular notch** is found at the base of the coracoid process on its medial side. Therefore, the coracoid process is located between the glenoid cavity and the scapular notch *(Figure 6–7)*.

When viewed from a lateral perspective, the scapula resembles the letter "Y," with the acromion and coracoid process forming the upper extensions and the body forming the lower vertical portion of the "Y." A lateral projection of the scapula can be helpful in the evaluation of shoulder dislocations. The head of the humerus is normally situated against the glenoid cavity; however, an anterior dislocation will demonstrate the head under the coracoid process, while a posterior dislocation shows it under the acromion *(Figure 6–8)*.

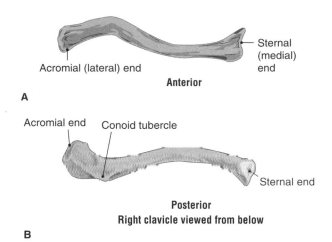

Anterior

A

Acromial (lateral) end

Sternal (medial) end

Acromial end   Conoid tubercle

Sternal end

Posterior
Right clavicle viewed from below

B

Figure 6–3. Clavicle: **(A)** anterior view, **(B)** posterior view.

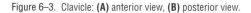

Borders

Superior border

Lateral border

Medial border

Right scapula, anterior aspect

Figure 6–4. Borders of the scapula demonstrated on an anterior view.

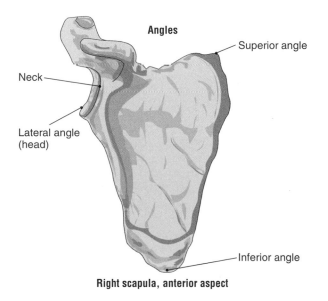

Angles

Superior angle

Neck

Lateral angle
(head)

Inferior angle

Right scapula, anterior aspect

Figure 6–5. Angles of the scapula demonstrated on an anterior view.

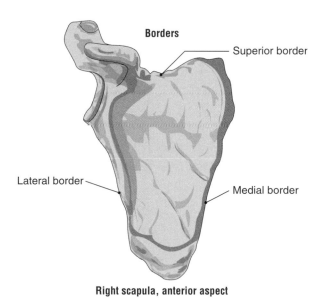

Surfaces

Dorsal (posterior)
surface

Ventral (anterior or
costal) surface

Right scapula, lateral aspect

Figure 6–6. Surfaces of the scapula demonstrated on a lateral view.

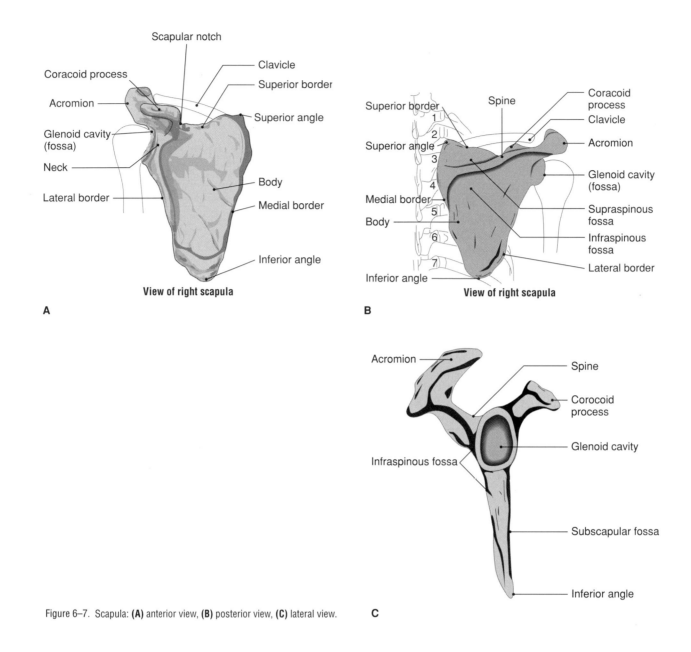

Figure 6–7. Scapula: **(A)** anterior view, **(B)** posterior view, **(C)** lateral view.

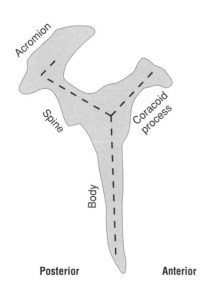

Figure 6–8. A lateral scapula resembles the letter "Y."

ARTHROLOGY

The bones of the shoulder girdle are involved in the formation of three pairs of joints: right and left sternoclavicular, acromioclavicular, and shoulder joints. All of these joints are synovial in structure.

The only articulation between the bones of the shoulder girdle occurs at each **acromioclavicular joint.** This joint is formed by the acromion of the scapula and the acromial or lateral end of the clavicle. It is a diarthrodial joint with gliding movement. A direct blow to this joint can result in a separation injury.

The clavicle articulates with the axial skeleton at the **sternoclavicular joint.** The sternal end of the clavicle forms a joint with the manubrium or upper portion of the sternum. This is also a diarthrodial joint with gliding movement.

The shoulder joint is formed by the articulation of the glenoid cavity of the scapula with the head of the humerus. Thus, the anatomic name for this joint is the **glenohumeral joint.** It is a diarthrodial joint with ball-and-socket type of movement (head of humerus = ball, glenoid cavity = socket). Because the glenoid cavity is so shallow, the shoulder joint has a wide range of motion but is relatively unstable, causing it to dislocate easily on a direct blow *(Figure 6–9).*

Table 6–2 summarizes the joints of the shoulder girdle.

Table 6–2. Summary of Joints of the Shoulder Girdle

Name of Joint	Classification	Structure	Movement Type
Sternoclavicular	Diarthrodial	Synovial	Gliding
Acromioclavicular	Diarthrodial	Synovial	Gliding
Glenohumeral (shoulder)	Diarthrodial	Synovial	Ball-and-socket

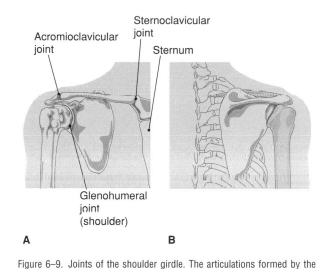

A   **B**

Figure 6–9. Joints of the shoulder girdle. The articulations formed by the bones of the shoulder girdle are illustrated on **(A)** anterior and **(B)** posterior views.

► PROCEDURAL CONSIDERATIONS

The shoulder joint, clavicle, scapula, and acromioclavicular joints of the shoulder girdle may all be radiographed to evaluate injury or pain of unknown origin. Because of proximity with the bony thorax, patient rotation and/or central ray angulation may be necessary to demonstrate some of the anatomy free of superimposition. Even with these technical manipulations, it is impossible to demonstrate the entire AP scapula without some superimposition of the thorax and lungs.

PATIENT PREPARATION

Following identification of the patient, the patient should be instructed to remove all clothing and jewelry from the waist up, including any dangling earrings. If the patient's arm is in a sling, the sling should not be removed without prior approval from a physician. Rotational movement of the arm, as done for nontraumatic examinations, could cause fracture fragments to move and damage nerves, vessels, and/or soft tissue. The projections performed to demonstrate the shoulder joint depend on the reason for examination; it is the radiographer's responsibility to obtain a relevant patient history, as described in Chapter 4. Failure to do so could result in further injury to the patient. Because radiographic examination of the shoulder girdle can be performed using an upright wall unit or the radiographic table, the patient's condition also has a significant impact on room preparation.

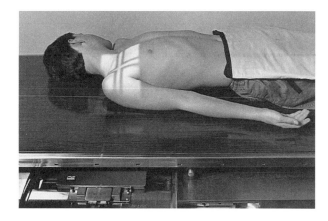

Figure 6–10. Recumbent AP shoulder.

POSITIONING CONSIDERATIONS

Radiographic examination of the shoulder is performed to rule out a fracture or identify calcium deposits or other pathology related to the shoulder. Although routines may vary, nontraumatic examination of the shoulder generally includes two AP projections: one with the arm externally rotated and one with the arm internally rotated (Table 6–3). These projections may be performed with the patient supine on the table or sitting or standing erect in front of an upright grid device (Figures 6–10, 6–11).

Table 6–3. Routine/Optional Projections: Shoulder Girdle

Shoulder	Scapula
AP with external rotation	AP
AP with internal rotation	Lateral
Inferosuperior axial (Lawrence)[a]	
PA oblique "Y"[a]	
Transthoracic lateral[a]	Acromioclavicular Joints
AP oblique (Grashey)[a]	AP erect with weights
	AP erect without weights
Clavicle	
AP/PA	
AP/PA axial	

Note. Although routines may vary between departments, this table summarizes some of the more common routine and optional projections.
[a]Optional projections; may be routine in some departments

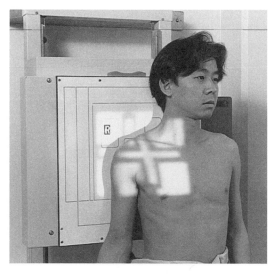

Figure 6–11. Erect AP shoulder.

▶ **_Trauma Shoulder Series_**

- _AP shoulder, neutral position_

- _Transthoracic lateral humerus_

- _Upright position preferred when possible_

▶ **_A–C Joints_**

- _72-in. SID reduces magnification_

- _Bilateral examination_

- _Must be performed upright_

Whenever a fracture is suspected, the arm should **not** be internally or externally rotated. Most fractures of the shoulder girdle involve the proximal humerus. Internal or external rotation of fracture fragments could cause additional damage to muscles, vessels, or nerves. If a fracture is suspected, the arm should not be moved. Two projections, 90° from each other, should be obtained. Generally, a neutral AP projection and a transthoracic lateral humerus to demonstrate the shoulder joint and proximal humerus, as described in Chapter 5, are acquired. Because shoulder injuries can be painful, the upright position should be used whenever possible to allow the weight of the arm to act as traction on the fracture, thereby minimizing the pain.

To adequately demonstrate the clavicle, two projections are taken; however, they are not 90° apart. Illustration of the clavicle on end, in a lateral position, would not be helpful in identifying a fracture or other pathology. Therefore, AP or PA and axial projections of the clavicle are obtained.

Radiographic examination of the scapula includes AP and lateral projections that may be obtained with the patient recumbent or upright. Although the AP projection is easily performed in either position, the lateral is frequently easier to obtain with the patient upright. Because most of the scapula is superimposed by the thorax on a frontal view, the arm is abducted for the AP projection, helping to pull the scapula out from under the rib cage.

Acromioclavicular (A–C) joints are radiographed to evaluate soft tissue damage evidenced by increased joint separation when weights are used to apply gentle traction. This is a bilateral study in which both joints are examined via weight-bearing and non-weight-bearing projections (both joints are always radiographed for comparison). The examination is performed with the patient in the upright position. A 72-in. SID is used to minimize magnification and increase the probability of including both joints on one 7 × 17-in. or 14 × 17-in. film. If the patient's size does not allow for the inclusion of both joints on one film, separate exposures of each joint must be made using 8 × 10-in. or 9 × 9-in. cassettes.

ALTERNATE PROJECTIONS

Two additional projections can be obtained to demonstrate the glenohumeral relationship. The lateral scapular plane position, more commonly called the "Y" or "Neer" view, demonstrates the glenohumeral joint in a true lateral position by rotating the patient to a 45° to 60° LAO or RAO upright position. In the resulting radiograph, the scapula is superimposed over the humerus and appears as a "Y." This projection is particularly beneficial in assessing dislocations of the shoulder joint.

The inferosuperior axial projection is obtained with the patient supine and the affected arm abducted. A horizontal beam is directed toward the acromioclavicular joint. This projection clearly demonstrates the relationship between the humeral head and glenoid cavity.

Although discussed in Chapter 5, the transthoracic lateral projection may also be included in the radiographic examination of the injured shoulder when a fracture is suspected. In addition to demonstrating displacement of fracture fragments, this projection also shows the glenohumeral relationship.

BREATHING INSTRUCTIONS

For AP projections of the shoulder (with varying degrees of arm rotation) and the AP clavicle projection, instructing the patient to stop breathing or to hold the breath is adequate. To elevate the clavicle for the axial clavicle projection, the patient should be instructed to suspend breathing after inhalation. Because part of the scapula is seen through the lung and thorax on an AP projection, quiet breathing with a long exposure time can be used to blur lung and rib detail. For acromioclavicular joints, the exposure should be made during suspended expiration. When a patient exhales, the shoulders and arms are more likely to relax, allowing for a more accurate assessment of acromioclavicular injuries.

EXPOSURE FACTORS

For most projections of the shoulder girdle, 60 to 75 kVp penetrates the part without compromising radiographic quality. The lower kVp should be used on osteoporotic patients; a higher kVp is necessary for extremely muscular patients. This kilovoltage assumes the use of a grid. Some projections, such as those of the inferosuperior axial shoulder and acromioclavicular joints, may be obtained without a grid and require an appropriate reduction in kilovoltage; 55 to 65 kVp should produce an adequate nongrid radiograph of these structures. The mAs needed depends on the type of equipment generator, film/screen speed, use and type of grid, and pathology.

EQUIPMENT CONSIDERATIONS

Most radiographs of the shoulder girdle are obtained using a grid. This may be accomplished by using an upright wall unit or flat or erect radiographic table. Because the grids in tables and wall units often differ, it is important for the radiographer to know the grid ratios and be able to convert techniques appropriately (see Chapter 4 for grid conversions). To improve overall radiographic density, a wedge filter can be used to compensate for the difference in tissue thickness between the areas of the coracoid and acromion processes. Mobile radiography of the shoulder girdle is frequently performed using a nongrid technique to minimize the risk of grid lines and reduce exposure to the patient and technologist.

6

RADIOGRAPHIC POSITIONING OF THE SHOULDER GIRDLE

- ▶ AP SHOULDER IN EXTERNAL ROTATION

- ▶ AP SHOULDER IN INTERNAL ROTATION

- ▶ INFEROSUPERIOR AXIAL SHOULDER JOINT
  (LAWRENCE POSITION)

- ▶ PA OBLIQUE "Y" SHOULDER JOINT

- ▶ AP CLAVICLE

- ▶ AP AXIAL CLAVICLE

- ▶ AP SCAPULA

- ▶ LATERAL SCAPULA

- ▶ AP ACROMIOCLAVICULAR JOINTS:
  WITH & WITHOUT WEIGHTS

► AP SHOULDER IN EXTERNAL ROTATION

Technical Considerations

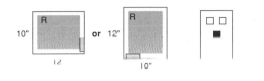

- Film size: 10 × 12 in. crosswise or lengthwise.
- Grid recommended for most patients.
- 60–75 kVp.
- Collimate to include soft tissue, clavicle (cw cassette), acromion, greater tubercle, and surgical neck of humerus.

CAUTION: Do NOT externally rotate the arm if a fracture of the humerus is suspected.

Shielding

- Gonadal shielding should be used on all patients, especially children and adults of reproductive age.

Patient Positioning

- Assist the patient to the supine position on the radiographic table or to the erect AP position in front of an upright grid unit. If supine, a small support may be placed under the patient's knees for comfort; a pillow under the patient's head should be positioned away from the shoulders to prevent unwanted artifacts.
- Adjust the patient's midsagittal plane to lie parallel with the long axis of the table.
- Rotate the patient slightly toward the affected side to place the shoulder parallel with the film plane. If supine, sponges or sandbags may be used to support the patient.
- Adjust the patient so the coracoid process is centered to the midline of the table or wall unit.

Part Positioning

- Externally rotate the arm so the hand is supinated. A sandbag may be placed over the supinated hand for immobilization when the patient is supine.
- Turn the patient's head away from the side of interest *(Figure 6–12)*.

Central Ray

- Direct the central ray perpendicular to the coracoid process.
- Adjust the centering of the cassette to coincide with the central ray.

Breathing Instructions

- Instruct the patient to suspend breathing during the exposure.

Image Evaluation

- The acromion, surgical neck of the humerus, greater tubercle of the humerus, and at least half of the clavicle should be included in the collimated area, depending on the radiologist's preference.
- The glenohumeral joint should be adequately penetrated and visible; bony trabeculae should be clearly seen.
- The greater tubercle should be demonstrated in profile laterally *(Figure 6–13)*.

1. Acromion process	4. Anatomical neck	7. Clavicle
2. Head of humerus	5. Lesser tubercle	8. Coracoid process
3. Greater tubercle	6. Surgical neck	9. Glenoid cavity

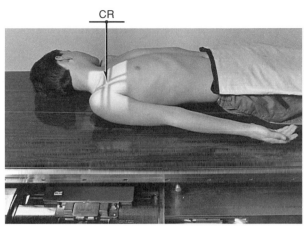

Figure 6–12. AP shoulder in external rotation.

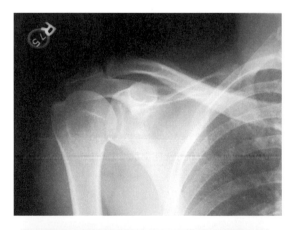

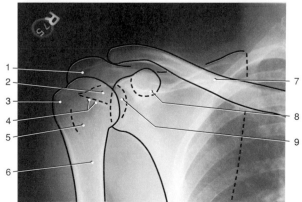

Figure 6–13. AP shoulder in external rotation.

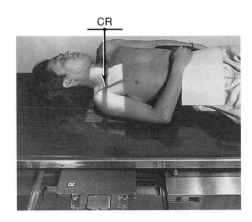

Figure 6–14. AP oblique glenoid cavity: Grashey method.

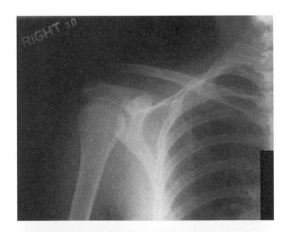

Figure 6–15. AP shoulder in internal rotation.

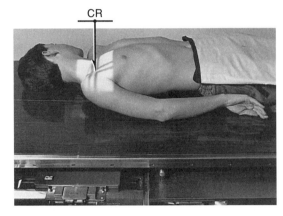

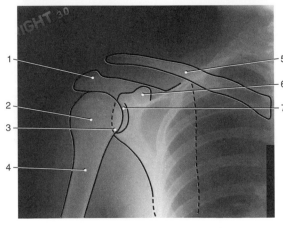

Figure 6–16. AP shoulder in internal rotation.

► AP SHOULDER IN INTERNAL ROTATION

Technical Considerations

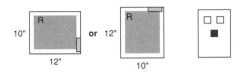

- Film size: 10 × 12 in. crosswise or lengthwise.
- Grid recommended for most patients.
- 60–75 kVp
- Collimate to include soft tissue, clavicle (cw cassette), acromion, greater tubercle, and surgical neck of humerus.

CAUTION: Do NOT rotate the arm if a fracture of the humerus is suspected.

Shielding

- Gonadal shielding should be used on all patients, especially children and adults of reproductive age.

Patient Positioning

- Assist the patient to the supine position on the radiographic table or to the erect AP position in front of an upright grid unit. If supine, a small support may be placed under the patient's knees for comfort; a pillow under the patient's head should be positioned away from the shoulders to prevent unwanted artifacts.
- Adjust the patient's midsagittal plane to lie parallel with the long axis of the table.
- Rotate the patient slightly toward the affected side to place the shoulder parallel with the film plane. If supine, sponges or sandbags may be used to support the patient. **Note:** To better demonstrate the glenoid cavity, the patient can be rotated 35° to 45° toward the affected side; the arm is internally rotated slightly and the palm of the hand is placed on the abdomen. This projection may be referred to as the *Grashey method* and may be routine in some departments *(Figure 6–14)*.
- Adjust the patient so the coracoid process is centered to the midline of the table or wall unit.

Part Positioning

- Internally rotate and adduct the arm so the back of the hand is resting along the lateral side of the patient's body; the elbow may be flexed slightly. A sandbag may be placed against the palm of the hand for immobilization when the patient is supine.
- Turn the patient's head away from the side of interest *(Figure 6–15)*.

Central Ray

- Direct the central ray perpendicular to the coracoid process.
- Adjust the centering of the cassette to coincide with the central ray.

Breathing Instructions

- Instruct the patient to suspend breathing during the exposure.

Image Evaluation

- The acromion, surgical neck of the humerus, lesser tubercle of the humerus, and at least half of the clavicle should be included in the collimated area, depending on radiologist's preference.
- The glenohumeral joint should be adequately penetrated and visible; bony trabeculae should be clearly seen.
- The lesser tubercle should be demonstrated in profile near the glenoid cavity *(Figure 6–16)*.

1. Acromion
2. Humeral head
3. Lesser tubercle, humerus
4. Surgical neck, humerus
5. Clavicle
6. Coracoid process, scapula
7. Glenoid cavity, scapula

▶ INFEROSUPERIOR AXIAL SHOULDER JOINT (LAWRENCE POSITION)

Technical Considerations

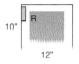

- Film size: 10 × 12 in., 8 × 10 in. crosswise, or 9 × 9 in.
- Grid cassette or nongrid.
- 55–65 kVp.
- Collimate to include soft tissue, glenoid cavity, acromion, coracoid process, and surgical neck of humerus.

Shielding

- Gonadal shielding should be used on all patients, especially children and adults of reproductive age.

Patient Positioning

- Assist the patient to the supine position on the radiographic table; a small support may be placed under the patient's knees for comfort, and a pillow under the patient's head should be positioned away from the shoulders to prevent unwanted artifacts.
- To facilitate centering the part to the cassette, a small radiolucent support can be positioned under the upper torso and head of thin patients.

Part Positioning

- Externally rotate and abduct the patient's affected arm; an arm board or other support may be needed.
- Immobilize the affected arm with sponges and sandbags, if necessary.
- Turn the patient's head away from the side of interest *(Figure 6–17)*.

Central Ray

- Position the cassette vertically against the superior aspect of the shoulder with the medial end of the cassette pushed as close to the neck as possible; support with sandbags.
- Direct the central ray horizontally and medially through the axilla to the acromioclavicular joint; the amount of medial angulation generally ranges from 15° to 30°.
- Adjust centering of cassette to include critical anatomy.

Breathing Instructions

- Instruct the patient to stop breathing during the exposure.

Image Evaluation

- The glenohumeral joint, acromion process, coracoid process, and surgical neck of the humerus should be included in the collimated area.
- The glenohumeral joint should be adequately penetrated and visible; bony trabeculae should be clearly seen.
- The coracoid process should be seen anteriorly and the acromion process should be visualized through the head of the humerus *(Figure 6–18)*.

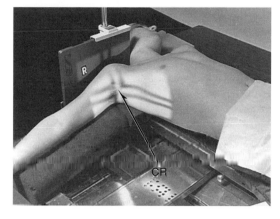

Figure 6–17. Inferosuperior axial shoulder joint: Lawrence method.

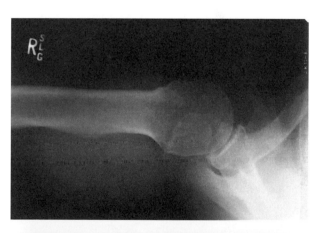

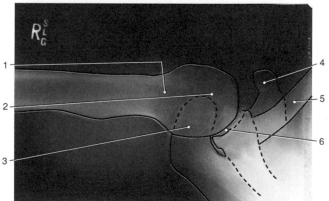

| 1. Surgical neck | 3. Acromion process | 5. Clavicle |
| 2. Head of humerus | 4. Coracoid process | 6. Glenoid cavity |

Figure 6–18. Inferosuperior axial shoulder joint: Lawrence method.

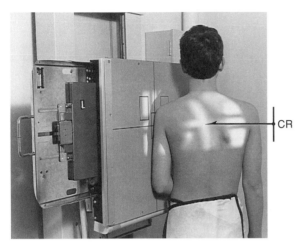

Figure 6–19. PA oblique, Y-view of the shoulder joint and scapula.

▶ PA OBLIQUE "Y" SHOULDER JOINT

Technical Considerations

- Film size: 10×12 in. lengthwise.
- Grid recommended.
- 70–80 kVp.
- Collimate to include soft tissue, acromion, coracoid process, and surgical neck of the humerus.

Shielding

- Gonadal shielding should be used on all patients, especially children and adults of reproductive age.

Patient Positioning

- Assist the patient to the anterior oblique (RAO or LAO) position with the shoulder of interest nearest the film; the patient may be recumbent on the radiographic table or erect in front of an upright grid unit.
- Center the humeral head of the side of interest to the grid device.

Part Positioning

- Adjust the rotation of the body so the midcoronal plane forms a 45° to 60° angle with the plane of the film; the plane of the dependent scapula should be perpendicular to the film plane.
- The affected arm should be positioned along side the body in a comfortable position (Figure 6–19).

Central Ray

- Direct the central ray horizontally through the midpoint of the vertebral border of the scapula to the glenohumeral joint.
- Adjust the centering of the cassette to coincide with the central ray.

Image Evaluation

- The acromion process, coracoid process, and inferior angle of the scapula should be included within the collimated area.
- Penetration and density should be sufficient to demonstrate the head of the humerus through the scapula; bony trabeculae should be visible and clear.
- The scapula should be superimposed over the humerus with the acromion, coracoid, and body of the scapula appearing as a "Y." **Note:** Location of the humeral head inferior to the coracoid process indicates anterior dislocation; the humeral head beneath the acromion process indicates posterior dislocation (Figure 6–20).

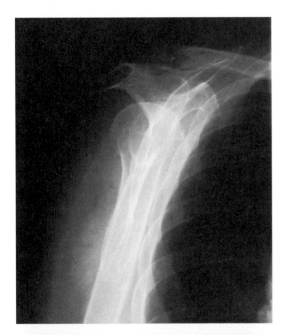

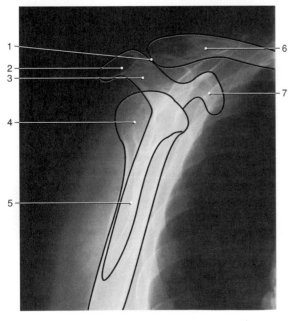

Figure 6–20. PA oblique, Y-view of the shoulder joint and scapula.

1. Acromioclavicular joint
2. Acromion, scapula
3. Scapular spine
4. Humeral head
5. Scapular body over humerus
6. Clavicle
7. Coracoid process, scapula

▶ AP CLAVICLE

Technical Considerations

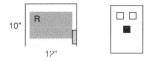

- Film size: 10 × 12 in. crosswise.
- Grid recommended.
- 60–75 kVp.
- Collimate to include soft tissue, acromioclavicular joints, and sternoclavicular joint.

Shielding

- Gonadal shielding should be used on all patients, especially children and adults of reproductive age.

Patient Positioning

- Assist the patient to the supine position on the radiographic table or to the erect position in front of an upright grid unit. If supine, a small support may be placed under the patient's knees for comfort; a pillow under the patient's head should be positioned away from the shoulders to prevent unwanted artifacts. **Note:** Although the PA projection may also be performed to reduce magnification, it is generally less comfortable for the recumbent patient with a suspected fracture.
- Center the midclavicle of the affected side to the midline of the grid device.
- Adjust the patient's midsagittal plane to lie parallel with the long axis of the table.

Part Positioning

- Position the patient's arms comfortably on the table and adjust the shoulders so they lie in a transverse plane parallel to the tabletop.
- Turn the patient's head away from the side of interest *(Figure 6–21)*.

Central Ray

- Direct the central ray perpendicular to the midclavicle; adjust crosswise centering to the grid, if necessary.
- Adjust the centering of the cassette to coincide with the central ray.

Breathing Instructions

- Instruct the patient to take in a breath and hold it in during the exposure to help elevate and angle the clavicle.

Image Evaluation

- The entire clavicle, sternoclavicular joint, and acromioclavicular joint should be included in the collimated area.
- Penetration and density should be such that the lateral end of the clavicle is not overexposed, yet the medial end is penetrated and clearly visible; bony trabeculae should be seen.
- The medial half of the clavicle will be superimposed over the thorax *(Figure 6–22)*.

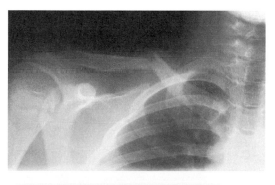

Figure 6–21. AP clavicle.

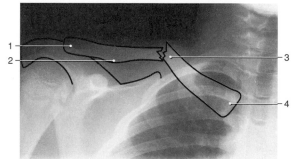

1. Acromial (lateral) end
2. Conoid tubercle
3. Body (shaft)
4. Sternal (medial) end

Figure 6–22. AP clavicle.

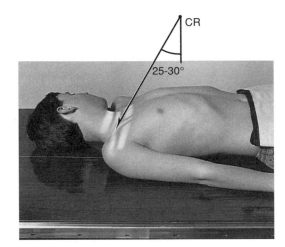

Figure 6–23. AP axial clavicle.

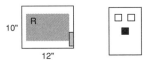

► AP AXIAL CLAVICLE

Technical Considerations

- Film size: 10 × 12 in. crosswise.
- Grid recommended.
- 60–75 kVp.
- Collimate to include soft tissue, acromioclavicular joints and sternoclavicular joints.

Shielding

- Gonadal shielding should be used on all patients, especially children and adults of reproductive age.

Patient Positioning

- Assist the patient to the supine position on the radiographic table or to the erect position in front of an upright grid unit. If supine, a small support may be placed under the patient's knees for comfort; a pillow under the patient's head should be positioned away from the shoulders to prevent unwanted artifacts. **Note:** Although the PA projection may also be performed to reduce magnification, it is generally less comfortable for the recumbent patient with a suspected fracture.
- Center the midclavicle of the affected side to the midline of the grid device.
- Adjust the patient's midsagittal plane to lie parallel with the long axis of the table.

Part Positioning

- Position the patient's arms comfortably on the table and adjust the shoulders so they lie in a transverse plane parallel to the tabletop.
- Turn the patient's head away from the side of interest *(Figure 6–23)*.

Central Ray

- Direct the central ray 25° to 30° cephalad to the midclavicle; thinner patients require a greater angle to project the clavicle above the thorax. Small pediatric patients may require a 35° to 40° angle. If performed with the patient prone for a PA projection, the central ray is directed caudally using the same angulation. **Note:** Depending on department routine, angulation may vary from 15° to 45°.
- Adjust the centering of the cassette to coincide with the central ray.

Breathing Instructions

- Instruct the patient to take in a breath, blow it out, then hold it out during the exposure.

Image Evaluation

- The entire clavicle, sternoclavicular joint, and acromioclavicular joint should be included in the collimated area.
- Penetration and density should be such that the lateral end of the clavicle is not overexposed, yet the medial end is penetrated and clearly visible; bony trabeculae should be seen.
- Most of the clavicle should be projected above the thorax *(Figure 6–24)*.

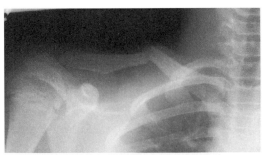

Figure 6–24. AP axial clavicle.

1. Acromial (lateral) end
2. Conoid tubercle
3. Body (shaft)
4. Sternal (medial) end

► AP SCAPULA

Technical Considerations

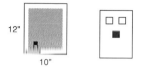

- Film size: 10 × 12 in. lengthwise.
- Grid recommended.
- 60–75 kVp.
- Collimate to include soft tissue, acromion, coracoid process, and inferior angle.

Shielding

- Gonadal shielding should be used on all patients, especially children and adults of reproductive age.

Patient Positioning

- Assist the patient to the supine position on the radiographic table or to the erect position in front of an upright grid unit. If supine, a small support may be placed under the patient's knees for comfort; a pillow under the patient's head should be positioned away from the shoulders to prevent unwanted artifacts.
- Center the plane passing through the coracoid process of the affected side to the midline of the grid device; the scapula should be centered to the grid.
- Adjust the patient's midsagittal plane to lie parallel with the long axis of the table (supine position); the shoulders should lie in a transverse plane parallel with the film.

Part Positioning

- Abduct the affected arm to a 90° angle with the long axis of the body to move the scapula laterally.
- Flex the elbow approximately 90° and supinate the hand; support the hand with sponges or sandbags at the level of the patient's head.
- Turn the patient's head away from the side of interest *(Figure 6–25)*.

Central Ray

- Direct the central ray perpendicular to the midscapula midway between the acromion and the inferior angle; adjust crosswise centering to the grid, if necessary.
- Adjust the centering of the cassette to coincide with the central ray.

Breathing Instructions

- Instruct the patient to breathe normally during the exposure to blur lung detail.

Image Evaluation

- The entire scapula should be included in the collimated area.
- Bony trabeculae should be seen while the lung detail should be blurred.
- The medial half of the scapula will be under the thorax.
- The arm should be at a 90° angle with the body *(Figure 6–26)*.

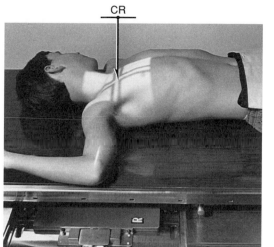

Figure 6–25. AP scapula.

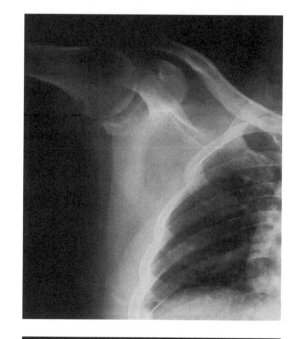

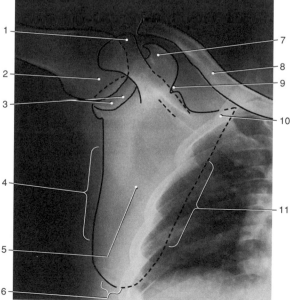

Figure 6–26. AP scapula.

1. Acromion
2. Humeral head
3. Glenoid cavity
4. Lateral, (axillary) border
5. Body
6. Inferior angle
7. Coracoid process
8. Clavicle
9. Scapular notch
10. Superior angle
11. Medial (vertebral) border

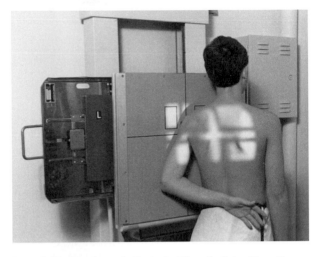

Figure 6–27. Lateral scapula. The back of the patient's hand is on the posterior thorax.

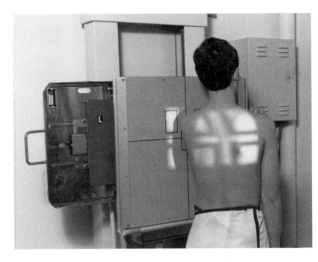

Figure 6–28. Lateral scapula with the patient in the LAO position.

▶ LATERAL SCAPULA

Technical Considerations

- Film size: 10 × 12 in. lengthwise.
- Grid recommended.
- 70–80 kVp.
- Collimate to include soft tissue, acromion, coracoid process, and inferior angle.

Shielding

- Gonadal shielding should be used on all patients, especially children and adults of reproductive age.

Patient Positioning

- Assist the patient to the anterior oblique (RAO/LAO) position in front of an upright grid unit or, if necessary recumbent on the radiographic table. Trauma patients may require the reverse oblique (LPO/RPO) to be performed; note that this will cause increased magnification of the part.
- Center the affected scapula to the midline of the grid device.

Part Positioning

- Position the arm according the area of interest: For the *body of the scapula,* either flex the elbow of the affected side and rest the back of the patient's hand behind the waist or palm on the abdomen at the waist level or extend the forearm across the upper chest *(Figures 6–27, 6–28).* For the *acromion and coracoid processes,* instruct the patient to extend the arm of the affected side above the head and rest the forearm on the head or opposite shoulder.
- Palpate the axillary and vertebral borders between the thumb and fingers of one hand and adjust the body rotation to place the wing of the scapula perpendicular to the film plane.
- Turn the patient's head away from the side of interest.

Central Ray

- Direct the central ray perpendicular to the film through the vertebral border, midway between the inferior angle and acromion.
- Adjust the center of the cassette to coincide with central ray.

Breathing Instructions

- Instruct the patient to suspend breathing during the exposure.

Image Evaluation

- The acromion, coracoid process, and inferior angle should be included in the collimated area.
- The glenoid cavity and body should be penetrated and adequately exposed; bony trabeculae should be seen.
- The vertebral and axillary borders should be superimposed; the body should be separated from the thorax *(Figure 6–29)*.

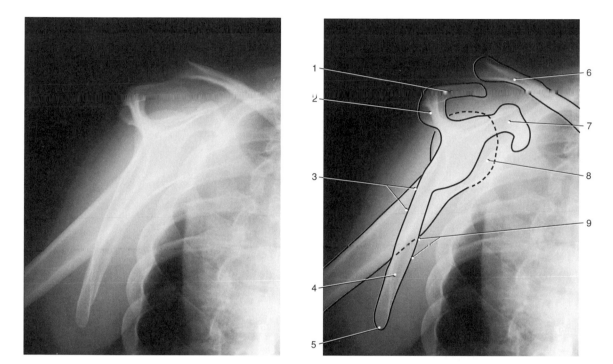

Figure 6–29. Lateral scapula. The patient's hand was positioned on the posterior thorax.

1. Acromion
2. Scapula spine
3. Dorsal surface
4. Body
5. Inferior angle
6. Clavicle
7. Coracoid process
8. Humeral head
9. Ventral surface

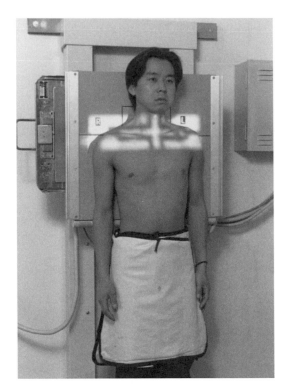

Figure 6–30. AP acromioclavicular joints without weights.

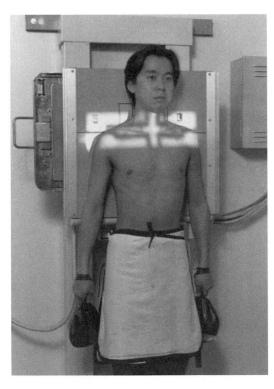

Figure 6–31. AP acromioclavicular joints with weights.

▶ AP ACROMIOCLAVICULAR JOINTS: WITH & WITHOUT WEIGHTS

Technical Considerations

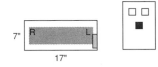

- Film size: 7 × 17 in., 14 × 17 in., or 2 to 8 × 10 in. crosswise.
- Grid recommended.
- 60–70 kVp.
- Collimate to include soft tissue, acromioclavicular joints.

CAUTION: A fracture of clavicle, shoulder, or arm should be ruled out before giving weights to any patient.

Shielding

- Gonadal shielding should be used on all patients, especially children and adults of reproductive age.

Patient Positioning

- Assist the patient to the standing or seated position with the back against an upright grid unit; if standing, the weight should be equally distributed on both feet.
- Center the midsagittal plane to the midline of the grid unit. Large patients may require four exposures and four cassettes to complete the examination; in this case, the acromioclavicular joint being examined is centered to the midline of the grid.

Part Positioning

- Position the patient's arms comfortably at the sides.
- Two bilateral projections are generally obtained: one without added weight and one with 5- to 10-pound weights hanging on the patient's wrists; holding the weights in each hand may cause the muscles to contract and prevent the diagnosis of small acromioclavicular separations. Markers should be used to indicate the use of weights. **Note:** Do not apply weights until ready to make the exposure *(Figures 6–30, 6–31)*.

Central Ray

- Using a 72-in. SID to minimize magnification, direct the central ray horizontally and perpendicular to a point midway between the acromioclavicular joints (bilateral examination); for single exposures (×4), the central ray is directed to the acromioclavicular joint of interest.
- Adjust the centering of the cassette to coincide with the central ray.

Breathing Instructions

- Instruct the patient to take in a breath, blow it out, and hold it out during the exposure to relax the shoulders.

Image Evaluation

Bilateral Exposure
- Both acromioclavicular joints should be included in the collimated area.
- The sternoclavicular joints should be equidistant from the spine.
- Penetration and density should be such that the lateral end of the clavicle and the acromion are not over-exposed; bony trabeculae should be clearly seen

Single Exposure
- The acromioclavicular joint of interest should be centered to the film.
- Penetration and density should be such that the lateral end of the clavicle and the acromion are not over-exposed; bony trabeculae should be clearly seen (Figure 6–32).

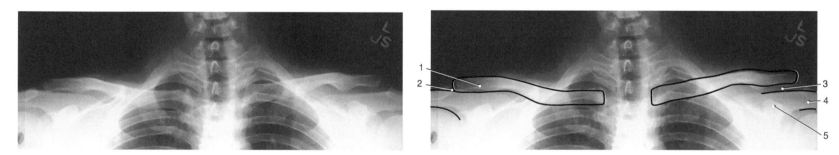

Figure 6–32. AP acromioclavicular joints with weights.

1. Clavicle
2. Right acromioclavicular joint
3. Left acromioclavicular joint
4. Acromion process
5. Coracoid process, scapula

SUMMARY

▶ Radiographic examinations of the shoulder girdle are frequently performed with the patient erect to minimize discomfort.

▶ When a fracture of the humerus is suspected, the arm should *not* be internally or externally rotated; when in doubt, an AP projection with the arm in neutral position can be obtained and checked first.

▶ In most cases, 60 to 75 kVp is appropriate for examinations of the shoulder girdle.

▶ Most examinations of the shoulder girdle are performed with the use of a grid; mobile radiography is usually performed using a nongrid technique.

▶ The glenohumeral relationship can be evaluated by the "Y" and inferosuperior views.

▶ Separation of the acromioclavicular joints can be evaluated by erect bilateral AP projections obtained with and without weights.

▶ To reduce magnification and increase the probability that both acromioclavicular joints will be included on one film, a 72-in. SID should be employed.

QUESTIONS FOR CRITICAL THINKING & APPLICATION

1. Why does the shape of the glenoid cavity permit dislocations of the shoulder joint to occur?

2. Identify several different contact sports in which clavicular injuries can occur. Explain why the clavicle is fractured more often than the scapula.

3. Palpate your right acromioclavicular joint as you shrug your shoulders. What type of movement are you feeling? How do the bones of the shoulder girdle work together during this action?

4. Your patient is an elderly woman who tripped over her throw rug and tried to catch herself on outstretched arms. Although she avoided a more serious injury, she did fracture her right clavicle. Explain why such a fracture occurred given this history.

5. What structures on the scapula can be palpated? Can you find them on yourself?

6. An elderly lady has fallen and injured her shoulder. Identify and describe the projections you would take to demonstrate a possible fracture or other injury.

7. A 20-year-old male athlete hurt his shoulder playing football. Describe the procedure you would follow to demonstrate a possible separation of the acromioclavicular joints.

8. Describe the patient preparation and list the questions you would ask as part of a pertinent patient history for a patient requiring radiographic examination of the shoulder.

9. A patient with an obvious dislocation of the shoulder has been admitted to the emergency room. Identify the best projections to adequately evaluate the injury.

10. How much would you angle the central ray for an axial projection of the clavicle to be performed on a thin 10-year-old? Explain your answer.

FILM CRITIQUE

Describe the patient positioning used in *Figure 6–33*. What structures are best demonstrated?

Is the centering accurate?

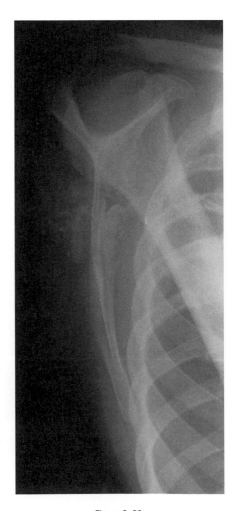

Figure 6–33.

7

LOWER LIMB (EXTREMITY)

► OBJECTIVES

Following the completion of this chapter the student will be able to:

- Given diagrams, radiographs, or dry bones, name and describe the bones of the lower limb, to include the foot, ankle, lower leg, knee, and femur.

- Locate the transverse and longitudinal arches in each foot and discuss their function.

- Classify the articulations in the lower limb and identify their type of movement.

- State the criteria used to determine positioning accuracy on radiographs of the lower limb and evaluate radiographs of the lower limb in terms of positioning, centering, image quality, radiographic anatomy, and pathology.

- Define terminology associated with the lower limb, to include anatomy, procedures, and pathology.

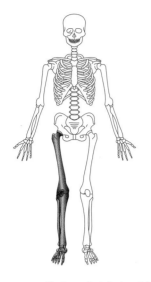

Figure 7–1. The lower limb (extremity).

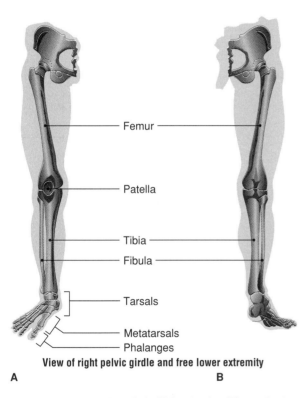

Femur

Patella

Tibia

Fibula

Tarsals

Metatarsals

Phalanges

View of right pelvic girdle and free lower extremity

A   B

Figure 7–2. Bones of the lower limb. **(A)** Anterior view, **(B)** posterior view.

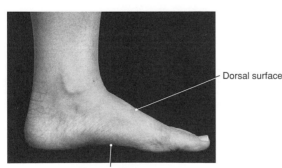

Dorsal surface

Plantar surface

Figure 7–3. Surfaces of the foot illustrated on a lateral view.

▶ ANATOMY OF THE LOWER LIMB (EXTREMITY)

The lower extremities or limbs function to support the weight of the body in the erect position. Because they are weight bearing and must be able to withstand force, especially during activities such as running and jumping, the bones of the lower limbs are generally larger and more stout than those of the upper limbs.

The skeletal design of the lower limbs is similar to that of the upper limbs *(Figure 7–1)*. That is, the lower limbs are suspended from the trunk. Each lower limb is composed of 30 bones *(Table 7–1)*. These include the phalanges, metatarsals, and tarsals of the foot, the tibia and fibula of the lower leg, the patella or kneecap, and the femur of each thigh *(Figure 7–2)*. In addition, small sesamoid bones may be present, particularly in the foot.

FOOT AND ANKLE

Surfaces of the Foot

The terms *plantar* and *dorsum pedis* are used to refer to the surfaces of the foot. The plantar surface is the sole of the foot. In the true anatomic position, this is the posterior aspect. The dorsum pedis, or simply dorsum, is the top of the foot or its anterior surface.

An AP projection of the foot is also known as a dorsoplantar projection as the x-ray beam is directed from the dorsum to the plantar surface *(Figure 7–3)*.

Phalanges

The foot is similar to the hand because it has 14 phalanges that constitute the digits or toes. Although still classified as miniature long bones, the phalanges of the foot are considerably smaller and less flexible than those of the hand; however, both the arrangement and structure of the phalanges of the foot resemble those

Table 7–1. Summary of the Lower Limb (Extremity)

Bones of Each Lower Limb	Description
Phalanges (14)	• Toes or digits • Distal, middle, proximal • Mini-long bones • Articulate with metatarsals
Metatarsals (5)	• Instep of foot • Mini-long bones • Articulate with phalanges and tarsals
Tarsals (7) 　Medial cuneiform 　Intermediate cuneiform 　Lateral cuneiform 　Cuboid 　Navicular 　Talus 　Calcaneus	• Posterior foot and ankle • Short bones • Anterior and posterior arrangement • Arch construction for support • Articulate with metatarsals and talus with tibia
Tibia (1)	• Medial bone of lower leg • Long bone • Weight bearing • Assists in formation of ankle and knee joints • Articulates distally with talus and fibula and proximally with fibula and femur
Fibula (1)	• Lateral bone of lower leg • Long bone • Non-weight bearing • Articulates distally with talus and tibia and proximally with tibia
Femur (1)	• Thigh • Long bone • Assists in formation of knee and hip joints • Articulates with tibia at knee joint and with acetabulum of the pelvis at hip joint
Patella (1)	• Kneecap • Sesamoid bone • Articulates with distal femur

of the hand. The 14 phalanges are arranged into three rows (distal, middle, and proximal) on the second through fifth digits and into two rows (distal and proximal) on the first digit. The first digit is usually referred to as either the **great toe** or the **hallux** (HAL-uks) and is situated on the medial side of the foot. Each phalanx has a head, shaft, and base. As in the phalanges of the hand, the head is found at the bone's distal end, and the base is at its proximal end *(Figure 7–4)*.

Metatarsals

The sole or instep of the foot is formed by the five metatarsals. These miniature long bones are similar in structure to the metacarpals of the hand, but arc longer and stronger to support the weight of the body. The first metatarsal is the largest, as it bears more weight than the other metatarsals. The base of the fifth metatarsal is very **prominent** and is often fractured as it lies on the exposed lateral margin of the foot. The heads of the metatarsals are found at their distal ends and articulate with the phalanges. They are very prominent and form what is referred to as the "ball" of the foot. The proximal end of each metatarsal articulates with the tarsal bones. A pair of sesamoid bones is commonly located on the plantar surface of the foot beneath the first metatarsophalangeal joint. Additional sesamoid bones might also be found in other areas of stress in the foot.

Tarsals

The term *tarsus* (TAR-sus) is sometimes used to refer to the ankle, but in fact denotes the proximal portion of the foot. This area is made up of seven tarsal bones, only one of which actually helps to form the ankle joint. Although they do not form two neat rows like the carpal bones of the wrist, the tarsal bones are grouped in a distal and proximal arrangement. The three cuneiforms and cuboid are distal, whereas the navicular, talus, and calcaneus are found in the proximal region of the foot. A mnemonic device such as the following suggested by a student can aid in learning the names of the tarsal bones: *3 Carribean cousins never take cruises (Table 7–2)*.

There are three cuneiform (kū-NĒ-i-form) bones which are located between the metatarsals and the navicular. These wedge-shaped bones are named according to their position in the foot. The **medial cuneiform** is also called the **first** or **internal cuneiform** as it is situated on the medial aspect of the foot. It articulates distally with the first metatarsal and proximally with the navicular. The middle cuneiform is the **intermediate** or **second cuneiform.** It is located just lateral to the first cuneiform. It articulates with the second metatarsal and the navicular. The **lateral** or **external cuneiform** is the **third** of the cuneiform bones and is situated between the second cuneiform and the cuboid, where it also articulates with the navicular and the third metatarsal.

As its name suggests, the **cuboid** (KŪ-boid) is a cube-shaped bone that is located on the lateral aspect of the foot. It articulates distally with the fourth and fifth metatarsals, proximally with the calcaneus, and medially with the navicular and third cuneiform.

The **navicular** (nah-VIK-ū-lar) is also known as the **scaphoid** (SKAF-oid). It is basically oval in shape and is located on the medial side of the foot. It articulates distally with the three cuneiforms, proximally with the talus, and laterally with the cuboid.

The **talus** (TĀ-lus) is also known as the **astragalus** (ah-STRAG-ah-lus). It is a large, posterior tarsal bone which articulates inferiorly with the calcaneus, anteriorly with the navicular, and superiorly with the tibia and fibula of the lower leg. It is the only tarsal bone involved in the formation of the ankle joint. The upper curved aspect of the talus is known as the **trochlea** (TROK-lē-ah). The concave inferior surface of the tibia fits over this part to form the ankle joint *(Figure 7–5)*.

The **calcaneus** (kal-KA-nē-us) or **os calcis** (OS KAL-sis) is the heel portion of the foot. It is the largest and strongest of the tarsal bones. The weight of the body is transmitted to the calcaneus via the talus. There are three articular facets on the superior surface of the calcaneus. The talus articulates with the

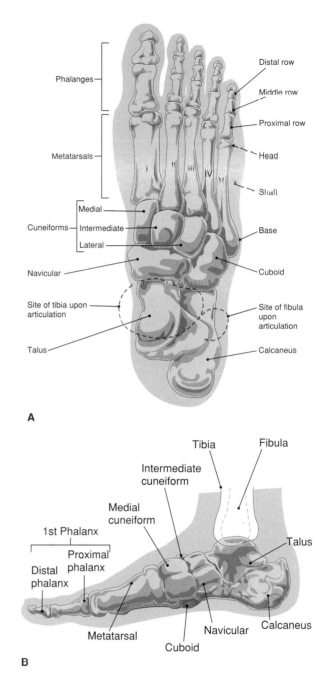

A

B

Figure 7–4. Foot. The position and relationship of the bones forming the foot are demonstrated on **(A)** superior and **(B)** lateral views.

Table 7–2. Mnemonic for the Tarsal Bones

Mnemonic	Tarsal Bones
*3 C*arribean	*3 C*uneiforms
	Medial (1st)
	Intermediate (2nd)
	Lateral (3rd)
*C*ousins	*C*uboid
*N*ever	*N*avicular
*T*ake	*T*alus
*C*ruises	*C*alcaneus

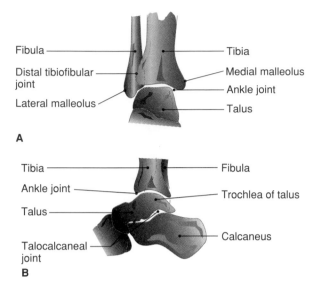

A

B

Figure 7–5. Ankle. The bones forming the ankle are demonstrated on **(A)** anterior and **(B)** lateral views.

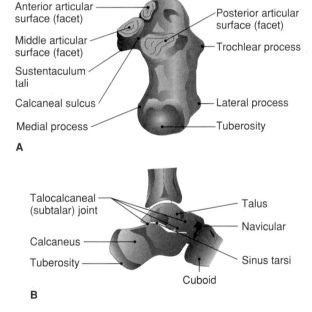

A

B

Figure 7–6. Calcaneus. **(A)** Superior view, **(B)** lateral view.

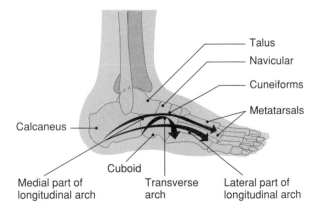

Figure 7–7. Arches of the foot illustrated on a lateral view.

calcaneus at these three points to form the **talocalcaneal** or **subtalar joint.** A small circular canal on this joint known as the **sinus tarsi** allows for the passage of blood vessels and ligaments. A projection of bone on the medial aspect of the calcaneus forms a shelf or support on which the talus rests. This bony process is called the **sustentaculum tali** (SUS-ten-TAK-ū-lum TĀ-lē). There are several other bony processes on the calcaneus which will be demonstrated radiographically on an axial projection. The large **tuberosity** of the calcaneus forms the "heel" of the foot. This is the roughened, posterior part of the bone. The Achilles tendon attaches to the posterior surface of the tuberosity. The **trochlear process** is a ridge of bone located on the distal, lateral side of the calcaneus. The **lateral** and **medial processes** are rounded bony processes found on either side of the tuberosity *(Figure 7–6).*

Arches of the Foot

To enable the foot to support the weight of the body, the tarsals and metatarsals are arranged into three arches. Strong ligaments and tendons in the foot form a half-dome shape that redistributes the weight among the bones of the foot. Like springs, the arches yield when a person is applying weight to the foot (ie, through standing, walking, jumping) to cushion shocks. The arches return to their normal shape when the weight is removed.

Two longitudinal arches run the length of each foot on its medial and lateral sides. The transverse arch is formed on the plantar surface by the bases of the metatarsals, the cuboid, cuneiforms, and calcaneus. It extends across the foot from its medial to lateral borders. The condition known as **pes planus** or **flatfoot** occurs when the ligaments and tendons of the longitudinal arches are excessively strained and weakened. An irregular prominence known as a **bunion** is formed when the transverse arch is weakened, causing an enlargement of the first metatarsophalangeal joint and displacement of the great toe *(Figure 7–7).*

LOWER LEG

Each lower leg is comprised of two long bones, the tibia (TIB-ē-ah) and the fibula (FIB-ū-lah) *(Figure 7–8).* These bones are roughly parallel to each other and extend from the knee joint to the ankle joint. They are held together by fibrous interosseous tissue. As a result of this arrangement, an injury to one bone might result in an injury to the other. For example, if the distal tibia is fractured as the result of a twisting type of injury, it is highly probable that the proximal fibula will also be fractured.

Tibia

The tibia is commonly referred to as the shinbone. It is the weight-bearing bone of the lower leg and, as such, is larger than the fibula. It is located medially to the fibula and assists in the formation of both the ankle and knee joints.

The distal extremity or end of the tibia articulates directly with the talus. The inferior surface of the tibia is slightly concave where it sits over the rounded trochlea of the talus. The **medial malleolus** (mah-LĒ-ō-lus) is a large process that can be palpated on the medial aspect of the ankle. It projects medially over the talus to provide stability to the medial side of the ankle joint. The **fibular notch** is situated on the distal lateral aspect of the tibia just opposite the medial malleolus. It is a smooth, depressed area that articulates with the fibula to form the distal tibiofibular joint. A slightly curved prominence on the posterior margin of the tibia is usually referred to as the **posterior malleolus.** It is important to be aware of this area as it can be involved in a trimalleolar fracture. This serious injury involves the medial and posterior malleoli of the tibia, as well as the lateral malleolus of the fibula.

The shaft or diaphysis of the tibia forms the body of the bone. It is large and sturdy and designed to bear weight. The **anterior crest** is a sharp ridge that runs the length of the shaft on its anterior surface. It is easily palpated (and bruised) as it lies just under the skin and is not covered by muscle tissue.

The proximal extremity or end of the tibia is expanded to provide for articulation with the femur. Large processes located on the medial and lateral aspects of the upper tibia are known respectively as the **medial** and **lateral condyles. Articular facets** on the superior aspect of the tibia are smooth and concave for articulation with the rounded condyles of the femur. These structures are referred to collectively as the **tibial plateau.** The **intercondylar (intercondyloid) eminence** or **tibial spine** is situated on the tibial plateau between the medial and lateral articular facets. It consists of two pointed tubercles which project upward into the intercondylar fossa of the femur. The **fibular facet** is a smooth articular surface on the posterolateral aspect of the lateral condyle of the tibia. The head of the fibula articulates with the tibia at this point to form the proximal tibiofibular joint.

The **tibial tuberosity** is a large roughened prominence that can be palpated on the anterior aspect of the proximal tibia just inferior to the condyles. It serves as the site of a muscle attachment. A sudden growth spurt during adolescence can result in the bones growing at a faster rate than the muscles. If this occurs, the patellar ligament, which attaches to the tibial tuberosity, is pulled tight and, in some cases, can actually pull the tibial tuberosity free from the shaft of the tibia. This condition, known as **Osgood–Schlatter disease,** can be demonstrated on a lateral projection of the lower leg or knee.

Fibula

The fibula, or calf bone, is a long, slender bone located laterally and slightly posteriorly to the tibia. The fibula acts as a splint or crutch for the tibia, but does not bear the weight of the body. It is the site for important muscle attachments.

At its distal end, the fibula has an expanded process on its lateral side called the **lateral malleolus.** This structure articulates with the talus at the ankle joint. Like the medial malleolus of the tibia, the lateral malleolus overhangs the talus to provide support to the ankle joint on its lateral side, with its inferior tip extending slightly lower and more posteriorly than the medial malleolus. The distal fibula articulates with the fibular notch of the tibia just above the ankle joint to form the distal tibiofibular joint.

The shaft or diaphysis forms the slender body of the fibula. This sticklike structure is parallel to the shaft of the tibia.

The head and neck of the fibula are found at its proximal end. The head is expanded and pointed on its superior aspect. This point is known as the **apex** or **styloid process.** The neck is the slightly constricted area just inferior to the head. The head of the fibula articulates with the proximal tibia on the posteroinferior aspect of the lateral tibial condyle. The fibula does not extend as high as the tibia and, therefore, does not assist in the formation of the knee joint.

UPPER LEG

The single bone of the upper leg or thigh is the **femur** (FĒ-mur). It extends from the hip joint to the knee joint and is the longest bone in the body, measuring approximately one fourth of the body's height. As a weight-bearing structure, it is also the body's strongest bone.

The femur articulates distally with the tibia to form the knee joint. The broadened distal extremity or end of the femur consists of two condyles, two epicondyles, an intercondylar fossa, and a patellar surface.

The **medial** and **lateral condyles** of the femur are rounded, knoblike processes found on the inferior portion of each femur. The smooth articular surfaces of the condyles articulate with the tibial plateau of the tibial condyles. A deep U-shaped notch on the posterior surface of the femur, the **intercondylar fossa,** separates the condyles from each other. The **medial** and **lateral epicondyles** are prominences found on the superior portion of the medial and lateral condyles, respectively. These rough areas serve as sites for muscle attachment. The medial epicondyle is the larger of the two processes, just as the medial condyle is slightly larger and extends more distally than the lateral condyle. The **patellar surface** is the smooth area located between the condyles on the anterior surface of the distal femur. It is directly anterior to the intercondylar fossa. The patella articulates with the femur at this surface.

Occasionally, a pea-shaped sesamoid bone known as a **fabella** (fah-BEL-ah) develops in the gastrocnemius muscle. This is located directly behind the lateral condyle of the femur and can be demonstrated radiographically (*Figure 7–9*).

The body of the femur is its shaft or diaphysis. It is long, smooth, and cylindrical. On the posterior surface of the femur, a vertical ridge called the **linea aspera** (LIN-ē-ah AS-per-ah) runs the length of the shaft. Abductor muscles of the thigh attach to this prominence. Instead of being truly vertical, the shaft of the femur is positioned in the leg at an approximate 10° medial angle. It is also slightly curved for added strength.

The proximal extremity or end of the femur articulates with the pelvis to form the hip joint. The **head** of the femur is a ball-like structure that fits into a cup-shaped socket on the pelvis called the **acetabulum** (as-ĕ-TAB-ū-lum). Together, these structures form the hip joint. A small pit on the center of the femoral head, the **fovea capitis** (FŌ-vē-ah KAP-i-tis), is often demonstrated on a radiograph of the hip. A ligament attaches the acetabulum to the femoral head at the fovea capitis. Blood vessels also enter the femoral head at this site.

Just inferior to the rounded head is the constricted neck of the femur. The **neck** essentially connects the head to the shaft. It is angled laterally and posteriorly from the head, and forms an angle of approximately 120° with the shaft. As the weakest area of the femur, the neck is a common site of fractures. When a patient is said to have a "hip" fracture, the area of injury is usually the femoral neck.

Two rough prominences are situated at the junction of the neck and shaft of the femur. The **greater trochanter** (trō-KAN-ter) is found on the lateral margin of the proximal femur. Because it is quite sizable and can be palpated on the upper thigh, it is a practical positioning landmark. The highest point of the greater trochanter lies approximately 1.5 in. (3.8 cm) above the symphysis pubis. The **lesser trochanter** is

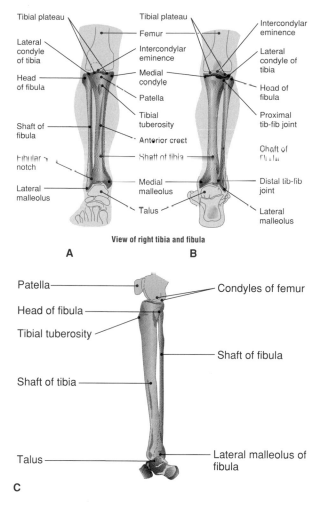

View of right tibia and fibula

A   **B**

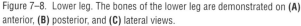

C

Figure 7–8. Lower leg. The bones of the lower leg are demonstrated on **(A)** anterior, **(B)** posterior, and **(C)** lateral views.

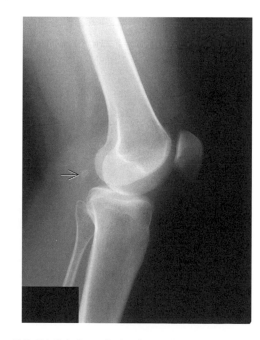

Figure 7–9. Fabella in the popliteal region on a lateral projection of the knee.

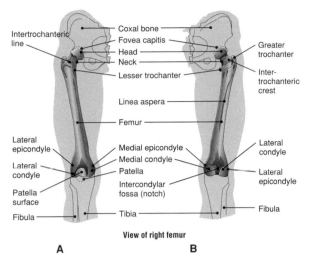

Figure 7–10. Femur. The single bone of the upper leg is demonstrated on **(A)** anterior and **(B)** posterior views.

smaller and lies on the posteromedial aspect of the proximal femur. Because of its location, it is not palpable. The greater and lesser trochanters both serve as attachment points for muscles of the buttock and thigh. The trochanters are connected on either side by a ridge of bone, the **intertrochanteric** (in-ter-trō-kan-TER-ic) **line** anteriorly and the **intertrochanteric crest** posteriorly *(Figure 7–10)*.

KNEECAP

Patella

Each leg has one patella (pah-TEL-ah), or kneecap. Classified as the largest sesamoid bone in the body, it develops in the tendon of the quadriceps femoris muscle, which attaches the anterior thigh muscles to the tibia. The patella is roughly a flat triangular bone, approximately 2 in. (5 cm) in diameter, designed to protect the knee joint and provide leverage to the muscle. The somewhat flat upper margin of the bone is called the **base;** the pointed inferior surface is termed the **apex.** The area between these two structures is the **body.** The patella has two surfaces. The **anterior surface** is the outer surface of the bone, in other words, the part that can be palpated under the skin. The **posterior surface** is the side that is adjacent to the femur. It is smooth and slightly curved to allow the patella to glide over the distal femur as the knee bends. The patella is easily palpated. With the knee in an extended position, it is somewhat movable. As the knee is flexed, the patella becomes fixed in position. Because of its location, it is subject to fracture or dislocation as the result of a direct blow to the anterior knee *(Figure 7–11)*.

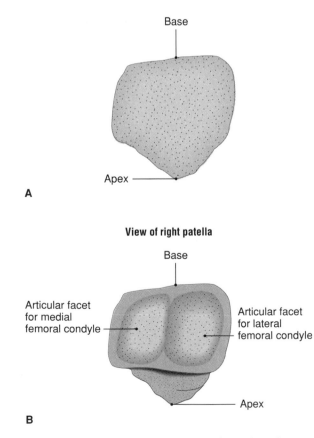

Figure 7–11. Patella. **(A)** Anterior surface, **(B)** posterior surface.

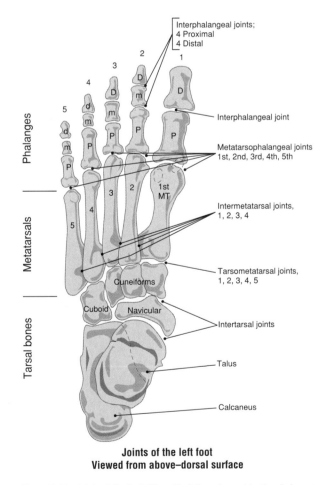

Figure 7–12. Joints of the foot. The articulations formed by the phalanges, metatarsals, and tarsals are illustrated on a superior view.

ARTHROLOGY OF THE LOWER LIMB (EXTREMITY)

The bones of the lower limb form many articulations which make it possible for the body to walk, run, dance, climb, and so on. For the most part, they are classified as diarthrodial joints that are synovial in structure. The only exception is the distal tibiofibular joint, which is a fibrous, amphiarthrodial joint.

The **interphalangeal joints** are formed between the phalanges of the toes. They are named according to their location and are classified as diarthrodial joints with hinge-type movements of flexion and extension. The **distal interphalangeal joints** are formed by the articulation of the distal phalanges with the middle phalanges. The **proximal interphalangeal joints** are formed by the articulation of the middle phalanges with the proximal phalanges. Like the first digit of the upper limb, the great toe only has one interphalangeal joint.

The **metatarsophalangeal joints** are formed by the articulation of the proximal phalanges with the heads of the metatarsals. There are five metatarsophalangeal joints in each foot. These diarthrodial joints have condylar or ellipsoidal movements of flexion, extension, abduction, and adduction. **Intermetatarsal joints** are formed by the articulation of the bases of the metatarsals with one another. There are four such joints in each foot, each having gliding movement.

There are five **tarsometatarsal joints** in each foot. They are located between the distal tarsal bones and the bases of the metatarsals. Specifically, the first metatarsal articulates with the medial cuneiform, the second metatarsal with the intermediate cuneiform, the third metatarsal with the lateral cuneiform, and the fourth and fifth metatarsals with the cuboid. These are diarthrodial joints with gliding movement.

The **intertarsal joints** are formed between adjacent tarsal bones. As gliding joints, they permit slight movement. The most movement occurs at the calcaneocuboid and talonavicular joints, which allow inversion and eversion movements of the foot. The talocalcaneal, or subtalar, joint is a three-faceted weight-bearing joint. As weight is transferred from the talus to the calcaneus, slight gliding movement occurs *(Figure 7–12)*.

The **ankle joint** is often referred to as the tibiotalar joint, which implies that the joint is formed between the tibia and talus. Actually, the tibia and fibula both articulate with the talus to form the ankle joint. The inferior margin of the tibia is slightly concave to articulate with the rounded trochlea of the talus, whereas the medial malleolus of the tibia articulates with the medial border of the talus. The lateral malleolus of the fibula articulates with the lateral margin of the talus. Together, the malleoli help to stabilize the joint by overlapping it on its sides. Along with the inferior surface of the tibia, the malleoli form a three-sided recess into which the talus fits securely. This construction resembles a mortise lock; hence, the ankle joint is also known as the **mortise joint.** To demonstrate this joint space radiographically, the lower limb must be internally rotated 15° *(Figure 7–13)*.

The ankle joint is a hinge joint, permitting flexion and extension movements or, more specifically, dorsiflexion and plantar flexion *(Figure 7–14)*. Strong ligaments are present to hold the bones of the ankle together. Inversion and eversion movements are not normal movements of the ankle joint. If an injury occurs that involves either of these movements (eg, ankle turns inward during ice skating), ligament damage usually takes place along with a possible bony injury.

There are two tibiofibular joints. The **distal tibiofibular joint** is formed by the articulation of the fibular notch of the tibia with the inferior portion of the fibula at a point just superior to the ankle joint. Ligaments bind the tibia and fibula together as a syndesmosis or fibrous joint. As the only amphiarthrodial joint in the lower extremity, it allows very slight "giving" movement. To demonstrate this joint radiographically, it is necessary to internally rotate the lower limb 45°. The **proximal tibiofibular joint** is formed by the head of the fibula articulating with the posterior aspect of the lateral condyle of the tibia. It is located inferiorly and laterally to the knee joint and is not part of the knee joint proper. This joint is a diarthrodial joint with gliding movement *(Figure 7–15)*.

As the largest joint in the body, the **knee joint** is also one of the most complex. It is actually composed of three separate articulations of the femur. The lateral and medial condyles articulate with their respective condyles of the tibia to collectively form the **tibiofemoral joint.** The patella also articulates with the patellar surface of the femur to form the **femoropatellar joint.**

Functionally, the knee joint appears to be a hinge joint. It allows flexion and extension movements. Because of its construction, however, it also permits some rotational movement when the knee is flexed. Movement occurs when the rounded condyles of the femur roll on the concave tibial plateau. As a weight-bearing joint, much stress is placed on the knee joint, particularly in jumping activities where the forces on it amount to almost seven times the weight of the body. To cushion the direct impact of the femur on the tibia, wedge-shaped fibrocartilage pads known as **menisci** are present within the joint and lie between the femoral and tibial condyles. The menisci are situated on the tibial plateau and are attached to the lateral margins of the tibial condyles. The knee joint is partially encapsulated on its lateral, medial, and posterior aspects. There are at least 12 bursae present in the area surrounding the joint. As stated in Chapter 4, the bursae are sacs that secrete synovial fluid to lubricate the joint and reduce friction between the articulating

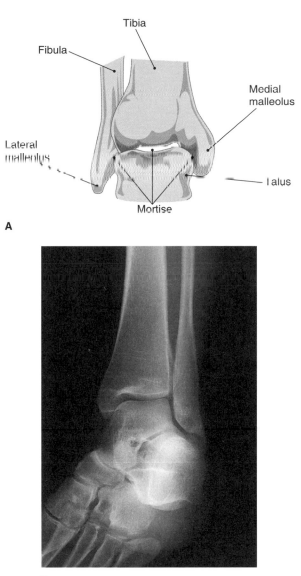

A

B

Figure 7–13. Ankle joint. The joint formed by the tibia, fibula, and talus is illustrated on a **(A)** frontal view and an **(B)** oblique projection.

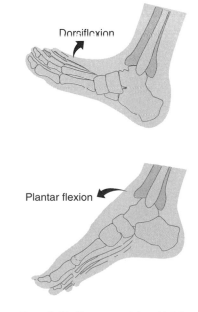

Figure 7–14. Movements of the ankle joint.

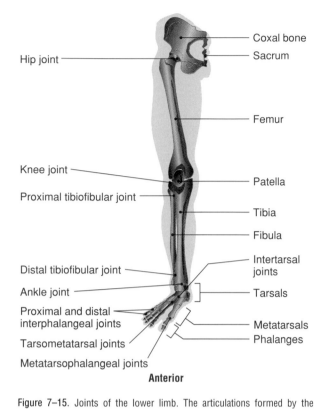

Anterior

Figure 7–15. Joints of the lower limb. The articulations formed by the bones of the lower limb are demonstrated on an anterior view.

Table 7–3. Summary of the Joints of the Lower Limb (Extremity)

Name of Joint	Classification	Structure	Movement
Interphalangeal	Diarthrodial	Synovial	Hinge
Metatarsophalangeal	Diarthrodial	Synovial	Condylar
Intermetatarsal	Diarthrodial	Synovial	Gliding
Tarsometatarsal	Diarthrodial	Synovial	Gliding
Intertarsal	Diarthrodial	Synovial	Gliding
Ankle (tibiotalar and fibulotalar)	Diarthrodial	Synovial	Hinge
Tibiofibular			
Distal	Amphiarthrodial	Syndesmosis	Slight give
Proximal	Diarthrodial	Synovial	Gliding
Knee			
Tibiofemoral	Diarthrodial	Synovial	Hinge
Femoropatellar	Diarthrodial	Synovial	Gliding
Hip		Synovial	Ball and socket

bones. The joint is stabilized by strong ligaments, tendons, and muscles. Of particular importance are the **cruciate ligaments** (*cruci* = "cross"), which attach to the anterior and posterior aspects of the tibial plateau. As they extend upward to attach to the femoral condyles, these ligaments cross each other to strengthen and stabilize the joint. Medial and lateral **collateral ligaments** bind the bones together. When the leg is extended, the knee "locks," with the collateral ligaments pulling tightly on the bones. When the knee is flexed, some slackness occurs in these ligaments, permitting some rotational movement. The **popliteal ligament** reinforces the posterior aspect of the joint capsule. Note that the area behind the knee is routinely referred to as the *popliteal region (Figure 7–16)*.

The **hip joint** is a ball-and-socket joint formed by the rounded head of the femur articulating with the socket, or acetabulum, of the pelvis. This joint is discussed more completely in Chapter 8.

Table 7–3 summarizes the joints of the lower limb and their movement type.

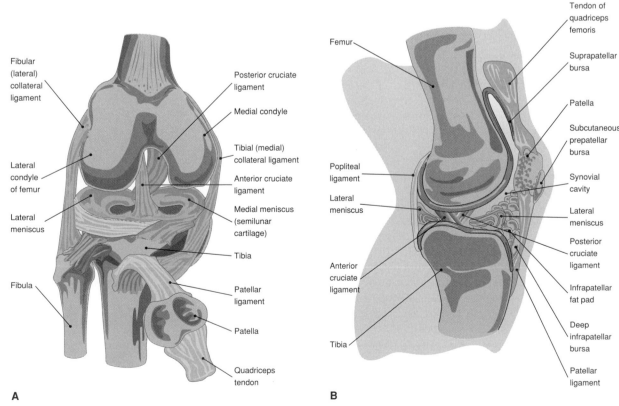

Figure 7–16. Knee joint. The structures forming the knee joint are illustrated on **(A)** anterior and **(B)** lateral views.

▶ PROCEDURAL CONSIDERATIONS

Although radiographs of the knees, feet, and ankles may be performed on request with the patient standing (weight bearing), most radiographic procedures of the lower limb are obtained with the patient sitting or lying on the radiographic table or stretcher. Radiographic examinations of the lower limb include those frequently performed, such as foot, ankle, and knee, as well as those infrequently performed or performed primarily in orthopedic clinics, such as special patella and intercondylar fossa projections.

PATIENT PREPARATION

To prevent unwanted artifacts on the radiographs, all articles of clothing should be removed from the area of interest. When radiographing the foot or ankle, the pantleg can usually be rolled or moved upward to eliminate it as a source of artifacts. For lower leg and knee radiography, it is sometimes impossible for the patient to move the pantleg above the knee, making it necessary for the patient to remove the pants and wear a patient gown. Radiographic examinations of the femur require the removal of all garments below the waist. Because shoes can elevate the legs from the table and increase object–image distance, shoes should be removed for all examinations of the lower limb.

Obtaining a pertinent patient history, as described in Chapter 4, can assist the radiographer in determining whether any changes in routine procedure, relative to film size, centering, or patient positioning, may be required. Some changes may need to be discussed with the radiologist or attending physician.

POSITIONING CONSIDERATIONS

Because the lower limb is made up primarily of long bones, it is important to remember several basic rules of positioning. Although both joints should be included in each projection, it is sometimes impossible to do this without making more than one exposure. In this situation, at least one complete joint should be included on each projection. For example, when the lower leg is radiographed, the ankle joint can be included on the longer films, with separate AP and lateral projections of the knee obtained using smaller films in the Bucky tray or tabletop, depending on patient size. Some department protocols dictate that the joint nearest the fracture be included on the larger film so the entire fracture is on one film. Because the lower leg is normally radiographed using a tabletop technique, the cassette can also be turned diagonally to include both joints on the same film. When the femur is radiographed, the longer films usually include the knee joint, with smaller films used to image the proximal femur and hip joint. There should be an overlap of at least 1 to 2 in. to allow the radiologist to match the films.

Because central ray angles are usually parallel to the long axis of the table, the part of interest should also be parallel to the long axis of the radiographic table. Failure to do so can produce unwanted distortion or partial closure of a joint space when using a central ray angle. Although patient condition may make it a challenge, the part should also be parallel to the film plane and the central ray should be perpendicular to the long axis of the structure of interest to minimize distortion (see Chapter 1). Radiographing the lower leg of a patient who could not fully extend the knee, for example, might require tilting the cassette and angling the central ray appropriately. As for all radiographic examinations, collimation is an important factor in reducing patient exposure and improving radiographic quality. Collimation should include all soft tissue and joints proximal and distal to the area of interest. Gonadal shielding can be used for all examinations of the lower limb.

As discussed in Chapter 4, at least two projections 90° apart should be obtained (Table 7–4). Normally, these projections are AP and lateral. Lateral projections of structures in the lower limb generally require the patient to turn either partially or totally onto the affected side. Because trauma or other conditions often preclude this, it may be necessary to obtain the lateral projections using a horizontal beam. In this situation, the cassette is supported vertically by sandbags or cassette holder adjacent to the part of interest. If possible, the part of interest should be elevated on a radiolucent support to center the structure to the cassette. If a fracture is apparent, no attempt should be made to rotate the part; obtaining two projections 90° apart will be acceptable.

Periodically, a special view of the intercondylar fossa may be requested. Commonly referred to as a **tunnel** or **notch view,** this projection can be obtained by one of several different methods. The patient can be prone, kneeling, or sitting with the knee flexed. A horizontal (transverse) fracture of the patella should be ruled out prior to flexing the knee, however, to prevent unnecessary pain and further damage.

Table 7–4. Routine and Optional* Projections: Lower Limb (Extremity)

Toes	Knee
AP	AP
Internal (medial) oblique	Medial (internal) oblique*
Lateral*	Lateral (external) oblique*
Foot	Lateral
AP	Patella
Medial (internal) oblique	PA/AP
Calcaneus (os calcis)	Tangential (Settegast [sunrise]/Hughston)
Plantodorsal/dorsoplantar	Lateral
Lateral	Intercondylar fossa
Ankle	PA/AP
AP	axial (Camp–Coventry/
Medial (internal) oblique	Homblad/Beclere)
Lateral	
Lower leg	Femur
AP	AP
Lateral	Lateral

Note. Although routine procedures vary according to department protocol, this table identifies some of the more common routine and optional projections.
*Optional projections; may be routine in some departments.

ALTERNATE PROJECTIONS

Following normal radiographic examination of the ankle or knee, it is sometimes necessary to obtain **stress views** to assist in the identification of possible partial or complete tears in the ligaments. To assess medial and lateral collateral ligament injury of the ankle, stress views are obtained with the patient positioned as for the routine AP ankle projection, remembering to dorsiflex the foot. Wearing a lead apron and gloves, a physician or other health professional holds the lower leg with one hand and inverts or everts the foot with the other hand, keeping the plantar surface of the foot perpendicular to the table *(Figure 7–17)*. Comparison views should be obtained because of the wide range of normal variation between patients. The lateral collateral ligament of the ankle is more frequently torn than the medial and is demonstrated by the widening of the lateral talotibial joint on the stressed inversion projection *(Figure 7–18)*.

Stress views of the knee may be indicated when either medial or lateral joint widening is seen on routine radiographs of the knee. These studies may be done unilaterally or bilaterally. Although it generally takes someone with considerable strength to apply the necessary stress, other techniques are available to assist in obtaining the desired images. With the patient positioned for an AP bilateral projection of the knees, a strap or belt is wrapped around the thighs to keep them together while lateral stress is applied to the lower legs to evaluate the medial collateral ligaments *(Figures 7–19)*. To assess the lateral collateral ligaments, a wooden block or other device is place between the knees while medial stress is applied to the lower legs *(Figure 7–20)*. Stress views can be very painful for the patient. Patients experiencing severe pain may require anesthesia for the procedure *(Figure 7–21)*.

To evaluate the arches in the feet, weight-bearing, or standing, projections may be requested. For this examination, the AP projection may be obtained either unilaterally or bilaterally with the patient standing on a cassette placed on the floor. A 15° cephalic central ray angle and 40-in. SID are used *(Figure 7–22)*. The lateral foot projections are obtained unilaterally with the patient standing on a firm support. The cassette is supported between the feet and the central ray is directed horizontally *(Figures 7–23, 7–24, 7–25)*.

Occasionally, weight-bearing AP or PA bilateral projections of knees are obtained to evaluate degenerative arthritis. Both knees are included on a single 14 × 17-in. cassette positioned crosswise in a vertical grid device for this examination. The patient should be standing straight with feet directed forward, heels positioned directly under the hips (if possible), and weight equally distributed on both feet. The central ray is directed horizontally through the knee joints *(Figures 7–26, 7–27)*.

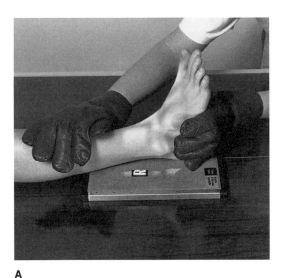

A

B

Figure 7–17. Lateral collateral ligament damage is evaluated by stress inversion **(A)** and eversion **(B)** of the foot.

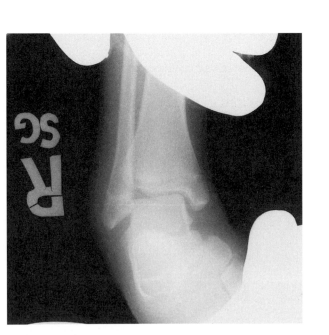

Figure 7–18. Stress was applied to evaluate the lateral collateral ligament of the ankle.

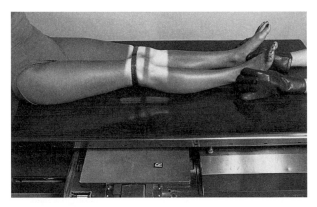

Figure 7–19. Bilateral stress views of the knees can be performed to evaluate the medial collateral ligaments.

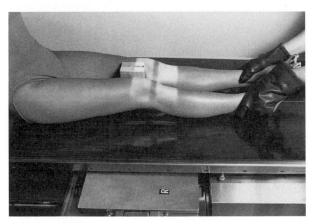

Figure 7–20. Bilateral stress applied to demonstrate the lateral collateral ligament.

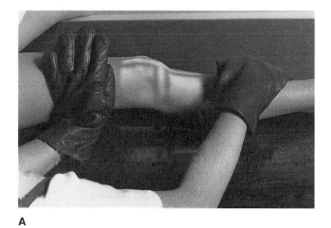

A

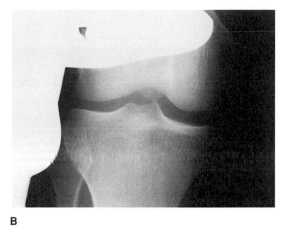

B

Figure 7–21. Unilateral study of the medial collateral ligament.

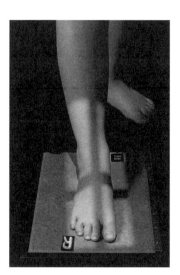

Figure 7–22. AP standing foot.

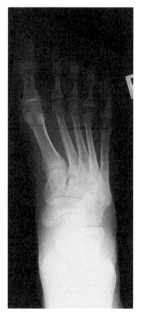

Figure 7–23. AP standing foot.

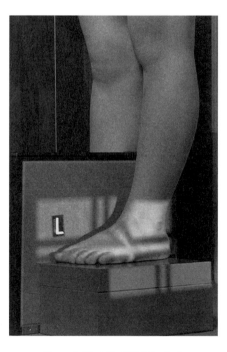

Figure 7–24. Lateral standing foot.

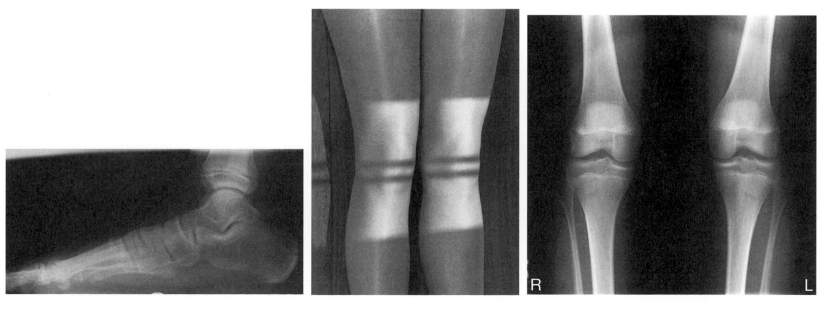

Figure 7–25. Lateral standing foot.

Figure 7–26. AP standing knees.

Figure 7–27. AP standing knees.

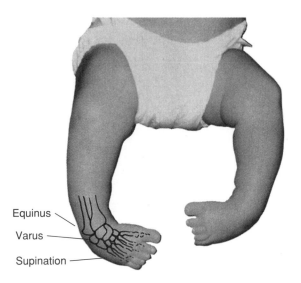

Figure 7–28. In a typical clubfoot, the bones are deviated from normal position. *(From Ball J, Bindler R. Pediatric Nursing. Stamford, CT: Appleton & Lange, 1995. Photo courtesy of Lynn T. Staheli, MD.)*

Equinus
Varus
Supination

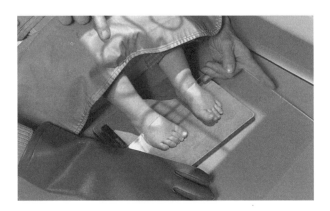

Figure 7–29. The patient may be standing or sitting for the AP projection; a plexiglass plate can be used for immobilization or to simulate the stress of standing when the patient is seated.

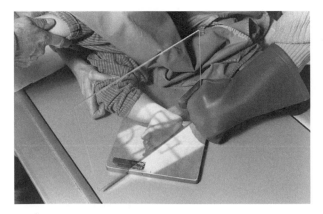

Figure 7–30. If the patient is unable to stand, a plexiglass strip held firmly against the plantar surface of the foot can be used to simulate standing.

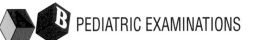 PEDIATRIC EXAMINATIONS

Although the positioning for most radiographic examinations of children is similar to that of adults, several procedures are performed primarily on children. Clubfoot (talipes equinovarus), one of the most common congenital deformities in infants, involves three deviations of the foot from normal alignment relative to the leg: plantar flexion with inversion of the calcaneus, medial displacement of the forefoot, and elevation of the medial border of the foot *(Figure 7–28)*. Weight-bearing views, if the patient is old enough to stand, should be obtained to determine the degree of deformity *(Figure 7–29)*. On younger patients, a plexiglass strip can be held against the plantar surface of the foot for a lateral projection with the foot in stressed dorsiflexion to simulate weight bearing *(Figure 7–30)*

Bone-length studies, or **scanograms,** are bilateral examinations performed to accurately illustrate discrepancy in length of the lower limbs; the legs can be radiographed simultaneously or separately. Although several methods are used to accomplish this examination, it is commonly performed using a radiopaque ruler and three exposures. Before the patient is positioned on the table, a radiopaque ruler is taped to the midline of the table *(Figure 7–31)*. Some facilities use two radiopaque rulers, taping them parallel to each other on the table and aligned approximately to each limb (keeping in mind that the patient will be centered to the table). The patient is then assisted to the supine position on the table, positioning the hips, knees, and ankles over the rulers. A single 14 × 17-in. cassette positioned lengthwise in the Bucky tray may be used *(Figure 7–32)*. The first exposure is made of the hips using the upper third of the cassette. Collimation and lead-impregnated vinyl placed directly over the lower two thirds of the cassette should eliminate concern of scatter radiation fogging the rest of the cassette. The second exposure is made of the knees using the middle third of the cassette, being sure to collimate and shield the remainder of the cassette. The last exposure is made of the ankles using the lower third of the cassette, while the upper two thirds of the cassette is shielded. Appropriate technical factors should be used for each body part and centering should be to the joint spaces *(Figure 7–33)*. Careful placement of gonadal shielding is important because of the number of examinations these patients often have. Surgery and follow-up studies may be required if the discrepancy is severe.

A bilateral AP projection of both knees may be requested to evaluate a child for lead poisoning. Although increased density at the epiphyseal plates of the femur and tibia is normal, dense bands seen at the growth plates of the proximal fibulas could indicate lead toxicity. Plain abdominal radiography may be performed to evaluate ingestion of leaded paint chips.

EXPOSURE FACTORS

The kilovoltage used for projections of the lower extremities ranges from 50 to 75 kVp. The appropriate mAs depends on the size of the part, type of equipment generator, film/screen speed, pathology, and presence or absence of a splint or cast, as discussed in Chapter 4.

EQUIPMENT CONSIDERATIONS

Although most radiographic examinations of the upper limb can be performed without a grid, the lower limb is larger and requires the use of a grid for imaging of the femur. Although radiography of the knee is performed either with or without a grid, the use of a grid is also recommended for most radiographic examinations of the knee to improve radiographic contrast. Children and small adults with knees measuring less than 10 cm can be radiographed without a grid. Lower legs, ankles, and feet are routinely radiographed using a nongrid technique.

The cassette size is determined by part size, number of projections on one film, availability, and department protocol. Detail, or slow speed, film/screen combinations are often used for radiographic examination of the toes, foot, calcaneus, and ankle. Radiolucent supports and sandbags should be used for immobilization as long as they do not interfere with the anatomy of interest.

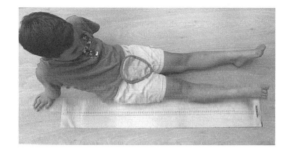

Figure 7–31. A ruler with radiopaque numbers is used to measure bone length.

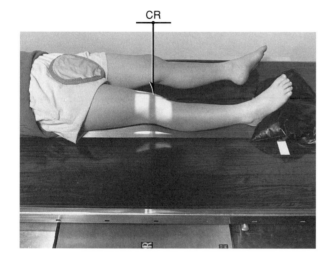

Figure 7–32. Gonadal shielding should be used when performing bone length studies of the legs.

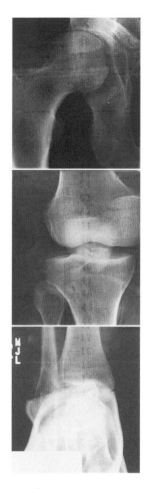

Figure 7–33. Scanogram of the right leg.

RADIOGRAPHIC POSITIONING OF THE LOWER LIMB (EXTREMITY)

- ► AP TOES

- ► MEDIAL OBLIQUE TOES

- ► LATERAL TOES (INDIVIDUAL)

- ► TANGENTIAL METATARSOPHALANGEAL SESAMOIDS

- ► AP FOOT

- ► MEDIAL OBLIQUE FOOT

- ► LATERAL FOOT

- ► AXIAL PLANTODORSAL CALCANEUS (OS CALCIS)

- ► LATERAL CALCANEUS (OS CALCIS)

- ► AP ANKLE

- ► MEDIAL OBLIQUE ANKLE

- ► LATERAL ANKLE

- ► AP LOWER LEG

- ► LATERAL LOWER LEG

- ► AP KNEE

- ► MEDIAL (INTERNAL) OBLIQUE KNEE

- ► LATERAL (EXTERNAL) OBLIQUE KNEE

- ► LATERAL KNEE

- ► PA AXIAL INTERCONDYLAR FOSSA (CAMP–CONVENTRY METHOD)

- ► PA AXIAL INTERCONDYLAR FOSSA (HOLMBLAD METHOD)

- ► AP AXIAL INTERCONDYLAR FOSSA (BECLERE METHOD)

- ► PA PATELLA

- ► LATERAL PATELLA

- ► TANGENTIAL PATELLA & FEMOROPATELLAR JOINT ("SUNRISE," "SKYLINE," SETTEGAST METHOD)

- ► TANGENTIAL PATELLA & FEMOROPATELLAR JOINT (HUGHSTON METHOD)

- ► AP FEMUR

- ► LATERAL FEMUR

► AP TOES

Technical Considerations

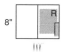

- Film size: 8 × 10 in. crosswise or 9 × 9 in. masked in half or thirds.
- Nongrid; detail cassette if available.
- 50 kVp.
- Collimate to include soft tissue, all toes, and up to one half of distal metatarsals.

Shielding

- Gonadal shielding should be used on all patients, especially children and adults of reproductive age.

Patient Positioning

- Assist the patient to a seated position on the radiographic table or stretcher; the patient's legs should be parallel with the long axis of the table.

Part Positioning

- Flex the knee of the affected side until the plantar surface of the foot rests firmly on the cassette.
- Center the second metatarsophalangeal joint to the unmasked half of the cassette. The toes should be in contact with the cassette (Figure 7–34).

Central Ray

- Direct the central ray perpendicular to the unmasked half of the cassette through the second metatarsophalangeal joint. **Note:** The toes may also be radiographed individually. In this situation, the central ray is directed perpendicular to the metatarsophalangeal joint of the affected toe.

Image Evaluation

- Soft tissue structures of the toe(s) and one third to one half of the metatarsals should be included in the collimated area.
- The cortex and trabeculae should be visualized and clear.
- The long axis of the foot should be parallel with the long axis of the unmasked portion of the cassette.
- The proximal interphalangeal joints and metatarsophalangeal joints should be open and well demonstrated.
- The proximal phalanges should exhibit symmetric curvatures on the medial and lateral sides (Figure 7–35).

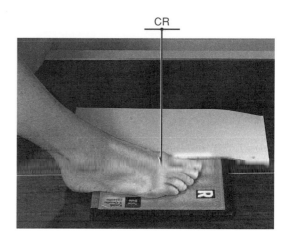

Figure 7–34. AP toes.

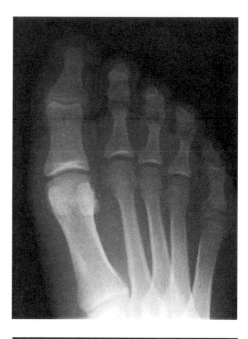

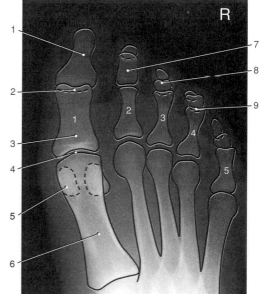

Figure 7–35. AP toes.

1. Distal phalanx, digits 1–5
2. Interphalangeal joint, 1st digit
3. Proximal phalanx, digits 1–5
4. Metatarsophalangal joint, 1–5
5. Sesamoid bone
6. Metatarsal, 1–5, distal
7. Middle phalanx, digits 2–5
8. Distal interphalangeal joint, digits 2–5
9. Proximal interphalangeal joint, digits 2–5

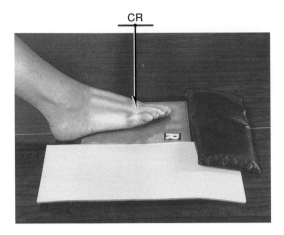

Figure 7–36. Medial oblique toes.

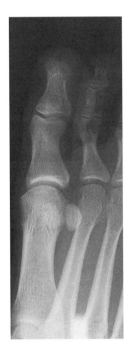

Figure 7–37. Medial oblique of the great toe.

► MEDIAL OBLIQUE TOES

Technical Considerations

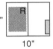

- Film size: 8 × 10 in. crosswise or 9 × 9 in. masked in half or thirds.
- Nongrid; detail cassette if available.
- 50 kVp.
- Collimate to include soft tissue, all toes, and one third to one half of distal metatarsals.

Shielding

- Gonadal shielding should be used on all patients, especially children and adults of reproductive age.

Patient Positioning

- Assist the patient to a seated position on the radiographic table or stretcher; the patient's legs should be parallel with the long axis of the table.

Part Positioning

- Flex the knee of the affected side until the plantar surface of the foot rests firmly on the table.
- Internally rotate the leg and foot until the plantar surface of the foot forms a 30° angle with the film plane; a sandbag can be used to immobilize the cassette.
- Center the third metatarsophalangeal joint to the unmasked half of the cassette *(Figure 7–36)*.

Central Ray

- Direct the central ray perpendicular to the unmasked half of the cassette through the second metatarsophalangeal joint. **Note:** The toes may also be radiographed individually. In this situation, the central ray is directed perpendicular to the metatarsophalangeal joint of the affected toe *(Figure 7–37)*.

Image Evaluation

- Soft tissue structures of all toes and one third to one half of the metatarsals should be included in the collimated area.
- The cortex and trabeculae should be visualized and clear.
- The long axis of the foot should be parallel with the long axis of the unmasked portion of the cassette.
- The proximal interphalangeal joints and metatarsophalangeal joints should be open and well demonstrated.
- The lateral aspect of the proximal phalanges should exhibit greater concavity than the medial side *(Figure 7–38).*

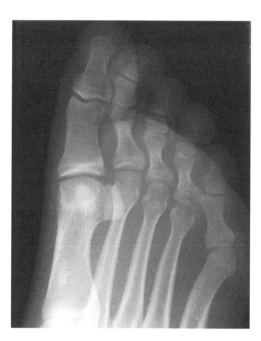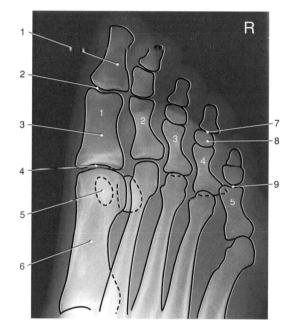

Figure 7–38. Medial oblique toes.

1. Distal phalanx, digits 1–5
2. Interphalangeal joint, 1st digit
3. Proximal phalanx, digits 1–5
4. Metatarsophalangeal joint, 1–5
5. Sesamoid bone
6. Metatarsal, 1 5
7. Distal interphalangeal joint, digits 2–5
8. Middle phalanx, digits 2–5
9. Proximal interphalangeal joint, digits 2–5

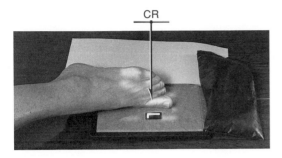

Figure 7–39. Lateral great toe (1st digit).

► LATERAL TOES (INDIVIDUAL)

Technical Considerations

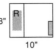

- Film size: 8 × 10 in. crosswise or 9 × 9 in. (can be divided for two or three projections)
- Nongrid; detail cassette if available.
- 50 kVp.
- Collimate to include soft tissue, toe of interest, and distal one third of metatarsal.

Shielding

- Gonadal shielding should be used on all patients, especially children and adults of reproductive age.

Patient Positioning

- Assist the patient to a seated position on the radiographic table or stretcher.

Part Positioning

- For the 1st (great toe) and 2nd digits, internally rotate the leg and foot to place the medial aspect of the foot on the cassette; for the 3rd to 5th digits, rotate the leg and foot laterally until the lateral side of the foot rests on the cassette.
- Adjust the rotation of the foot to place the injured toe in a true lateral position; the long axis of the affected toe should be parallel with the axis of the cassette.
- Using a tongue blade, tape, or gauze, move the unaffected toes away to prevent superimposition over the toe of interest; use care to avoid unnecessary pain.
- Center the metatarsophalangeal (1st digit) or proximal interphalangeal joint (2nd–5th digits) to the cassette *(Figure 7–39)*.

Central Ray

- Direct the central ray perpendicular to the cassette through the metatarsophalangeal joint (1st digit) or proximal interphalangeal joint (2nd–5th digits).

Image Evaluation

- Soft tissue structures of affected toe, metatarasophalangeal joint, and distal metatarsal should be included in the collimated area.
- The cortex and trabeculae should be visualized and clear.
- The long axis of the toe should be parallel with the axis of the unmasked portion of the cassette.
- The interphalangeal joint(s) should be open and well demonstrated.
- The posterior aspect of the proximal phalanx should exhibit greater concavity than the anterior surface *(Figure 7–40)*.

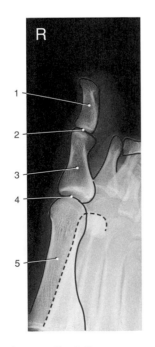

Figure 7–40. Lateral great toe (1st digit).

1. Distal phalanx	3. Proximal phalanx	5. 1st metatarsal
2. Interphalangeal joint	4. 1st metatarsophalangeal joint	

▶ TANGENTIAL METATARSOPHALANGEAL SESAMOIDS

Technical Considerations

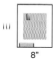

8"

- Film size: 8 × 10 in. lengthwise or 9 × 9 in.
- Nongrid; detail cassette if available.
- 50–55 kVp.
- Collimate to include soft tissue and heads of first, second, and third metatarsals.

Shielding

- Gonadal shielding should be used on all patients, especially children and adults of reproductive age.

Patient Positioning

- Assist the patient to a kneeling (or prone) position on the radiographic table or stretcher. **Note:** This projection can also be performed with the patient sitting; however, the increased OID will increase magnification of the sesamoids.
- Adjust patient's position so patient's legs are parallel to the long axis of the table.

Part Positioning

- Dorsiflex the foot and metatarsophalangeal joints of the affected side until the plantar surfaces of the toes rest firmly on the table.
- Center the first metatarsophalangeal joint to the cassette *(Figure 7–41)*.

Central Ray

- Direct the central ray perpendicular to the cassette through the first metatarsophalangeal joint.

Image Evaluation

- Heads of at least the first three metatarsals and the sesamoid bones should be included in the collimated area.
- The cortex and trabeculae should be visualized and clear.
- The long axis of the foot should be parallel with the long axis of the cassette.
- The joint spaces between the sesamoids and distal metatarsals should be open and clearly demonstrated *(Figure 7–42)*.

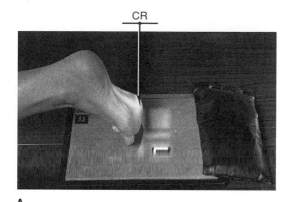

A

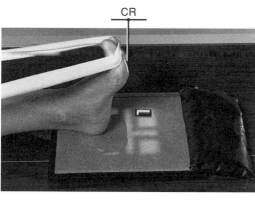

B

Figure 7–41. **(A)** Tangential metatarsophalangeal sesamoids. **(B)** Tangential sesamoids with patient seated.

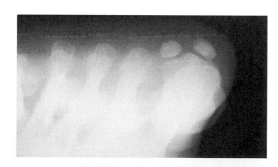

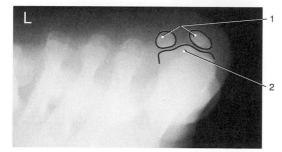

1. Sesamoid bones   2. 1st metatarsal, head

Figure 7–42. Tangential metatarsophalangeal sesamoids.

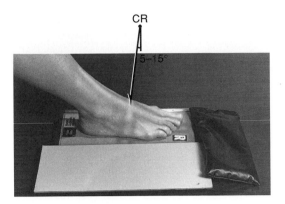

Figure 7–43. AP foot.

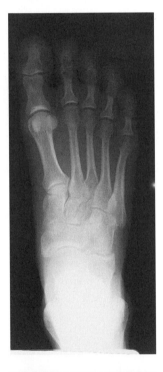

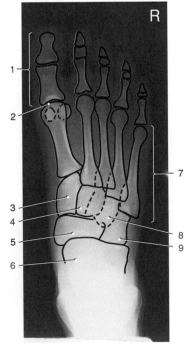

Figure 7–44. AP foot.

► AP FOOT

Technical Considerations

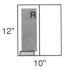

- Film size: 10 × 12 in. masked in half lengthwise.
- Nongrid; detail cassette if available.
- 50–55 kVp.
- Collimate to include soft tissue, all toes, and tarsals.

Shielding

- Gonadal shielding should be used on all patients, especially children and adults of reproductive age.

Patient Positioning

- Assist the patient to a seated position on the radiographic table or stretcher; the patient's legs should be parallel with the long axis of the table.

Part Positioning

- Flex the knee of the affected side until the plantar surface of the foot rests firmly on the table.
- Center the foot to the unmasked half of the cassette; the toes should be in contact with the cassette; a sandbag can be used to prevent the cassette from sliding (Figure 7–43).

Central Ray

- Direct the central ray 10° cephalad to the base of the third metatarsal. **Note:** The amount of central ray angulation can vary from 5° to 15°, depending on the size of the longitudinal arch. Some department protocols require a perpendicular central ray; a perpendicular central ray should be used when looking for a foreign body.

Image Evaluation

- Soft tissue structures of all toes and tarsals should be included in the collimated area.
- The cortex and trabeculae should be visualized and clear.
- The long axis of the foot should be parallel with the long axis of the unmasked portion of the cassette.
- The proximal interphalangeal joints, metatarsophalangeal joints, medial cuneiform, and navicular should be well demonstrated.
- The metatarsals should exhibit symmetrical curvatures on the medial and lateral sides (Figure 7–44).

1. Phalanges
2. Metatarsophalangeal joint
3. Medial cuneiform
4. Intermediate cuneiform
5. Navicular
6. Talus
7. Metatarsals
8. Lateral cuneiform
9. Cuboid

▶ MEDIAL OBLIQUE FOOT

Technical Considerations

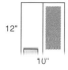

- Film size: 10 × 12 in. masked in half lengthwise.
- Nongrid; detail cassette if available.
- 50–55 kVp.
- Collimate to include soft tissue, all toes, and tarsals.

Shiolding

- Gonadal shielding should be used on all patients, especially children and adults of reproductive age.

Patient Positioning

- Assist the patient to a seated position on the radiographic table or stretcher; the patient's legs should be parallel with the long axis of the table.

Part Positioning

- Flex the knee of the affected side until the plantar surface of the foot rests firmly on the table.
- Internally rotate the leg and foot until the plantar surface of the foot forms a 30° angle with the film plane.
- Center the base of the third metatarsal to the unmasked half of the cassette *(Figure 7–45)*.

Central Ray

- Direct the central ray perpendicular to the unmasked half of the cassette through the base of the third metatarsal.

Image Evaluation

- Soft tissue structures of all toes and tarsals should be included in the collimated area.
- The cortex and trabeculae should be visualized and clear.
- The long axis of the foot should be parallel with the long axis of the unmasked portion of the cassette.
- The bases of the first and second metatarsals should be superimposed and the bases of the third, fourth, and fifth metatarsals should be free or nearly free of superimposition.
- The lateral intertarsal joints, cuboid, lateral cuneiform, and sinus tarsi should be well demonstrated.
- The lateral aspect of the metatarsals should exhibit greater concavity than the lateral side *(Figure 7–46)*.

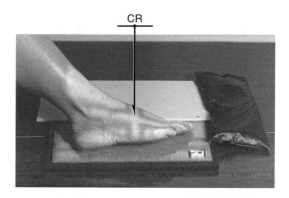

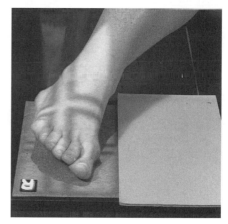

Figure 7–45. Medial oblique foot.

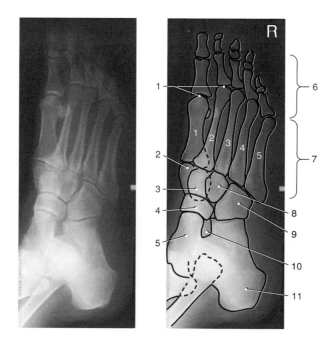

1. Metatarsophalangeal joint, 1–5	5. Talus	9. Cuboid
2. Medial cuneiform	6. Phalanges	10. Sinus tarsi
3. Intermediate cuneiform	7. Metatarsal, 3–5	11. Calcaneus
4. Navicular	8. Lateral cuneiform	

Figure 7–46. Medial oblique foot.

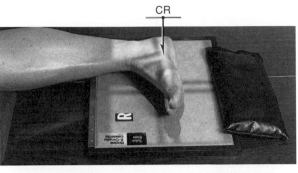

A

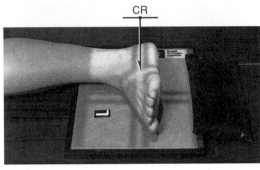

B

Figure 7–47. Lateral foot. The patient can be positioned with the lateral side nearest the film **(A)** or with the medial side against the cassette **(B)**.

▶ LATERAL FOOT

Technical Considerations

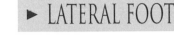

- Film size: 10 × 12 in. lengthwise with long axis of foot.
- Nongrid; detail cassette if available.
- 55–60 kVp.
- Collimate to include soft tissue, all toes, tarsals, ankle joint, and 1 in. of distal tibia and fibula.

Shielding

- Gonadal shielding should be used on all patients, especially children and adults of reproductive age.

Patient Positioning

- Assist the patient to the lateral recumbent position on the radiographic table or stretcher; the patient should be lying on the affected side.

Part Positioning

- Externally rotate the leg of the affected side until the patella is perpendicular to the film plane and the lateral aspect of the foot rests on the cassette. **Note:** The mediolateral projection, as described here, is usually performed because it is relatively comfortable for the patient. The lateromedial projection, with the medial surface adjacent to the cassette, is often preferred for those patients capable of assuming the position.
- Dorsiflex the foot and adjust the patient position so the plantar surface of the foot is perpendicular to the table; elevating the knee on a small support will help place the foot in the correct position.
- Center the cassette to the tarsometatarsal joints *(Figure 7–47)*.

Central Ray

- Direct the central ray perpendicular through the tarsometatarsal joints.

Image Evaluation

- Soft tissue structures of all toes, tarsals, ankle joint, and 1 in. of distal tibia and fibula should be included in the collimated area.
- The cortex and trabeculae of the tarsals and metatarsals should be visualized and clear.
- The long axis of the foot should be parallel with the long axis of the cassette (some departments permit angling the cassette diagonally to accommodate large feet).
- The metatarsals should be almost superimposed with the base of the fifth metatarsal extending slightly more inferiorly due to the transverse arch of the foot.
- The fibula should be under the posterior aspect of the tibia *(Figure 7–48)*.

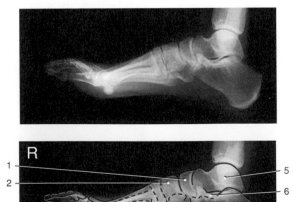

Figure 7–48. Lateral foot.

1. Navicular
2. Medial cuneiform
3. Sesamoid bone
4. 5th metatarsal, base
5. Talus
6. Subtalar joint
7. Calcaneus
8. Cuboid

► AXIAL PLANTODORSAL CALCANEUS (OS CALCIS)

Technical Considerations

- Film size: 8 × 10 in. or 10 × 12 in. masked in half crosswise.
- Nongrid; detail cassette if available.
- 60–65 kVp.
- Collimate to include calcaneus and subtalar joint.

Shielding

- Gonadal shielding should be used on all patients, especially children and adults of reproductive age.

Patient Positioning

- Assist the patient to a seated position on the radiographic table or stretcher; the patient's legs should be parallel with the long axis of the table. **Note:** The view can also be obtained with the patient prone, the cassette supported vertically against the plantar surface of the foot, and the central ray directed 40° caudally (dorsoplantar projection) *(Figure 7–49)*.

Part Positioning

- Center the unmasked half of the cassette to the malleoli of the ankle.
- Dorsiflex the affected foot.
- Position a long strip of tape or gauze around the ball of the foot and instruct the patient to gently pull back on the ends to immobilize the foot in 90° dorsiflexion.
- Center the base of the third metatarsal to the unmasked half of the cassette *(Figure 7–50)*.

Central Ray

- Direct the central ray 40° cephalad to the midplantar surface at the level of the base of the fifth metatarsal.

Image Evaluation

- Soft tissue structures of calcaneus and the subtalar joint should be included in the collimated area.
- The cortex and trabeculae should be visualized and clear; density and penetration should be sufficient to demonstrate the subtalar joint.
- The long axis of the calcaneus should be parallel with the long axis of the unmasked portion of the cassette.
- Metatarsals should not be visualized lateral to the foot *(Figure 7–51)*.

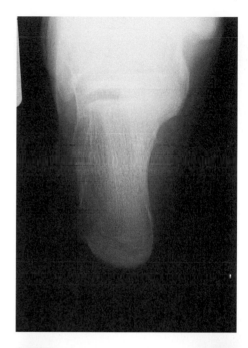

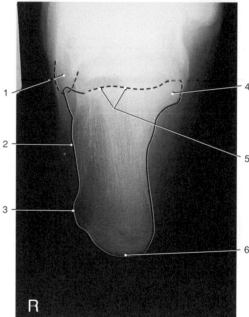

Figure 7–51. Axial plantodorsal calcaneus.

1. 5th metatarsal
2. Trochlear process
3. Lateral process
4. Sustentaculum tali
5. Talocalcaneal joint
6. Tuberosity

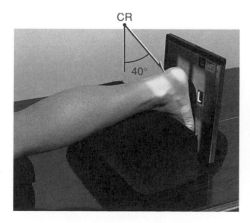

Figure 7–49. Axial dorsoplantar calcaneus.

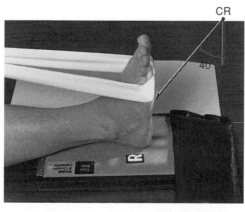

Figure 7–50. Axial plantodorsal calcaneus.

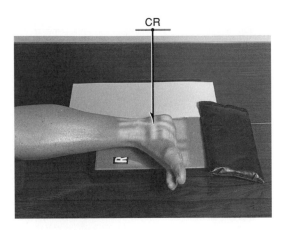

Figure 7–52. Lateral calcaneus.

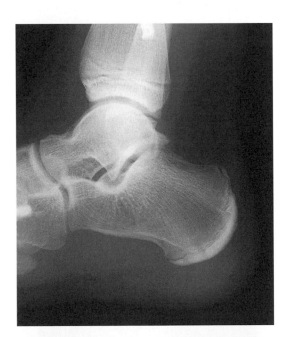

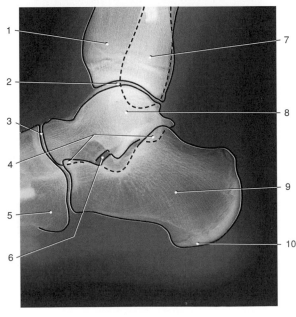

Figure 7–53. Lateral calcaneus.

▶ LATERAL CALCANEUS (OS CALCIS)

Technical Considerations

- Film size: 8 × 10 in. or 10 × 12 in. masked in half crosswise.
- Nongrid, detail cassette if available.
- 55–60 kVp.
- Collimate to include calcaneus and talus.

Shielding

- Gonadal shielding should be used on all patients, especially children and adults of reproductive age.

Patient Positioning

- Assist the patient to the lateral recumbent position on the radiographic table or stretcher; the patient should be lying on the affected side.

Part Positioning

- Rotate the leg of the affected side until the patella is perpendicular to the film plane and the lateral aspect of the foot rests on the cassette; the leg should be parallel with the long axis of the table.
- Dorsiflex the foot and adjust the patient position so the plantar surface of the foot is perpendicular to the table; elevating the knee on a small support will help place the foot in the correct position.
- Center the unmasked half of the cassette to the midpoint of the calcaneus approximately 1 to 1.5 in. distal to the medial malleolus *(Figure 7–52)*.

Central Ray

- Direct the central ray perpendicular to a point 1 to 1.5 in. distal to the medial malleolus.

Image Evaluation

- Soft tissue structures of the calcaneus, talus, and navicular and 1 in. of distal tibia and fibula should be included in the collimated area.
- The cortex and trabeculae of the calcaneus, talus, and navicular should be visualized and clear.
- The long axis of the lower leg should be parallel with the long axis of the unmasked portion of the cassette.
- The fibula should be seen under the posterior aspect of the tibia *(Figure 7–53)*.

1. Tibia
2. Tibiotalar joint
3. Talonavicular joint
4. Talocalcaneal (subtalar) joint

5. Cuboid
6. Sinus tarsi
7. Fibula

8. Talus
9. Calcaneus
10. Tuberosity, calcaneus

► AP ANKLE

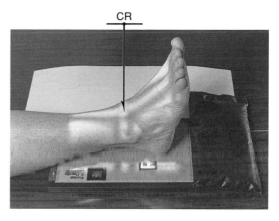

Figure 7–54. AP ankle.

Technical Considerations

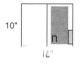

10" 12"

- Film size: 10 × 12 in. masked in half crosswise.
- Nongrid; detail cassette if available.
- 55–60 kVp.
- Collimate to include proximal talus, medial and lateral malleoli, and distal one fourth of lower leg.

Shielding

- Gonadal shielding should be used on all patients, especially children and adults of reproductive age.

Patient Positioning

- Assist the patient to a seated position on the radiographic table or stretcher; the patient's legs should be parallel to the long axis of the table.

Part Positioning

- Center the affected ankle joint to the unmasked half of the cassette; if more of the lower leg must be visualized, the joint can be centered lower on the film.
- Dorsiflex the foot so the plantar surface forms a 90° angle with the lower leg *(Figure 7–54)*.

Central Ray

- Direct the central ray perpendicular to the ankle joint, located about 0.5 in. above the bottom of the malleoli and midway between the malleoli. If the joint is centered lower on the cassette, the central ray will be off centered to the film.

Image Evaluation

- Soft tissue structures of the distal tibia and fibula and the proximal talus should be included in the collimated area.
- The cortex and trabeculae should be visualized and clear.
- The long axis of the lower leg should be parallel with the long axis of the unmasked portion of the cassette.
- The distal fibula and tibia will be slightly superimposed *(Figure 7–55)*.

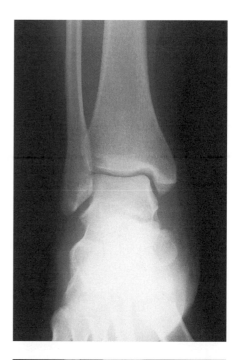

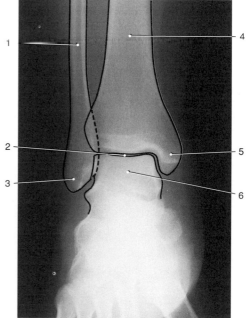

1. Fibula, distal
2. Tibiotalar joint
3. Lateral malleolus
4. Tibia, distal
5. Medial malleolus
6. Talus, proximal

Figure 7–55. AP ankle.

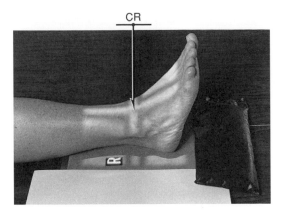

Figure 7–56. Medial oblique ankle.

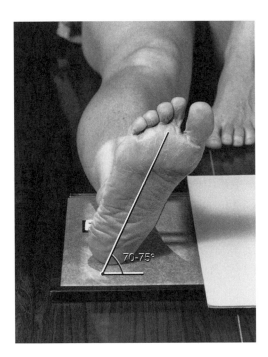

Figure 7–57. To demonstrate the mortise joint, the longitudinal plane of the foot and the table should form an angle of 70° to 75°.

► MEDIAL OBLIQUE ANKLE

Technical Considerations

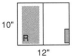

- Film size: 10 × 12 in. masked in half crosswise.
- Nongrid; detail cassette if available.
- 55–60 kVp.
- Collimate to include soft tissue of distal one fourth of tibia and fibula and proximal talus.

Shielding

- Gonadal shielding should be used on all patients, especially children and adults of reproductive age.

Patient Positioning

- Assist the patient to a seated position on the radiographic table or stretcher; the patient's legs should be parallel with the long axis of the table.

Part Positioning

- Internally rotate the leg and foot 15° to 20° to demonstrate the mortise joint (a line between the malleoli should be parallel to the film plane); internally rotate the leg and foot 45° to demonstrate the distal tibiofibular joint.
- Center affected ankle joint to the unmasked half of the cassette; if more of the lower leg must be visualized, the joint can be centered lower on the film.
- Dorsiflex the foot to form a 90° angle with the lower leg.
- Adjust the cassette so a point midway between the malleoli is centered to the unmasked half of the cassette *(Figures 7–56, 7–57).*

Central Ray

- Direct the central ray perpendicular to the ankle joint, located at the level about 0.5 in. above the tip of the malleoli and midway between the malleoli. If the joint is centered lower on the cassette, the central ray will be off centered to the film.

Image Evaluation

- Soft tissue structures of the distal tibia and fibula and the proximal talus should be included in the colli-mated area.
- The cortex and trabeculae should be visualized and clear; the distal tibia and proximal talus should be penetrated.
- The long axis of the lower leg should be parallel with the long axis of the unmasked portion of the cassette.
- When the leg is rotated 15° to 20°, the mortise joint between the proximal talus and distal tibia and fibula should be demonstrated (Figure 7–58).
- When the leg is rotated 45°, the distal tibiofibular joint should not be demonstrated (Figure 7–59).

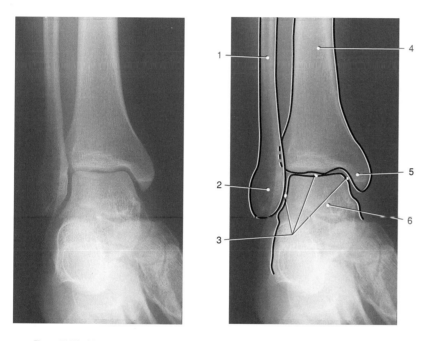

Figure 7–58. Medial oblique ankle with 15° to 20° rotation to demonstrate the mortise joint.

1. Fibula
2. Lateral malleolus
3. Mortise joint
4. Tibia
5. Medial malleolus
6. Talus, proximal

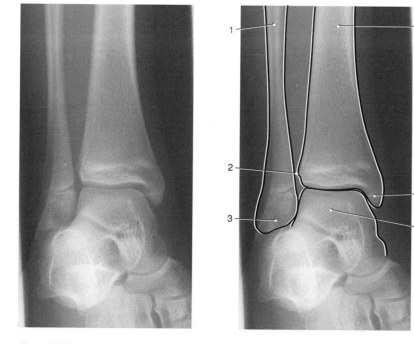

Figure 7–59. Medial oblique ankle with 45° rotation to demonstrate the distal tibiofibular articulation.

1. Fibula
2. Distal tibiofibular joint
3. Lateral malleolus
4. Tibia
5. Medial malleolus
6. Talus, proximal

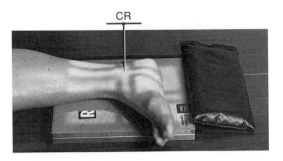

Figure 7–60. Lateral ankle.

► LATERAL ANKLE

Technical Considerations

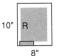

- Film size: 8 × 10 in. lengthwise or 9 × 9 in.
- Nongrid; detail cassette if available.
- 55–60 kVp.
- Collimate to include soft tissue of distal one fourth of tibia and fibula and proximal talus.

Shielding

- Gonadal shielding should be used on all patients, especially children and adults of reproductive age.

Patient Positioning

- Assist the patient to a seated position on the radiographic table or stretcher; the patient's legs should be parallel with the long axis of the table.

Part Positioning

- Externally rotate the leg of the affected side until the patella is perpendicular to the film plane and the lateral aspect of the ankle rests on the cassette; a small support may be needed under the knee.
- Center the affected ankle joint to the cassette; if more of the lower leg must be visualized, the joint can be centered lower on the film; the leg should be parallel with the long axis of the cassette.
- Dorsiflex the foot and adjust the patient position so the foot and leg form a 90° angle (Figure 7–60).

Central Ray

- Direct the central ray perpendicular to the ankle joint, located 0.5 in. above the tip of the lateral malleolus. If the joint is centered lower on the film, the central ray may be off-centered to the cassette.

Image Evaluation

- Soft tissue structures of distal tibia and fibula and the proximal talus should be included in the collimated area.
- The cortex and trabeculae should be visualized and clear; the distal tibia and fibula should be penetrated.
- The long axis of the lower leg should be parallel with the long axis of the cassette.
- The fibula should be demonstrated over the posterior portion of the tibia (Figure 7–61).

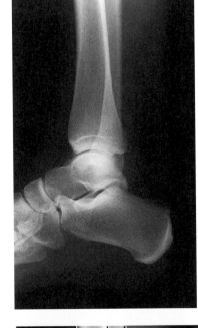

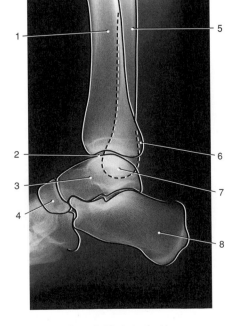

Figure 7–61. Lateral ankle.

1. Tibia
2. Tibiotalar joint
3. Talus
4. Navicular
5. Fibula
6. Posterior malleolus, tibia
7. Lateral malleolus, fibula
8. Calcaneus

▶ AP LOWER LEG

Technical Considerations

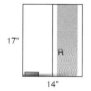

- Film size: 14 × 17 in. masked in half lengthwise or 7 × 17 in.
- Nongrid; detail cassette may be used.
- 60–65 kVp.
- Collimate to include 1 in. of talus, at least 1 in. of femur, and all soft tissue.

Shielding

- Gonadal shielding should be used on all patients, especially children and adults of reproductive age.

Patient Positioning

- Assist the patient to a seated position on the radiographic table or stretcher; the patient's legs should be parallel with the long axis of the table.

Part Positioning

- Center the affected lower leg to the unmasked half of the cassette; the cassette should extend at least 1 to 1.5 in. beyond both the ankle and knee joints. **Note:** To include both joints, it is sometimes necessary to make two exposures or use one 14 × 17-in. cassette diagonally *(Figure 7–62)*.
- Adjust the leg so a line between the femoral condyles is parallel with the film plane.
- Dorsiflex the foot to form a 90° angle with the lower leg; a sandbag placed against the plantar surface of the foot can be used for immobilization *(Figure 7–63)*.

Central Ray

- Direct the central ray perpendicular to the midpoint of the leg.

Image Evaluation

- Soft tissue structures of the lower leg and at least 1 in. of the distal femur and proximal talus should be included in the collimated area.
- The cortex and trabeculae should be visualized and clear.
- The long axis of the lower leg should be parallel with the long axis of the film (unless using one cassette diagonally to include both joints).
- Both the proximal and distal fibula and tibia will be slightly superimposed while the shafts of the tibia and fibula will be separated.
- The medial and lateral condyles of the femur should be symmetrical *(Figure 7–64)*.

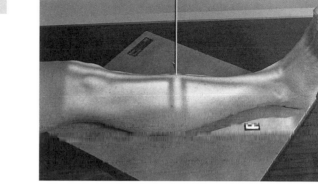

Figure 7–62. AP lower leg, with the cassette positioned diagonally to include both joints.

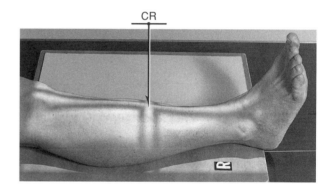

Figure 7–63. AP lower leg, positioning the cassette to include two projections.

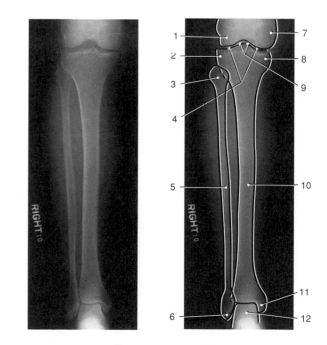

Figure 7–64. AP lower leg.

1. Lateral condyle, femur
2. Lateral condyle, tibia
3. Fibular head
4. Tibial plateau
5. Fibula, body (shaft)
6. Lateral malleolus, fibula
7. Medial condyle, femur
8. Medial condyle, tibia
9. Intercondylar eminence
10. Tibia, body (shaft)
11. Medial malleolus, tibia
12. Talus

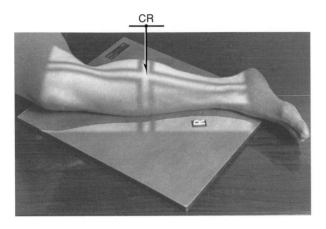

Figure 7–65. Lateral lower leg, with the cassette turned diagonally to include both joints.

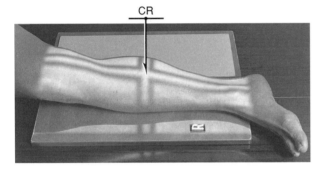

Figure 7–66. Lateral lower leg, with the cassette positioned to include two projections.

► LATERAL LOWER LEG

Technical Considerations

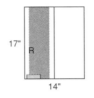

- Film size: 14 × 17 in. masked in half lengthwise or 7 × 17 in.
- Nongrid; detail cassette may be used.
- 60–65 kVp.
- Collimate to include 1 in. of talus, at least 1 in. of femur, and all soft tissue.

Shielding

- Gonadal shielding should be used on all patients, especially children and adults of reproductive age.

Patient Positioning

- Assist the patient to a seated or recumbent position on the radiographic table or stretcher; the patient's legs should be parallel to the long axis of the table.

Part Positioning

- Externally rotate the leg of the affected side until a line passing through the condyles is perpendicular to the film plane and the lateral aspect of the leg rests on the cassette; the knee can be flexed slightly.
- Center the affected leg to the unmasked half of the cassette (remembering that the bones are anterior to the large calf muscle; the cassette should extend at least 1 to 1.5 in. beyond both the ankle and knee joints. **Note:** To include both joints, it is sometimes necessary to make two exposures on two cassettes or use one 14 × 17-in. cassette diagonally (*Figure 7–65*).
- Dorsiflex the foot and adjust the patient position so the foot and leg form a 90° angle; a sandbag placed against the plantar surface of the foot can be used for immobilization (*Figure 7–66*).

Central Ray

- Direct the central ray perpendicular to the midpoint of the leg.

Image Evaluation

- Soft tissue structures of the lower leg and at least 1 in. of the distal femur and proximal talus should be included in the collimated area.
- The cortex and trabeculae should be visualized and clear.
- The long axis of the lower leg should be parallel with the long axis of the unmasked portion of the film (unless using one cassette diagonally to include both joints).
- Both the proximal and distal fibula and tibia will be slightly superimposed while the shaft of the tibia will be anterior and separate from the shaft of the fibula.
- The medial and lateral condyles of the femur should be superimposed (*Figure 7–67*).

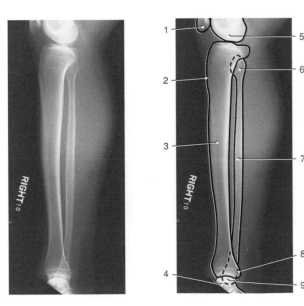

Figure 7–67. Lateral lower leg.

1. Patella
2. Tibial tuberosity
3. Tibia, body (shaft)
4. Talus
5. Femoral condyles, superimposed
6. Fibular head
7. Fibula, body (shaft)
8. Posterior malleolus, tibia
9. Lateral malleolus, fibula

► AP KNEE

Technical Considerations

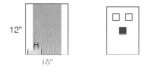

- Film size: 10 × 12 in. or 8 × 10 in. lengthwise.
- Grid or nongrid.
- 60–70 kVp.
- Collimate to include soft tissue crosswise and to film size lengthwise.

Shielding

- Gonadal shielding should be used on all patients, especially children and adults of reproductive age.

Patient Positioning

- Assist the patient to a seated or supine position on the radiographic table; the patient's legs should be parallel with the long axis of the table.

Part Positioning

- Center the affected knee to the midline of the table; the leg should remain parallel with the table.
- Position the leg so a line between the femoral condyles is parallel with the film plane; the leg may be slightly inverted to accomplish this *(Figure 7–68).*

Central Ray

- Direct the central ray 5° cephalad to a point 0.5 in. distal to the apex of the patella to demonstrate the joint space; center the cassette to the central ray. **Note:** To demonstrate the distal femur or proximal lower leg, the central ray is directed perpendicular to the joint space.

Image Evaluation

- Soft tissue structures of the distal femur and proximal lower leg should be included in the collimated area.
- The cortex and trabeculae should be visualized and clear; the distal femur and patella should be penetrated.
- The long axis of the leg should be parallel with the long axis of the film.
- The knee joint should be seen in the middle of the collimated area and film.
- Both the proximal fibula and tibia will be slightly superimposed.
- The medial and lateral condyles of the femur should be symmetrical *(Figure 7–69).*

1. Femur
2. Lateral condyle, femur
3. Lateral condyle, tibia
4. Tibial plateau
5. Fibular head
6. Patella
7. Medial condyle, femur
8. Medial condyle, tibia
9. Intercondylar eminence
10. Tibia

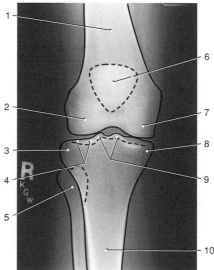

Figure 7–68. AP knee.

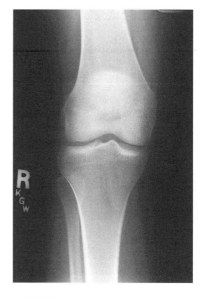

Figure 7–69. AP knee.

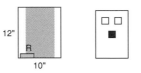

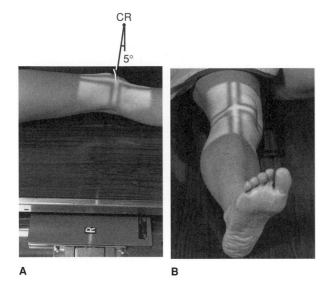

A   **B**

Figure 7–70. **(A)** Medial oblique internal knee (from side). **(B)** Medial oblique (internal) knee from foot of table.

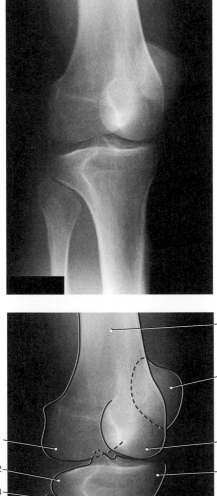

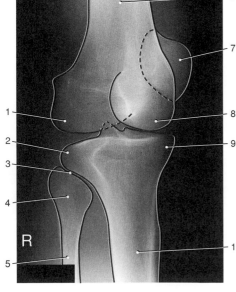

Figure 7–71. Medial oblique knee.

▶ MEDIAL (INTERNAL) OBLIQUE KNEE

Technical Considerations

- Film size: 10 × 12 in. or 8 × 10 in. lengthwise.
- Grid or nongrid.
- 60–70 kVp.
- Collimate to include soft tissue crosswise and to film size lengthwise

Shielding

- Gonadal shielding should be used on all patients, especially children and adults of reproductive age.

Patient Positioning

- Assist the patient to a seated or supine position on the radiographic table; the patient's legs should be parallel with the long axis of the table.

Part Positioning

- Center the affected knee to the midline of the table; the leg should remain parallel with the table.
- Rotate the leg medially so a line between the femoral condyles is at a 45° angle with the film plane; the hip of the affected side can be elevated and supported for patient comfort *(Figure 7–70)*.

Central Ray

- Direct the central ray perpendicular or 5° cephalad to a point just distal to the apex of the patella to demonstrate the joint space; degree of angle depends on amount of hip elevation and department routine.
- Center the cassette to the central ray.

Image Evaluation

- Soft tissue structures of the distal femur and proximal lower leg should be included in the collimated area.
- The cortex and trabeculae should be visualized and clear; the distal femur and patella should be penetrated.
- The long axis of the leg should be parallel with the long axis of the film.
- The knee joint should be seen in the middle of the collimated area and film.
- Approximately one third to one half of the patella should be projected medial to the distal femur.
- The proximal tibiofibular articulation should be visualized *(Figure 7–71)*.

1. Lateral condyle, femur
2. Lateral condyle, tibia
3. Proximal tibiofibular joint
4. Fibular head
5. Fibula
6. Femur
7. Patella
8. Medial condyle, femur
9. Medial condyle, tibia
10. Tibia

► LATERAL (EXTERNAL) OBLIQUE KNEE

Technical Considerations

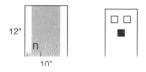

- Film size: 10 × 12 in. or 8 × 10 in. lengthwise.
- Grid or nongrid.
- 60–70 kVp
- Collimate to include soft tissue crosswise and to film size lengthwise.

Shielding

- Gonadal shielding should be used on all patients, especially children and adults of reproductive age.

Patient Positioning

- Assist the patient to a seated or supine position on the radiographic table; the patient's legs should be parallel with the long axis of the table.

Part Positioning

- Center the affected knee to the midline of the table; the leg should remain parallel with the table.
- Rotate the leg laterally so a line between the femoral condyles is at a 45° angle with the film plane; the hip of the unaffected side can be elevated and supported for patient comfort *(Figure 7–72)*.

Central Ray

- Direct the central ray perpendicular or 5° cephalad to a point just distal to the apex of the patella to demonstrate the joint space; the degree of angle depends on department routine.
- Center the cassette to the central ray.

Image Evaluation

- Soft tissue structures of the distal femur and proximal lower leg should be included in the collimated area.
- The cortex and trabeculae should be visualized and clear; the distal femur and patella should be penetrated.
- The long axis of the leg should be parallel with the long axis of the film.
- The knee joint should be seen in the middle of the collimated area and film.
- Approximately one third to one half of the patella should be projected lateral to the distal femur.
- The fibula should be superimposed over the proximal tibia *(Figure 7–73)*.

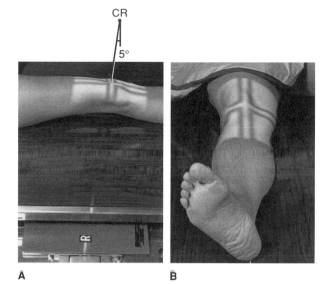

Figure 7–72. **(A)** Lateral oblique external knee (from side). **(B)** Lateral oblique (external) knee from foot of table.

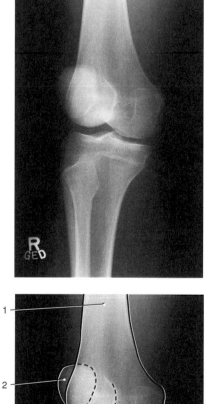

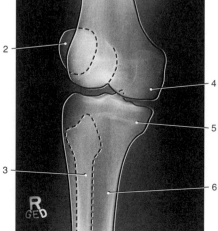

Figure 7–73. Lateral oblique knee.

1. Femur	3. Fibula	5. Medial condyle, tibia
2. Patella	4. Medial condyle, femur	6. Tibia

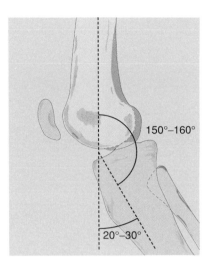

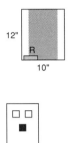

Figure 7–74. When the knee is correctly flexed for a lateral knee projection, the angle between the tibia and femur will be approximately 150° to 160°.

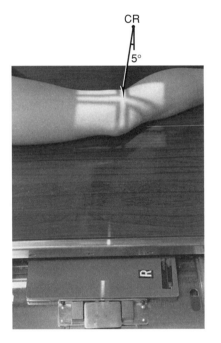

Figure 7–75. Lateral knee, with the unaffected leg behind the knee of interest.

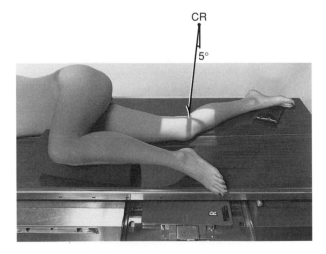

Figure 7–76. By bringing the unaffected leg anterior to the knee of interest, the entire body can be in a lateral position, minimizing the possibility of rotation of the affected knee.

▶ LATERAL KNEE

Technical Considerations

- Film size: 10 × 12 in. or 8 × 10 in. lengthwise.
- Grid or nongrid.
- 60–70 kVp.
- Collimate to include soft tissue crosswise and to film size lengthwise.

Shielding

- Gonadal shielding should be used on all patients, especially children and adults of reproductive age.

Patient Positioning

- Assist the patient to the lateral recumbent position on the radiographic table with the affected side down.
- The unaffected leg may be brought behind the affected leg or, with knee flexed, brought in front of the affected leg and supported to prevent rotation.

Part Positioning

- Center the affected femur to the midline of the table; the femur should be parallel with the table.
- Flex the affected knee 20° to 30° from full extension to form a 150° to 160° angle between the lower leg and femur *(Figure 7–74);* this degree of flexion will relax the muscles and demonstrate a maximum amount of joint space.
- Adjust the patient position so a line drawn through the femoral epicondyles is perpendicular to the film plane; the condyles should be superimposed *(Figures 7–75, 7–76).*

Central Ray

- Direct the central ray 5° cephalad to the knee joint, approximately 1 in. below the medial condyle of the femur.
- Center the cassette to the central ray.

Image Evaluation

- Soft tissue structures of the distal femur and proximal lower leg should be included in the collimated area.
- The cortex and trabeculae should be visualized and clear; the distal femur should be adequately penetrated.
- The long axis of the femur should be parallel with the long axis of the film.
- The knee joint should be seen in the middle of the collimated area and film.
- The patella should be projected anterior to the distal femur and in a lateral position.
- There should be a 150° to 160° angle between the lower leg and femur.
- The femoral condyles should be superimposed (Figure 7-77).

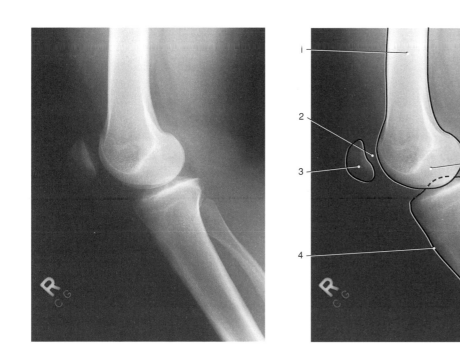

Figure 7–77. Lateral knee.

1. Femur	4. Tibial tuberosity	6. Fibular head
2. Femoropatellar joint	5. Femoral condyles, superim-	7. Fibular
3. Patella	posed	8. Tibia

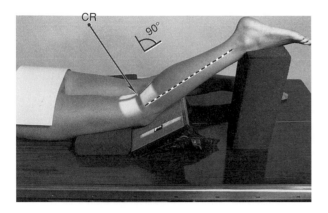

Figure 7–78. PA axial intercondylar fossa, with elevated distal femurs and angled cassette to minimize distortion.

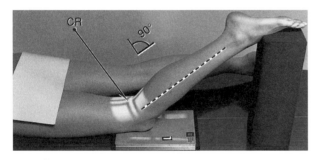

Figure 7–79. PA axial intercondylar fossa without elevation of distal femur and cassette angulation.

▶ PA AXIAL INTERCONDYLAR FOSSA (CAMP-COVENTRY METHOD)

Technical Considerations

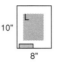

- Film size: 8 × 10 in. lengthwise or crosswise or 9 × 9 in.
- Nongrid or grid.
- 60–70 kVp.
- Collimate to include soft tissue crosswise and to film size lengthwise.

Caution: A horizontal fracture of the patella should be ruled out before flexing the knee.

Shielding

- Gonadal shielding should be used on all patients, especially children and adults of reproductive age.

Patient Positioning

- Assist the patient to the prone position on the radiographic table; position the patient so the affected leg is parallel to the long axis of the table.

Part Positioning

- Position the proximal half of the cassette under the knee joint; the cassette can also be centered in the Bucky tray. **Note:** This projection can also be performed by elevating the distal femurs on radiolucent supports. The cassette can then be angled and supported by sandbags. This positioning reduces the angle between the central ray and cassette, reducing distortion of the intercondylar fossa *(Figure 7–78)*.
- Flex the affected knee so the lower leg forms an angle of approximately 40° to 50° with the table and rest the foot on a sponge or other support; check to be sure the leg is not rotated *(Figure 7–79)*.

Central Ray

- Direct the central ray perpendicular to the long axis of the tibia and to the popliteal depression; the central ray will pass through the knee joint (if the lower leg forms a 40° angle with the table, the central ray should be directed 40° caudally).
- Adjust the centering of the cassette to the central ray, if necessary.

Image Evaluation

- Soft tissue structures of the distal femur and proximal lower leg should be included in the collimated area.
- The cortex and trabeculae should be visualized and clear; the distal femur should be adequately penetrated in the area of the fossa.
- The long axis of the femur should be parallel with the long axis of the film.
- The knee joint should be seen in the middle of the collimated area and film.
- The medial and lateral condyles of the femur should be symmetrical *(Figure 7–80)*.

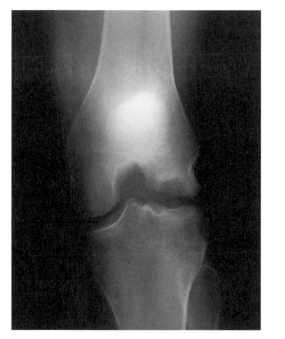 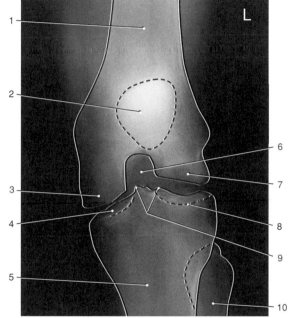

Figure 7–80. PA axial intercondylar fossa: Camp–Coventry method.

1. Femur	5. Tibia	8. Articular facet (tibial plateau)
2. Patella	6. Intercondylar fossa	9. Intercondylar eminence
3. Medial condyle, femur	7. Lateral condyle, femur	10. Tibia
4. Articular facet (tibial plateau)		

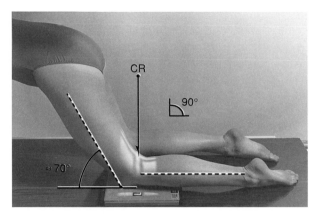
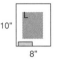

Figure 7–81. PA axial intercondylar fossa: Holmblad method.

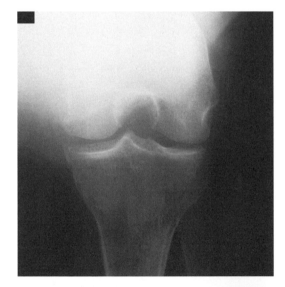

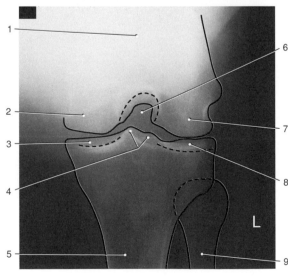

Figure 7–82. PA axial intercondylar fossa: Holmblad method.

▶ PA AXIAL INTERCONDYLAR FOSSA (HOLMBLAD METHOD)

Technical Considerations

- Film size: 8 × 10 in. lengthwise or 9 × 9 in.
- Nongrid or grid.
- 60–70 kVp.
- Collimate to include soft tissue crosswise and to film size lengthwise.

Caution: A horizontal fracture of the patella should be ruled out before flexing the knee.

Shielding

- Gonadal shielding should be used on all patients, especially children and adults of reproductive age.

Patient Positioning

- Assist the patient to the kneeling position on the radiographic table; position the patient so the lower leg of the affected side is parallel with the long axis of the table. **Note:** This position is uncomfortable, so speed is important.

Part Positioning

- Center the cassette under the affected knee joint.
- Adjust the patient position so the angle between the femur and table is approximately 70°; check foot and lower leg for rotation *(Figure 7–81)*.

Central Ray

- Direct the central ray perpendicular to the long axis of the tibia through the knee joint; the central ray will enter at the popliteal depression.
- Adjust the centering of the cassette to the central ray, if necessary.

Image Evaluation

- Soft tissue structures of the distal femur and proximal lower leg should be included in the collimated area.
- The cortex and trabeculae should be visualized and clear; the distal femur should be adequately penetrated in the area of the fossa.
- The long axis of the femur should be parallel with the long axis of the film.
- The knee joint should be seen in the middle of the collimated area and film.
- The medial and lateral condyles of the femur should be symmetrical *(Figure 7–82)*.

1. Femur
2. Medial condyle, femur
3. Articular facet, (tibial plateau)
4. Intercondylar eminence
5. Tibia
6. Intercondylar fossa
7. Lateral condyle, femur
8. Articular facet (tibial plateau)
9. Fibula

► AP AXIAL INTERCONDYLAR FOSSA (BECLERE METHOD)

Technical Considerations

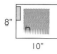

- Film size: 8 × 10 in. crosswise, 9 × 9 in., or curved cassette.
- Nongrid.
- 60–70 kVp.
- Collimate to include soft tissue crosswise and to film size lengthwise.

Caution: A horizontal fracture of the patella should be ruled out before flexing the knee.

Shielding

- Gonadal shielding should be used on all patients, especially children and adults of reproductive age.

Patient Positioning

- Assist the patient to the supine position on the radiographic table; position the patient so the affected leg is parallel with the long axis of the table.

Part Positioning

- Flex the knee so there is approximately a 120° angle between the femur and lower leg; support the knee on sponges or sandbags.
- Position the cassette under the knee on the supports; center the distal end of the cassette under the affected knee joint.
- Adjust the leg so there is no rotation; a sandbag can be positioned under the foot for immobilization *(Figure 7–83)*.

Central Ray

- Direct the central ray perpendicular to the long axis of the tibia to a point 0.5 in. distal to the apex of the patella; adjust the centering of the cassette to the central ray, if necessary.

Image Evaluation

- Soft tissue structures of the distal femur and proximal lower leg should be included in the collimated area
- The cortex and trabeculae should be visualized and clear; the distal femur should be adequately penetrated in the area of the fossa.
- The long axis of the femur should be parallel with the long axis of the film.
- The knee joint should be seen in the middle of the collimated area and film.
- The medial and lateral condyles of the femur should be symmetrical *(Figure 7–84)*.

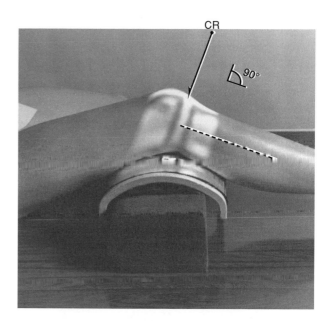

Figure 7–83. AP axial intercondylar fossa: Beclere method.

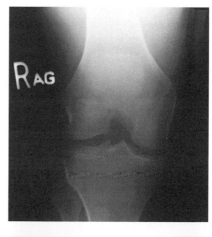

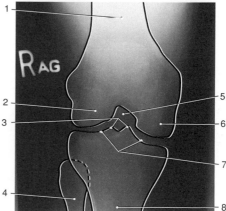

1. Femur	4. Fibula	7. Articular facets, tibial plateau
2. Lateral condyle, femur	5. Intercondylar fossa	8. Tibia
3. Intercondylar eminence	6. Medial condyle, femur	

Figure 7–84. AP axial intercondylar fossa: Beclere method.

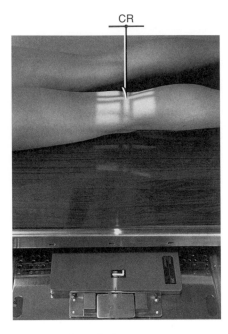

Figure 7–85. PA patella.

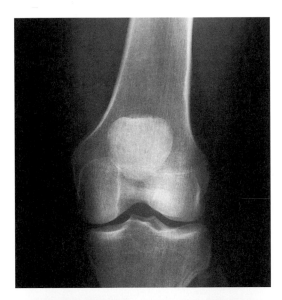

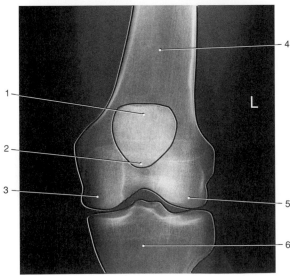

Figure 7–86. PA patella.

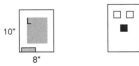

▶ PA PATELLA

Technical Considerations

- Film size: 8 × 10 in. lengthwise or 9 × 9 in.
- Grid.
- 60–70 kVp.
- Collimate to include soft tissue of patella, distal femur, and proximal lower leg.

Shielding

- Gonadal shielding should be used on all patients, especially children and adults of reproductive age.

Patient Positioning

- Assist the patient to the prone position on the radiographic table; position the patient so the affected leg is parallel with the long axis of the table.

Part Positioning

- Center the affected knee to the midline of the table; the leg should remain parallel with the table.
- Position the leg so the patellar plane is parallel with the film plane; the leg may be laterally rotated 5° to 10° to accomplish this (Figure 7–85).

Central Ray

- Direct the central ray perpendicular to the midpoint of the patella through the popliteal region.
- Center the cassette to the central ray.

Image Evaluation

- Soft tissue structures of the distal femur and proximal lower leg should be included in the collimated area.
- The cortex and trabeculae should be visualized and clear; the distal femur and patella should be penetrated.
- The long axis of the leg should be parallel with the long axis of the film.
- The patella should be seen in the middle of the collimated area and film and superimposed over the distal femur.
- Both the proximal fibula and tibia will be slightly superimposed.
- The medial and lateral condyles of the femur should be symmetrical (Figure 7–86).

1. Patella, base	3. Medial condyle, femur
2. Patella, apex	4. Femur
5. Lateral condyle, femur	6. Tibia

► LATERAL PATELLA

Technical Considerations

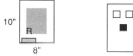

- Film size: 8 × 10 in. lengthwise or 9 × 9 in.
- Grid or nongrid.
- 60–70 kVp.
- Collimate to include soft tissue of patella, distal femur, and proximal lower leg.

Shielding

- Gonadal shielding should be used on all patients, especially children and adults of reproductive age.

Patient Positioning

- Assist the patient to the lateral recumbent position on the radiographic table with the affected side down.
- The unaffected leg may be brought behind the affected leg or, with knee flexed, brought in front of the affected leg and supported to prevent rotation.

Part Positioning

- Center the affected leg to the midline of the table; the femur should be parallel with the table.
- Flex the affected knee only 5° to 10° to maximize the femoropatellar joint space and minimize the chance of separating fracture fragments.
- Adjust the patient position so a line drawn through the femoral epicondyles is perpendicular to the film plane; the condyles should be superimposed and the plane of the patella should be perpendicular to the film (Figure 7–87).

Central Ray

- Direct the central ray perpendicular to the femoropatellar joint space, just anterior to the medial condyle of the femur.
- Center the cassette to the central ray.

Image Evaluation

- Soft tissue structures of the patella, distal femur, and proximal lower leg should be included in the collimated area.
- The cortex and trabeculae should be visualized and clear; the patella should be adequately penetrated.
- The long axis of the femur should be parallel with the long axis of the film.
- The patella should be seen in the middle of the collimated area and film.
- The patella should be projected anterior to the distal femur and in a lateral position.
- There should be a 170° to 175° angle between the lower leg and femur.
- The femoral condyles should be superimposed (Figure 7–88).

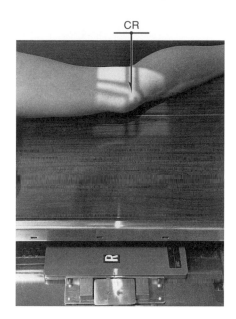

Figure 7–87. Lateral patella.

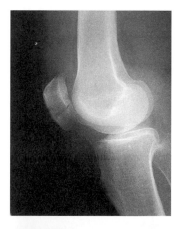

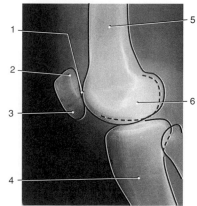

Figure 7–88. Lateral patella; note the transverse fracture.

1. Femoropatellar joint
2. Patella, base
3. Patella, apex
4. Tibia
5. Femur
6. Femoral condyles, superimposed

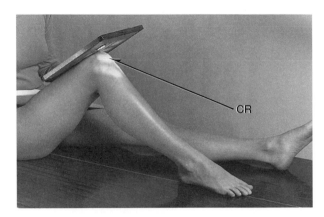
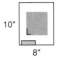

Figure 7–89. The sitting or supine position can also be used to produce a tangential projection.

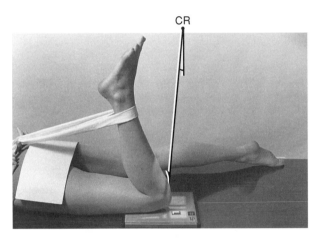

CR

Figure 7–90. Tangential patella: Settegast method.

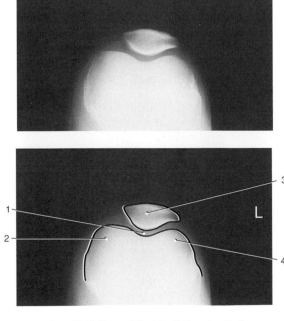

1. Femoropatellar joint
2. Medial condyle, femur
3. Patella
4. Lateral condyle, femur

Figure 7–91. Tangential patella: Settegast method.

► TANGENTIAL PATELLA & FEMOROPATELLAR JOINT ("SUNRISE," "SKYLINE," SETTEGAST METHOD)

Technical Considerations

- Film size: 8 × 10 in. lengthwise or 9 × 9 in.
- Nongrid.
- 60–70 kVp.
- Collimate to include soft tissue of patella and distal femur.

Caution: A horizontal fracture of the patella should be ruled out before flexing the knee.

Shielding

- Gonadal shielding should be used on all patients, especially children and adults of reproductive age.

Patient Positioning

- Assist the patient to the prone position on the radiographic table; adjust the affected leg so it is parallel with the long axis of the table. **Note:** This projection can also be obtained with the patient in the supine or sitting position *(Figure 7–89)*. Because this position can be uncomfortable to maintain, technical factors should be set before further positioning.

Part Positioning

- Slowly flex the knee slightly more than 90°; position the leg so there is no medial or lateral rotation; the leg can be immobilized by looping a long strip of tape or gauze bandage around the patient's foot or ankle and instructing the patient to hold the ends.
- Center the cassette under the patella *(Figure 7–90)*.

Central Ray

- Direct the central ray through the joint space between the patella and femoral condyles, angling the tube so the central ray is parallel with the plane of the patella (usually 5°–10° cephalad); the more the knee is flexed, the less the central ray must be angled.
- Adjust centering of the cassette to correspond with the central ray.

Image Evaluation

- Soft tissue structures of the patella, distal femur, and proximal lower leg should be included in the collimated area.
- The cortex and trabeculae should be visualized and clear; the distal femur should be adequately penetrated.
- The long axis of the femur should be parallel with the long axis of the film.
- The patella should be seen in the middle of the collimated area and film.
- The patella should be projected anterior to the distal femur.
- The joint space between the patella and condyles should be well demonstrated *(Figure 7–91)*.

► TANGENTIAL PATELLA & FEMOROPATELLAR JOINT (HUGHSTON METHOD)

Technical Considerations

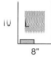

- Film size: 8 × 10 in. lengthwise
- Grid or nongrid.
- 60–70 kVp.
- Collimate to include soft tissue of patella and distal femur.

Caution: A horizontal fracture of the patella should be ruled out before flexing the knee.

Shielding

- Gonadal shielding should be used on all patients, especially children and adults of reproductive age.

Patient Positioning

- Assist the patient to the prone position on the radiographic table; adjust the affected leg so it is parallel with the long axis of the table. Because this position can be uncomfortable to maintain, technical factors should be set before further positioning. **Note:** This projection can also be performed bilaterally, demonstrating both patellae for comparison. In this case, a 14 × 17-in. cassette would be positioned crosswise under the patellae.

Part Positioning

- Center the cassette under the patella; the center of the cassette should be approximately at the level of the base(s) of the patella.
- Slowly flex the knee(s) to form a 45° to 55° angle between the lower leg and table; ensure there is no medial or lateral rotation; the foot can rest on the collimator for immobilization (make sure it is not hot enough to burn the patient) *(Figure 7–92)*.

Central Ray

- Direct the central ray 45° cephalad through the patellofemoral joint space.

Image Evaluation

- Soft tissue structures of the patella, distal femur, and proximal lower leg should be included in the collimated area.
- The cortex and trabeculae should be visualized and clear; the distal femur should be adequately penetrated.
- The long axis of the femur should be parallel with the long axis of the film.
- The patella should be seen in the middle of the collimated area and film.
- The patella should be projected anterior to the distal femur.
- The joint space between the patella and femoral condyles should be well demonstrated *(Figure 7–93)*.

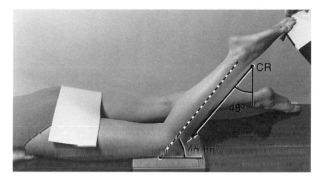

Figure 7–92. Tangential patella: Hughston method.

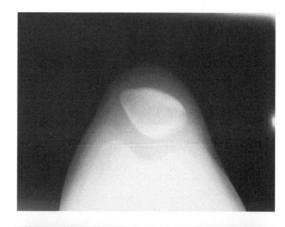

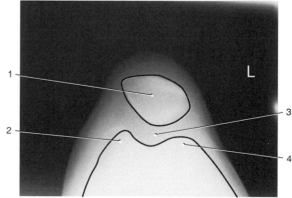

1. Patella
2. Medial condyle, femur
3. Femoropatellar joint
4. Lateral condyle, femur

Figure 7–93. Tangential patella: Hughston method.

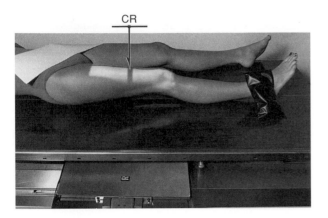

Figure 7–94. AP femur, to include the knee joint.

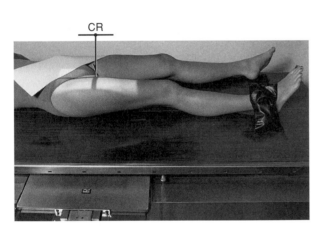

Figure 7–95. AP femur, to include the hip joint.

► AP FEMUR

Technical Considerations

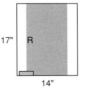

- Film size: 14 × 17 in. or 7 × 17 in. lengthwise; because two films are needed to include both joints on most adults, a 10 × 12-in. cassette will also be needed.
- Grid (nongrid for mobile radiography).
- 65–75 kVp.
- Collimate to include soft tissue crosswise and 1 to 2 in. beyond joints.

Caution: If a fracture is suspected, the leg should not be inverted; an AP projection with the leg in a neutral position should be obtained.

Shielding

- Gonadal shielding should be used on all patients, especially children and adults of reproductive age.

Patient Positioning

- Assist the patient to the supine position on the radiographic table; the patient's affected leg should be parallel with the long axis of the table.

Part Positioning

Mid- and Distal Femur
- Center the affected femur to the midline of the table, remembering that the proximal femur is located laterally in the thigh.
- Internally rotate the leg approximately 5°; position a sandbag over the ankle for immobilization.
- Center the 14 × 17-in. cassette so the distal margin is 2 in. below the knee joint to compensate for the diverging rays *(Figure 7–94)*.

Proximal Femur
- Internally rotate the leg approximately 15° to 20° to compensate for the natural curvature of the femur and prevent forshortening of the femoral neck.
- Center the 10 × 12-in. cassette to the level of the greater trochanter, which is palpable on the proximal, lateral aspect of the femur *(Figure 7–95)*. **Note:** Some department protocols may require using the larger film to include the hip joint or joint nearest the fracture.

Central Ray

- Direct the central ray perpendicular to the midpoint of the cassette.

Image Evaluation

- Soft tissue structures of the femur and 1 to 2 in. beyond the associated joints should be included in the collimated area.
- The cortex and trabeculae should be visualized and clear; the proximal femur should be penetrated.
- The long axis of the leg should be parallel with the long axis of the film and centered crosswise on the film.

Mid- and Distal Femur
- The medial and lateral condyles of the femur should be symmetrical *(Figure 7–96)*.

Proximal Femur
- The greater trochanter should be seen in profile laterally; the lesser trochanter should be barely or not seen medially *(Figure 7–97)*.

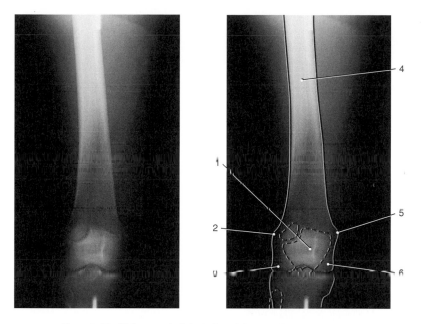

Figure 7–96. AP femur, to include the knee joint; note the bipartite patella.

1. Patella, bipartite
2. Lateral epicondyle
3. Lateral condyle
4. Femur, body (shaft)
5. Medial epicondyle
6. Medial condyle

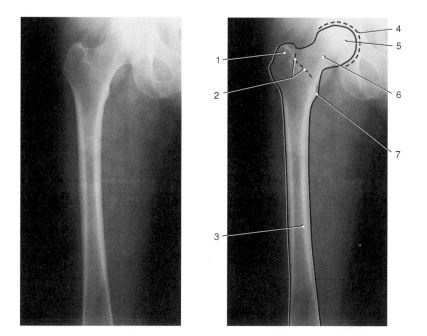

Figure 7–97. AP femur, to include the hip joint; a 14 × 17 in. cassette was used, per routine.

1. Greater trochanter
2. Intertrochanteric crest
3. Femur, body (shaft)
4. Acetabulum
5. Femoral head
6. Femoral neck
7. Lesser trochanter

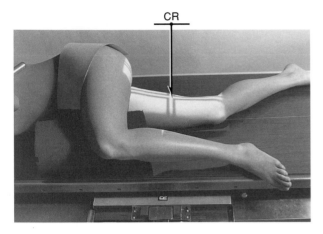

Figure 7–98. Lateral femur to include the knee joint.

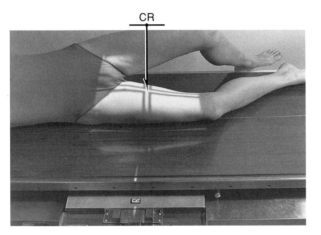

Figure 7–99. Lateral femur, to include the hip joint.

► LATERAL FEMUR

Technical Considerations

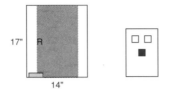

- Film size: 14 × 17 in. or 7 × 17 in. lengthwise; because two films are needed to include both joints on most adults, a 10 × 12-in. cassette may also be used.
- Grid (nongrid for mobile radiography).
- 65–75 kVp
- Collimate to include soft tissue crosswise and 1 to 2 in. beyond joints.

Caution: If a fracture is suspected, the patient should not be moved; a transfemoral lateral projection(s) using a horizontal beam should be obtained without rotating the leg.

Shielding

- Gonadal shielding should be used on all patients, especially children and adults of reproductive age.

Patient Positioning

- Assist the patient to the lateral recumbent position on the radiographic table with the affected side down.
- Center the affected thigh to the midline of the table.

Mid- and Distal Femur

- Bring the unaffected leg, with knee flexed, in front of the affected leg and support it to prevent rotation.
- Adjust the leg so a line through the femoral condyles is perpendicular to the table.
- Center the 14 × 17-in. cassette so the distal margin is 2 in. below the knee joint to compensate for the diverging rays *(Figure 7–98)*.

Proximal Femur

- Support the unaffected leg behind the affected leg and rotate the patient posteriorly just enough to prevent superimposition of the unaffected leg over the affected leg.
- Center the 10 × 12-in. cassette to the level of the greater trochanter, which is palpable on the proximal, lateral aspect of the femur *(Figure 7–99)*. **Note:** Some department protocols may require using the larger film to include the hip joint or joint nearest the fracture.

Central Ray

- Direct the central ray perpendicular to the midpoint of the cassette.

Image Evaluation

- Soft tissue structures of the femur and 1 to 2 in. beyond the associated joints should be included in the collimated area.
- The cortex and trabeculae should be visualized and clear; the proximal femur should be penetrated.
- The long axis of the leg should be parallel with the long axis of the film and centered crosswise on the film.

Mid- and Distal Femur

- The medial and lateral condyles of the femur should be superimposed *(Figure 7–100)*.

Proximal Femur

- The greater trochanter should be superimposed over the femoral neck; the lesser trochanter should be seen in profile *(Figure 7–101)*.

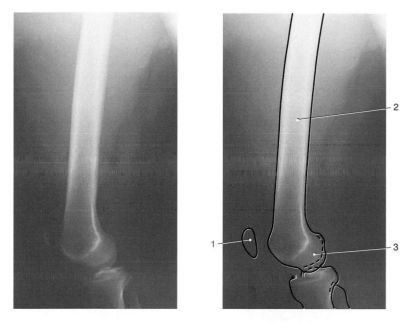

Figure 7–100. Lateral femur, to include the knee joint.

1. Patella
2. Femur, body (shaft)
3. Femoral condyles, superimposed

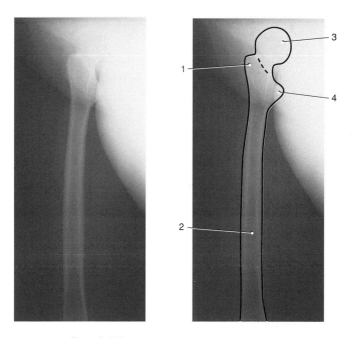

Figure 7–101. Lateral femur, to include the hip joint.

1. Greater trochanter
2. Femur, body (shaft)
3. Femoral head
4. Lesser trochanter

$\mathscr{S}$UMMARY

▶ Most radiographic images of the lower limb are obtained with the patient sitting or lying on the radiographic table or mobile stretcher.

▶ For all radiographic examinations of the lower limb, at least two projections, 90° from each other, should be obtained.

▶ Radiographic examinations of the foot and ankle generally require a minimum of three projections, AP, medial oblique, and lateral, whereas examination of the knee includes only AP and lateral projections in many departments.

▶ Kilovoltages for imaging the lower limb range from 50 to 75 kVp.

▶ Although detail or slow-speed film/screen combinations are preferred for small structures, such as the foot and ankle, faster-speed screens are recommended for the lower leg, knee, and femur.

▶ A grid is recommended for any structure measuring more than 10 cm.

▶ To prevent foreshortening or elongation, the central ray should be directed perpendicular to long bones.

▶ The lower limb should be aligned parallel to the long axis of the radiographic table to prevent closure of joints when angling the central ray.

▶ When radiographing long bones, more than one cassette may be required for each projection to include both joints in the examination.

▶ Rotation of the leg is contraindicated when a hip or femur fracture is suspected.

▶ To demonstrate the intercondylar fossa, the central ray is always directed perpendicular to the long axis of the tibia.

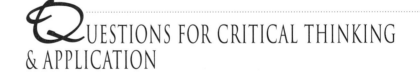

$\mathscr{Q}$UESTIONS FOR CRITICAL THINKING & APPLICATION

1. (A) With respect to the feet, why might a person with plantar warts have difficulty walking? (B) What activities could contribute to the occurrence of flatfeet?

2. Develop a chart summarizing the surface markings of the bones of the lower limb.

3. Which bones in the lower extremity are frequently the site of stress fractures? What occupations would have the highest incidence of this problem?

4. Mr. Edwards developed a large cyst on his fibula. As a result, the orthopedic surgeon needed to remove a significant portion of the shaft of the fibula. Discuss the implications this type of procedure might have on the patient's ability to walk. What happens to the muscles that normally attach to the fibula?

5. Many sporting activities involve jumping. Discuss the effects jumping might have on the joints of the lower extremity, particularly the knee.

6. Your patient was brought to the emergency room by ambulance following a downhill skiing accident. When transported to the radiology department, the patient has sandbags on either side of her head. You are instructed to obtain radiographic images of her lower leg without moving your patient's head. Describe how you will obtain these images.

7. While standing on a chair to hang curtains, a friend slipped and landed on the lateral aspect of her foot. She visits the emergency room for evaluation. A radiographic examination of the foot is ordered. If a fracture is present, which projection do you think would *best* demonstrate this fracture?

8. Several months following a sports injury, a young man is admitted to the emergency room with knee pain. The attending physician suspects a possible foreign body behind the knee joint. Identify and describe the projection(s) you would obtain to rule out a foreign body in this region.

9. You and a technologist are sent to obtain portable images of a femur on a patient who is in an orthopedic bed. As a result of a car accident, the patient has an oblique fracture of the distal femur and has the leg suspended in traction with the knee flexed about 40°. Describe how you would obtain AP and lateral projections, including the positioning of mobile unit, cassette positioning, film size, cassette type, and technical factors.

10. A patient wearing a leg splint is sent to radiology from the emergency room. Your orders are to radiograph the ankle and lower leg; however, the doctor has not indicated whether or not you can remove the splint prior to making the exposures. You know that parts of the splint will be seen on the images. What should you do?

11. Following a car accident, a patient has been brought to the emergency department with severe trauma to the right leg. Although a femur fracture is suspected, the doctor has ordered radiographic examinations of the femur, lower leg, ankle, and foot. Describe how you will obtain the required projections.

FILM CRITIQUE

After studying this oblique ankle radiograph *(Figure 7–102)*, describe how the patient was positioned. How did you determine positioning accuracy or error?

According to the routine in your department, how should the patient be positioned for an oblique projection of the ankle?

How much should the leg be rotated and what should be demonstrated?

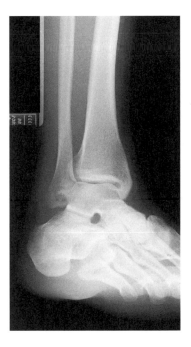

Figure 7–102.

Name this projection *(Figure 7–103)*. Describe how the patient was positioned for this projection.

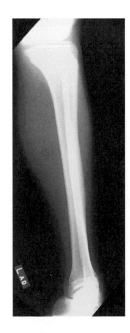

Figure 7–103.

8

PELVIC GIRDLE

▶ OBJECTIVES

Following the completion of this chapter the student will be able to:

- Given diagrams, radiographs, or dry bones, name and describe the bones of the pelvic girdle, to include the ilium, ischium, pubis, sacrum, coccyx, and proximal femur.

- Describe the locations and relationships of specific structures and positioning landmarks of the pelvic girdle (ie, ischial tuberosity is posterior and 1.5 in. inferior to symphysis pubis).

- Differentiate between the true and false divisions of the pelvis, to include structures and function.

- Identify the structural differences on a male pelvis versus a female pelvis, and differentiate between the sexes on radiographs of the pelvis.

- Classify the articulations of the pelvic girdle and identify their type of movement.

- Describe procedural modifications for patients suspected of having a hip fracture.

- State the criteria used to determine positioning accuracy on radiographs of the pelvic girdle and evaluate radiographs of the pelvic girdle in terms of positioning, centering, image quality, radiographic anatomy, and pathology.

- Define terminology associated with the pelvic girdle, to include anatomy, procedures, and pathology.

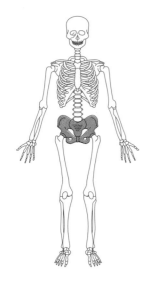

Figure 8–1. The pelvic girdle.

▶ ANATOMY OF THE PELVIC GIRDLE

The pelvic girdle is formed by the paired ossa coxae (AH-sah KOK-sē), which are commonly referred to as the hip bones *(Figure 8–1, Table 8–1)*. The coxal *(coxa* = hip) bones articulate with each other anteriorly and with the sacrum of the vertebral column posteriorly to form a basin that is known as the bony pelvis. The pelvis supports the visceral organs of the lower abdomen. In addition, the pelvic girdle functions to attach the lower limbs to the trunk of the body. As the weight of the upper body is transmitted to the lower limbs via the pelvis, strong ligaments firmly secure the pelvic girdle to the axial skeleton.

OSSA COXAE

The ossa coxae are also known as the **innominate** (i-NOM-i-nāt) **bones.** Each of these large, irregular-shaped hip bones is actually formed by the fusion of three bones. In infancy, the ilium, ischium, and pubis are separate bones *(Figure 8–2)*. They fuse together in the area of the acetabulum (as-e-TAB-ū-lum) during late adolescence, approximately ages 18 to 20. The acetabulum is a deep cup-shaped depression located on either lower lateral margin of the pelvis. The head of the femur fits into this socket to form the hip joint *(Figure 8–3)*.

ILIUM

The ilium (IL-ē-um) is the largest segment of the hip bone, located superior to the acetabulum and forming the upper two fifths of the socket. The bone consists of two main portions: the ala and the body.

The upper flared portion of the ilium is called the **ala** (A-lah). This winglike structure has a sightly concave inner surface termed the **iliac fossa.** The ala is thin but broad, allowing for the attachment of abdominal muscles. The curved upper margin of the ala is known as the **iliac crest.** It can be palpated at the lateral aspect of the waistline and is a commonly used positioning and centering landmark for abdominal radiography. The iliac crest extends from the **anterior superior iliac spine (ASIS)** anteriorly to the **posterior superior iliac spine (PSIS)** posteriorly. The ASIS can also be palpated as a positioning landmark. The **anterior inferior iliac spine (AIIS)** is a smaller, nonpalpable structure located approximately 1 in. (2.5 cm) inferior to the ASIS. The PSIS cannot be readily palpated but is marked on a person's backside by the appearance of a dimple in the skin caused by the attachment of deep muscles. The **posterior inferior iliac spine (PIIS)** lies approximately 1 in. (2.5 cm) inferior to the PSIS and also cannot be palpated. The **greater sciatic** (sī-AT-ik) **notch** is a deep indentation on the posterior aspect of the ilium just below the PIIS. The sciatic nerve passes through this area as it travels to the leg. A smaller indentation, the **lesser sciatic notch,** is located more inferiorly on the ischium. The posterolateral surface of the ilium may also be referred to as the **gluteal** (GLOO-tē-al) **surface.** On the posterior surface of the ilium, there are three arched ridges known as the posterior, anterior, and inferior **gluteal lines,** which serve as the attachment site for the gluteal muscles of the buttock.

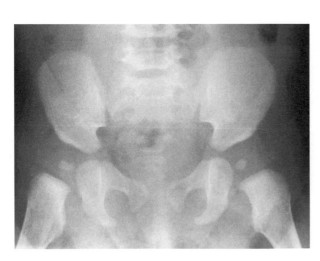

Figure 8–2. Radiograph of an infant's pelvis. Notice the hip bones are not fused in the area of the acetabulum.

Table 8–1 Summary of the Pelvic Girdle

Bones of Each Os Coxa	Description
Ilium (2)	Body Winglike ala Landmarks: iliac crest, ASIS Two fifths of acetabulum
Ischium (2)	Body and ramus L-shaped Landmark: ischial tuberosity Two fifths of acetabulum
Pubis (2)	Body and two rami V-shaped Landmark: symphysis pubis One fifth of acetabulum

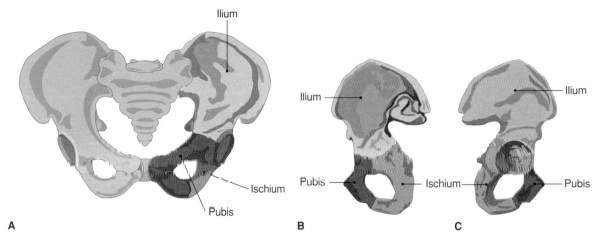

Figure 8–3. Hip bone. The locations of the ilium, ischium, and pubis are illustrated on **(A)** anterior, **(B)** medial, and **(C)** lateral views.

Each ilium attaches to the sacrum posteriorly. The **auricular** (aw-RIK-u-lar) **surface** of the ilium is an ear-shaped area located posterior to the iliac fossa. It articulates with a similarly shaped area on the sacrum to form the sacroiliac joint. The **arcuate** (AR-kū-at) **line** is a ridge of bone on the anterior surface of the ilium extending medially and inferiorly from the auricular surface to the symphysis pubis.

The body of the ilium is the inferior aspect of the bone. It is thicker than the ala and forms the upper two fifths of the acetabulum *(Figure 8–4)*.

ISCHIUM

The ischium (ISH-ē-um or IS-kē-um) is smaller than the ilium and constitutes the posteroinferior portion of the hip bone. It is basically L-shaped and consists of a body and ramus.

The thick upper part of the body makes up the lower, posterior two fifths of the acetabulum. The **ischial spine** is a triangular bony structure projecting posteriorly from the acetabulum and medially into the pelvic cavity. It is located at the lower border of the greater sciatic notch. The **lesser sciatic notch** is found on the ischium just below the ischial spine. It serves as a passageway for blood vessels and nerves of the pelvis and leg. The rounded, roughened process on the posteroinferior aspect of the body is the **ischial tuberosity.** It can be palpated just below the gluteal folds and lateral to the anus. It can be used as a positioning landmark for a PA projection of the abdomen because it lies approximately 1.5 in. (3.8 cm) below the level of the symphysis pubis. The ischial tuberosities are sturdy structures, as together they bear most of the body's weight in a sitting position.

The **ramus** is that part of the ischium that extends anteriorly, interiorly, and medially from the body to adjoin the inferior ramus of the pubis. It is thinner and flatter than the body (see *Figure 8–4*).

PUBIS

The anteroinferior aspect of each hip bone is formed by the pubis (PŪ-bis), or pubic bone. It is essentially a V-shaped bone, consisting of a body and two rami.

The body of the pubis constitutes the anterior one fifth of the acetabulum. It extends anteriorly and medially as the **superior ramus.** The superior rami of the right and left pubic bones meet at the midsagittal plane to form the **symphysis pubis.** A small ridge of bone on the anterior border of the superior ramus is known as the **pubic crest.** It extends between the symphysis pubis and the **pubic tubercle,** a small bony process located slightly lateral to the symphysis pubis. The **inferior ramus** of the pubis extends inferiorly from the superior ramus and angles laterally to join the ramus of the ischium. The inferior rami of the right and left pubic bones form an inverted V-shaped area known as the **pubic arch.**

Each hip bone has a large opening on its inferior aspect. The rami of the ischium and pubis join to form a bony loop. The loop encircles an opening called the **obturator** (ob-tū-RĀ-tor) **foramen** through which nerves and blood vessels pass. The opening is generally covered with a fibrous tissue providing for a site of muscle attachments. It also serves to lighten the weight of the pelvis (see *Figure 8–4*).

▶ *Makeup of the Acetabulum*

- ⅖ *Ilium*

- ⅖ *Ischium*

- ⅕ *Pubis*

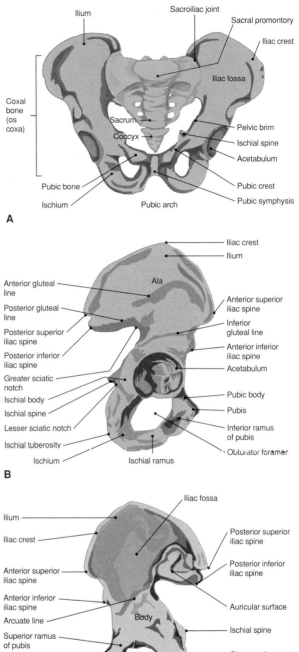

A

B

C

Figure 8–4. Hip bone. Structures on the ilium, ischium, and pubis are demonstrated on **(A)** anterior, **(B)** medial, and **(C)** lateral views.

BONY PELVIS

As previously stated, the bony pelvis is a basinlike structure. It is divided into the false, or greater, pelvis and the true, or lesser, pelvis at the pelvic brim. This is a bony ridge that passes obliquely from the upper margin of the symphysis pubis and through the arcuate lines to the sacral promontory, which is the prominent projection on the upper anterior part of the sacrum.

The **false pelvis** is located above the pelvic brim. It is bounded posteriorly by the lower lumbar spine, laterally by the ilia, and anteriorly by the muscles of the abdominal wall. The false pelvis supports organs of the abdomen, as well as the developing fetus during pregnancy.

The **true pelvis** begins at the pelvic brim and continues as that area beneath the brim. It is actually a cavity surrounded by bony walls. The urinary bladder and rectum are contained within the true pelvis, as are the vagina and uterus in a female. The pelvic brim is also known as the pelvic inlet, as it forms the upper border of the pelvic cavity. The opening at the lower end of the cavity is known as the pelvic outlet. It is bounded posteriorly by the tip of the coccyx, laterally by the ischial spines and tuberosities, and anteriorly by the pubic arch *(Figure 8–5)*. During childbirth, the baby passes through the inlet, cavity, and outlet of the true pelvis. In an ultrasound examination conducted during pregnancy, measurements can be taken of the inlet and outlet of the maternal pelvis, as well as the head of the fetus. If the mother's pelvis is too narrow or the baby too large, the obstetrician may perform a cesarean section to avoid potential complications during delivery. The measurements can also be determined radiographically through a pelvimetry examination; however, this procedure is rarely performed today because of the radiation exposure to the fetus.

DIFFERENCES BETWEEN MALE AND FEMALE PELVES

There are distinct structural differences between the male and female pelves. The female pelvis demonstrates definite adaptations for pregnancy and childbearing. It is tilted forward; the male pelvis is not. Overall, the bones of the female pelvis are smoother and lighter than those of the male pelvis. The ilia are broader, less curved, and more shallow on the female pelvis. The pelvic inlet is larger and more rounded. The sacrum is broader, shorter, and less curved on the female pelvis, which causes the pelvic cavity to be wider. The pelvic outlet is also wider on the female pelvis because the ischial spines and ischial tuberosities are further apart. This structure allows the baby's head to pass through easily during childbirth. The pubic arch or angle is also greater than 90°. The hips appear more prominent on a female because there is greater distance between the anterior superior iliac spines and ischial tuberosities. *Table 8–2* summarizes the structural differences between the female and male pelves.

ARTHROLOGY OF THE PELVIC GIRDLE

The bones of the pelvic girdle articulate to form the paired sacroiliac and hip joints, the single symphysis pubis, and the fused joints in the acetabula.

The **sacroiliac** (sā-krō-IL-ē-ak) **joints** are commonly referred to as the S-I joints. They are formed by the articulation of the ilia with the sacrum. Each joint is wedge-shaped and positioned in the pelvis at an oblique angle. This is due to the shape of the sacrum and ilium, requiring the auricular surface of the sacrum to overlap the auricular surface of the ilium. Structurally, it is an unusual joint which has two joint classifications to reflect this fact. The upper portion of the joint is fibrous (syndesmosis) and permits very little movement; therefore, it is classified as amphiarthrodial. It is very strong to support the weight of the upper body. The lower part of the joint is slightly weaker. It is diarthrodial (synovial) with gliding-type movement; however, the movement is slight and takes place primarily in a female during late pregnancy and delivery.

The **hip joints** are also known as the **coxofemoral,** or **coxal, joints.** Each coxal joint is formed by the ball-like head of the femur articulating with the cup-shaped acetabulum of the pelvis. It is classified as a diarthrodial joint with ball-and-socket type of movement. Although a wide range of motion is permitted (rotation, circumduction, flexion, extension, abduction, and adduction), strong ligaments and the depth of the acetabulum place limitations on the joint movement. Thus, it is not as freely movable as the shoulder joint, although it has the same type of movement.

The **symphysis pubis** is a single joint formed when the rami of the right and left pubic bones meet at the midline. It is cartilaginous in structure, as articular cartilage is present on each articular surface and a pad of fibrocartilage is situated between the bones. Ligaments hold the pubic bones securely together. Only slight movement is permitted at the joint; thus, it is classified as amphiarthrodial.

Each **acetabulum** is formed by the fusion of the ilium, ischium, and the pubis. Because the acetabulum must be a sturdy structure, the articulations permit no movement and are classified as synarthrodial. Initially, they are synchondroses because cartilage is present; however, the bones fuse together completely in the adult, forming synostoses *(Figure 8–6)*. *Table 8–3* summarizes the joints of the pelvic girdle.

Table 8–2. Structural Differences Between Female and Male Pelves

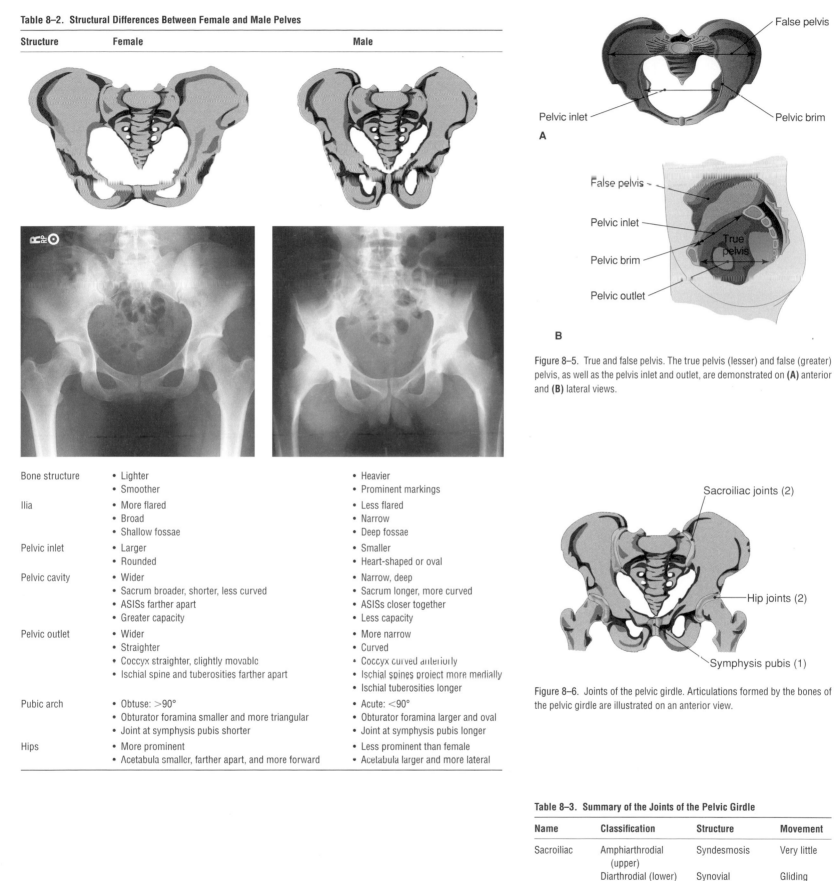

Structure	Female	Male
Bone structure	• Lighter • Smoother	• Heavier • Prominent markings
Ilia	• More flared • Broad • Shallow fossae	• Less flared • Narrow • Deep fossae
Pelvic inlet	• Larger • Rounded	• Smaller • Heart-shaped or oval
Pelvic cavity	• Wider • Sacrum broader, shorter, less curved • ASISs farther apart • Greater capacity	• Narrow, deep • Sacrum longer, more curved • ASISs closer together • Less capacity
Pelvic outlet	• Wider • Straighter • Coccyx straighter, slightly movable • Ischial spine and tuberosities farther apart	• More narrow • Curved • Coccyx curved anteriorly • Ischial spines project more medially • Ischial tuberosities longer
Pubic arch	• Obtuse: >90° • Obturator foramina smaller and more triangular • Joint at symphysis pubis shorter	• Acute: <90° • Obturator foramina larger and oval • Joint at symphysis pubis longer
Hips	• More prominent • Acetabula smaller, farther apart, and more forward	• Less prominent than female • Acetabula larger and more lateral

Figure 8–5. True and false pelvis. The true pelvis (lesser) and false (greater) pelvis, as well as the pelvis inlet and outlet, are demonstrated on **(A)** anterior and **(B)** lateral views.

Figure 8–6. Joints of the pelvic girdle. Articulations formed by the bones of the pelvic girdle are illustrated on an anterior view.

Table 8–3. Summary of the Joints of the Pelvic Girdle

Name	Classification	Structure	Movement
Sacroiliac	Amphiarthrodial (upper)	Syndesmosis	Very little
	Diarthrodial (lower)	Synovial	Gliding
Coxal (hip)	Diarthrodial	Synovial	Ball and socket
Symphysis pubis	Amphiarthrodial	Symphysis	Slight give
Acetabulum	Synarthrodial	Synchondrosis → synostosis	None

223

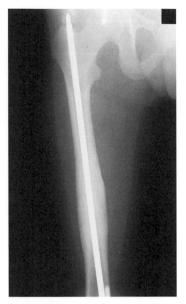

A

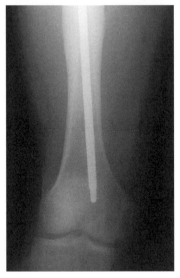

B

Figure 8–7. Although a hip series was ordered on this patient, 14 × 17-in. **(A)** and 10 × 12-in. **(B)** cassettes were needed to include the entire intramedullary rod in the femur.

▶ PROCEDURAL CONSIDERATIONS

Although radiographic examination of the pelvis and hips is usually performed to identify fractures or arthritic conditions on adults, these procedures can also be performed to assess congenital hip dislocations and other developmental conditions in children. Radiography of the pelvis and hips is usually performed with the patient recumbent on the radiographic table; however, weight-bearing pelvis and hip examinations may be done on request.

PATIENT PREPARATION

After the patient is correctly identified, he or she should be instructed to remove everything below the waist, except socks and shoes, and dress in a patient gown. After assisting or moving the patient to the radiographic table, the shoes should be removed to facilitate accurate positioning and eliminate distortion caused by elevation of the legs. As discussed in Chapter 4, a patient history should be obtained to determine the reason for examination and any previous surgery that may impact the procedure. If a patient has had previous hip surgery, any prosthetic device should be included entirely within the collimated area. Because some hip prostheses have very long plates or intramedullary rods, it is important to check previous films or ask the patient specific questions relative to the type and size of the device *(Figure 8–7)*.

POSITIONING CONSIDERATIONS

Radiographic examinations of the pelvis and hips are fairly common procedures, especially for the older patient. An exception to the rule of obtaining at least two projections, the routine examination of the pelvis usually includes only one projection: the AP *(Table 8–4)*. This projection is obtained with the patient lying supine on the radiographic table, with no rotation of the pelvis and the legs internally rotated 15° to 20° to compensate for the anteversion of the femoral necks. To ensure that the patient is internally rotating more than the toes, the radiographer should grasp the patient's heels and internally rotate both entire legs. Sandbags should be positioned against the distal legs for immobilization. When the legs are adequately rotated, the greater trochanters will not be superimposed over the femoral necks and the lesser trochanters will be minimally demonstrated or not seen at all. As previously stated, however, the legs should not be internally rotated when a fracture of the femur is suspected.

One of the most difficult aspects of hip radiography is often the localization of the hip joint and femoral neck. The traditional method requires drawing an imaginary line from the ASIS to the upper border of the symphysis pubis, bisecting that line, and drawing a line perpendicular to the bisection *(Figure 8–8)*. The head of the femur is approximately 1.5 in. distal to the bisection, whereas the femoral neck is approximately 2.5 in. distal to the bisection. Using another method, the central ray is directed to a point 2 in. medial to the ASIS at the level of the superior aspect of the greater trochanter, or inguinal crease *(Figure 8–9)*.

When the hip is radiographed, two projections are generally taken. The initial projection is usually an AP pelvis, taken to include both hips. Subsequent examinations may include an AP projection of the af-

Table 8–4 Routine/Optional Projections: Pelvic Girdle

Pelvis	Sacroiliac joints	Acetabulum
AP	AP obliques	AP oblique (Judet method)
	PA/AP axial[a]	PA axial oblique
		(Teufel method)
Hip	Anterior pelvic bones[a]	
AP (unilateral or bilateral)	AP axial (Taylor method)	
AP oblique (modified Cleaves method)	Superoinferior axial	
Lateral (Lauenstein method)	(Lilienfeld method)	
Transfemoral lateral		

Note. Although routines may vary between departments, this table summarizes some of the more common routine and optional projections and examinations.
[a]Optional projections or examinations; may be routine in some departments.

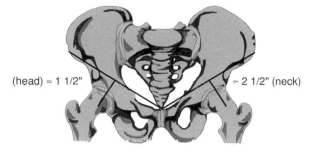

(head) ≈ 1 1/2"   ≈ 2 1/2" (neck)

Figure 8–8. Using the ASIS and symphysis pubis as landmarks, the femoral head and neck can be located.

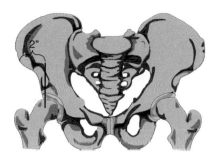

Figure 8–9. Alternate method of locating the hip joint uses the ASIS and upper border of the greater trochanter as landmarks.

fected side only, depending on department routine. The second projection is either the AP oblique (modified Cleaves or "frog-leg"), a lateral (Lauenstein), or a transfemoral lateral. The first two projections are somewhat similar relative to patient position. For the frog-leg projection, the patient's pelvis is supine. For the lateral hip projection, however, the patient is rotated toward the affected side. Because the affected leg is abducted in both of these projections, they are contraindicated when a pelvis or hip fracture is suspected. When a fracture is suspected, an AP projection with the affected leg in neutral position and a transfemoral lateral projection should be obtained. The transfemoral lateral projection may also be requested as part of a postoperative hip examination.

If a fractured hip is suspected because of foreshortening or unnatural position of the limb, the leg should NOT be internally rotated. In addition to causing severe pain because of muscle or nerve injury, internal rotation of a fractured hip could also cause unnecessary vascular damage that might lead to blood clot formation and possible pulmonary embolism.

Because the sacroiliac joints are positioned obliquely within the body, the patient must be rotated to "open" or fully demonstrate the joint. The patient is typically positioned in a 25° to 30° posterior oblique with the affected side elevated. Both joints are examined for comparison. The PA axial projection, obtained with the patient prone and central ray directed 30° caudad, may also be used to demonstrate the sacroiliac joints. Because of the anteroposterior angle of the joints, the prone projection uses the diverging central ray to more clearly demonstrate the joints and should be used if the patient is able to lie in this position. Keep in mind, however, there is increased object–image receptor distance with the PA projection. When the patient is unable to lie prone, the reverse of this, the AP axial, may be performed with a 30° to 35° cephalic angle.

ALTERNATE PROJECTIONS

Although not used on a regular basis, special projections can be obtained to demonstrate the anterior pelvic bones and acetabulum to evaluate suspected fractures or other pathology. The AP axial projection elongates and opens up the obturator foramina and can also be used to evaluate the pelvic outlet, whereas the superoinferior projection superimposes the superior rami of the pubic bones over the inferior rami of the pubic bones and ischia and is sometimes used to examine the pelvic inlet. Because acetabular fractures may be difficult to diagnose, AP oblique and PA axial projections of the acetabulum may also be performed.

For patients with bilateral hip fractures, bilateral hip arthroplasty, or inability to elevate the unaffected leg, an axiolateral projection (Clements–Nakayama method) can be used. The patient is supine on the radiographic table with the legs in a neutral or slightly externally rotated position. A grid cassette is positioned lengthwise along the side of the hip, parallel to the femoral neck, and tilted backward 15°. The central ray is directed 15° posteriorly and perpendicularly to the femoral neck and cassette *(Figure 8–10)*.

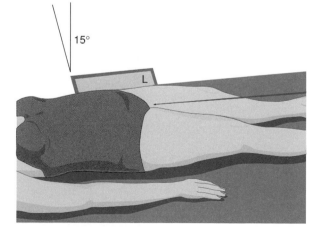

Figure 8–10. Axis lateral hip (Clements–Nakayama method). The central ray is directed 15° posteriorly and perpendicular to the femoral neck.

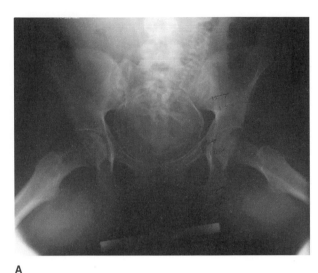

A

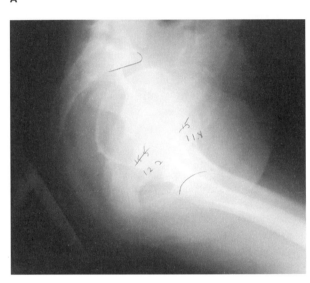

B

Figure 8–11. AP **(A)** and lateral **(B)** pelvimetry projections were at one time fairly common, but have been replaced by ultrasound today.

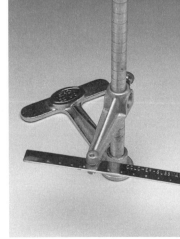

Figure 8–12. Colcher–Sussman pelvimeter.

Although rarely performed today, pelvimetries were performed to measure the pelvic inlet and outlet relative to the fetal head *(Figure 8–11)*. This information provided vital information regarding the possibility of a gravid woman's ability to deliver a child naturally. The most common method included anteroposterior and lateral projections of the mother's pelvis with a special ruler called a Colcher–Sussman pelvimeter *(Figure 8–12)*. This ruler was positioned at the level of the ischial tuberosities for the AP projection and the midsagittal plane for the lateral projection. Because of the possible risk of radiation exposure to the fetus, however, diagnostic medical sonography has become the preferred method for examining the gravid female.

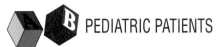 PEDIATRIC PATIENTS

In addition to trauma, other diseases or conditions may necessitate pelvic or hip radiography of children. Developmental dysplasia of the hip (DDH), formerly called congenital dislocation of the hip, is a fairly common abnormality, occurring in 1.5 to 10 per 1000 live births. Although some of the factors contributing to DDH are still unknown, intrauterine position of the fetus, a shallow acetabulum, and/or hormonal influences may contribute to this problem in the newborn. Bilateral radiographic imaging of the hips can be performed to measure the angle of the acetabular roof and the degree of dislocation. Although debate continues regarding the best method to demonstrate DDH, one technique used is the von Rosen method, which involves abducting the legs 45° and fully rotating the legs and hips internally. To obtain a reliable study, however, the radiographer must ensure that the legs and hips are symmetrically positioned for comparison. Because of the difficulty of immobilizing infants, sonography is preferred for children less than 1 year of age.

Legg–Calvé–Perthes disease, commonly called Perthes' disease, is an idiopathic condition usually diagnosed in children between the ages of 3 and 12. This disease, technically termed avascular necrosis, is caused by a loss of blood supply to the femoral head, resulting in abnormal growth and bone necrosis. Eventually, as revascularization occurs, necrotic tissue is reabsorbed and the femoral head can develop normally following treatment. Although initial radiographs may appear normal (living bone and dead bone look the same on radiographs), follow-up radiographs illustrate deterioration of the femoral head and may be required to evaluate the progress of the disease.

As with all radiography of children, radiation protection is vitally important when radiographing the pelvis or hips. Because of the location of the gonads and the likelihood of follow-up examinations, it is an even more important factor. High-speed film/screen combinations, collimation, and appropriate shielding minimize the dose to the patient's gonads and active bone marrow.

BREATHING INSTRUCTIONS

Although specific instructions relative to inspiration or expiration are not necessary, the patient should be instructed to suspend respiration for all projections of the pelvic girdle. Suspending respiration minimizes patient motion and alerts the patient to the exposure.

EQUIPMENT CONSIDERATIONS

Most radiographs of the pelvic girdle are obtained using a grid. Mobile radiography, however, can be performed without a grid when the patient is small to eliminate the risk of grid lines and reduce exposure to the patient and technologist.

A grid holder or sandbag is needed to immobilize the cassette for the transfemoral or axiolateral projection of the hip. Sandbags should be used to immobilize the legs for AP projections of the pelvis or hip when no fracture is suspected.

EXPOSURE FACTORS

Because of the location of the gonads, radiation protection is an important factor in pelvis and hip radiography. As the use of gonadal shielding could compromise the examination, technical factor selection is one of the few options available to minimize gonadal dose. To visualize bony trabeculae within the bones, therefore, 70 to 75 kVp should be used for most radiographic examinations of the pelvis and hips to produce the highest quality radiographs. Patient condition, however, may require upward or downward adjustment of this range. For example, very thin, elderly patients may require decreasing the kilovoltage to 65 kVp to compensate for the decreased calcium in the bones, while an 80-kVp technique might be used to reduce the exposure time for patients who are unable to hold still. When mobile radiography of the pelvis or hip is performed on very small adults or children, a nongrid technique can be employed using 65 to 70 kVp. The mAs needed depends on the size of the patient, type of equipment generator, film/screen speed used, type of grid, and pathology.

RADIOGRAPHIC POSITIONING OF THE PELVIC GIRDLE

► AP PELVIS

Technical Considerations

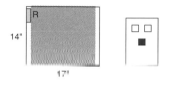

- Film size: 14 × 17 in. crosswise.
- Grid required.
- 65–80 kVp.
- Collimate to include iliac crests and femoral trochanters crosswise and lengthwise.

Note: To avoid placing the ID blocker over the anatomy of interest, position the blocker up when radiographing the hips and down when the right ilium must be demonstrated.

Caution: Do NOT internally rotate the legs if a fracture is suspected.

Shielding

- Gonadal shielding may be used on male patients, especially children and adults of reproductive age, as long as it does not compromise the examination.

Patient Positioning

- Assist the patient to the supine position on the radiographic table; the patient's legs should be extended, if possible.
- Center the midsagittal plane to the midline of the table.
- Adjust the patient's midsagittal plane to lie parallel with the long axis of the table.

Part Positioning

- Adjust the patient's body so the distances between the ASISs and tabletop are equal to ensure there is no rotation; sponges may be needed to support and position very thin patients.
- Center the cassette to the midpoint of the pelvis, approximately halfway between the iliac crests and symphysis pubis; the top edge of the cassette should be about 1.5 to 2 in. above the iliac crests.
- Grasping the patient's heels, internally rotate the patient's legs 15° to 20°; immobilize by placing sandbags against the lower legs and ankles *(Figure 8–13)*.

Central Ray

- Direct the central ray perpendicular to the center of the cassette, the central ray should enter approximately 2 in. above the symphysis pubis. **Note:** This projection is also performed in many departments as part of the routine hip examination. In this situation, centering may be slightly lower to include more of the proximal femurs.

Breathing Instructions

- Instruct the patient to stop breathing during the exposure.

Image Evaluation

- The iliac crests and greater and lesser trochanters should be included in the collimated area.
- The ilia and hip joints should be adequately penetrated; bony trabeculae should be clearly seen.
- The obturator foramina and iliac crests should be symmetrical in size and shape.
- The femoral necks should be free of superimposition by the greater trochanters, and the lesser trochanters should be minimally demonstrated or not seen *(Figure 8–14)*.

1. Sacrum
2. Ischial spine
3. Acetabulum
4. Greater trochanter
5. Ischial tuberosity
6. Symphysis pubis
7. Iliac crest
8. Anterior superior iliac spine
9. Superior ramus of pubis
10. Femoral head
11. Femoral neck
12. Obturator foramen

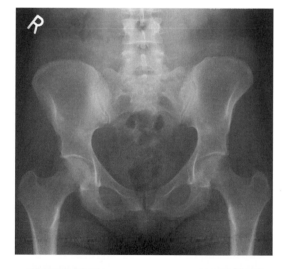

Figure 8–13. AP pelvis.

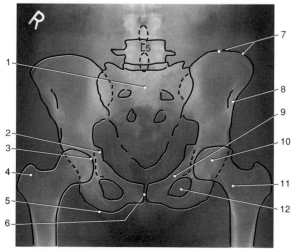

Figure 8–14. Female AP pelvis with legs rotated internally 15° to 20°.

229

► AP HIP

Technical Considerations

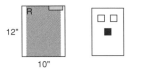

- Film size: 10 × 12 in. lengthwise.
- Grid required.
- 65–80 kVp.
- Collimate to include the ASIS, symphysis pubis, and greater trochanter.

Caution: Do NOT internally rotate the legs if a fracture is suspected.

Shielding

- Gonadal shielding may be used on all patients, especially children and adults of reproductive age, as long as it does not compromise the examination.

Patient Positioning

- Assist the patient to the supine position on the radiographic table; the patient's legs should be extended, if possible.
- Center the sagittal plane 2 in. medial to the ASIS of the affected side to the midline of the table. **Note:** For the initial hip examination, the AP projection of the entire pelvis is usually obtained. Follow-up studies may include only the affected side.
- Adjust the patient's midsagittal plane to lie parallel with the long axis of the table.

Part Positioning

- Adjust the patient's body so the distances between the ASISs and tabletop are equal to ensure there is no rotation; sponges may be needed to support and position very thin patients.
- Grasping the patient's heel, internally rotate the patient's leg 15° to 20°; immobilize by placing a sandbag against the lower leg and ankle *(Figure 8–15)*. **Note:** External rotation or neutral position of the leg will demonstrate the lesser trochanter.

Central Ray

- Using one of the localization techniques previously described, direct the central ray perpendicular to the cassette through the femoral neck; the central ray should enter at the inguinal crease (where the leg bends).
- Center the cassette to the central ray.

Breathing Instructions

- Instruct the patient to stop breathing during the exposure.

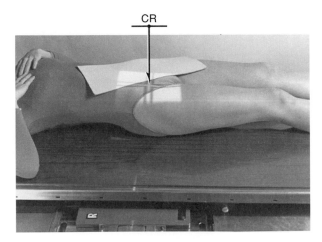

Figure 8–15. AP hip.

Image Evaluation

- The inferior portion of the iliac crest, acetabulum, greater and lesser trochanters, and approximately one third of the proximal femur, including any prosthetic device, should be included in the collimated area.
- The femoral head and acetabulum should be adequately penetrated; bony trabeculae should be clearly seen.
- The femoral neck should be centered to the film and seen free of superimposition by the greater trochanter, without any foreshortening; the lesser trochanter should be minimally demonstrated or not seen (*Figure 8–16*).

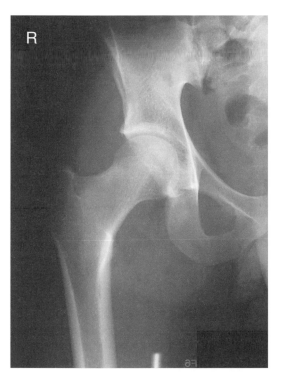
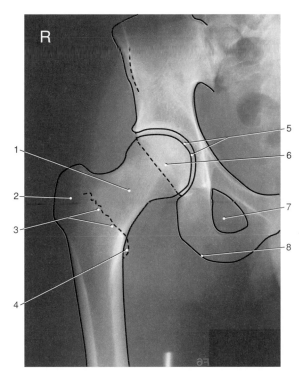

Figure 8–16. Unilateral right AP hip.

1. Femoral neck
2. Greater trochanter
3. Intertrochanteric crest
4. Lesser trochanter
5. Acetabulum
6. Femoral head
7. Obturator foramen
8. Ischial tuberosity

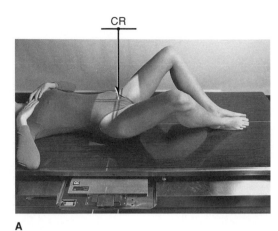

A

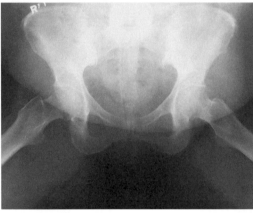

B

Figure 8–17. Bilateral AP oblique hip.

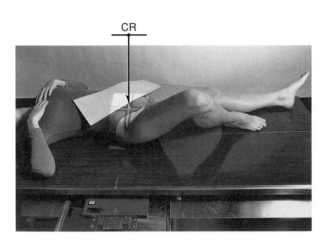

Figure 8–18. Unilateral AP oblique (frog-leg) hip.

▶ AP OBLIQUE HIP (MODIFIED CLEAVES METHOD—"FROG-LEG" LATERAL)

Technical Considerations

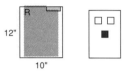

- Film size: 10 × 12 in. lengthwise or crosswise.
- Grid required.
- 65–80 kVp.
- Collimate to include ASIS, acetabulum, and proximal one third of femur.

Caution: Do NOT perform this projection if a fracture is suspected.

Shielding

- Gonadal shielding may be used on all patients, especially children and adults of reproductive age, as long as it does not compromise the examination.

Patient Positioning

- Assist the patient to the supine position on the radiographic table; the patient's legs should be extended, if possible.
- Center the sagittal plane passing through the ASIS of the affected side to the midline of the table. **Note:** This projection can also be performed bilaterally, with the patient's midsagittal plane centered to the midline of the grid device *(Figure 8–17)*.
- Adjust the patient's midsagittal plane to lie parallel with the long axis of the table.

Part Positioning

- Adjust the patient's body so the distances between the ASISs and tabletop are equal to ensure there is no rotation; sponges may be needed to support and position very thin patients.
- Flex the hip and knee of the affected side, resting the foot near the knee of the opposite leg; move the patient slowly as this position may be somewhat painful.
- Keeping the knee and hip flexed, abduct the flexed leg 40° *(Figure 8–18)*.

Central Ray

- Using one of the localization techniques previously described, direct the central ray perpendicular through the femoral neck; the central ray should enter at the inguinal crease (where the leg bends).
- Center the cassette to the central ray.

Breathing Instructions

- Instruct the patient to stop breathing during the exposure.

Image Evaluation

- The inferior portion of the ilium, acetabulum, greater and lesser trochanters, and approximately one third of the proximal femur, including any prosthetic device, should be included in the collimated area.
- The femoral head and acetabulum should be adequately penetrated; bony trabeculae should be clearly seen.
- The femoral neck should be in the center of the film and seen without any unnecessary foreshortening.
- The greater trochanters should be superimposed over the femoral neck (*Figure 8–19*).

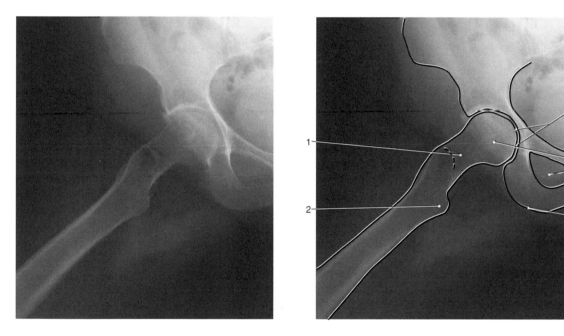

Figure 8–19. Unilateral AP oblique hip.

1. Femoral neck	3. Acetabulum	5. Obturator foramen
2. Lesser trochanter	4. Femoral head	6. Ischial tuberosity

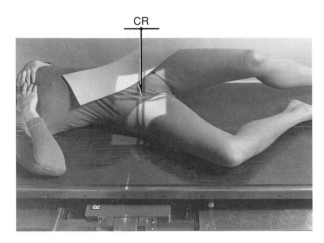

Figure 8–20. Lateral hip using Lauenstein method.

► LATERAL HIP (LAUENSTEIN METHOD)

Technical Considerations

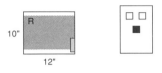

- Film size: 10 × 12 in. crosswise or lengthwise.
- Grid required.
- 65–80 kVp.
- Collimate to include acetabulum and proximal one third of femur.

Caution: Do NOT perform this projection if a fracture is suspected.

Shielding

- Gonadal shielding may be used on all patients, especially children and adults of reproductive age, as long as it does not compromise the examination.

Patient Positioning

- Assist the patient to the supine position on the radiographic table.
- Rotate the patient slightly toward the side of interest; use a sponge to support the elevated side.
- Center the sagittal plane passing midway between the ASIS and symphysis pubis to the midline of the table.

Part Positioning

- Flex the hip and knee of the affected side, bringing the thigh to almost a 60° angle with the body; abduct the thigh until it is resting on the tabletop *(Figure 8–20)*.

Central Ray

- Using one of the previously described localization techniques, direct the central ray perpendicular to the hip joint; the central ray should enter approximately midway between the ASIS and symphysis pubis.
- Center the cassette to the central ray.

Breathing Instructions

- Instruct the patient to stop breathing during the exposure.

Image Evaluation

- The inferior portion of the ilium, acetabulum, greater and lesser trochanters, and approximately one third of the proximal femur, including any prosthetic device, should be included in the collimated area.
- The femoral head and acetabulum should be adequately penetrated; bony trabeculae should be clearly seen.
- The hip joint should be centered to the film.
- The femoral neck should be seen without any foreshortening.
- The greater and lesser trochanters should be partially superimposed over the femoral neck and femoral shaft, respectively *(Figure 8–21)*.

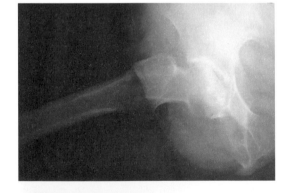

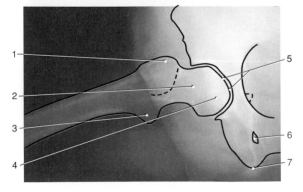

Figure 8–21. Lateral hip using Lauenstein method; note the appearance of the obturator foramen.

1. Greater trochanter
2. Femoral neck
3. Lesser trochanter
4. Femoral head
5. Acetabulum
6. Obturator foramen
7. Ischial tuberosity

► TRANSFEMORAL (SURGICAL, CROSS-TABLE) LATERAL HIP

Technical Considerations

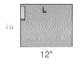

- Film size: 10 × 12 in. lengthwise.
- Grid required.
- 80–90 kVp.
- Collimate to include acetabulum, proximal one third of femur, and ischial tuberosity.

Caution: Do NOT internally rotate the legs if a fracture is suspected.

Shielding

- Gonadal shielding may be used on female patients, especially children and adults of reproductive age, as long as it does not compromise the examination.

Patient Positioning

- Assist the patient to the supine position on the radiographic table; a radiolucent support can be placed under the pelvis of thin patients to place the hip in the center of the film.
- Adjust the patient's midsagittal plane to lie parallel with the long axis of the table.
- Support the grid cassette in the vertical position next to the affected hip with the side nearest the patient's head at the level of the iliac crest; angle the opposite end away from the patient until the cassette is parallel with the femoral neck. Use a cassette holder or sandbags to immobilize the cassette.

Part Positioning

- Adjust the patient's body so the distances between the ASISs and tabletop are equal to ensure there is no rotation; sponges may be needed to support and position very thin patients.
- Flex the hip and knee of the unaffected leg and elevate the leg; rest the foot on sandbags or other support to remove the leg from the field of view.
- Unless contraindicated because of the patient's condition, internally rotate the patient's leg by grasping the patient's heel and internally rotating 15° to 20°; immobilize by placing sandbags against the lower legs and ankles *(Figures 8–22, 8–23)*.

Central Ray

- Direct the central ray horizontally and at right angles to the femoral neck; use the localization techniques previously described to identify the location and angle of the femoral neck. Adjust the cassette to coincide with the central ray.

Breathing Instructions

- Instruct the patient to stop breathing during the exposure.

Image Evaluation

- The acetabulum, ischial tuberosity, greater and lesser trochanters, and approximately one third of the proximal femur, including any prosthetic device, should be included in the collimated area.
- The femoral head and acetabulum should be adequately penetrated; bony trabeculae should be seen.
- The femoral neck should be demonstrated without any foreshortening or elongation; the greater and lesser trochanters will be partially superimposed over the proximal femur when the leg is inverted *(Figure 8–24)*.

1. Femoral head
2. Acetabulum
3. Ischial tuberosity
4. Femoral neck
5. Lesser trochanter
6. Greater trochanter

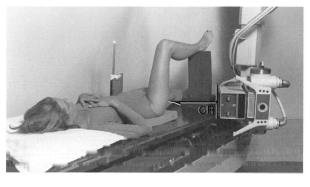

Figure 8–22. To obtain a transfemoral lateral hip projection, the patient's unaffected leg must be elevated above the path of the central ray.

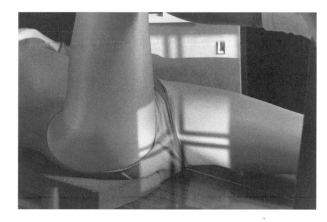

Figure 8–23. When positioning for the transfemoral lateral hip projection, the central ray is directed horizontally and perpendicular to the femoral neck and film.

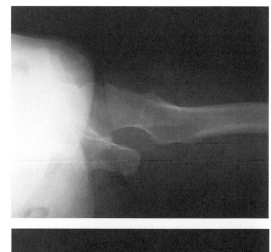

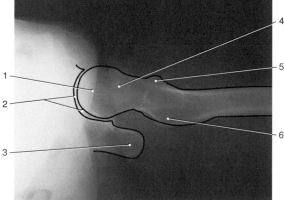

Figure 8–24. Transfemoral lateral hip.

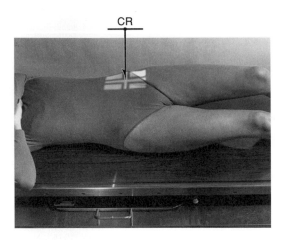

Figure 8–25. RPO position to demonstrate the left sacroiliac joint.

► AP OBLIQUE SACROILIAC JOINTS

Technical Considerations

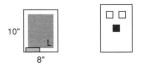

- Film size: 8 × 10 in. lengthwise, 9 × 9 in. or 10 × 12 in. lengthwise.
- Grid required.
- 65–80 kVp.
- Collimate to include sacroiliac joint furthest from the film.

Shielding

- Gonadal shielding may be used on all patients, especially children and adults of reproductive age, as long as it does not compromise the examination.

Patient Positioning

- Assist the patient to the supine position on the radiographic table.
- Adjust the patient's midsagittal plane to lie parallel with the long axis of the table.

Part Positioning

- Rotate the patient's body to a 25° to 30° posterior oblique position; the arm of the elevated side should be brought across the chest and a sponge or other radiolucent support should be positioned behind the patient for immobilization. The shoulders should be rotated the same degree as the hips.
- Center the plane passing 1 in. medial to the ASIS of the side up to the midline of the table; the joint furthest from the film will be demonstrated *(Figure 8–25)*.
- Examine the opposite side in the same manner for comparison.

Central Ray

- Direct the central ray perpendicular to a point 1 in. medial to the ASIS of the elevated side; center the cassette to the central ray.

Breathing Instructions

- Instruct the patient to stop breathing during the exposure.

Image Evaluation

- The sacroiliac joint, ASIS, and ilium of the elevated side should be included in the collimated area.
- The sacroiliac joint should be adequately penetrated; bony trabeculae should be clearly seen.
- The sacroiliac joint of the elevated side should be clearly demonstrated; RPO and LPO projections should be mirror images of each other *(Figure 8–26)*.

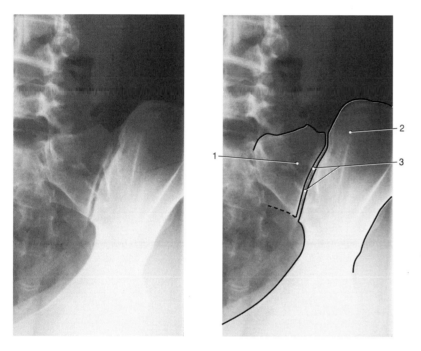

Figure 8–26. Left sacroiliac joint demonstrated with the patient in a 25° to 30° RPO position.

1. Sacrum   2. Ilium   3. Left sacroiliac joint

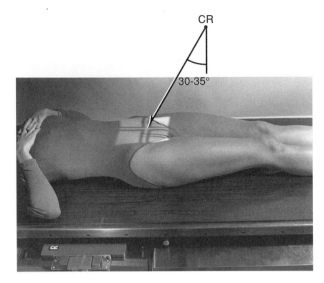

Figure 8–27. An AP axial sacroiliac joint projection can be obtained when the patient is unable to lie in the prone position.

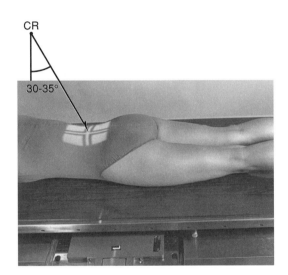

Figure 8–28. PA axial sacroiliac joints.

► PA AXIAL SACROILIAC JOINTS

Technical Considerations

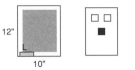

- Film size: 10 × 12 in. lengthwise.
- Grid required.
- 65–80 kVp.
- Collimate to include sacroiliac joints.

Shielding

- Gonadal shielding may be used on male patients, especially children and adults of reproductive age, as long as it does not compromise the examination.

Patient Positioning

- Assist the patient to the prone position on the radiographic table. **Note:** This view can also be obtained with the patient supine and the central ray directed 30° to 35° cephalad, entering approximately 1.5 to 2 in. below the level of the ASIS *(Figure 8–27)*.
- Adjust the patient's midsagittal plane to lie parallel with the long axis of the table.

Part Positioning

- Adjust the patient's body so there is no rotation; sponges may be needed to support and position some patients *(Figure 8–28)*.

Central Ray

- Direct the central ray 30° to 35° caudad through the lumbosacral junction; shallow pelves (female) usually require a steeper angle than deep pelves (male). The central ray enters slightly above the iliac crests; center the cassette to the central ray.

Breathing Instructions

• Instruct the patient to stop breathing during the exposure.

Image Evaluation

• The sacroiliac joints, fifth lumbar vertebra, and superior border of the symphysis pubis should be included in the collimated area.
• The sacroiliac joints should be adequately penetrated; bony trabeculae should be clearly seen *(Figure 8–29)*.

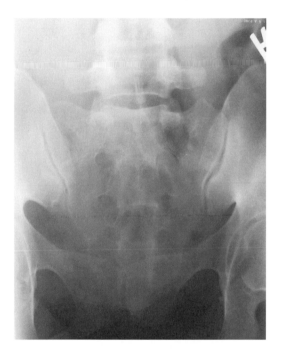 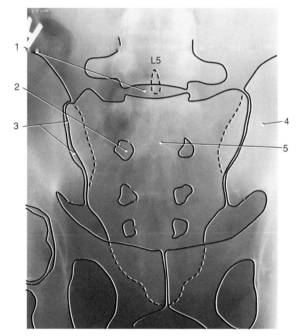

Figure 8–29. PA axial sacroiliac joints, bilateral examination.

1. L5–S1 junction   3. Sacroiliac joint   5. Sacrum
2. Sacral foramen   4. Ilium

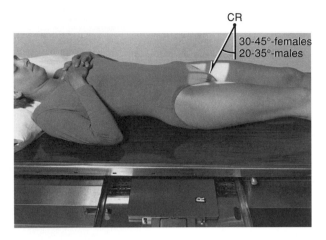

Figure 8–30. AP axial anterior pelvic bone projection (Taylor method).

▶ AP AXIAL ANTERIOR PELVIC BONES (TAYLOR METHOD)

Technical Considerations

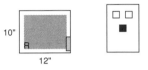

- Film size: 10 × 12 in. crosswise.
- Grid required.
- 65–80 kVp.
- Collimate to include acetabula and ischial tuberosities crosswise and lengthwise.

Note: This projection may also be performed to evaluate the pelvic outlet. A 14 × 17-in. cassette is positioned crosswise to include the entire pelvis.

Shielding

- Carefully placed gonadal shielding may be used when examining the anterior pelvic bones, especially for children and adults of childbearing age, as long as it does not obscure the structures of interest.

Patient Positioning

- Assist the patient to the supine position on the radiographic table; the patient's legs should be extended, if possible.
- Center the midsagittal plane to the midline of the table.
- Adjust the patient's midsagittal plane to lie parallel with the long axis of the table.

Part Positioning

- Adjust the patient's body so the distances between the ASISs and tabletop are equal to ensure there is no rotation; sponges may be needed to position and support very thin patients *(Figure 8–30)*.

Central Ray

- Direct the central ray cephalad (the degree of angulation depends on the depth of the pelvis; thin, shallow pelves require a greater angle): *Females:* 30° to 45° cephalad to a point 2 in. distal to the upper border of the symphysis pubis; center the cassette to the central ray. *Males:* 20° to 35° cephalad to a point 2 in. distal to the upper border of the symphysis pubis; center the cassette to the central ray.

Note: When obtaining this projection to examine the pelvic outlet, centering should be slightly higher to include the entire pelvis.

Breathing Instructions

- Instruct the patient to stop breathing during the exposure.

Image Evaluation

- The hip joints, pubic and ischial rami, and ischial tuberosities should be included in the collimated area.
- The hip joints, ischia, and pubic bones should be adequately penetrated; bony trabeculae should be clearly seen.
- The obturator foramina should be clearly demonstrated, symmetrical in size and shape, and somewhat elongated *(Figure 8–31)*.

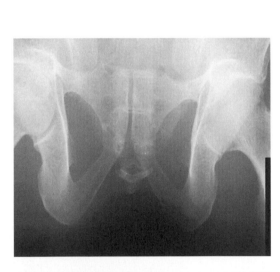

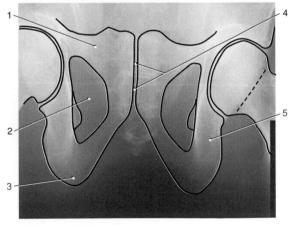

Figure 8–31. AP axial anterior pelvic bones.

1. Superior ramus of pubis
2. Obturator foramen
3. Ischial tuberosity
4. Symphysis pubis
5. Ischium

► SUPEROINFERIOR AXIAL ANTERIOR PELVIC BONES (LILIENFELD METHOD)

Technical Considerations

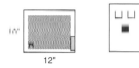

- Film size: 10 × 12 in. crosswise.
- Grid required.
- 70–80 kVp.
- Collimate to include hip joints and ischial tuberosities.

Note: This projection can also be performed to evaluate the pelvic inlet, using a 14 × 17-in. cassette crosswise and centering slightly higher to include the entire pelvis.

Shielding

- Carefully placed gonadal shielding may be used for male patients, especially children and adults of childbearing age, as long as it does not obscure the structures of interest.

Patient Positioning

- Assist the patient to the seated erect position on the radiographic table; the patient's knees may be flexed and supported for comfort.
- Center the midsagittal plane to the midline of the table.
- Adjust the patient's midsagittal plane to lie parallel with the long axis of the table.

Part Positioning

- Adjust the patient's body so the distances between the ASISs and tabletop are equal to ensure there is no rotation; sponges may be needed to support and position very thin patients.
- Center the cassette to the level of the greater trochanter.
- Instruct the patient to lean backward 45° to 50°, using the arms for support; the patient should arch the back, if possible, to help position the pubic arch perpendicular to the film plane *(Figure 8–32)*. **Note:** This projection may also be obtained by positioning the patient supine and the central ray directed 35° to 40° caudally *(Figure 8–33)*.

Central Ray

- Direct the central ray perpendicular to a point approximately 1.5 in. above the symphysis pubis; centering must be slightly higher to include the entire pelvic outlet.
- Center the cassette to the central ray.

Breathing Instructions

- Instruct the patient to stop breathing during the exposure.

Image Evaluation

- The hip joints, pubic and ischial rami, and ischial tuberosities should be included in the collimated area.
- The hip joints, ischia, and pubic bones should be adequately penetrated; bony trabeculae should be clearly seen.
- The obturator foramina should be nearly or completely closed; the pubic rami should be superimposed medially, and the pubic and ischial rami should be almost superimposed laterally *(Figure 8–34)*.

1. Ischium   2. Pubis   3. Symphysis pubis

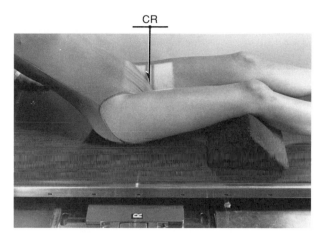

Figure 8–32. Superoinferior axial anterior pelvic bones (Lilienfeld method) with the patient semisitting and back arched forward.

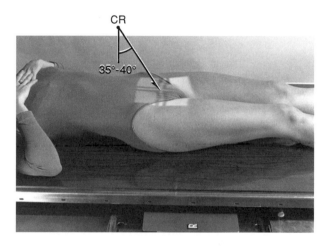

Figure 8–33. Superoinferior axial anterior pelvic bones with the patient supine and central ray directed 35° to 40° caudad.

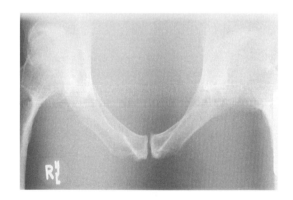

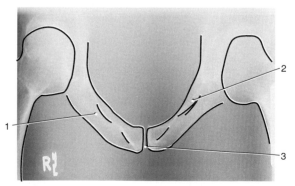

Figure 8–34. Superoinferior axial anterior pelvic bones (Lilienfeld method).

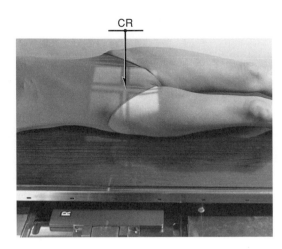

Figure 8–35. RPO position for the right acetabulum (Judet method).

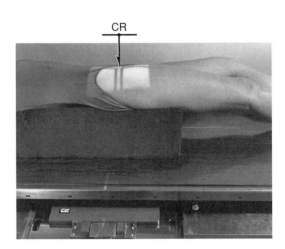

Figure 8–36. LPO position for the right acetabulum (Judet method).

► AP OBLIQUE ACETABULUM (JUDET METHOD)

Technical Considerations

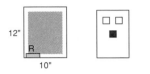

- Film size: 10 × 12 in. lengthwise.
- Grid required.
- 70–80 kVp.
- Collimate to include hip joint.

Shielding

- Gonadal shielding may be used, especially for children and adults of reproductive age, as long as it does not compromise the examination.

Patient Positioning

- Assist the patient to the supine position on the radiographic table.
- Adjust the patient's midsagittal plane to lie parallel with the long axis of the table.

Part Positioning

First Projection
- Rotate the patient to a 45° oblique with the unaffected hip elevated from the table; radiolucent supports should be positioned under the elevated hip and shoulder for immobilization.
- Adjust crosswise centering of the patient so the affected hip is centered to the midline of the grid *(Figure 8–35)*.

Second Projection
- Rotate the patient to a 45° oblique with the affected side elevated from the table; radiolucent supports should be positioned under the elevated hip and shoulder for immobilization.
- Adjust crosswise centering of the patient so the affected hip is centered to the midline of the grid *(Figure 8–36)*.

Central Ray

- Direct the central ray perpendicular to the femoral head of the affected side.
- Center the cassette to the central ray.

Breathing Instructions

- Instruct the patient to stop breathing during the exposure.

Image Evaluation

- The acetabulum, femoral head and neck, and greater trochanter should be included in the collimated area.
- The acetabulum and femoral head should be adequately penetrated; bony trabeculae should be clearly seen *(Figures 8–37, 8–38)*.

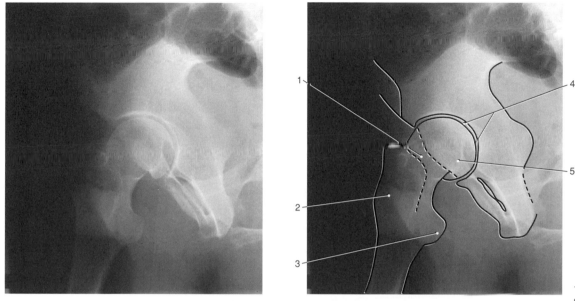
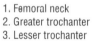

Figure 8–37. RPO position for the right acetabulum (Judet method).

1. Femoral neck
2. Greater trochanter
3. Lesser trochanter
4. Acetabulum
5. Femoral head

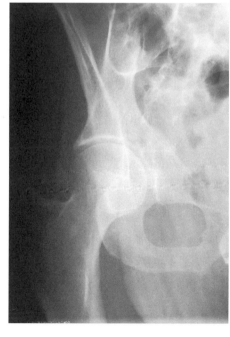
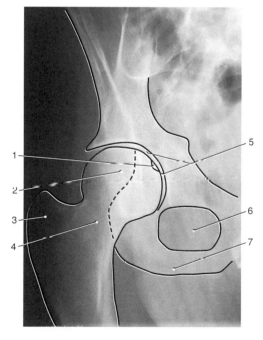

Figure 8–38. LPO position for the right acetabulum (Judet method).

1. Fovea capitis
2. Femoral head
3. Greater trochanter
4. Femoral neck
5. Acetabulum
6. Obturator foramen
7. Ischium

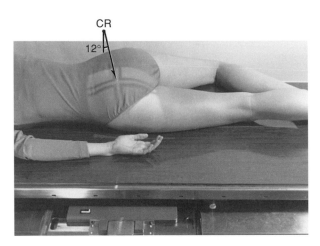

Figure 8–39. LAO position for the left acetabulum (Teufel method).

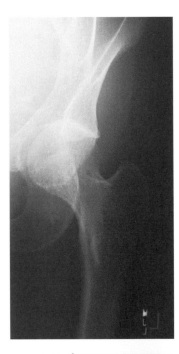

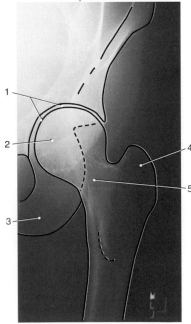

Figure 8–40. LAO position for the right acetabulum (Teufel method).

► PA AXIAL OBLIQUE ACETABULUM (TEUFEL METHOD)

Technical Considerations

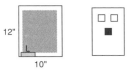

- Film size: 10 × 12 in. lengthwise.
- Grid required.
- 70–80 kVp.
- Collimate to include hip joint of affected side.

Shielding

- Gonadal shielding may be used, especially for children and adults of reproductive age, as long as it does not compromise the examination.

Patient Positioning

- Assist the patient to the semiprone position on the radiographic table; the affected side should be nearest the table.
- Adjust the patient's crosswise centering so the affected hip is centered to the midline of the grid.
- Adjust the patient's longitudinal plane to lie parallel with the long axis of the table.

Part Positioning

- Adjust the patient rotation so the coronal plane forms a 38° angle with the table; the patient may use the arm and leg of the unaffected side for support *(Figure 8–39)*.

Central Ray

- Direct the central ray 12° caudad through the hip joint at the level of the inferior aspect of the coccyx; center the cassette to the central ray.

Breathing Instructions

- Instruct the patient to stop breathing during the exposure.

Image Evaluation

- The acetabulum, femoral head and neck, and greater trochanter should be included in the collimated area.
- The acetabulum and femoral head should be adequately penetrated; bony trabeculae should be clearly seen *(Figure 8–40)*.

1. Acetabulum
2. Femoral head
3. Ischium
4. Greater trochanter
5. Femoral neck

SUMMARY

▶ Radiographic examinations of the pelvis and hip are usually performed with the patient recumbent on the radiographic table.

▶ If a fractured hip is suspected, the affected leg should *not* be internally rotated.

▶ Routine examination of the pelvis usually requires only the single view AP projection.

▶ When the patient is correctly positioned for an AP projection of the pelvis, the ilia and obturator forum ina are symmetrical and the lesser trochanters are barely visible.

▶ Radiography of the hip requires AP and oblique, lateral, or transfemoral lateral projections, depending on patient condition and department protocol

▶ When the posterior oblique projections (RPO and LPO) are used to evaluate the sacroiliac joints, both sides are examined for comparison.

▶ Congenital or developmental conditions often require radiographic hip examinations of the pediatric patient.

▶ Although radiation protection can be challenging when obtaining radiographs of the pelvis and hips, collimation and shielding should be used to minimize patient dose as long as they do not compromise the examination.

▶ Respiration should be suspended during the exposure for all radiography of the pelvic girdle.

▶ Depending on patient condition and position, kilovoltage ranges from 65 to 80.

QUESTIONS FOR CRITICAL THINKING & APPLICATION

1. Explain why the ischial tuberosity is considered to be the strongest part of the hip bone.

2. On a recent dig, an archeologist found a human skeleton. Discuss the process she will use to determine the sex of the person. Will she be able to ascertain the age of the skeleton? Explain your answer.

3. Discuss the similarities and differences between the hip and shoulder joints, to include structure, classification of joint, and type of movement. Why does the shoulder joint permit more freedom of movement than the hip joint?

4. Explain how the joint composition of each acetabulum contributes to the strength of the structure, rather than weakens it

5. You have a request to perform a hip examination on an elderly female patient. When taking her history, you learn that she had complete hip replacement surgery approximately 1 year ago. What bony structures have been replaced? What types of materials are used as replacements? Are they radiolucent or radiopaque? How are these parts demonstrated radiographically? Are there implications for centering and film size when radiographing the hip on this patient?

6. A patient admitted to the emergency room requires a radiographic examination of the left hip. State the questions that should be asked as part of a relevant patient history.

7. A 3-year-old child with chronic hip pain has entered the radiology department as an outpatient. Describe the approach you will take toward the patient and parents and the techniques you would use to immobilize the patient when obtaining routine AP and frog-leg lateral projections.

8. A 66-year-old woman has recently had bilateral hip replacement surgery. Her surgeon has ordered AP and lateral projections of each hip. Keeping the patient's condition in mind, describe the projections you will obtain to accomplish this task.

9. In addition to the AP projection of the hip, a second projection must be obtained. Given that there are several alternatives, how do you determine which other projection should be performed?

10. You must radiograph the pelvis and hips of an asthenic, 85-year-old man. Identify the kVp that would produce the best radiographic quality and describe how you would position him for the projections.

FILM CRITIQUE

Evaluate the AP pelvis radiograph relative to patient positioning *(Figure 8–41)*. What criteria did you use to determine whether the patient was correctly or incorrectly positioned?

Does the pelvis belong to a male or female patient?

What criteria did you use to make this determination?

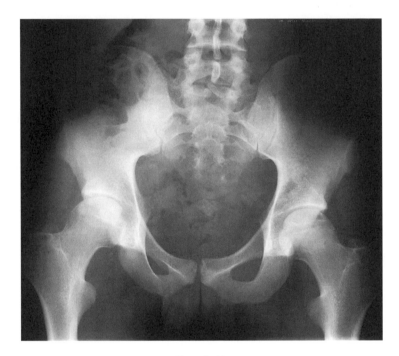

Figure 8–41.

9

BONY THORAX

► OBJECTIVES

Following the completion of this chapter the student will be able to:

- Given diagrams, radiographs, or dry bones, name and describe the bones of the bony thorax, to include the ribs and sternum.

- Classify the articulations of the bony thorax and identify their type of movement, if applicable.

- State the criteria used to determine positioning accuracy on radiographs of the bony thorax and evaluate radiographs of the bony thorax in terms of positioning, centering, image quality; radiographic anatomy, and pathology.

- Define terminology associated with the bony thorax, to include anatomy, procedures, and pathology.

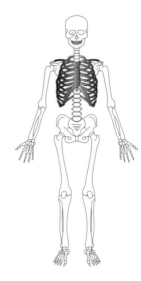

Figure 9–1. The bony thorax.

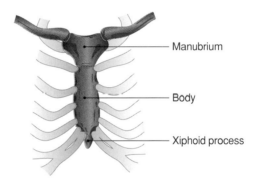

Manubrium

Body

Xiphoid process

Figure 9–2. Three components of the sternum.

► ANATOMY OF THE BONY THORAX

The bony thorax constitutes the upper portion of the trunk of the body *(Figure 9–1, Table 9–1)*. The sternum and 12 pairs of ribs, along with the 12 thoracic vertebrae, form a bony cage that surrounds and protects the vital organs of the thoracic cavity. In addition to affording protection, the bony thorax provides sites for the attachment of shoulder, chest, and back muscles and supports the bones of the shoulder girdle. The construction of the bony thorax allows for continuous expansion and contraction of the lungs during respiration.

STERNUM

In layman's terms, the sternum (STER-num) is known as the **breastbone.** It is a flat bone that can be compared in shape to either a sword or a man's necktie. It is approximately 6 in. (15 cm) long and is located on the midline of the body, forming the most anterior part of the bony thorax. The sternum has three distinct components—manubrium, body, and xiphoid process—all of which fuse into one bony structure in adulthood. As red blood cells are produced in the red bone marrow of the sternum, the bone marrow can be harvested from this site for transfusion, although the ilium of the pelvis is a more common site *(Figure 9–2)*.

The **manubrium** (mah-NŪ-brē-um) is the most superior portion of the sternum. It is broad, triangular, and, depending on the comparison made above, shaped roughly like the handle on the sword or the knot on the necktie. A slight depression on the superior border of the manubrium is known as the **jugular notch.** Alternate names for this area are suprasternal notch and manubrial notch. The jugular notch is a palpable bony landmark located at the level of the disk space between the second and third thoracic vertebrae. To either side of the jugular notch is a slight depression called the **clavicular notch.** Each clavicle articulates with the sternum at the clavicular notch to form a sternoclavicular joint. Directly below each sternoclavicular joint on the manubrium is a slight depression or facet (FAS-et) for articulation with the costocartilage of the first rib.

The second component of the sternum is the **body;** it is also called the **gladiolus** (glah-DI-ō-lus), which is derived from the Latin word for "sword." This structure is elongated and therefore forms the longest segment of the sternum. It is analogous to the blade of the sword or the length of the necktie. During childhood, the body is actually composed of four separate segments. They fuse into one solid structure around the age of 25. The juncture between the manubrium of the sternum and the body is known as the **sternal angle** or manubriosternal joint. For most of one's lifetime, it is a cartilaginous joint that allows the body of the sternum to move very slightly during respiration. In later life, the joint forms a bony fusion and

Table 9–1. Summary of the Bony Thorax

Bones of the Bony Thorax	Description

Sternum (1)	• Breastbone
	• Flat bone with three components
	    Manubrium
	    Body
	    Xiphoid process
	• Source of red bone marrow
	• Articulates with ribs and clavicles

Ribs (12 pairs)	• Flat bones but elongated and curved in shape
	• Curve anteriorly and inferiorly
	• Vertebral extremity
	    Head: forms costovertebral joint
	    Neck
	    Tubercle: forms costotransverse joint
	• Shaft = body
	• Sternal extremity
	    Costocartilage
	• True ribs = 1st through 7th pairs
	• False ribs = 8th through 12th pairs
	• Floating ribs = 11th and 12th pairs
	• Articulates with thoracic vertebrae and sternum

Thoracic vertebrae (12)	• Not considered part of the bony thorax, but forms posterior aspect of bony cage • Articulates with heads and tubercles of the ribs

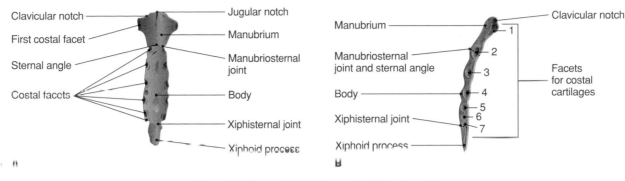

Figure 9–3. Sternum: **(A)** anterior aspects, **(B)** lateral aspect.

thus becomes immovable. The sternal angle is located approximately at the level of the disk space between the fourth and fifth thoracic vertebrae and can be palpated as a transverse ridge on the anterior aspect of the sternum. The sternal angle is a useful landmark when counting a person's ribs because the costocartilage of the second pair of ribs attaches to the sternum at this level. The third through seventh ribs attach via cartilage to the body of the sternum. Facets are present on the lateral surfaces of the sternal body for articulation with the costocartilage (*costo* = "rib").

The third segment and inferior tip of the sternum is known as the **xiphoid** (ZĪ-foid) **process.** An older term for this structure is **ensiform process.** This structure is composed of hyaline cartilage until approximately age 40, at which time it undergoes ossification and fuses to the sternal body. The xiphoid process articulates only with the body of the sternum and does not have any rib attachments; however, it does act as the attachment site for the diaphragm and some abdominal muscles. The liver and heart are located posteriorly to the xiphoid process. Forceful impact on the tip of the sternum can sever the xiphoid process from the sternal body and seriously lacerate these organs *(Figure 9–3).*

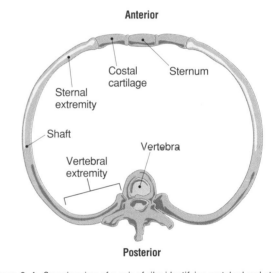

Figure 9–4. Superior view of a pair of ribs identifying vertebral and sternal extremities.

RIBS

Twelve pairs of ribs form the lateral portions of the bony cage of the thorax. Twelve thoracic vertebrae constitute the posterior aspect of the bony thorax. Each rib attaches posteriorly to its corresponding thoracic vertebra. The typical rib has a vertebral (dorsal) extremity and a sternal extremity. It is classified as a flat bone, although it is also elongated and curved in shape *(Figure 9–4).*

The **vertebral extremity** is located at the posterior end of the rib. It consists of a head, neck, and tubercle. The head is expanded and somewhat wedge-shaped. It has either one or two flattened articular facets for articulation with similar surfaces on the corresponding thoracic vertebra. The 2nd through 9th ribs articulate with two adjacent vertebrae, and the 1st, 10th, 11th, and 12th ribs articulate with the correspondingly numbered vertebral bodies. The neck of the rib is the short, constricted area just distal to the head. The tubercle is a small bump found on the posteroinferior surface of the rib between the neck and shaft. It articulates with a facet on the transverse process of the correspondingly numbered thoracic vertebra *(Figure 9–5).*

The **shaft** or **body** is that portion of the rib between the vertebral and sternal extremities. The point at which the shaft curves forward is termed the costal angle. The **costal groove** is a furrow on the inner curved surface of each shaft. As blood vessels and a nerve are housed in this site, a fractured rib can be quite painful and/or cause hemorrhage.

The **sternal extremity** is at the anterior end of the rib. This part of each rib attaches to costocartilage (costal cartilage), which is a flat band of hyaline cartilage. The cartilage is translucent and is not demonstrated radiographically unless calcified because of age. The costocartilage of the first seven ribs attaches directly to the sternum. Therefore, these ribs are known as **true ribs** or more accurately as **vertebrosternal** (ver-tē-brō-STER-nal) **ribs.** The lower five pairs of ribs are designated as **false ribs** because they do not directly articulate with the sternum. On the 8th through 10th ribs, the costocartilage of each attaches to the cartilage of the rib above it. As they are indirectly attached to the sternum via the cartilage of the 7th rib, the 8th through 10th ribs are also called **vertebrochondral** (ver-tē-brō-KON-dral) **ribs** (*chondro* = "cartilage"). The **costal arch** is the curved margin formed by the costocartilage of the 1st through 10th ribs on each side with the xiphoid process inbetween. The arch can be palpated on the anterior surface of the

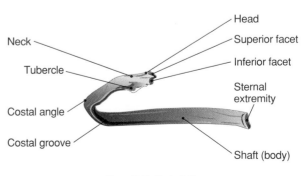

Figure 9–5. Typical rib.

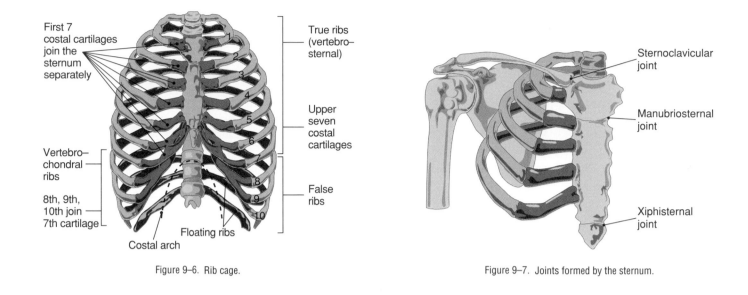

First 7 costal cartilages join the sternum separately

True ribs (vertebro–sternal)

Upper seven costal cartilages

Vertebro–chondral ribs

8th, 9th, 10th join 7th cartilage

False ribs

Floating ribs

Costal arch

Figure 9–6. Rib cage.

Sternoclavicular joint

Manubriosternal joint

Xiphisternal joint

Figure 9–7. Joints formed by the sternum.

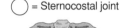

= Sternocostal joint

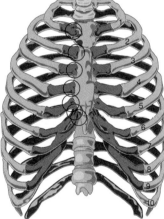

Figure 9–8. Sternocostal joints.

= Costochondral joint

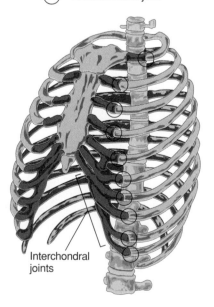

Interchondral joints

Figure 9–9. Rib cage is seen in a slight oblique position to demonstrate the costochondral and interchondral joints.

upper abdomen *(Figure 9–6)*. The 11th and 12th ribs do not have any sternal attachments. As a result, they are called **floating,** or **vertebral, ribs.** They do not actually float, however, as their short costocartilage is embedded in the muscle of the abdominal wall.

The area between adjacent ribs is known as an **intercostal space.** As discussed in Chapter 2, the intercostal muscles are located between the ribs in the intercostal spaces. They are important muscles of respiration because they elevate the ribs during breathing, which in turn increases both the width of the chest and lung volume.

Occasionally, extra ribs may attach on either side of the last cervical vertebra. They are known simply as **cervical ribs.** Their presence may cause pain as they exert pressure on the nerves that pass to the upper extremities. Short ribs may also be seen on the first lumbar vertebra.

ARTHROLOGY

The sternum and ribs articulate with each other and additional structures to form a large number of joints in the bony thorax.

There are two **sternoclavicular** (ster-nō-klah-VIK-ū-lar) **joints,** each of which is formed by the articulation of the sternal end of a clavicle with the manubrium of the sternum. Structurally they are synovial joints that are classified as diarthrodial with gliding-type movement *(Figure 9–7)*.

As previously discussed, the sternum consists of three parts that eventually fuse to become one structure. The **manubriosternal** (mah-nū-brē-ō-STER-nal) **joint** is a cartilaginous joint formed by the manubrium and the body of the sternum at the sternal angle. It is a synchondrosis, allowing some flexibility until it ossifies at a point late in life, at which time it then becomes a synostosis, permitting no movement at all. The **xiphisternal** (zīf-i-STER-nal) **joint** is found between the body of the sternum and the xiphoid process. It is the same structurally as the manubriosternal joint, although it generally ossifies around age 40. It is a palpable bony landmark located approximately at the level of the disk space between the 9th and 10th thoracic vertebrae.

There are a total of 14 **sternocostal** (ster-nō-KOS-tal) **joints.** They are formed by the articulation of the manubrium and body of the sternum with the costocartilage of the first seven pairs of ribs. The sternocostal joints found between the sternum and first pair of ribs are synchondroses. They are cartilaginous in form and are classified as synarthrodial joints with no movement. The second through seventh pairs of sternocostal joints are synovial. They are diarthrodial in classification and allow gliding movement *(Figure 9–8)*.

The sternal extremities of the ribs articulate with their corresponding costocartilage to form the **costochondral** (kos-tō-KON-dral) **joints.** There are a total of 24 such joints in the bony thorax. They are synarthrodial joints permitting no movement.

The **interchondral joints** are formed by the costocartilages of the 7th through 10th ribs articulating with the adjacent rib cartilage. These diarthrodial joints permit gliding movement *(Figure 9–9)*.

Table 9–2. Summary of Joints of the Bony Thorax

Name of Joint	Classification	Structure	Movement
Sternoclavicular	Diarthrodial	Synovial	Gliding
Manubriosternal	Amphiarthrodial → synarthrodial	Synchondrosis → synostosis	Immovable
Xiphisternal	Synarthrodial	Synchondrosis → synostosis	Immovable
Sternocostal			
1st pair	Synarthrodial	Synchondrosis	Immovable
2nd–7th pairs	Diarthrodial	Synovial	Gliding
Costochondral	Synarthrodial	Synchondrosis	Immovable
Interchondral	Diarthrodial	Synovial	Gliding
Costovertebral	Diarthrodial	Synovial	Gliding
Costotransverse	Diarthrodial	Synovial	Gliding

The posterior extremity of each rib is involved in the formation of two joints. The **costovertebral joint** is formed by the articulation of the head of the rib with the body of the adjacent thoracic vertebra. The **costotransverse joint** is formed by the articulation of the tubercle of the rib with the transverse process of the adjacent thoracic vertebra. These joints are classified as diarthrodial joints. They are synovial in structure with gliding movement *(Figure 9–10)*.

Although no single joint allows more than gliding movement, the joints work together to move the bony thorax, particularly in the form of expansion and contraction during respiration. *Table 9–2* summarizes the joints of the bony thorax.

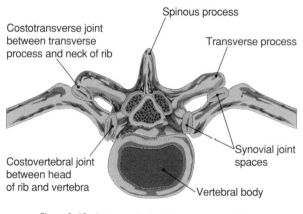

Figure 9–10. Costovertebral and costotransverse joints.

▶ PROCEDURAL CONSIDERATIONS

Rib and sternum radiography can be very frustrating examinations for radiographers. Although the patient positioning is not necessarily that difficult, obtaining high-quality films can be challenging.

PATIENT PREPARATION

Patients should be instructed to remove all clothing and jewelry between the neck and hips and wear a patient gown. A pertinent patient history should provide information relative to the exact location of the pain. This information is necessary to determine which projections should be performed and the breathing instructions to be used.

POSITIONING CONSIDERATIONS

Although many projections included in the radiographic examinations of the ribs and sternum are performed with the patient recumbent, they can also be performed with the patient upright in front of a vertical grid device or a dedicated chest unit. Because of the nerves that pass along the internal and inferior borders of the ribs, rib injuries can be very painful. Upright radiography may be preferred for those patients in severe pain who are able to sit or stand. For patients radiographed on the table, support should be provided to minimize discomfort when moving to or from the table or when changing position.

Routine examination of the ribs generally includes a frontal AP or PA projection and at least one oblique rib projection of the area of interest, in addition to a PA or AP projection of the chest *(Figure 9–11, Table 9–3)*. Department routines may require two AP or PA projections: one for the ribs above and one for the ribs below the diaphragm. Depending on department protocol and patient condition, the patient may be positioned prone when the anterior ribs are of interest and supine when the posterior ribs are affected. When the oblique projection is obtained, the patient should be rotated to place the area of interest roughly parallel to the film plane. Right axillary ribs, therefore, are best demonstrated with the patient in the RPO position for pain radiating posteriorly or the LAO position for pain radiating anteriorly. The left axillary

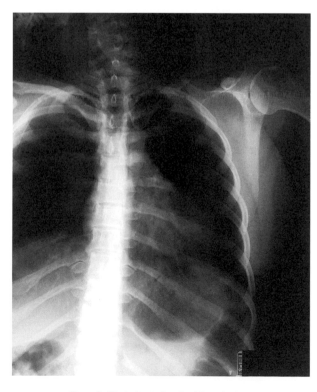

Figure 9–11. Left anterior ribs, PA projection.

Table 9–3. Routine/Optional Projections: Bony Thorax

Ribs	Sternoclavicular joints
AP/PA: above/below diaphragm	RAO and LAO
Oblique: above/below diaphragm	PA[a]
PA/AP chest (see Chapter 2)	
Sternum	
RAO	
Lateral	

Note. Although routines may vary between departments, this table summarizes some of the more common routine and optional projections.
[a]Optional projection; may be routine in some departments.

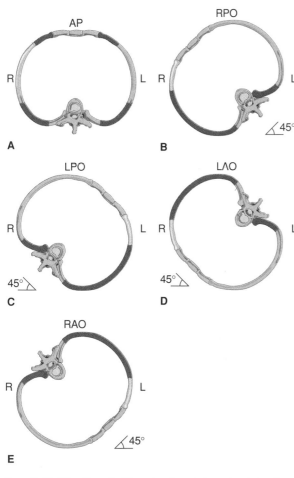

A

B

C

D

E

Figure 9–12. When the patient is supine, the anterior and posterior ribs are demonstrated **(A)**. When the patient is positioned for the posterior oblique projections (RPO/LPO), the axillary ribs nearest the film **(B)** and the vertebral ribs furthest from the film **(C)** are seen. The anterior obliques (RAO/LAO) demonstrate the axillary ribs furthest from the film **(D)** and vertebral ribs nearest the film **(E)**.

ribs are demonstrated with the patient in the LPO position for pain radiating posteriorly or in the RAO position for pain radiating anteriorly *(Table 9–4)*. When the patient is in the RPO position, the vertebral end of the right ribs is perpendicular to the film and superimposed by the spine, and the vertebral end of the left ribs is parallel to the film plane and lateral to the spine. If the vertebral end of the ribs is of interest, therefore, the opposite oblique must be performed *(Figure 9–12)*; both obliques of the affected side must be done to demonstrate the entire length of the ribs. Patient centering for rib projections may be done bilaterally, to include both sides, or unilaterally, to demonstrate only the side of interest, depending on patient size and department protocol. A frontal (PA/AP) chest radiograph is often included as part of the rib series to evaluate soft tissue damage and to identify any pneumothorax or hemothorax caused by fractured ribs.

The RAO and lateral projections are routinely performed when radiographing the sternum. Because the sternum is a thin bone and would be superimposed by the spine when the patient is prone, the patient must be rotated just enough to free the sternum from that superimposition. Although thinner patients must be rotated more than larger patients to accomplish this, the normal rotation is approximately 15° to 20° from the true prone position. By use of the RAO position, the sternum is projected over the heart shadow to the left of the spine. Because the heart and mediastinum are homogeneous in density, the sternum can be better visualized.

The lateral sternum projection can be obtained with the patient either upright next to an upright grid device or recumbent on the table. Because of the object–image receptor distance, the upright position is generally preferred when possible, as it allows for a 72-in. source–image receptor distance to minimize magnification. When the upright position is not possible because of the patient's condition, the patient can be positioned laterally on the table or supine with the central ray directed horizontally. The latter method is also beneficial for female patients with large breasts.

Although it is not a commonly performed examination, the sternoclavicular joints can be demonstrated by assisting the patient to shallow (10° to 15°) RAO and LAO positions on the radiographic table. The joint nearest the table will be demonstrated. A true PA projection of the sternoclavicular joints is sometimes included in the department protocol. Both joints are generally examined for comparison.

Table 9–4. Structures Demonstrated on Oblique Projections

LPO/RAO	RPO/LAO
Left axillary ribs	Right axillary ribs
Right vertebral ribs (heads and necks)	Left vertebral ribs (heads and necks)

BREATHING INSTRUCTIONS

Because the rib cage extends both above and below the diaphragm, different breathing instructions and technical factors must be used to produce optimum images of the ribs. The breathing instructions given will depend on the location of the injury or pain. To demonstrate the ribs above the diaphragm, the patient must be instructed to suspend respiration following a deep inspiration. Doing so allows visualization of the maximum number of ribs above the diaphragm. For ribs below the diaphragm, the patient should be instructed to suspend respiration on expiration, after inhaling and exhaling. Because breathing may be painful, it is important to allow time for the patient to breathe slowly.

To blur overlying lung markings, a breathing technique is preferred when radiographing the sternum in the RAO position. If the patient is panting or having difficulty breathing, the breathing technique may be inappropriate; the exposure should then be made during suspended expiration. When the sternum is radiographed in the lateral position, it is important to try to move the sternum anterior to the surrounding thoracic structures. Making the exposure during suspended deep inspiration can help accomplish this. The breathing instructions for radiography of the bony thorax are summarized in *Table 9–5*.

Table 9–5. Summary of Breathing Instructions

Upper ribs	Deep inspiration
Lower ribs	Full expiration
RAO sternum	Breathing technique or full expiration
Lateral sternum	Full inspiration
Sternoclavicular joints	Expiration

EXPOSURE FACTORS

Producing rib films with sufficient radiographic contrast is a common problem. Patient age and pathology can have a significant effect on radiographic quality. Many older patients have little calcium in their bones, which can detract from image quality. Because the bones of the bony thorax are fairly thin, a low to moderate kilovoltage should be used to prevent overexposure and low-contrast films. It is recommended that the kilovoltage for upper ribs and the RAO sternum be 60 to 65, and that for lower ribs, 65 to 70.

The lateral sternum can be radiographed using 70 to 80 kVp. By decreasing the kilovoltage of a lateral chest technique by 15% intervals and doubling the mAs for each interval, an acceptable lateral sternum technique can be calculated.

EQUIPMENT CONSIDERATIONS

A grid is recommended for most radiography of the bony thorax. When the sternum is radiographed in the lateral position, however, the object–image receptor distance produces somewhat of an air gap. Acceptable radiographs of the lateral sternum can, therefore, be obtained without a grid. To minimize magnification of the lateral sternum, a 72-in. SID should be used whenever possible.

To enhance visualization of the sternum in the RAO position, the SID can be reduced to 30 in. Doing so will increase the blurring effect of the ribs and lung detail that are further from the film. To keep the skin dose within safe limits, however, it is important to maintain a minimum distance of 6 in. (15 cm) between the collimator and the skin.

RADIOGRAPHIC POSITIONING OF THE BONY THORAX

- ▶ AP RIBS (ABOVE & BELOW DIAPHRAGM)

- ▶ AP OBLIQUE RIBS

- ▶ RAO STERNUM

- ▶ LATERAL STERNUM

- ▶ PA OBLIQUE STERNOCLAVICULAR JOINTS

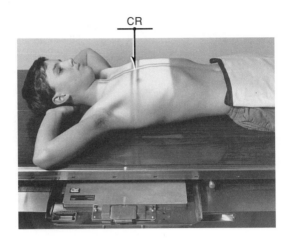

Figure 9–13. AP ribs above the diaphragm using a 14 × 17-in. cassette crosswise.

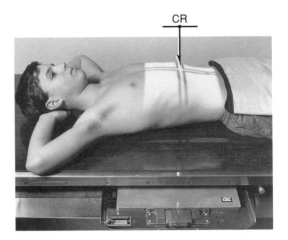

Figure 9–14. AP ribs below the diaphragm using a 14 × 17-in. cassette crosswise.

▶ AP RIBS (ABOVE & BELOW DIAPHRAGM)

Technical Considerations

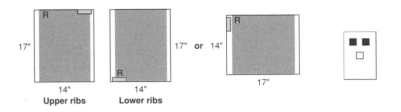

- Film size: 14 × 17 in. lengthwise or crosswise.
- Grid required.
- 60–65 kVp, upper ribs.
- 65–70 kVp, lower ribs.
- Collimate to include lateral ribs and C7 for upper ribs and the iliac crests for lower ribs.

Shielding

- Gonadal shielding should be used on all patients, especially children and adults of reproductive age.

Patient Positioning

- Assist the patient to the supine position on the radiographic table, making sure to move the pillow away from the upper thorax; the patient's legs may be flexed to relieve the stress on the back. **Note:** If the upper, anterior ribs are of interest, the patient should be positioned prone; either projection may also be obtained with the patient erect in front of an upright grid device. When the patient is in the upright position, gravity helps lower the diaphragm allowing better visualization of the upper ribs through the lungs.
- Center the midsagittal plane (bilateral examination) or sagittal plane midway between the spine and lateral margin of the thorax (unilateral examination) to the midline of the table.
- Adjust the patient's midsagittal plane to lie parallel with the long axis of the table.

Part Positioning

- Adjust the patient's body so the distances between the shoulders and tabletop are equal to ensure there is no rotation; the patient should be looking straight ahead with the chin elevated slightly.
- Position the patient's arms above the head or alongside the body with the palms turned outward to move the scapulae away from the ribs.

Ribs Above the Diaphragm
- Position the cassette so the upper border is 2 in. above the top of the shoulders *(Figure 9–13)*.

Ribs Below the Diaphragm
- Position the cassette so the lower border is approximately 1 in. below the level of the iliac crests *(Figure 9–14)*.

Central Ray

- Direct the central ray perpendicular to the midpoint of the cassette; when both upper and lower rib projections are obtained, there should be at least 2 in. of overlap between the two films.

Breathing Instructions

Ribs Above the Diaphragm

- Instruct the patient to take in a deep breath; make the exposure during suspended deep inspiration.

Ribs Below the Diaphragm

- Instruct the patient to take in a breath and blow it out; make the exposure during suspended deep expiration.

Image Evaluation

Ribs Above the Diaphragm

- The upper 8 to 10 ribs (depending on film orientation) should be included in the collimated area.
- The sternoclavicular joints should be symmetrical.
- The ribs should be clearly seen without overexposure through the lungs and heart *(Figure 9–15)*.

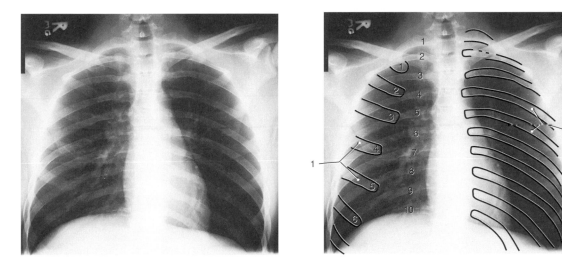

1st through 10th ribs   2. Posterior ribs
1. Sternal extremities,
   anterior ribs

Figure 9–15. AP ribs above the diaphragm, bilateral examination.

Ribs Below the Diaphragm

- The lower 4–6 ribs (depending on film orientation) and the top 0.5 in. of the iliac crests should be included in the collimated area.
- For bilateral examinations, the right and left ribs should look symmetrical; the spine should not appear rotated.
- The ribs should be clearly seen without overexposure through the abdomen *(Figure 9–16)*.

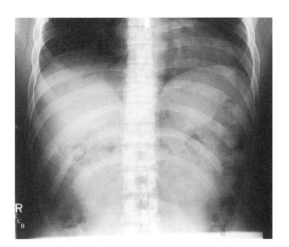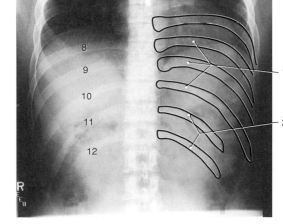

8th through 12th ribs
1. False ribs
2. Floating ribs

Figure 9–16. AP ribs below the diaphragm, bilateral examination.

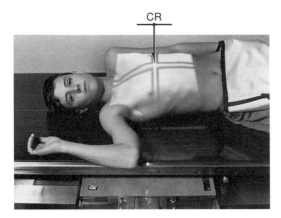

Figure 9–17. RPO ribs, right axillary ribs.

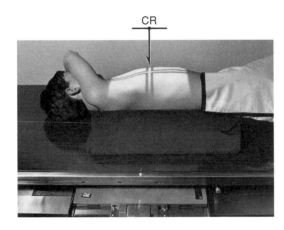

Figure 9–18. LPO ribs, right posterior ribs.

▶ AP OBLIQUE RIBS

Technical Considerations

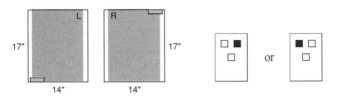

- Film size: 14 × 17 in. lengthwise.
- Grid required.
- 60–65 kVp, upper ribs.
- 65–70 kVp, lower ribs.
- Collimate to include lateral ribs and C-6 for upper ribs and the iliac crests for lower ribs.

Shielding

- Gonadal shielding should be used on all patients, especially children and adults of reproductive age.

Patient Positioning

- Assist the patient to the supine position on the radiographic table, making sure to move the pillow away from the upper thorax; if the upper anterior ribs are of interest, the patient should be positioned prone for the PA oblique (RAO/LAO) projection(s). **Note:** The oblique projections may also be obtained using an upright grid device with the patient standing or sitting. When the patient is in the upright position, gravity helps lower the diaphragm, allowing better visualization of the upper ribs through the lungs.
- Adjust the patient's midsagittal plane to lie parallel with the long axis of the table.

Part Positioning

- Rotate the patient to a 45° RPO or LPO position with the affected side nearest the table; use a sponge to support the patient's shoulders and hips. **Note:** When the RAO or LAO position is used for anterior rib pain, the side of interest is furthest from the film; the patient's arm and leg of the elevated side can be used for support.
- Raise the arm of the side down above the head and rest it on the table to move the scapula away from the rib cage; the arm of the elevated side should be positioned behind the thorax *(Figures 9–17, 9–18)*.

Ribs Above the Diaphragm
- Position the cassette so the upper border is 2 in. above the top of the shoulder.

Ribs Below the Diaphragm
- Position the cassette so the lower border is approximately 1 in. below the level of the iliac crests.

Central Ray

- Direct the central ray perpendicular to the midpoint of the cassette; when both upper and lower rib projections are obtained, there should be at least 2 in. of overlap between the two films.

Breathing Instructions

Ribs Above the Diaphragm
- Instruct the patient to take in a deep breath; make the exposure during suspended deep inspiration.

Ribs Below the Diaphragm
- Instruct the patient to take in a breath and blow it out; make the exposure during suspended deep expiration.

Image Evaluation

Ribs Above the Diaphragm

- The upper 10 ribs should be included in the collimated area.
- The distance between the lateral margin of the ribs and the spine of the side of interest should be approximately twice as great as that of the unaffected side.
- The axillary ribs should be demonstrated free of superimposition.
- The ribs should be clearly seen without overexposure through the lungs and heart *(Figure 9–19)*.

Ribs Below the Diaphragm

- The lower four to nine ribs and the top 0.5 in. of the iliac crests should be included in the collimated area.
- The distance between the lateral margin of the ribs and the spine of the affected side should be approximately twice as great as that of the unaffected side.
- The axillary ribs should be demonstrated free of superimposition.
- The ribs should be clearly seen without overexposure through the abdomen *(Figure 9–20)*.

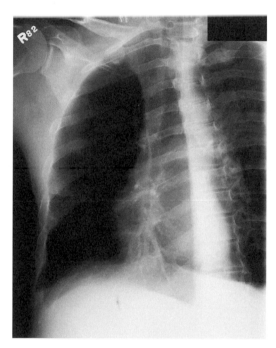
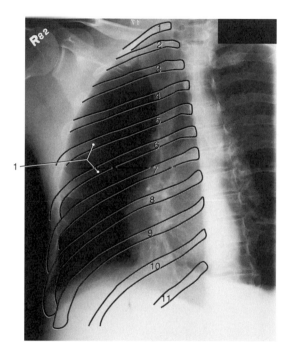

1. Axillary ribs

Figure 9–19. RPO, right axillary ribs.

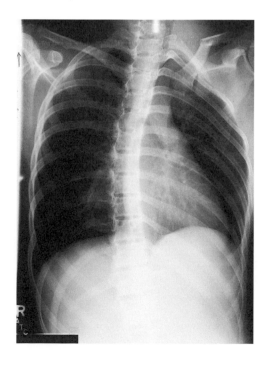
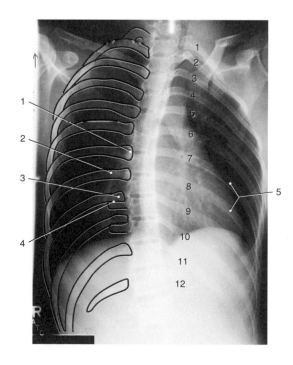

Vertebral ribs of elevated side and axillary ribs of side down
1. Costovertebral joint, T7
2. Neck of 8th rib, right

3. Head of 9th rib, right
4. Costotransverse joint of T9, right
5. Axillary ribs

Figure 9–20. LPO, right vertebral and left axillary ribs; because of patient size, both sides are demonstrated. Note the rib fractures on the left side.

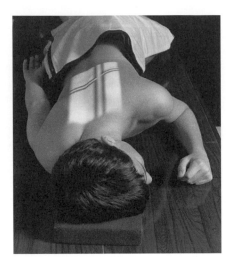

Figure 9–21. For the RAO sternum projection, a thin patient must be rotated more than a large, barrel-chested patient.

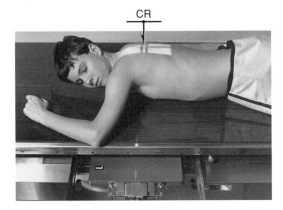

Figure 9–22. RAO sternum.

► RAO STERNUM

Technical Considerations

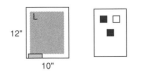

- Film size: 10 × 12 in. lengthwise.
- Grid required.
- 60–65 kVp.
- Collimate to include the sternal ends of clavicles and entire sternum.

Shielding

- Gonadal shielding should be used on all patients, especially children and adults of reproductive age.

Patient Positioning

- Assist the patient to the semiprone position on the radiographic table, making sure to move the pillow away from the upper thorax. **Note:** This projection may also be obtained with the patient standing or sitting, facing an upright grid device.
- Adjust the patient's midsagittal plane to lie parallel with the long axis of the table.
- Align the top edge of the cassette to the level of the spinous process of C7.

Part Positioning

- With the patient's right arm at the side and the left arm raised with the hand near the head, rotate the patient to form a 15° to 20° right anterior oblique position; the patient should be rotated just enough to separate the sternum and vertebral column (position one hand on the sternum and the other on the spinous processes to help evaluate positioning accuracy). **Note:** Thin-chested patients must be rotated more than large, barrel-chested patients.
- Center the sternum to the midline of the table *(Figures 9–21, 9–22)*.

Central Ray

- Direct the central ray perpendicular to the midpoint of the sternum at the level of T5–6.
- Center the cassette to the central ray (a 30-in. SID can be used to blur the ribs and lung detail).

Breathing Instructions

- Instruct the patient to breathe slowly (breathing technique) or take in a breath, blow it out, and make the exposure during suspended deep expiration.

Image Evaluation

- The sternal ends of the clavicles and entire sternum should be included in the collimated area.
- The sternum should be seen separated from the vertebral column with minimal obliquity of the sternum.
- The sternum should be superimposed over the cardiac shadow.
- The right sternoclavicular joint will be open and the left will be closed.
- The sternum will be adequately penetrated; bony detail should be clearly seen (*Figure 9–23*).

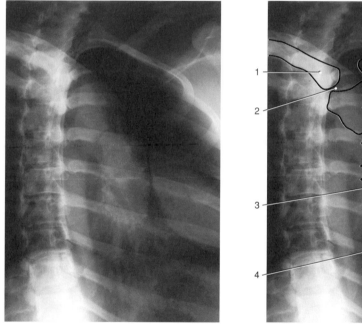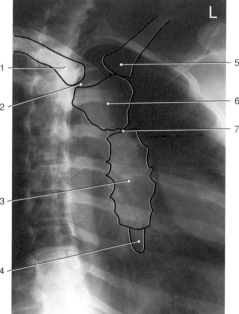

Figure 9–23. RAO sternum.

1. Right clavicle
2. Right sternoclavicular joint
3. Body
4. Xiphoid process
5. Left clavicle
6. Manubrium
7. Sternal angle

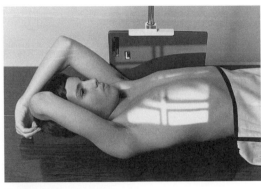

A

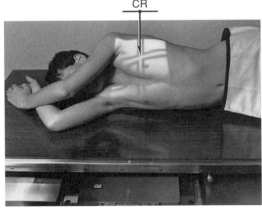

B

Figure 9–24. **(A)** The lateral sternum projection can also be obtained with the patient supine, using a horizontal beam, or **(B)** in the lateral recumbent position.

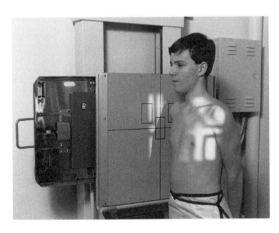

Figure 9–25. Lateral sternum.

► LATERAL STERNUM

Technical Considerations

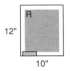

- Film size: 10 × 12 in. lengthwise.
- Grid required.
- 70–80 kVp.
- Collimate to include manubrium and xiphoid process.

Shielding

- Gonadal shielding should be used on all patients, especially children and adults of reproductive age.

Patient Positioning

- Assist the patient to the erect, lateral position in front of an upright grid device; the patient may be standing or sitting. **Note:** This projection may also be obtained with the patient in the lateral recumbent position or the supine position with a horizontal beam *(Figure 9–24)*.

Part Positioning

- Rotate the shoulders backward and place the patient's hands behind the back.
- Adjust the patient's position so the midcoronal plane is perpendicular to the film plane.
- Center the sternum to the midline of the grid device. *(Figure 9–25)*.
- Center the cassette so the upper border is approximately 1½ in. above the jugular notch.

Central Ray

- Direct the central ray perpendicular (horizontally) to the midpoint of the sternum using a 72-in. SID.

Breathing Instructions

- Instruct the patient to take in a deep breath; make the exposure during suspended deep inspiration.

Image Evaluation

- The entire sternum should be included in the collimated area.
- The sternal ends of the clavicles should be seen superimposed.
- The sternum should be seen separated from the ribs and soft tissue of the shoulders.
- The sternum will be adequately penetrated; bony detail should be clearly seen *(Figure 9–26)*.

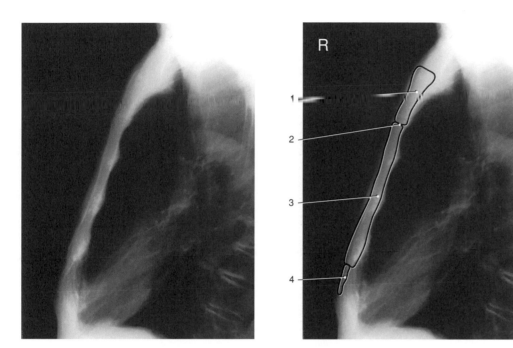

Figure 9–26. Lateral sternum, obtained with the patient erect.

1. Manubrium
2. Sternal angle

3. Body

4. Xiphoid process

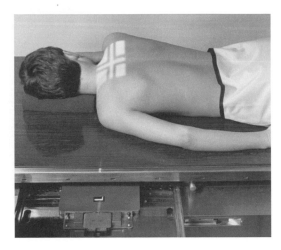

Figure 9–27. LAO for the left sternoclavicular joint.

► PA OBLIQUE STERNOCLAVICULAR JOINTS

Technical Considerations

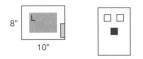

- Film size: 8 × 10 in. crosswise or 9 × 9 in.
- Grid required.
- 60–70 kVp.
- Collimate to include the sternal ends of clavicles and the manubrium.

Shielding

- Gonadal shielding should be used on all patients, especially children and adults of reproductive age.

Patient Positioning

- Assist the patient to the prone position on the radiographic table, making sure to move the pillow away from the upper thorax. **Note:** Although the joints are not opened, some department protocols include a true PA projection as part of the routine examination of the sternoclavicular joints; centering is to the jugular notch. Care must be taken to ensure the patient's head is not rotated for this projection.
- Adjust the patient's midsagittal plane to lie parallel with the long axis of the table.

Part Positioning

- Rotate the patient 10–15°, keeping the side of interest nearest the table; the patient should be rotated only enough to position the interested sternoclavicular joint anterior to the vertebral column (thin patients need to be rotated more than large patients). The dependent arm should be positioned near the body with the palm of the hand up, and the opposite arm should be raised to support the body; both joints are routinely examined for comparison.
- Center the affected joint to the midline of the table (Figure 9-27).

Central Ray

- Direct the central ray perpendicular to the level of the jugular notch.
- Center the cassette to the central ray.

Breathing Instructions

- Instruct the patient to take in a breath, blow it out, and make the exposure during suspended expiration.

Image Evaluation

- The sternal ends of the clavicles and manubrium should be included in the collimated area.
- The sternoclavicular joint nearest the film should be open and clearly demonstrated.
- The sternoclavicular joint should be adequately penetrated; bony detail should be clearly seen (Figure 9–28).

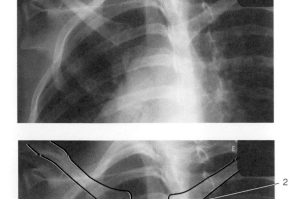

Figure 9–28. LAO, left sternoclavicular joint.

1. Manubrium   2. Left clavicle   3. Left sternoclavicular joint

SUMMARY

▶ Radiographic examinations of the bony thorax can be obtained with the patient recumbent or erect.

▶ Because of the curvature of the ribs, it is necessary to obtain both obliques of the affected side to see the entire length of the ribs, from their sternal to vertebral ends.

▶ Because of the relationship of the spine and sternum, it is necessary to oblique the patient slightly to visualize the sternum in a 15° to 20° RAO position.

▶ To magnify, and therefore blur, the posterior ribs overlying the sternum when the patient is in the RAO position, the SID can be reduced to 30 in.

▶ Although a 40-in. SID is used for most radiography, a 72-in. SID should be used when radiographing the sternum in the lateral position to minimize magnification, whenever possible.

▶ When the ribs are radiographed, appropriate breathing instructions must be given to maximize the number of ribs seen.

▶ A grid is recommended for radiography of the bony thorax.

▶ Because the bones of the bony thorax are relatively thin, a low to moderate kilovoltage, 60 to 70, is recommended to prevent overexposure and enhance the ribs and sternum.

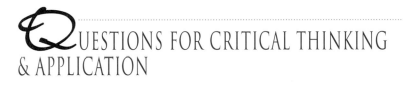

QUESTIONS FOR CRITICAL THINKING & APPLICATION

1. What part of the sternum is used when performing CPR (cardiopulmonary resuscitation)? How much do you depress the sternum on each compression? What possible complications might occur if you performed compressions too low on the sternum?

2. Why is the sternum a good source of red bone marrow during a marrow transplant? Your explanation should include a description of the physical characteristics of the sternum.

3. During a recent jumping competition, Jillian fell from her horse, breaking several ribs. Because she is in a great deal of pain, she spends most of the day lying down. She must take shallow breaths as deep breathing is uncomfortable. Why would her physician be concerned about pneumonia? What complications could have occurred if a rib had punctured the lung?

4. You received a requisition to take a portable chest film on a patient involved in a motor vehicle accident. Although the patient appeared alert and was sitting upright, he was hooked up to a cardiac monitor because he had an irregular heartbeat. He complained of a "bruised chest" and said he was not wearing his seatbelt. What is the connection between the mechanism of injury and the patient's condition? What structure(s) do you suppose is (are) injured?

5. Discuss the relationship of the sternum, ribs, and thoracic spine to one another, including the types of articulations they form. How is the combined movement of the joints important to the process of respiration?

6. If the patient's condition permitted either, would it be better to radiograph the 7th and 8th ribs with the patient in the upright or the recumbent position? Why?

7. While not wearing a seat belt, your patient had been in a car accident and was forced forward onto the steering wheel. In addition to cervical spine injuries, her sternum is badly bruised. Describe how you would obtain the oblique and lateral projections of the sternum while keeping the patient supine.

8. Your patient fell backward off a porch step onto a pipe projecting out of the ground. The patient experienced severe pain immediately left of the spine. Describe the projection(s) that would best demonstrate the ribs in this region.

9. When evaluating a routine chest x-ray, the radiologist discovered a suspicious density on the fourth rib near the axilla. Describe the rib projections you would obtain to further evaluate this area.

10. A rather broad, 7-ft man has come to the radiology department for radiography of his ribs. He has been suffering some generalized chest pain across the left side of his back and under his arm. Describe the projections you would obtain to ensure all ribs are included.

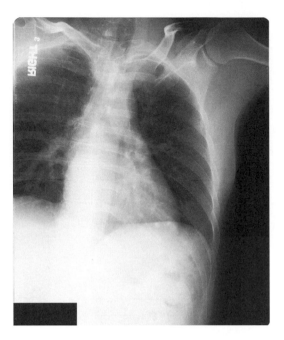

Figure 9–29.

FILM CRITIQUE

Evaluate the oblique projection *(Figure 9–29)* of the ribs for patient positioning and technique. Was the patient correctly positioned?

What criteria did you use in this evaluation?

Was the film correctly marked?

Were proper technical factors used?

Why or why not?

Discuss your answer in terms of radiographic contrast and density. Which ribs (if any) are well demonstrated? What could have been done differently?

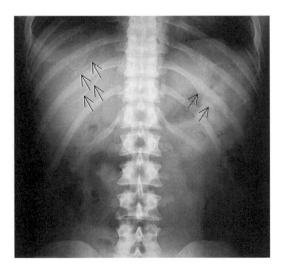

Figure 9–30.

When assessing this AP rib radiograph *(Figure 9–30)*, you will notice some structures not always seen radiographically. What are they and why are they visible on the film?

10

VERTEBRAL COLUMN

▶ OBJECTIVES

Following the completion of this chapter the student will be able to:

- Given diagrams, radiographs, or dry bones, name and describe the bones of the vertebral column.

- Identify the topographical landmarks associated with specific vertebrae.

- Differentiate between the curves of the vertebral column, to include primary curves, compensatory curves, lordosis, kyphosis, and scoliosis.

- Describe the structural differences between the cervical, thoracic, and lumbar vertebrae.

- Classify the articulations in the vertebral column according to structure and identify their type of movement, if applicable.

- Describe the procedural adaptations necessary for radiography of the spine in a trauma situation.

- State the criteria used to determine positioning accuracy on radiographs of the vertebral column and evaluate radiographs of the vertebral column in terms of positioning, centering, image quality, radiographic anatomy, and pathology.

- Define terminology associated with the vertebral column, to include anatomy, procedures, and pathology.

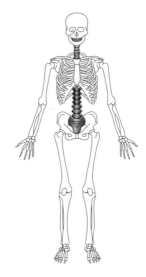

Figure 10–1. The vertebral column.

▶ ANATOMY OF THE VERTEBRAL COLUMN

The vertebral column is commonly referred to as the *spine (Figure 10–1)*. It is located posteriorly on the midsagittal plane of the body and extends inferiorly from the base of the skull to the tailbone to constitute the longitudinal axis, or "backbone," of the axial skeleton. A group of 33 bones known as *vertebrae* (VER-te-bre) stack on each other to form a column which is approximately 28 in. (71 cm) long *(Table 10–1)*. This sturdy column supports the head, surrounds and protects the spinal cord, transmits the weight of the trunk to the lower limbs, serves as the site of articulation for the ribs of the bony thorax, and allows for the attachment of many muscles of the back. One might expect such a bony structure to be rigid; however, a variety of joints makes it flexible enough to bend forward, backward, and from side to side.

REGIONAL DIVISIONS

The vertebral column is divided into regions according to location and structure of the vertebrae. There are seven cervical (SER-vi-kal) vertebrae, which are located in the neck (*cervico* = "neck"). Twelve thoracic (tho-RAS-ik) vertebrae constitute the posterior thorax or chest (*thoraco* = "chest"). Five lumbar (LUM-bar) vertebrae are located posteriorly to the abdomen and form the lower back (*lumbo* = "loin"). The sacrum (SA-krum) and coccyx (KOK-siks) are both located in the pelvis. The sacrum is formed by the fusion of five sacral vertebrae, whereas an average of four coccygeal segments fuse in adulthood to comprise the single coccyx. Although the average adult vertebral column usually consists of 26 vertebrae, the vertebral column of a child contains 33 separate vertebrae *(Figure 10–2)*.

CURVATURES OF THE VERTEBRAL COLUMN

The spine is not a straight, inflexible column of bone. There are four normal anteroposterior curves in the vertebral column, which are characteristically demonstrated as an elongated "S" shape on a lateral view *(Figure 10–3)*.

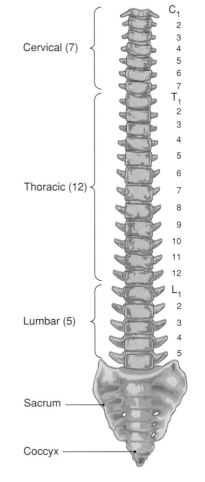

Figure 10–2. Cervical, thoracic, lumbar, sacral, and coccygeal regions of the vertebral column.

Cervical (7)
C1 2 3 4 5 6 7

Thoracic (12)
T1 2 3 4 5 6 7 8 9 10 11 12

Lumbar (5)
L1 2 3 4 5

Sacrum

Coccyx

Table 10–1. Summary of the Vertebral Column

Bones of the Vertebral Column	Description
Cervical vertebrae (7)	• Neck • C1, C2, and C7 are atypical • Bifid tips on spinous processes • Transverse foramina • Concave posterior (lordotic) curve
Thoracic vertebrae (12)	• Upper back • Facets and demifacets on body for articulation with ribs • Costal facets on transverse processes • Convex posterior (kyphotic) curve
Lumbar vertebrae (5)	• Lower back • Largest vertebral body • Concave posterior (lordotic) curve
Sacrum (1)	• Five fused sacral segments • Base, apex, and alae • Sacral foramina • Forms posterior pelvis • Articulates with ilia to form sacroiliac joints • Sacral cornua (horns) • Convex posterior (kyphotic) curve
Coccyx (1)	• Tailbone • Three to five fused coccygeal segments • Base and apex • Cornua (horns) • Curves anteriorly and inferiorly

The curves in the thoracic and sacral regions are denoted as **primary curves** as they appear in the later stages of fetal development and are present at birth. They serve to increase the flexibility and strength of the spine, much like the curved arches of the foot. While the posterior surface of the spine is convex, the anterior surface is concave. Therefore, they are considered to be convex posterior curves. The thoracic curve begins about the level of the second thoracic vertebra and extends to the end of the thoracic region of the vertebral column. The sacral curve is sometimes referred to as the *pelvic curve* because it is formed by both the sacrum and the coccyx in the pelvis. This curve extends from the superior portion of the sacrum to the inferior tip of the coccyx.

The **cervical** and **lumbar curves** are known as **secondary** or **compensatory curves** because they develop after birth. They function to stabilize the spine in an upright position and provide balance. The cervical and lumbar curves develop in the opposite direction of the thoracic and sacral curves. Consequently, they can be described as concave posterior curves. The cervical curve extends from the second cervical vertebra to the second thoracic vertebra. It develops when the infant begins to hold his or her head erect around the age of 3 or 4 months. The lumbar curve extends through the lumbar region of the vertebral column to the articulation with the sacrum. It is usually acquired around 1 year of age when the child begins to stand erect and walk. This curve is normally more pronounced in females, especially during advanced stages of pregnancy.

On occasion, the normal curves of the vertebral column may become distorted as the result of disease, poor posture, trauma, or a congenital condition. An exaggerated thoracic curvature is known as **kyphosis** (ki-FŌ-sis). With this condition, a person develops a "hunchback" from the increased posterior convexity of the spine. This is typically seen in individuals suffering from osteoporosis. If the lumbar curve becomes exaggerated and more concave, a condition called **lordosis** (lor-DŌ-sis) occurs. Carrying an excessively heavy weight in front of the body, being very obese, as well as wearing shoes with very high heels, may result in lordosis. Because they affect the anteroposterior curves, kyphosis and lordosis are best demonstrated on a lateral projection of the vertebral column. An abnormal lateral curvature of the spine is called **scoliosis** (sko-lē-Ō-sis). *Scolio-* means "bent" or "crooked." In this condition, the spine forms an S-shaped curvature as it curves toward one side of the body and then forms a compensating curve in the opposite direction. A severe case of scoliosis can affect the thoracic and abdominal organs, and may also cause the person to walk with a limp as one side of the pelvis is tilted. Because a person's muscles are often stronger on either the right or left side of the body, depending on which extremity is dominant, a slight lateral deviation may develop in the spine, which is considered normal. In this situation, the upper thoracic vertebrae will curve convexly toward the dominant side *(Figure 10–4)*.

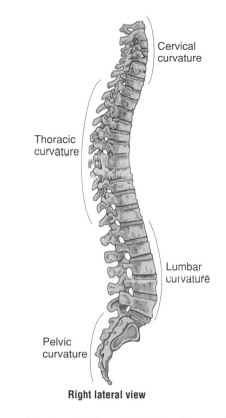

Right lateral view

Figure 10–3. Lateral aspect of the vertebral column demonstrating the four normal curves.

CHARACTERISTICS OF THE TYPICAL VERTEBRA

Although vertebrae possess characteristics unique to a particular region of the vertebral column, their overall general structure is similar. Each vertebra is an irregularly shaped bone composed of two main parts: a body and a vertebral arch.

The **body** or **centrum** (CEN-trum) is the anterior, weight-bearing portion of the vertebra. It is roughly cylindrical in shape with a slightly flattened posterior surface. The body is a large, solid structure composed of cancellous bone covered with a layer of compact bone. There are several small nutrient foramina located on the anterior and lateral aspects of the body. The superior and inferior surfaces of the body are flat and rough to allow for the attachment of intervertebral disks.

The **vertebral arch** is the posterior ringlike portion of the vertebra and, like the body, is composed of cancellous bone covered by compact bone. It attaches to the body to enclose an opening known as the **vertebral foramen.** When the vertebrae are stacked in succession to form the vertebral column, the vertebral foramina form a channel through which the spinal cord passes. This bony passage, called the **vertebral canal,** completely surrounds and protects the spinal cord.

The vertebral arch is formed by two pedicles and two laminae. The **pedicles** (PED-i-kulz) are two short, thick structures that attach to either posterolateral margin of the body. In essence, they attach the arch to the body. Each pedicle is notched on its superior and inferior surface. These notches are known respectively as the **superior** and **inferior vertebral notches.** When the vertebrae articulate with each other, the inferior vertebral notches on the pedicles of one vertebrae and the superior vertebral notches of the vertebrae directly below it form circular openings on either side of the vertebral column. The **intervertebral foramina,** as these openings are called, allow for the passage of blood vessels and nerves from the spinal cord. As each vertebra has two pedicles, there are two intervertebral foramina formed between adjacent vertebrae.

The **laminae** (LAM-i-nē) (singular, lamina) are broad, flat plates of bone that extend posteriorly and medially from each pedicle. The two laminae meet posteriorly at the midline to complete the arch. If the laminae fail to unite at this point, leaving a gap in the vertebral arch, a congenital anomaly known as **spina**

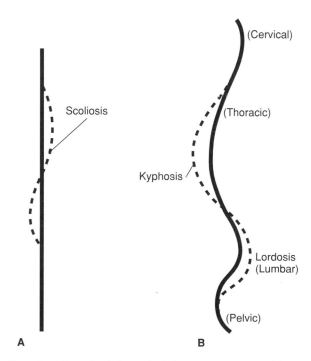

Figure 10–4. Normal and abnormal spinal curvatures as seen on **(A)** anterior and **(B)** lateral views. The solid lines represent the normal curvatures; the broken lines represent abnormal curvatures.

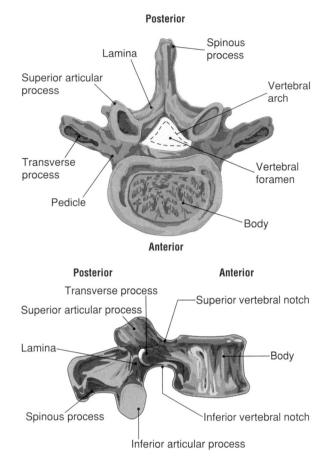

Figure 10–5. Typical vertebra: **(A)** superior view, **(B)** lateral view.

bifida (SPI-nah BIF-i-dah) occurs. Depending on the vertebra affected, this can be a serious condition as the spinal cord can herniate through the resultant opening and cause neurologic damage.

Seven processes originate from the vertebral arch. There are two **transverse processes,** each of which projects laterally from the junction of a pedicle and lamina. The single **spinous process** is situated posteriorly on the midline of the arch. It is formed at the point of fusion of the two laminae. The spinous processes can often be palpated down the middle of an individual's back and will appear more prominently as "bumps" on a thinner person. The transverse processes and spinous process serve as the sites of muscle attachments. The remaining four processes function to adjoin adjacent vertebrae and are known as **articular processes** or **zygapophyses** (zi-gah-POF-i-sez). Two **superior articular processes** project upward from the junctions of the pedicles and laminae with their articular surfaces facing posteriorly. The two **inferior articular processes** also originate at the junction of each pedicle and lamina; however, they project downward and their articular surfaces face anteriorly. The inferior articular processes of one vertebra articulate with the superior articular processes of the vertebra directly below it when the vertebrae are stacked in succession *(Figure 10–5).*

Regional differences can be seen in the vertebral column. Although the vertebrae in each of the regions share common features, there are individual differences. Each of these regions is discussed in detail.

CERVICAL VERTEBRAE

The seven cervical vertebrae form the upper part of the vertebral column. They differ from the typical vertebra more than those of the thoracic or lumbar regions. The body of a typical cervical vertebra is smaller than average in its anteroposterior dimension but is broad from side to side. It slants inferiorly toward its anterior aspect at an approximate 15° angle, causing slight overlap of the cervical bodies in the articulated skeleton. The vertebral arch, and therefore the vertebral foramen, is also larger than average and roughly triangular in shape to accommodate the spinal cord, which is more expanded in this region. The pedicles arise from the body and are at a 45° angle in the body. Therefore, the intervertebral foramina are best seen on a 45° oblique projection. The two transverse processes are more forward as they originate from the junction of the body and pedicle instead of arising from the junction between the pedicle and lamina as in the typical vertebra. A transverse foramen is present on each of the transverse processes through which the vertebral artery and vein pass along with nerve fibers. An articular pillar is located directly posterior to each transverse process. The superior articular process is located on the top of this short column of bone; the inferior articular process is on the inferior surface. The articular processes slant posteriorly from a horizontal position. In the articulated vertebral column, the articular pillars stack on top of each other to form a column or pillar of bone on each side of the cervical spine which helps to support the head. The spinous processes of the second through sixth cervical vertebrae are short and directed almost horizontally. They have bifid (BĪ-fid) tips, meaning the tips of the spinous processes are split or forked. The spinous process of C7 is more pronounced than those of the other cervical vertebrae. It is larger and projects horizontally, making it palpable at the base of the neck. Because the spinous process is so prominent, C7 is also known as the **vertebra prominens** *(Figure 10–6).*

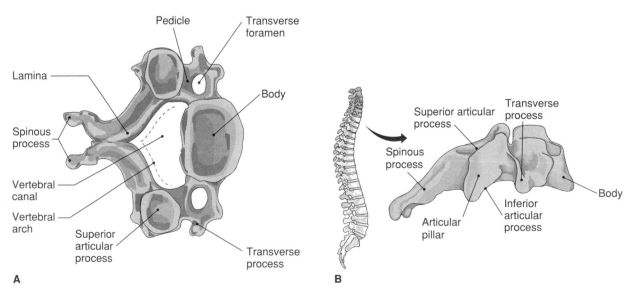

Figure 10–6. Typical cervical vertebra: **(A)** superior view, **(B)** lateral view.

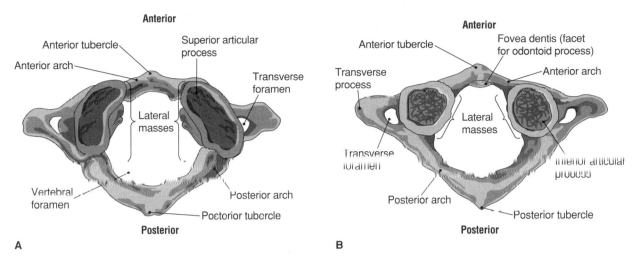

Figure 10–7. Atlas (C1): **(A)** superior view, **(B)** inferior view.

C1

The first cervical vertebra supports the head. Hence, it is also known as the **atlas** after the mythologic Atlas who carried the world on his shoulders. The atlas is ringlike in structure. It has neither a body nor a spinous process. The anterior arch forms the anterior part of the vertebra, and the posterior arch completes the ring posteriorly. There is a posterior tubercle on the midline of the posterior arch in lieu of a spinous process. The large vertebral foramen is enclosed within the ring. The dens of C2 will extend upward into the anterior portion of the foramen. A ligament extends transversely between the two lateral masses to separate the anterior part of the foramen from the posterior portion through which the spinal cord passes. The lateral mass is a solid area of bone situated on either side of the vertebral foramen between the anterior and posterior arches. The superior articular process, an oval, concave area, is situated on the superior surface of each lateral mass. The corresponding condyle on the occipital bone of the skull articulates at this point. The inferior articular process is located on the inferior surface of the lateral mass. It articulates with the corresponding superior articular process of C2. A transverse process extends off of each lateral mass. A transverse foramen is present on each of the transverse processes *(Figure 10–7)*.

C2

Rotational movement of the head takes place between C1 and C2. It can be compared with the revolution of the earth around an axis. This is actually an appropriate analogy as C2 is also called the **axis.** A tooth-shaped process known as the **dens** (denz) or **odontoid** (o-DON-toyd) **process** projects upward from the top of the vertebral body through the anterior arch of the atlas. It acts as a pivot to allow rotation of the head and atlas on the axis. Some scientists theorize that the dens is actually the body of C1, but during embryologic development it fuses with the body of C2. Like the typical cervical vertebra, the axis has transverse foramina on its transverse processes and a bifid spinous process. The superior articular processes are flattened areas on the superior surface of the transverse processes. They are located more anteriorly than on other cervical vertebrae to correspond with the position of the inferior articular processes on the atlas. The inferior articular processes are situated more posteriorly under the lamina *(Figure 10–8)*.

THORACIC VERTEBRAE

The thoracic vertebrae become progressively larger from T1 through T12. Therefore, the thoracic vertebrae are larger than the cervical but not quite as massive as the lumbar vertebrae. The fifth through eighth thoracic vertebrae are considered the most typical of this region of the vertebral column. The body of a thoracic vertebra is more heart-shaped rather than cylindrical. It is unique compared with other vertebral bodies because it bears at least one **costal facet** (KOS-tal FAS-et) on each posterolateral aspect. This is a smooth, round depression for articulation with the head of a rib. Some of the thoracic bodies have **demifacets** (dem-ē-FAS-ets), which are semicircular. In this case, the head of a rib articulates with demifacets

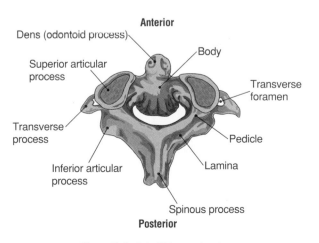

Figure 10–8. Axis (C2): superior view.

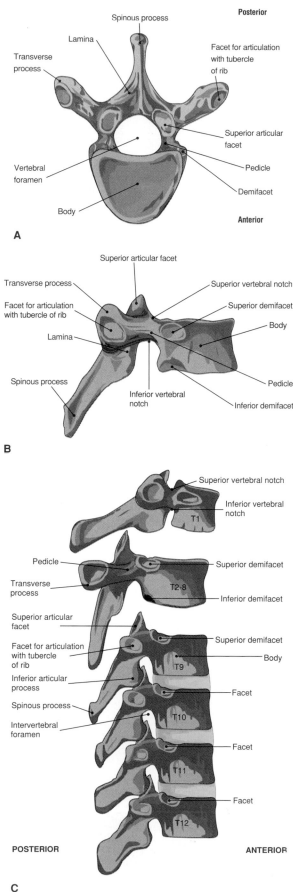

on two adjacent vertebrae. T1 has a full facet on each side of the body at its superior edge. It also has a demifacet on each side of the body at its inferior edge. The bodies of T2 through T9 bear demifacets, whereas T10 through T12 each have a full facet on either side. The vertebral foramen is smaller on a thoracic vertebra than on a cervical vertebra and more circular. The pedicles extend posteriorly. In the articulated spine, the intervertebral foramina of the thoracic vertebrae are demonstrated between the pedicles. As these structures are at a 90° angle to the midline, the intervertebral foramina are best demonstrated on a lateral projection of the thoracic spine. The transverse processes of the first through tenth thoracic vertebrae have facets that articulate with the tubercles of the corresponding ribs. The spinous process of each thoracic vertebra is long and slender, pointing caudally to overlap the vertebral body beneath *(Figure 10–9)*.

LUMBAR VERTEBRAE

The five lumbar vertebrae are under more stress than other vertebrae because they bear the weight of the body; therefore, they are the largest and most sturdy of the vertebrae. The body of a typical lumbar vertebra is large and cylindrical. The vertebral foramen is somewhat triangular and not as large as the other regions. The pedicles are short, sturdy structures extending posteriorly from the body. The intervertebral foramina formed between the pedicles are best demonstrated on a lateral projection. The transverse processes are somewhat smaller than those of the thoracic spine. They have neither transverse foramina nor costal facets. The lamina are short and thick *(Figure 10–10)*. The area on each lamina between the superior and inferior articular processes is known as the **pars interarticularis** (pars in-ter-ar-tik-ū-LAR-is). If a congenital defect or fracture occurs in this area, the body of the vertebra may slip forward over the vertebra beneath it. This condition is known as **spondylolisthesis** (spon-di-lō-lis-THĒ-sis). The articular facets on the superior and inferior articular processes are oriented at an average angle of 45° to the midline of the vertebra. On a 45° oblique projection, a lumbar vertebra takes on the appearance of a "scotty dog." Bony structures on one side of the vertebra correspond to various parts of the dog *(Figure 10–11)*. Table 10–2 illustrates the relationship of the bony structures to the parts of the dog.

SACRUM

The sacrum is a triangular structure situated in the posterior pelvis. The broad upper border of the sacrum is the base; the apex is located at its inferior end. The sacrum is formed by the union of five sacral vertebrae. Prior to fusion, the segments are separated by cartilage. After fusion is completed between ages 20 and 30, there are four **transverse lines (ridges)** that delineate the sacral segments. The first sacral segment is somewhat similar in structure to the fifth lumbar vertebra. Two superior articular processes extend upward from its upper border to articulate with the inferior articular processes of the fifth lumbar vertebra. Occasionally, the body of L5 fuses to the body of S1. This condition is known as **sacralization** (sā-kral-i-ZĀ-shun). When **lumbarization** (lum-bar-i-ZĀ-shun) occurs, the first and second sacral segments fail to fuse, resulting in a sixth lumbar vertebra.

The body of the sacrum is the large, curved central portion of the bone. It is formed by the fused bodies of the sacral segments. The **sacral promontory** (PROM-on-tor-e) is the anterior margin of the first sacral segment. This prominent ridge extends into the pelvis to form the posterosuperior portion of the pelvic brim and inlet of the pelvis. It is best seen when viewed from the side. The **alae** are the broad wing-like areas situated laterally to the body of the first sacral segment. A rough, ear-shaped auricular surface is seen on the posterolateral side of each ala. This area articulates with a similarly shaped area on the ilium to form a sacroiliac joint. The **sacral canal** is a continuation of the vertebral canal. Nerves, blood vessels, and

Table 10–2. Correlation of Bony Structures With the "Scotty Dog"

Lumbar Vertebra	"Scotty Dog"
Transverse process	Nose
Pedicle	Eye
Superior articular process	Ear
Pars interarticularis	Neck
Inferior articular process	Front leg

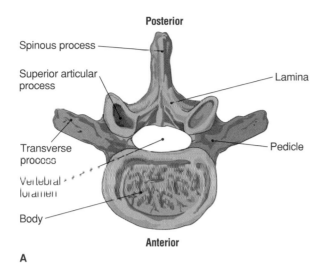

A

Posterior

Spinous process

Superior articular process

Lamina

Transverse process

Pedicle

Vertebral foramen

Body

Anterior

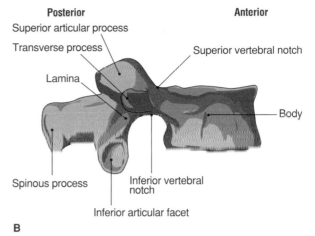

B

Posterior

Anterior

Superior articular process

Transverse process

Superior vertebral notch

Lamina

Body

Spinous process

Inferior vertebral notch

Inferior articular facet

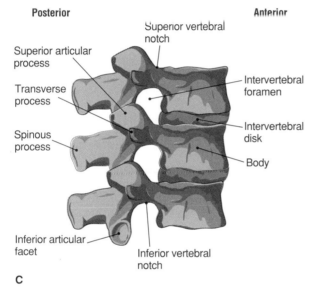

C

Posterior

Anterior

Superior vertebral notch

Superior articular process

Intervertebral foramen

Transverse process

Intervertebral disk

Spinous process

Body

Inferior articular facet

Inferior vertebral notch

Figure 10–10. Typical lumbar vertebra: **(A)** superior view, **(B)** lateral view. **(C)** Lateral view of articulated lumbar vertebrae.

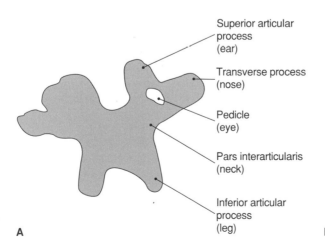

A

Superior articular process (ear)

Transverse process (nose)

Pedicle (eye)

Pars interarticularis (neck)

Inferior articular process (leg)

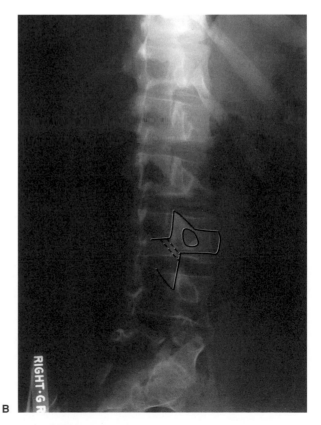

B

Figure 10–11. **(A)** "Scotty dog" as seen on an LPO projection. **(B)** LPO projection of lumbar spine with "scotty dog" outlined.

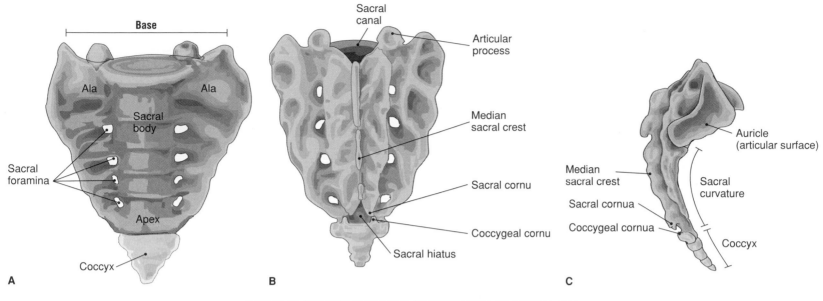

Figure 10–12 Sacrum: **(A)** lateral surface, **(B)** anterior surface, **(C)** posterior surface.

connective tissue are transmitted through this passage, which begins at the base of the sacrum between the articular processes and ends in an opening known as the **sacral hiatus** (hi-A-tus). This opening is located on the lower end of the posterior sacrum and is generally covered by connective tissue. There are four pairs of holes on the anterior aspect of the sacrum which can be seen at either end of a transverse line. Known as the anterior sacral (pelvic) foramina, they communicate with the posterior (dorsal) sacral foramina on the posterior aspect of the sacrum. Nerves and blood vessels pass through the foramina from the sacral hiatus. The posterior sacral surface has a rough appearance due to the presence of the **median sacral crest,** a ridge of bone running down the midline of the sacrum. It is formed by the fused spinous processes of the sacral segments. There are two **sacral cornua,** which are horn-shaped projections extending inferiorly on each side of the sacral hiatus. These bony projections represent the inferior articular processes of the last sacral segment. They articulate with similar structures on the coccyx. The cornua are often used as landmarks to localize the sacral hiatus for administration of epidural anesthesia *(Figure 10–12).*

COCCYX

The coccyx or tailbone is also a triangular structure, but it is significantly smaller than the sacrum. It is fairly superficial, and can be palpated below the surface of the skin. On the average, the coccyx is formed from the fusion of four coccygeal segments, although the number of segments varies from 3 to 5. The fusion of these segments usually occurs between the ages of 20 and 30. Each coccygeal segment is actually an incompletely developed vertebra. Like the sacrum, the upper margin of the coccyx is the base and the inferior tip is known as the apex. The first or upper segment has two cornua (horns), which project upward to articulate with the cornua of the sacrum. This is also the only segment to have transverse processes, which project laterally. The coccyx generally curves anteriorly to point toward the symphysis pubis. In females, however, the coccyx is usually directed more inferiorly and is less curved so that it does not project into the birth canal *(Figure 10–13).*

Table 10–3 summarizes the differences that can be seen in the various regions of the vertebral column.

ARTHROLOGY

Each vertebra articulates with contiguous vertebrae. Joints are formed between adjacent vertebral bodies and also between adjacent vertebral arches. The range of motion between any two vertebrae is restricted; however, there are many articulations in the vertebral column that work together to permit a fair amount of mobility and flexibility in the spine.

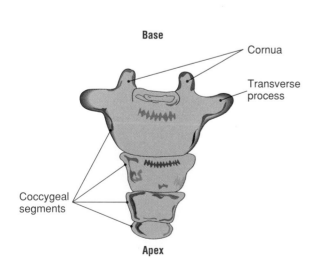

Figure 10–13. Anterior aspect of the coccyx.

Table 10–3. Summary of Regional Differences of the Vertebral Column

	Cervical	Thoracic	Lumbar
Location	Neck	Upper back	Lower back
Number	7	12	5
Body	Small C1: none	Heart-shaped	Large and cylindrical
Vertebral Foramen	Triangular Large	Circular Smaller	Somewhat triangular Smallest
Transverse Processes	Transverse foramina	Costal facets	Neither foramina nor facets
Spinous Process	Short Bifid tips (C2–6) C1: none	Long Slender Point inferiorly	Thick Blunt Point posteriorly
Intervertebral Foramina	Demonstrated on 45° oblique projection	Demonstrated on 90° (lateral) projection	Demonstrated on 90° (lateral) projection
Zygapophyseal Joints	C1–2: demonstrated on 0° (AP open-mouth) projection C2–7: demonstrated on 90° (lateral) projection	T1–12: demonstrated on 70° oblique projection	L1–5: demonstrated on 45° oblique projection L5–S1: demonstrated on 30° oblique projection

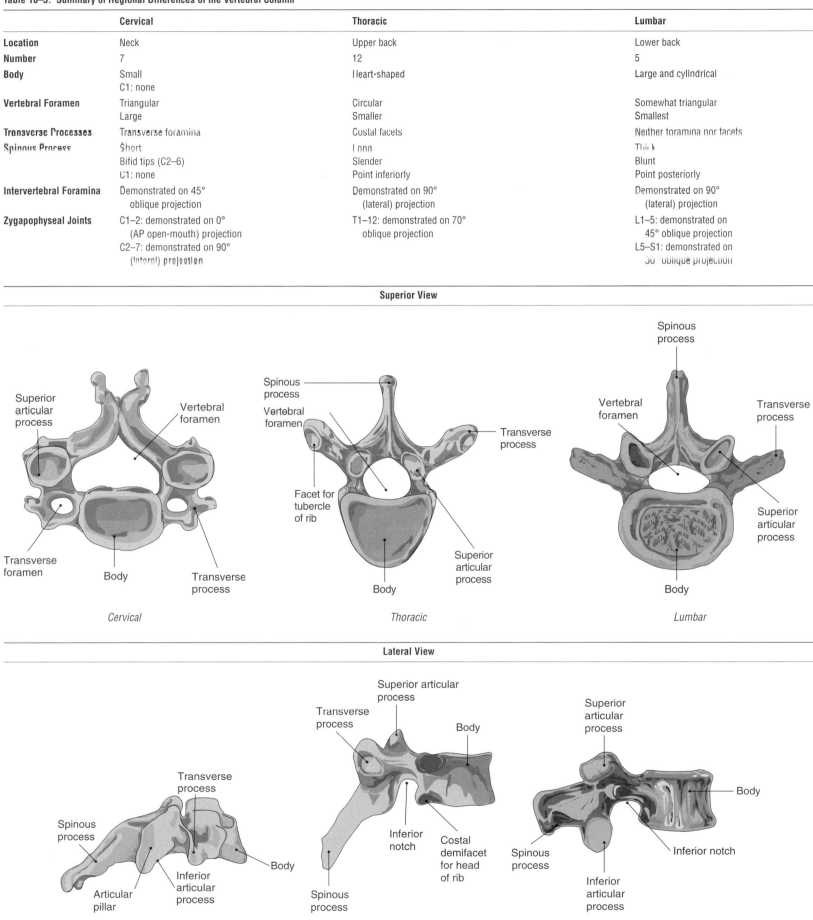

Superior View

Cervical

Thoracic

Lumbar

Lateral View

Cervical

Thoracic

Lumbar

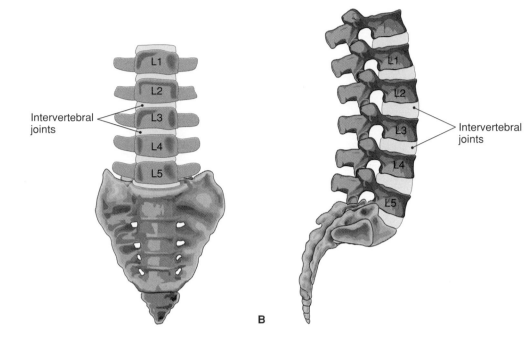

Figure 10–14. Intervertebral joints between the lumbar vertebrae are demonstrated on **(A)** anterior and **(B)** lateral views.

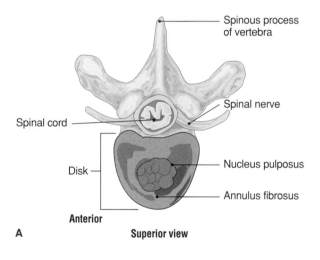

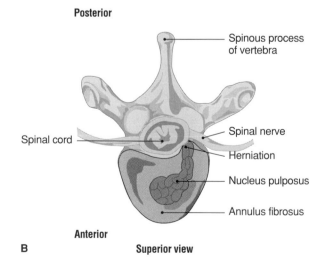

Figure 10–15. Superior views of intervertebral disk: **(A)** normal appearance, **(B)** herniated nucleus pulposus.

Intervertebral Joints

An intervertebral joint is a symphysis formed between the bodies of two adjoining vertebrae *(Figure 10–14)*. It is an amphiarthrodial joint that is cartilaginous in structure. As such, it permits only slight movement. The intervertebral joints between adjoining regions of the spine are particularly vulnerable to injury and are therefore important radiographically. These joints are the cervicothoracic, thoracolumbar, lumbosacral, and sacrococcygeal articulations.

A fibrocartilaginous disk known as an **intervertebral disk** acts as a cushion or shock absorber between the vertebral bodies to prevent the bones from hitting or scraping against each other during movement. This pad or disk is constructed much like a jelly donut. The tough, fibrous outer ring called the **annulus fibrosis** (AN-ū-lus fī-BRŌ-sis) surrounds the **nucleus pulposus** (NŪ-klē-us pul-PŌ-sus), which is a semifluid, gelatinous substance that makes the disk compressible. Because the posterior portion of the annulus fibrosis is thinner than the anterior side, it is subject to tearing or rupturing from excess strain or injury. If this occurs, the nucleus pulposus may protrude through the tear to press on the spinal cord or nerve roots. This condition is accurately termed a **herniated nucleus pulposus,** although it is often referred to as a "slipped disk" *(Figure 10–15)*.

The intervertebral disks account for approximately one fourth of the length of the vertebral column. They are found between most of the vertebrae. The exceptions are between C1 and C2 and between the sacral and coccygeal segments after synostosis has taken place. The disks are thicker and more resilient in the cervical and lumbar regions of the vertebral column, where movement is greater, and thinner in the thoracic region, where movement is more restricted. They tend to lose their resiliency and cushion with age, and as a result, an individual loses height as he or she grows older.

Interarticular Joints

The interarticular joints are formed between the vertebral arches of adjacent vertebrae and are known as the **zygapophyseal** (zi-gah-POF-i-se-al) **joints.** Each joint is formed by the articulation of a superior articular process of one vertebra and the inferior articular process of the vertebra directly above it. Structurally, the zygapophyseal joint is synovial and is classified as diarthrodial with gliding movement. The amount of movement permitted depends on the relationship of the articular processes to one another.

In the cervical region of the vertebral column, the articular processes are located on the superior and inferior surface of each vertebra, allowing more movement than in other regions of the vertebral column. Therefore, flexion, extension, abduction (side-to-side bending), and rotation are possible. The zygapophyseal joints formed by C2 through T1 are best demonstrated on a lateral (90°) projection *(Figure 10–16),*

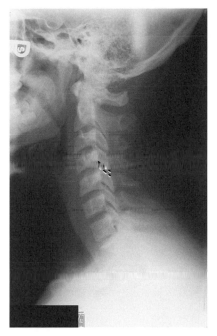

Figure 10–16. Lateral projection demonstrating articular processes and zygapophyseal joints between two adjacent cervical vertebrae.

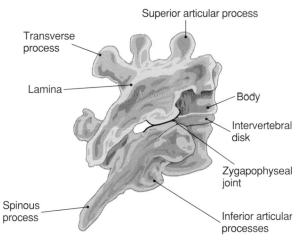

Figure 10–17. AP open-mouth projection demonstrating the zygapophyseal joints between C1 and C2.

whereas the C1–C2 zygapophyseal joint is seen on an AP (open-mouth) projection *(Figure 10–17)*. The **atlantoaxial joint,** as it is known, lets the head and C1 rotate on C2 because it is a diarthrodial joint allowing pivot movement. The atlas also articulates with the occipital bone of the skull to form the **atlanto-occipital joint.** The superior articular surface on each lateral mass articulates with a corresponding occipital condyle to form a synovial joint, which is classified as diarthrodial with condyloid movement. It permits flexion, extension, and some lateral flexion.

The articular processes of the thoracic region are positioned on the vertebra at an angle of 15° to 20°. The articular surfaces of the superior articular processes face obliquely anterior, and the articular surfaces of the inferior articular processes face obliquely posterior. The zygapophyseal joints of the thoracic spine allow the same movements as the cervical spine but on a more limited basis. They are best visualized when the patient is obliqued approximately 70° to 75° from a true AP or PA position *(Figure 10–18)*.

In the lumbar spine, the articular processes are positioned obliquely on the vertebra at a 45° angle. The articular surfaces of the superior articular processes face posteromedially, and the articular surfaces of the inferior articular processes face anterolaterally. Although very little rotation is possible, flexion and extension are greater in this area of the vertebral column. The zygapophyseal joints of the lumbar spine are best seen on a 45° oblique projection. The exception is the zygapophyseal joint between the fifth lumbar vertebra and the first sacral segment, which is angled 60° in the body. It is demonstrated on a 30° oblique projection *(Figure 10–19)*.

Costovertebral and Costotransverse Joints

As discussed in Chapter 9, the thoracic vertebrae are involved in the formation of costovertebral and costotransverse joints. A **costovertebral joint** is formed by the articulation of the head of a rib with a single facet or two demifacets on the vertebral body(s). A **costotransverse joint** is formed by the tubercle of the rib and the transverse process of the vertebra. Both of these joints are synovial in structure and are classified as diarthrodial with gliding movement *(Figure 10–20)*.

The joints of the vertebral column are summarized in Table 10–4.

Topographical Landmarks

Particular vertebrae can be localized by palpating either the spinous process or other body structures. C1 is at the level of the hard palate or the mastoid tips. C3 corresponds to the angle of the mandible (gonion). C4 is at the superior margin of the thyroid cartilage. The spinous process of C7 is palpable on the posterior aspect of the neck.

Superior articular process

Transverse process

Lamina

Body

Intervertebral disk

Zygapophyseal joint

Spinous process

Inferior articular processes

A

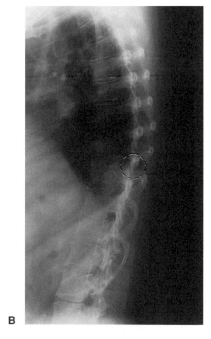

B

Figure 10–18. Articular processes and zygapophyseal joints of adjacent thoracic vertebrae are demonstrated on **(A)** posterolateral view and **(B)** 70°—75° oblique projection

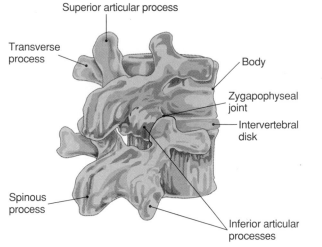

A

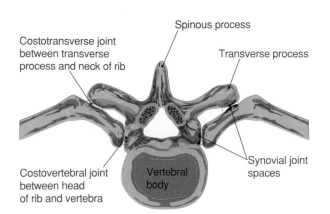

B

Figure 10–19. Zygapophyseal joints between adjacent lumbar vertebrae are demonstrated on **(A)** posterolateral view and **(B)** 45° oblique projection.

Figure 10–20. Costovertebral and costotransverse joints demonstrated on a superior view.

Table 10–4. Summary of Joints of the Vertebral Column

Name of Joint	Classification	Structure	Movement
Intervertebral	Amphiarthrodial	Cartilaginous	Slight
Interarticular	Diarthrodial	Synovial	
Atlanto-occipital			Condyloid
Atlantoaxial			Pivot
Zygapophyseal C2–S1			Gliding
Costovertebral	Diarthrodial	Synovial	Gliding
Costotransverse	Diarthrodial	Synovial	Gliding

The sternum is often used for localization of thoracic vertebrae. The T2–3 disk space is at the level of the jugular (suprasternal) notch. The T4–5 disk space corresponds to the level of the sternal angle, whereas the xiphoid process is a very prominent landmark used to find T10. The inferior angle or tip of the scapula can be used to find the midthoracic margin, which corresponds to the T6–7 disk space.

The L23 disk space is at the level of the lower costal margin (subcostal plane). The disk space between L2 and L3 corresponds approximately with the umbilicus whereas L4–5 is at the level of the iliac crest. The second sacral segment (S2) is at the level of the ASIS. The coccyx is directly posterior to the symphysis pubis *(Figure 10–21).*

► PROCEDURAL CONSIDERATIONS

Although radiographs are also obtained as part of a preemployment physical, traumatic injury and chronic pain are the primary reasons for performing radiographic examinations of the vertebral column. Because spinal problems can impair sensory function in the limbs and organs in the thorax and abdomen, good patient care and the production of the highest quality radiographs is imperative for accurate diagnosis.

PATIENT PREPARATION

After the patient is correctly identified, he or she should be instructed to remove all articles of clothing and metallic objects that could result in artifacts on the radiographs. Patient preparation depends on the specific area of the spine to be examined and the condition of the patient.

- *Cervical spine:* A patient preparing for a radiographic examination of the cervical spine should be instructed to remove any earrings, necklaces, eyeglasses, oral appliances (dentures, removable partial plates, orthodontic retainers, etc), and clothing with zippers, buttons, hooks, or clasps above the level of the axillae prior to patient positioning. It may be necessary for the patient to remove clothing above the waist and wear a patient gown.
- *Thoracic spine:* For radiography of the thoracic spine, patients must remove all clothing and jewelry above the waist and dress in a patient gown that is open in the back, if possible. The ability to examine the spine when positioning for the lateral projection can improve positioning accuracy.
- *Lumbosacral spine:* Lumbar spine radiography requires removal of all clothing above and below the waist to eliminate the possibility of artifacts on the film. Patients preparing for only radiographic examination of the sacrum or coccyx need to only remove clothing below the waist. Again, a gown that is open in the back is preferred to facilitate patient positioning for the lateral projection.
- *Trauma care:* If an accident victim arrives in the radiology department on a stretcher, extreme care must be taken when moving the patient onto the radiographic table. Although the trauma patient's condition may have been stabilized prior to being sent to radiology, frequently this is not the case. Extreme care must be taken to monitor the patient closely at all times. If not already done, any clothing that interferes with the procedure may have to be carefully removed or cut away.

Because the ribs help provide stability to the thoracic spine, most spinal injury occurs in the cervical and lumbar regions. Because of the potential for damage to the spinal cord, immobilization is critical. Although the abdominal muscles help immobilize the lumbar vertebrae, the cervical vertebrae have insufficient inherent immobilization and require external immobilization devices such as sandbags, neck brace, and collar. When the patient's head is immobilized, at least four people should participate in moving the patient smoothly and gently, using a sheet, striker frame, or other appropriate device. Extreme care must be taken to prevent movement of the head which could contribute to spinal cord damage. Sandbags positioned on either side of the head may be removed for the initial lateral projection, but should be replaced immediately following the exposure. **Do not remove collars or other immobilization devices until a diagnosis has been confirmed and a physician supervises the removal.**

When the injury is in the thoracic or lumbosacral regions, patients often prefer to log roll (roll the entire body in one movement) onto the table after sliding toward the edge of the stretcher. Patients usually know which movements cause the greatest distress and can avoid them to minimize pain. At least two people should be available to assist the patient, if necessary.

As for all radiographic examinations, a pertinent patient history is very valuable in assessing the patient's ability to assume specific radiographic positions, determining the best technical factors for the procedure, and assisting the radiologist in diagnosis. This information should be communicated in writing or verbally to the radiologist.

POSITIONING CONSIDERATIONS

Routine examination of the cervical spine virtually always includes AP, AP odontoid, and lateral projections. Although some departments do not perform oblique cervical projections routinely, the majority do *(Table 10–5)*. While most cervical spine projections can be performed with the patient upright, the AP cervical and odontoid views are often obtained with the patient recumbent. Because the patient is lying on his back, he is less likely to sway to one side and can be better immobilized, eliminating movement during or prior to the exposure. The oblique and lateral projections are usually obtained with the patient in the upright position. The patient position for these projections produces a large OID, requiring a 72-in. SID to minimize magnification. This distance cannot usually be obtained when the patient is recumbent.

Because the C7–T1 junction may not be adequately demonstrated on a person with a short neck or large muscular shoulders, the patient is generally instructed to hold two sandbags of equal weight, one in each hand, during the exposure to depress the shoulders. A lateral cervicothoracic (swimmer's) projection may be taken to more adequately demonstrate the C7–T1 junction.

Radiographic examinations of the thoracic and lumbosacral regions are usually performed with the patient recumbent. The thoracic spine series always includes the AP and lateral projections; the lateral cervicothoracic projection is also often included. Because of the difference in tissue thickness between the upper and lower thoracic spine, the AP projection should be obtained with the patient positioned on the table so the head is nearest the anode end of the tube, using the anode–heel effect and producing a more uniform density. Routine examination of the lumbosacral spine includes AP and lateral projections, including a lateral spot of the L5–S1 junction. Although some radiology departments include oblique lumbar projections in the routine lumbar spine series, they are usually optional.

One projection that is frequently repeated is the AP open-mouth odontoid. A common positioning error is incorrect head flexion resulting in inadequate demonstration of the odontoid process and additional

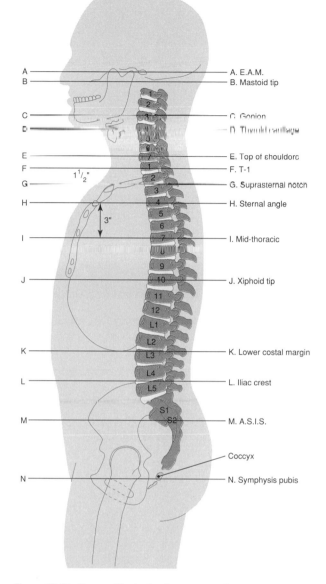

Figure 10–21. Topographic landmarks corresponding to the vertebral column.

A. E.A.M.
B. Mastoid tip
C. Gonion
D. Thyroid cartilage
E. Top of shoulders
F. T-1
G. Suprasternal notch
H. Sternal angle
I. Mid-thoracic
J. Xiphoid tip
K. Lower costal margin
L. Iliac crest
M. A.S.I.S.
Coccyx
N. Symphysis pubis

1½"

3"

Table 10–5. Routine/Optional Projections: Vertebral Column

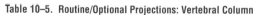

Cervical spine	Sacrum
AP	AP
AP atlas and axis (odontoid)	Lateral
RPO/LPO or LAO/RAO	
Lateral	
Lateral flexion/extension[a]	
Thoracic spine	Coccyx
AP	AP
Lateral	Lateral
Lateral cervicothoracic[a]	
Lumbosacral spine	Scoliosis
AP	AP
RPO/LPO or LAO/RAO[a]	Lateral
Lateral	
AP L5–S1 junction[a]	
Lateral L5–S1 junction	
Lateral flexion/extension[a]	

Note. Although routines may vary between departments, this table summarizes some of the more common routine and optional projections and examinations.
[a]Optional projections; may be routine in some departments.

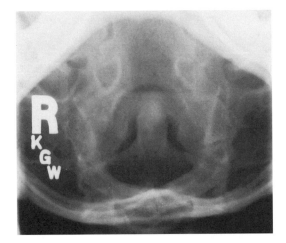

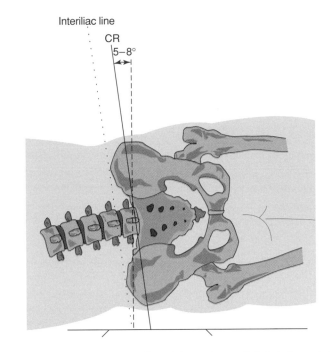

Figure 10–24. Without radiolucent supports, a 5° to 8° caudal central ray angle is typically used. *(With permission from Francis, Charles. Method Improves Consistency in LS–S1 Joint Space Films. Radiologic Technology, 1992; 63(S).)*

Figure 10–22. Reverse parietoacanthal (Water's) projection for the odontoid process.

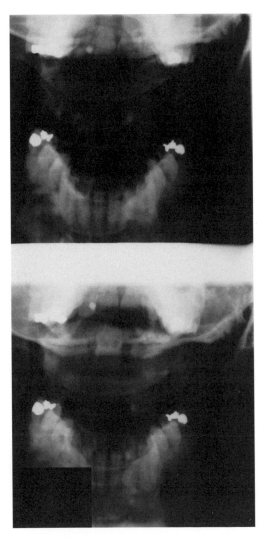

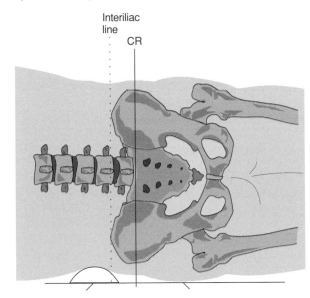

Figure 10–25. If radiolucent supports are used to ensure the entire spine is parallel with the tabletop, a perpendicular central ray can be used. *(With permission from Francis, Charles. Method Improves Consistency in LS–S1 Joint Space Films. Radiologic Technology, 1992; 63(S).)*

Figure 10–23. AP open-mouth odontoid projection with no central ray angle (top) and with 5° cephalic angle (bottom) can be obtained at the same time to ensure demonstration of the zygapophyseal joints and odontoid process.

exposures. If the projection is repeated because the initial film demonstrates the C1–2 zygapophyseal joints but not the entire dens, a reverse parietoacanthial (Water's) projection (as described in Chapter 12) can then be taken to demonstrate the entire odontoid process *(Figure 10–22)*. An alternative is to obtain two initial projections, one with the central ray directed perpendicular to the film, the second with the patient in the same position and the central ray directed 5° cephalad; both projections can be included on one film *(Figure 10–23)*. When following this procedure, all necessary anatomy is almost always demonstrated on one of the two projections, resulting in fewer repeats.

Another difficult area to demonstrate can be the intervertebral disk space between L5 and S1 when the patient is in the lateral position. Several different techniques can be used to accomplish this goal. One of the more common methods is to direct the central ray 5° or 8° caudad for men and women, respectively *(Figure 10–24)*. This method, however, does not take into consideration the broad variation in patient build and the need to increase or decrease tube angle accordingly.

An alternative method is to use radiolucent supports to position the entire spine parallel with the film plane *(Figure 10–25)*. The spinous processes can be palpated to determine the thickness and placement of supports. If the plane passing through the spine is truly parallel with the film, no angle is needed. Although both of these methods work most of the time, the second method does not require as much guesswork.

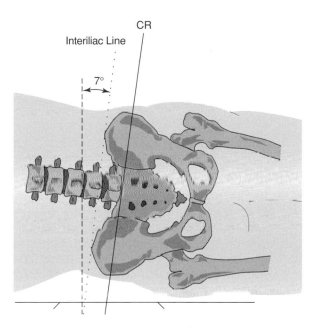

Figure 10–26. When the thorax is wider than the hips, a cephalic angle may be used when employing the Francis method. *(With permission from Francis, Charles. Method Improves Consistency in LS–S1 Joint Space Flms.* Radiologic Technology, *1992; 63(S).)*

Neither of the above methods, however, takes into account the patient with a unique L5–S1 disk space. A third technique, described by Charles Francis, requires determination of the angle of the L5–S1 joint space by determining the tilt of the pelvis (the sacrum tilts with the pelvis and affects the angle of the joint). When the patient is in the lateral position, an imaginary line is drawn between the iliac crests. The central ray should then be directed parallel to this line *(Figure 10–26)*. For most patients, the central ray will be directed caudally, however, some patients may require a cephalic central ray angle.

TRAUMA CONSIDERATIONS

When a patient enters the emergency room following a traumatic injury, one of the first assessments performed by the physician is an evaluation of the spine. Because the cervical region is the least stable area of the vertebral column, it is frequently the site of injury and the patient's head should be immobilized. Cervical spine injuries can range from minor soft tissue and ligament damage to complete fracture, dislocation, and spinal cord injury. A cross-table lateral cervical projection, used to detect up to 90% of significant injuries, should be performed first and cleared by a physician prior to moving the patient or removing any brace or collar. This initial film is often obtained using a mobile unit to prevent unnecessary movement of the patient. Although radiolucent immobilization devices should remain in place for this initial projection, sandbags, if used, need to be removed for the exposure and immediately replaced afterward. All seven cervical and the first thoracic vertebrae should be included within the collimated area. To demonstrate the lower cervical and first thoracic, it is often necessary to move the arms downward to eliminate superimposition of the shoulders; this can be accomplished by instructing the patient to gently pull on a strap wrapped around his or her feet or by a nonradiation worker pulling gently on the patient's hands. Please note that although this technique may be very effective, it also causes some hyperextension of the cervical spine and should be used only if there is little clinical indication for injury and no neurologic deficit. *Figure 10–27* provides a recommended course of action.

The AP, open-mouth odontoid, and oblique (if requested) projections can be obtained on the direction of the physician. All can be performed with the patient supine, if necessary *(Figure 10–28)*. Although the AP projections are performed in the same manner as for nontraumatic patients, the oblique projection is performed using a nongrid, tabletop technique and requires a double angle of the central ray: 45° crosstable and 15° to 20° cephalad.

Cervical spine evaluation

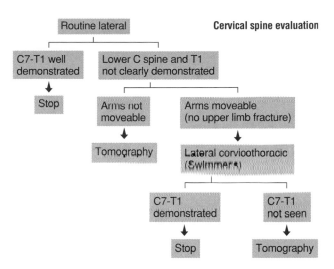

Figure 10–27. Typical order of study of the lower cervical spine. *(Adapted from Berquist TH. Diagnostic Imaging of the Acutely Injured Patient. Baltimore, MD: Urban & Schwarzenberg. Copyright 1995 by the Mayo Foundation, Rochester, MN.)*

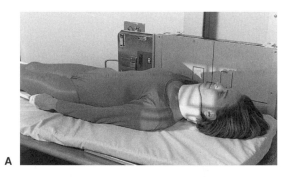

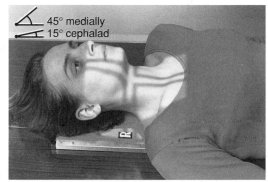

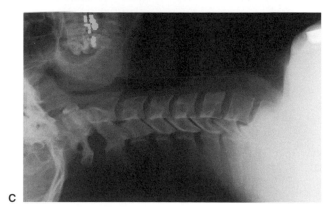

Figure 10–28. Lateral **(A)** and AP oblique **(B)** cervical spine projections can be obtained on the trauma patient in the supine position. **(C)** Cross-table lateral cervical spine.

Although cervical spine injuries are less common in infants and children than in adolescents and adults, head trauma can cause injury to the upper cervical spine. In infants, a cervical spine injury tends to involve the upper three vertebrae, whereas the lower five vertebrae are more likely to be affected in older children and adults. Because an infant or small child's head is disproportionately larger than the shoulders and thorax, lying supine on a backboard or radiographic table thrusts the head and neck forward. Care must be taken to ensure that the head and body are aligned; the thorax should be elevated with padding to prevent potential damage to the spinal cord.

ALTERNATE PROJECTIONS

Hyperflexion/Hyperextension Studies

In order to evaluate the degree of anteroposterior mobility, ligament injuries, or potential instability, hyperflexion/hyperextension projections of the cervical spine are performed. Limited movement in the cervical spine may be the result of trauma, surgery, or disease. **Hyperflexion/hyperextension examinations of the cervical spine should not be performed prior to ruling out a fracture.** Any fracture should be treated prior to checking for instability. Performing these projections within 48 hours of the injury may also result in false-negative studies due to muscle spasm.

Hyperflexion/hyperextension studies may also be performed on the lumbar spine to localize a herniated disk or, following surgery, to evaluate motion at the site of a spinal fusion.

Scoliosis

Scoliosis, the abnormal lateral rotary curvature of the vertebral column, may be a result of abnormal chondrification and ossification, or a neuromuscular disorder, such as cerebral palsy, tumor, paralysis, or trauma; the condition may also be idiopathic (no known origin). Scoliosis can be classified as either nonstructural, due to extrinsic factors such as leg shortening and hip dysplasia, or structural, relating directly to the vertebrae. Nonstructural scoliosis disappears when the patient is recumbent, whereas structural scoliosis involves a lateral curvature and vertebral rotation that do not disappear when the patient is lying down. Although curve progression can be monitored in other ways, radiographs of the vertebral column provide more accurate measurements and are necessary for initial evaluation of structural anatomy and deformity; they may also be obtained periodically during the puberty years. In addition to the spinal radiographs, a PA projection of the left hand and wrist may be obtained to assess skeletal maturity.

The most common projection for evaluating scoliosis is the erect PA projection; because most scoliosis patients are young women, the PA projection, rather than the AP, is recommended to minimize the dose to the radiosensitive breast tissue. The erect lateral projection may also be requested on initial examination or prior to surgery. Both recumbent and erect projections may be requested to differentiate between nonstructural and structural scoliosis. To further evaluate the natural ability of the spine to correct curvature and vertebral rotation, right and left lateral side bending projections may be requested prior to surgery; these are usually performed with the patient supine, however, they may be obtained with the patient erect

▶ *Scoliosis Series*

Minimize patient dose by:

- *Using PA instead of AP projections.*

- *Collimating to the spine.*

- *Shielding gonads and breasts.*

- *Using high speed film/screen systems.*

- *Using high kVp, low mAs techniques.*

Improve radiographic quality by using compensating filters.

Table 10–6. Summary of Breathing Instructions

Cervical Spine Projections	
AP open-mouth atlas and axis	Phonate soft "ah"
AP	Suspended respiration
Oblique	Suspended respiration
Lateral	Suspended expiration
Lateral with flexion/extension	Suspended expiration
Thoracic spine projections	
AP	Shallow breathing or suspended expiration
Lateral	Shallow breathing or suspended expiration
Lateral cervicothoracic	Suspended respiration
Lumbar spine projections	
AP	Suspended expiration
Oblique	Suspended expiration
Lateral	Suspended expiration
Lateral with flexion/extension	Suspended expiration
Sacrum/coccyx projections	
AP	Suspended expiration
Lateral	Suspended expiration

if so directed by the physician. Although orthopedic surgeons may wish to see the entire rib cage on initial films to evaluate rib deformity, it is recommended that close collimation and breast shields be used to minimize patient dose on subsequent films; collimation on initial films should be done according to department routine. To minimize magnification, a 72-in. SID should be used. The first cervical vertebrae through the level of the ASISs should be included within the collimation field.

Because of the potential for follow-up examinations, radiation protection is critical. Collimation, use of the PA projection, shielding of the breasts and gonads, high-speed film/screen combinations, and high-kVp techniques all help to minimize the patient's dose.

BREATHING INSTRUCTIONS

Different breathing techniques can be used for a variety of reasons: to minimize blurring of the radiographic image, to blur some structures to better visualize others, or to ensure that the patient simply holds still. For most cervical spine projections, the latter is true. For the AP atlas and axis projection, however, the patient should be instructed to phonate a soft "ah" during the exposure. Doing so will prevent movement of the mandible and immobilize the tongue on the floor of the mouth, preventing its shadow from being superimposed over the atlas and axis. For the lateral cervical spine projection, the exposure should be made during suspended expiration, to help relax the shoulders and move them inferiorly *(Table 10–6)*.

When obtaining the AP thoracic projection, a shallow breathing technique may be used, if the patient's breathing is not labored. Suspended expiration can also be used for the this projection to produce a more uniform density between the spine and lungs. Shallow, quiet breathing is recommended for the lateral projection of the thoracic spine to blur lung and rib detail, allowing for better visualization of the vertebrae. When the patient is unable to breathe quietly, however, the exposure should be made during suspended expiration. To minimize tissue thickness and produce a more uniform radiographic density, all projections of the lumbosacral region should be obtained during suspended expiration.

EXPOSURE FACTORS

Because there is wide variation in tissue thickness and density between the cervical, thoracic, and lumbar regions, the optimum kVps for these regions will also vary. In general, the cervical spine is usually radiographed using 60 to 75 kVp. The AP projections of the thoracic and lumbar vertebrae should be obtained using 70 to 80 kVp to minimize patient dose, yet produce films with an acceptable scale of contrast. Because of increased tissue thickness, the lateral projections require 80 to 90 kVp, with the lateral L5–S1 spot possibly needing as much as 100 kVp for penetration. Because of the small size of the coccyx, 60 to 70 kVp is recommended for the AP projection and 65 to 75 kVp for the lateral projection to produce the optimum radiographic contrast. In all cases, patients with advanced arthritis or osteoporosis require the use of kVps at the low end of the ranges—and possibly lower—to produce radiographs of the highest quality. The mAs required depends on the patient size, type of equipment generator, film/screen speed, type of grid, and pathologic conditions present. Although automatic exposure control may be used for most projections of the vertebral column, it is not recommended for hyperextension/hyperflexion studies or those projections requiring very close collimation, such as that of the lateral coccyx.

EQUIPMENT CONSIDERATIONS

Although most radiography of the vertebral column is produced with the use of a grid, the lateral and oblique projections of the cervical spine can be obtained without a grid. Because of the increased OID with these projections, the air gap produces an effect similar to that of a grid (this technique is more fully discussed in Chapter 2).

Although a horizontal radiographic table is adequate for most radiography of the thoracic and lumbar spine, a vertical grid device is usually used for the oblique and lateral cervical projections. Scoliosis films are also obtained with the patient in the upright position. In departments where scoliosis radiography is performed frequently, a special 36-in. cassette may be available to include the entire spine with one exposure. A high-speed film/screen system is recommended, as spinal curvature rather than bony detail is being evaluated. Compensating filters may be strategically attached to the collimator to decrease the radiographic density of the lower cervical/upper thoracic region on the AP thoracic spine projection (wedge filter) and the midthoracic region on the lateral projection, producing more consistent density throughout.

For lateral projections of the thoracic and lumbar spines, sacrum, and coccyx, a lead shield or glove can be placed on the table behind the patient to reduce the amount of scattered radiation reaching the film.

A cassette holder or upright grid device is needed for cross-table lateral spine projections. A sheet, rope, or strip of tape may be used to help the patient depress the shoulders for the lateral projection of the cervical spine.

ALTERNATE IMAGING PROCEDURES

Myelography is an invasive procedure used to demonstrate the spinal canal, spinal cord, and nerve roots. It is performed to evaluate cord tumors, posterior protrusion of herniated disks, degenerative diseases of the central nervous system, and malformation of the spinal cord. Because of the risk of infection, aseptic technique is followed and the injection site is surgically scrubbed.

The examination is generally performed by a radiologist or orthopedic surgeon, with the assistance of fluoroscopy. To accomplish the procedure, either an oil-based or water-soluble contrast medium is injected into the subarachnoid space under fluoroscopic guidance. Although the oil-based contrast medium was used for many years, it had to be removed from the spinal canal with a needle after the examination. A water-soluble contrast media is generally preferred today because of its ability to coat the nerve roots and to be absorbed by the surrounding tissues. Although it does not have to be removed, it is absorbed rapidly; filming, therefore, must be accurate and quick. After the contrast has been administered, the physician tilts the table head down and feet down and observes the flow of contrast media fluoroscopically; spot films are obtained as needed. When the patient is in the Trendelenburg position, the head must be in acute hyperextension to prevent flow of contrast media through the cisterna magna and into the head. Following fluoroscopy, a cross-table lateral of the area of interest is obtained with the patient prone; PA and oblique projections may also be requested *(Figure 10–29)*. After the procedure, the patient is usually instructed to remain on bedrest for 8 to 24 hours and to drink plenty of fluids.

Although cervical myelography can be done, most myelography performed today is of the lumbar region. Computed tomography (CT) and magnetic resonance imaging (MRI), which are noninvasive examinations, are frequently performed in place of the myelogram.

Discography may be performed to evaluate internal disk lesions that cannot be visualized by myelography. A local anesthetic is used to numb the area of injection and may also be added to the contrast media. By use of a technique similar to myelography, water-soluble contrast media is injected directly into the intervertebral disk. In addition to fluoroscopic spot films, overhead films are obtained as requested by the physician.

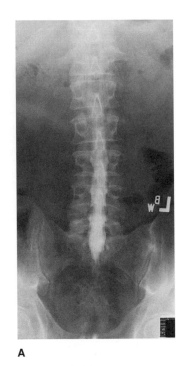

A

B

Figure 10–29. PA **(A)** and cross-table **(B)** lateral projections of the lumbar spine; myelography.

RADIOGRAPHIC POSITIONING OF THE VERTEBRAL COLUMN

- ► AP CERVICAL SPINE

- ► AP ATLAS AND AXIS (OPEN-MOUTH ODONTOID)

- ► AP AXIAL OBLIQUE CERVICAL SPINE

- ► LATERAL CERVICAL SPINE

- ► HYPERFLEXION/HYPEREXTENSION LATERAL CERVICAL SPINE

- ► LATERAL CERVICOTHORACIC SPINE (SWIMMER'S POSITION)

- ► AP THORACIC SPINE

- ► PA OBLIQUE THORACIC SPINE

- ► LATERAL THORACIC SPINE

- ► AP LUMBAR SPINE

- ► AP OBLIQUE LUMBAR SPINE

- ► LATERAL LUMBAR SPINE

- ► HYPERFLEXION/HYPEREXTENSION LATERAL LUMBAR SPINE

- ► AP AXIAL LUMBOSACRAL JUNCTION

- ► LATERAL LUMBOSACRAL JUNCTION

- ► AP SACRUM

- ► LATERAL SACRUM

- ► AP COCCYX

- ► LATERAL COCCYX

- ► PA SCOLIOSIS

- ► LATERAL SCOLIOSIS

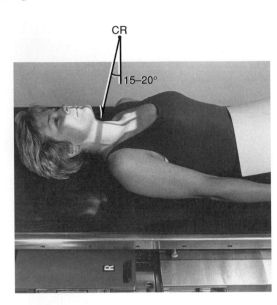

Figure 10–30. AP cervical spine.

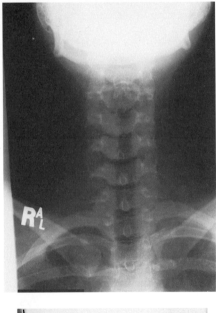

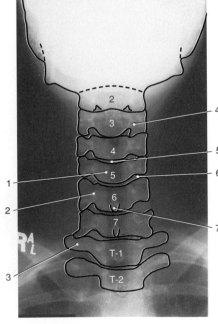

Figure 10–31. AP cervical spine.

▶ AP CERVICAL SPINE

Technical Considerations

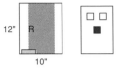

- Film size: 10 × 12 in. or 8 × 10 in. lengthwise.
- Grid required.
- 65–75 kVp.
- Collimate to the soft tissue of the neck crosswise and to film size lengthwise.

Shielding

- Gonadal shielding should be used on all patients, especially children and adults of reproductive age.

Patient Positioning

- Assist the patient to the supine position on the radiographic table; the patient may flex the knees and hips, placing the plantar surface of the feet flat against the table for comfort. **Note:** This projection may also be obtained with the patient standing or sitting in front of an upright grid device.
- Center the midsagittal plane of the patient to the midline of the table; check for rotation of the head and shoulders.
- Adjust the long axis of the patient parallel with the long axis of the table; pull gently on the patient's legs or under the patient's arms to straighten the patient.

Part Positioning

- Extend the patient's head so that a line between the upper occlusal plane and the mastoid tips (base of the skull) is perpendicular to the film plane *(Figure 10–30)*.

Central Ray

- Direct the central ray 15° to 20° cephalad to a point slightly inferior to the most prominent point of the thyroid cartilage and through the fourth cervical vertebra; the degree of angulation depends on the amount of cervical spine curvature.
- Center the cassette to the central ray.

Breathing Instructions

- Instruct the patient to stop breathing during the exposure. **Note:** An AP projection of all seven cervical vertebrae can be obtained by instructing the patient to open and close the mouth during the exposure; a 2- to 3-second exposure time is needed to produce an acceptable image.

Image Evaluation

- Soft tissue structures of the neck, lower five cervical vertebrae, and upper two thoracic vertebrae should be included in the collimated area.
- Bony trabeculae should be seen within the vertebral bodies.
- The fourth cervical body should be in the middle of the film.
- The mastoid tips should be symmetrical; the gonia should also be symmetrical.
- The mandible should be superimposed over the base of the skull and upper one to two cervical bodies.
- The intervertebral disk spaces should be clearly demonstrated *(Figure 10–31)*.

1. Vertebral body
2. Pedicle
3. Transverse process, T1
4. Articular pillar
5. Intervertebral disk space
6. Interpediculate space
7. Spinous process

► AP ATLAS AND AXIS (OPEN-MOUTH ODONTOID)

Technical Considerations

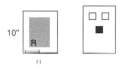

- Film size: 8 × 10 in. lengthwise or 9 × 9 in.
- Grid required.
- 65–75 kVp.
- Collimate to a 5 × 5-in. field size.

Shielding

- Gonadal shielding should be used on all patients, especially children and adults of reproductive age.

Patient Positioning

- Assist the patient to the supine position on the radiographic table; the patient may flex the knees and hips, placing the plantar surface of the feet flat against the table for comfort. **Note:** This projection may also be obtained with the patient standing or sitting in front of an upright grid device.
- Center the midsagittal plane of the patient to the midline of the table; check for rotation of the head and shoulders.
- Adjust the long axis of the patient parallel with the long axis of the table; pull gently on the patient's legs or under the patient's arms to straighten the patient.
- Set the technical factors, as this position may be difficult for the patient to maintain.

Part Positioning

- Instruct the patient to open the mouth as wide as possible.
- Position the patient's head so that a line between the lower margin of the upper incisors and the base of the skull (level of the mastoid tips) is perpendicular to the film plane; sandbags on either side of the head or tape drawn across the chin can be used to immobilize the head to prevent rotation *(Figure 10–32)*.

Central Ray

- Direct the central ray perpendicular to C1 through the open mouth; 30- to 32-in. SID (with an appropriate reduction in mAs) may be used to magnify the open mouth and allow better visualization of the atlas and axis.
- Center the cassette to the central ray.

Breathing Instructions

- Instruct the patient to maintain the wide-open mouth and say "ah" during the exposure.

Image Evaluation

- The entire atlas and axis should be included in the collimated area.
- Bony trabeculae should be seen within the lateral masses of C1, the dens, and the vertebral body of C2.
- C1 should be in the middle of the film.
- The lateral masses should be equal distances from the rami of the mandible.
- The lower edge of the upper incisors should be even with the base of the skull.
- The zygapophyseal joints between C1 and C2 should be clearly demonstrated *(Figure 10–33)*.

1. Transverse process, C1
2. Zygapophyseal joint, C1–2
3. Spinous process, C2
4. Dens, C2
5. Lateral mass, C1
6. Body, C2

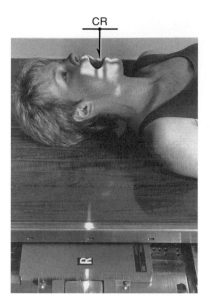

Figure 10–32. AP, open-mouth odontoid.

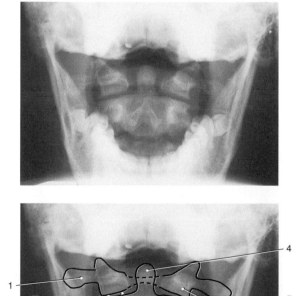

Figure 10–33. AP, open-mouth odontoid.

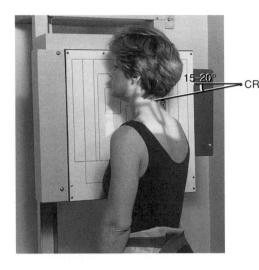

Figure 10–34. RAO cervical spine.

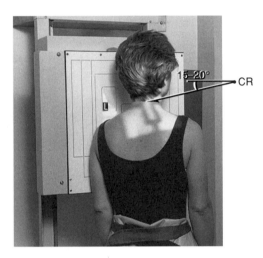

Figure 10–35. LAO cervical spine.

► AP AXIAL OBLIQUE CERVICAL SPINE

Technical Considerations

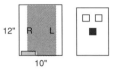

- Film size: 10 × 12 in. or 8 × 10 in. lengthwise.
- Grid or nongrid.
- 65–75 kVp.
- Collimate to the soft tissue of the neck crosswise and to film size lengthwise.

Shielding

- Gonadal shielding should be used on all patients, especially children and adults of reproductive age.

Patient Positioning

- Assist the patient to the AP seated or standing position in front of the upright grid device. **Note:** The RAO and LAO projections may be substituted for the LPO and RPO projections *(Figures 10–34, 10–35).* This projection may also be obtained with the patient recumbent on the radiographic table.

Part Positioning

- Rotate the entire body and head to form a 45° angle between the coronal plane and the film; the shoulder nearest the film should be firmly positioned against the upright grid device.
- Center the cervical spine to the midline of the upright grid device; the gonion of the side furthest from the film should coincide with the midline of the grid.
- Elevate the patient's chin slightly to minimize superimposition of the mandible over the spine; both obliques are obtained *(Figures 10–36, 10–37).*

Positioning Tip. To ensure accurate and consistent patient rotation, position tape or paint lines on the floor at 45° angles and instruct the patient to place one foot on either side of the line! Square tiles on the floor can also be used as a guide—instruct the patient to point the toes toward the corner for a perfect oblique!

Central Ray

- Using a 72-in. SID, direct the central ray 15° to 20° cephalad to a point slightly inferior to the level of the most prominent point of the thyroid cartilage and through the fourth cervical vertebra; the degree of angulation depends on the amount of cervical spine curvature.
- Center the cassette to the central ray.

Breathing Instructions

- Instruct the patient to stop breathing during the exposure.

Image Evaluation

- Soft tissue structures of the neck and seven cervical and the first thoracic vertebrae should be included in the collimated area.
- Bony trabeculae should be seen within the vertebral bodies.
- The fourth cervical body should be in the middle of the film.
- The intervertebral foramina furthest from the film should be clearly demonstrated.
- C1 should be demonstrated without superimposition of the occipital bone.
- The intervertebral disk spaces should be clearly demonstrated.
- The rami and gonia of the mandible should not be superimposed over the cervical vertebrae *(Figures 10–38, 10–39).*

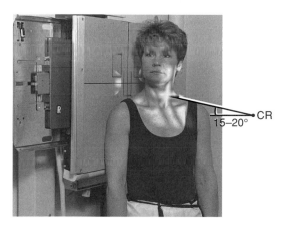

Figure 10–36. RPO cervical spine.

15–20° CR

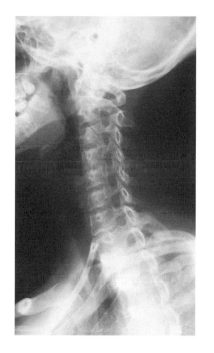
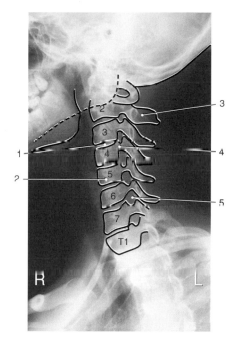

Figure 10–38. RPO cervical spine.

1. Intervertebral disk space
2. Vertebral body
3. Spinous process
4. Pedicle, left
5. Intervertebral foramen, left

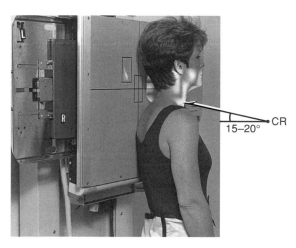

Figure 10–37. LPO cervical spine.

15–20° CR

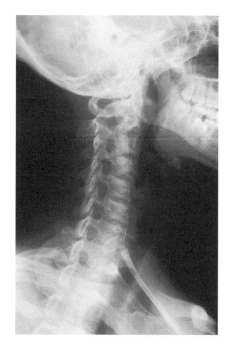
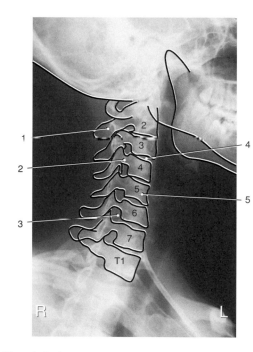

Figure 10–39. LPO cervical spine.

1. Spinous process
2. Pedicle, right
3. Intervertebral foramen, right
4. Intervertebral disk space
5. Vertebral body

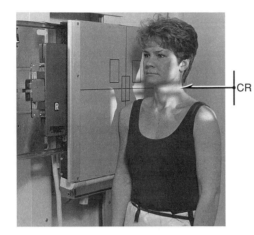

Figure 10–40. Lateral cervical spine.

▶ LATERAL CERVICAL SPINE

Technical Considerations

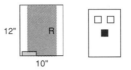

- Film size: 10 × 12 in. or 8 × 10 in. lengthwise.
- Grid or nongrid.
- 65–75 kVp.
- Collimate to the soft tissue of the neck crosswise and to film size lengthwise.

Shielding

- Gonadal shielding should be used on all patients, especially children and adults of reproductive age.

Patient Positioning

- Assist the patient to the lateral erect position in front of the upright grid device with the arms positioned comfortably at the sides; either lateral may be performed, depending on department protocol. **Note:** This projection may also be obtained using a horizontal beam with the patient supine on the radiographic table or stretcher.

Part Positioning

- Center the coronal plane passing through the external auditory meatus (EAM) to the midline of the upright grid device.
- Adjust the entire patient's body to a true lateral position, with the shoulder nearest the film firmly against the upright grid device; a line drawn between the shoulders should be perpendicular to the film plane.
- Elevate the patient's chin slightly to prevent superimposition of the mandible over the anterior arch of C1 *(Figure 10–40)*.
- Depress the shoulders as much as possible and suspend small sandbags of equal weight from each wrist for immobilization.

Positioning Tip. To prevent head rotation, instruct the patient to stare at an appropriately placed object during the exposure; a piece of tape affixed to the wall works!

Central Ray

- Using a 72-in. SID, direct the central ray perpendicular to C4, located at the level of the uppermost part of the thyroid cartilage.
- Center the cassette to the central ray.

Breathing Instructions

- Instruct the patient to take in a breath, blow it out, then hold it out during the exposure.

Image Evaluation

- Soft tissue structures of the neck and C1 through C7 should be included in the collimated area. **Note:** If C7 and/or the intervertebral disk space between C7 and T1 are not demonstrated, a lateral cervicothoracic projection should be obtained.
- Bony trabeculae should be seen within the vertebral bodies and spinous processes.
- The fourth cervical body should be in the middle of the film.
- The zygapophyseal joints, intervertebral disk spaces, and spinous processes of C2 through C7 should be clearly demonstrated.
- The first two cervical vertebrae should be seen free of superimposition by the rami of the mandible. The EAMs should be superimposed (Figure 10–41).

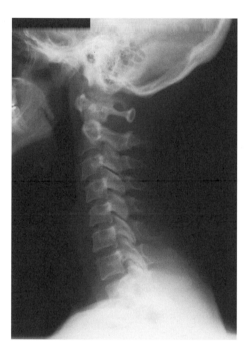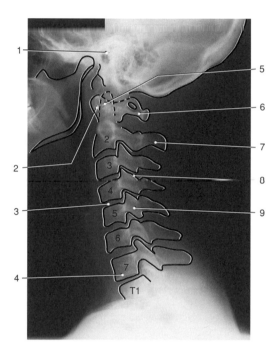

Figure 10–41. Lateral cervical spine.

1. External acoustic meatus (EAM)	4. Vertebral body	7. Spinous process
2. Anterior arch, C1	5. Dens, C2	8. Zygapophyseal joint
3. Intervertebral disk space	6. Posterior arch, C1	9. Articular pillars

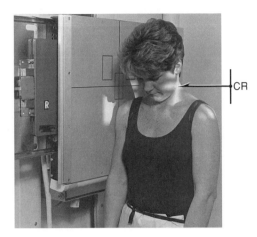

Figure 10–42. Hyperflexion lateral cervical spine.

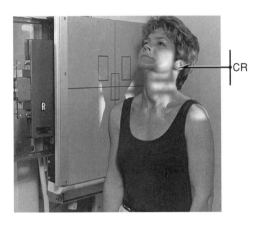

Figure 10–43. Hyperextension lateral cervical spine.

► HYPERFLEXION/HYPEREXTENSION LATERAL CERVICAL SPINE

Technical Considerations

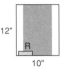

- Film size: 10 × 12 in. lengthwise.
- Grid or nongrid.
- 65–75 kVp.
- Collimate to the soft tissue of the neck crosswise and to film size lengthwise.

Caution: These patient positions should never be attempted unless a fracture of the cervical spine has been ruled out.

Shielding

- Gonadal shielding should be used on all patients, especially children and adults of reproductive age.

Patient Positioning

- Assist the patient to the lateral erect position in front of the upright grid device with the arms positioned comfortably at the sides; either lateral may be performed depending on department protocol.

Part Positioning

- Adjust the entire patient's body to a true lateral position, with the shoulder nearest the film firmly against the upright grid device; a line drawn between the shoulders should be perpendicular to the film plane.
- Set the technical factors; the patient position may be difficult to maintain.

Hyperflexion
- Instruct the patient to bend the head forward, bringing the chin as close to the chest as possible without rotating the head; center the cervical vertebrae to the midline of the cassette or grid *(Figure 10–42)*. A sandbag may be suspended from each wrist.

Hyperextension
- Instruct the patient to bend the head backward, elevating the chin as much as possible without rotating the head; center the cervical vertebrae to the midline of the cassette or grid *(Figure 10–43)*. A sandbag may be suspended from each wrist.

Central Ray

- Using a 72-in. SID, direct the central ray perpendicular to C4, located at the level of the uppermost part of the thyroid cartilage.
- Center the cassette to the central ray.

Breathing Instructions

- Instruct the patient to take in a breath, blow it out, then hold it out during the exposure.

Image Evaluation

- Soft tissue structures of the neck and C1 through C7 should be included in the collimated area.
- Bony trabeculae should be seen within the vertebral bodies and spinous processes.
- The fourth cervical body should be in the middle of the film.
- The zygapophyseal joints, intervertebral disk spaces, and spinous processes of C2 through C7 should be clearly demonstrated.
- The EAMs should be superimposed; the head should not be rotated.

Hyperflexion

- The spinous processes should be separated.
- The body of the mandible should be angled toward the lower anterior corner of the film *(Figure 10–44)*.

Hyperextension

- The spinous processes will be close together.
- The body of the mandible should be at a 45° angle with the horizontal axis of the film, pointing toward the upper anterior corner of the film *(Figure 10–45)*.

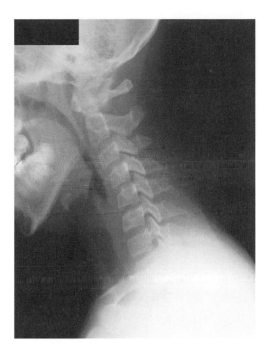

Figure 10–44. Hyperflexion lateral cervical spine.

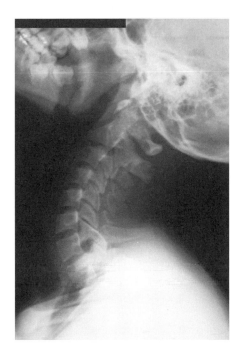

Figure 10–45. Hyperextension lateral cervical spinc.

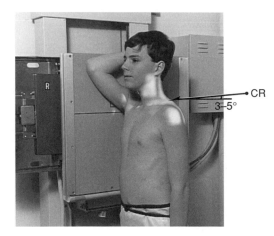

Figure 10–46. Lateral cervicothoracic spine, upright.

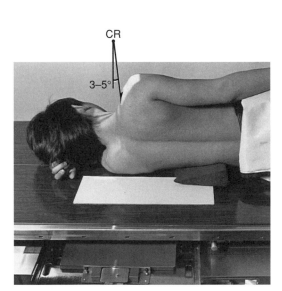

Figure 10–47. Lateral cervicothoracic spine, recumbent.

▶ LATERAL CERVICOTHORACIC SPINE (SWIMMER'S POSITION)

Technical Considerations

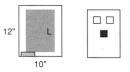

- Film size: 10 × 12 in. lengthwise.
- Grid required.
- 70–85 kVp.
- Collimate to the soft tissue of the neck crosswise and to film size lengthwise.

Shielding

- Gonadal shielding should be used on all patients, especially children and adults of reproductive age.

Patient Positioning

- Assist the patient to the lateral recumbent position on the radiographic table. **Note:** This projection may also be obtained with the patient erect, making sure the patient's side is positioned firmly against the upright grid device *(Figure 10–46)*, or by positioning the patient supine and using a horizontal beam, as would be necessary in the case of a suspected fracture.

Part Positioning

- Center the midaxillary plane to the midline of the table.
- Adjust the entire patient's body to a true lateral position, with the arm nearest the film raised above the head and the shoulder moved slightly anteriorly; the forearm or sponge should be used to support the patient's head, keeping the spine parallel to the tabletop.
- Adjust the head so it is in a true lateral position.
- Depress the shoulder furthest from the film and rotate it slightly posteriorly to prevent superimposition of the shoulders over the spine; the thoracic spine should remain lateral for this projection.
- Place a sheet of leaded rubber on the table behind the patient to reduce the amount of scatter reaching the film and improve radiographic quality *(Figure 10–47)*.

Central Ray

- Direct the central ray 3° to 5° caudad through T1, located at the level of the vertebra prominens; the central ray should be angled only enough to separate the humeral heads. **Note:** If the shoulder away from the film can be appropriately depressed, no central ray angle is needed.
- Center the cassette to the central ray.

Breathing Instructions

- Instruct the patient to take in a breath, blow it out, and hold it out during the exposure.

Image Evaluation

- Soft tissue structures of the neck and C5 through T4 should be included in the collimated area.
- Bony trabeculae should be seen within the vertebral bodies and spinous processes.
- The first C7–T1 interspace should be in the middle of the film.
- The intervertebral disk spaces of C5 through T4 should be clearly demonstrated.
- The vertebral bodies should appear boxlike; no rotation should be evident.
- The humeral heads should be separated *(Figure 10–48)*.

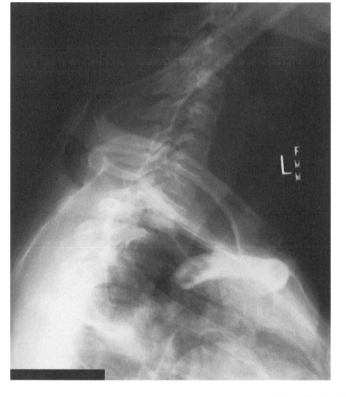 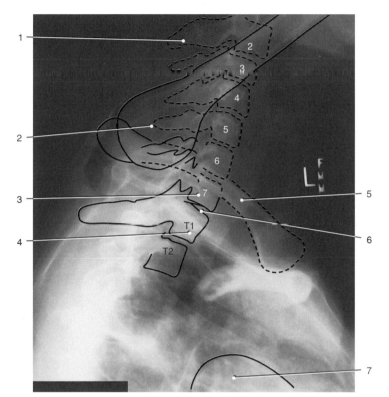

Figure 10–48. Lateral cervicothoracic spine.

1. Spinous process, C2
2. Humeral head, left
3. Vertebral body, C7

4. Vertebral body, T1
5. Clavicle

6. Intervertebral disk space,
   C7–T1
7. Humeral head, right

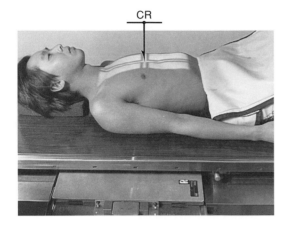

Figure 10–49. AP thoracic spine.

► AP THORACIC SPINE

Technical Considerations

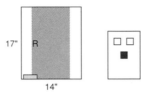

- Film size: 14 × 17 in. or 7 × 17 in. lengthwise.
- Grid required.
- 70–80 kVp.
- Collimate to the spine crosswise and to film size lengthwise.

Shielding

- Gonadal shielding should be used on all patients, especially children and adults of reproductive age.

Patient Positioning

- Assist the patient to the supine position on the radiographic table. The patient may flex the knees and hips; the legs can rest on a suitable support, or the plantar surface of the feet can be placed flat against the table for comfort. If a pillow is used, it should be thin to avoid enhancing dorsal kyphosis. (**Note:** To use the "anode–heel" effect, the patient should be positioned on the table with the head near the anode end of the table.)

Part Positioning

- Center the midsagittal plane of the patient to the midline of the table; check for rotation of the head and shoulders.
- Adjust the long axis of the patient to lie parallel with the long axis of the table; pull gently on the patient's legs or under the patient's arms to straighten the patient.
- Position the patient's arms comfortably on the radiographic table (*Figure 10–49*).

Central Ray

- Direct the central ray perpendicular to the film through T7; the central ray should enter approximately 3 in. inferior to the jugular notch.
- Center the cassette to the central ray; the top edge of the cassette should be at least 1.5 to 2 in. above the top of the shoulders.

Breathing Instructions

- Instruct the patient either to take slow, shallow breaths or to take a breath in, blow it out, and hold it out during the exposure.

Image Evaluation

- The vertebral bodies of C7 through L1 should be included in the collimated area.
- Bony trabeculae should be seen within the vertebral bodies.
- The seventh thoracic body should be in the middle of the film.
- The sternoclavicular joints should be symmetrical.
- Spinous processes should be seen at the midline of the vertebrae.
- The intervertebral disk spaces should be clearly demonstrated *(Figure 10–50)*.

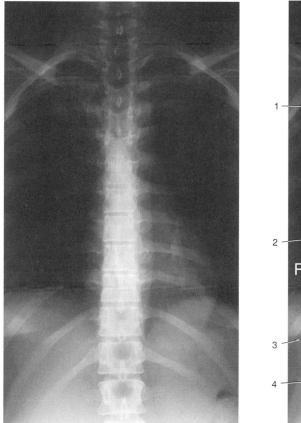 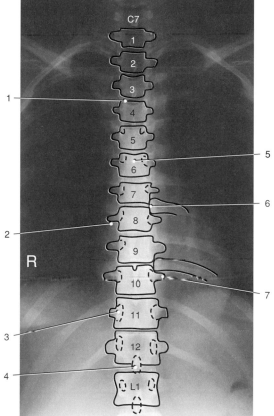

Figure 10–50. AP thoracic spine.

1. Vertebral body
2. Transverse process
3. Pedicle

4. Spinous process
5. Intervertebral disk space

6. Costovertebral joint
7. Costotransverse joint

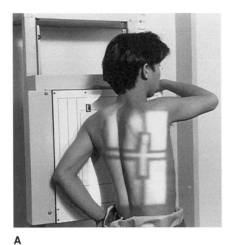

A

B

Figure 10–51. LAO **(A)** and RAO **(B)** thoracic spine.

► PA OBLIQUE THORACIC SPINE

Technical Considerations

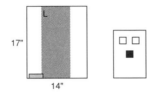

- Film size: 14 × 17 in. or 7 × 17 in. lengthwise.
- Grid required.
- 70–85 kVp.
- Collimate to the spine crosswise and to film size lengthwise.

Shielding

- Gonadal shielding should be used on all patients, especially children and adults of reproductive age.

Patient Positioning

- Assist the patient to the left lateral position in front of an upright grid device for the LAO projection. **Note:** The RAO projection must also be obtained; both sides are examined for comparison. The posterior or AP oblique, RPO and LPO, positions can also be used; the oblique projections can be obtained with the patient recumbent.

Part Positioning

- Rotate the patient 20° toward the film to form a 70° angle between the coronal plane and film. The right arm should be elevated with the hand supported on the top of the grid device; the left arm should be positioned with the elbow flexed and the back of the hand resting on the hip.
- Center the thoracic spine to the midline of the upright grid device; the shoulder nearest the film should be positioned firmly against the upright grid device.
- Adjust the rotation of the head so the midsagittal plane is perpendicular to the coronal plane of the body.
- The opposite oblique should be obtained in a similar manner for comparison *(Figure 10–51)*.

Central Ray

- Direct the central ray perpendicular to the film through T7; the central ray should enter approximately 3 to 4 in. inferior to the level of the jugular notch.
- Center the cassette to the central ray; the top edge of the cassette should be at least 1.5 to 2 in. above the top of the shoulders.

Breathing Instructions

- Instruct the patient to take a breath in, blow it out, and hold it out or to take slow, shallow breaths during the exposure.

Image Evaluation

- The vertebral bodies of C7 through L1 should be well visualized within the collimated area.
- Bony trabeculae should be seen within the vertebral bodies.
- The 7th thoracic body should be in the middle of the film.
- The 1st through 12th vertebral bodies should be adequately penetrated.
- The zygapophyseal joints nearest the film should be clearly demonstrated (Figure 10–52).

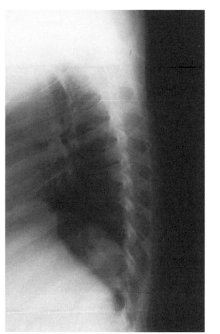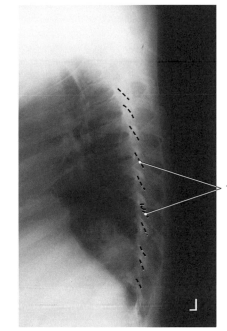

Figure 10–52. LAO thoracic spine.

1. Zygapophyseal joints, left

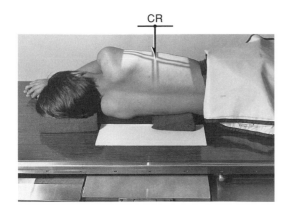

Figure 10–53. Lateral thoracic spine.

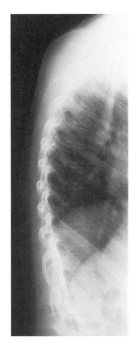

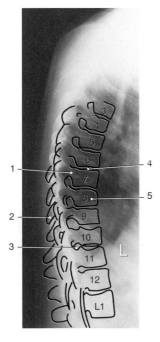

Figure 10–54. Lateral thoracic spine.

► LATERAL THORACIC SPINE

Technical Considerations

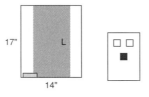

- Film size: 14 × 17 in. or 7 × 17 in. lengthwise.
- Grid required.
- 70–85 kVp.
- Collimate to the spine crosswise and to film size lengthwise.

Shielding

- Gonadal shielding should be used on all patients, especially children and adults of reproductive age.

Patient Positioning

- Assist the patient to the left lateral position on the radiographic table; the patient may flex the knees and hips for comfort and balance. **Note:** This projection can also be obtained with the patient erect.
- Position a firm pillow under the head and radiolucent supports under the waist and lower thoracic area so the spine is parallel with the tabletop.

Part Positioning

- Center the midaxillary plane to the midline of the table; position the arms at a right angle with the body.
- Adjust the long axis of the spine to lie parallel with the long axis of the table; the right leg should be directly over the left leg.
- Adjust the body so a line through the shoulders and another through the hips are perpendicular to the film plane.
- Place a sheet of leaded rubber on the table behind the patient to reduce the amount of scatter reaching the film and improve radiographic quality *(Figure 10–53)*.

Central Ray

- Direct the central ray perpendicular to the film through T7; the central ray should enter approximately 3 to 4 in. inferior to the level of the jugular notch. **Note:** If radiolucent supports are not used under the lower thorax and waist, the central ray may require a cephalic angle to make it parallel to the intervertebral joints.
- Center the cassette to the central ray; the top edge of the cassette should be at least 1.5 to 2 in. above the top of the shoulders.

Breathing Instructions

- Instruct the patient either to take slow, shallow breaths during the exposure, or to take a breath in, blow it out, and hold it out; quiet breathing is generally preferred to blur the rib and lung detail.

Image Evaluation

- The vertebral bodies of T3 through L1 should be well visualized within the collimated area.
- Bony trabeculae should be seen within the vertebral bodies.
- The 7th thoracic body should be in the middle of the film.
- The 3rd through 12th vertebral bodies should be adequately penetrated.
- The vertebral bodies should appear boxlike; posterior ribs should be superimposed.
- The intervertebral disk spaces and pedicles should be clearly demonstrated *(Figure 10–54)*.

1. Pedicles, superimposed
2. Spinous process
3. Intervertebral foramina, superimposed
4. Intervertebral disk space
5. Vertebral body

► AP LUMBAR SPINE

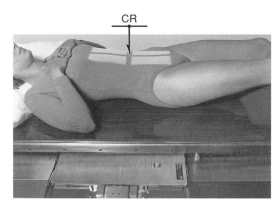

Figure 10–55. AP lumbar spine.

Technical Considerations

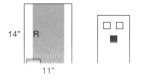

- Film size: 14 × 17 in. or 11 × 14 in. lengthwise.
- Grid required.
- 70–80 kVp.
- Collimate to include the kidneys crosswise and to film size lengthwise.

Shielding

- Gonadal shielding should be used on male patients, especially children and adults of reproductive age.

Patient Positioning

- Assist the patient to the supine position on the radiographic table; the patient may flex the knees and hips. The legs can rest on a suitable support, or the plantar surface of the feet can be placed flat against the table for comfort.

Part Positioning

- Center the midsagittal plane of the patient to the midline of the table; check for rotation of the head and shoulders.
- Adjust the long axis of the patient to lie parallel with the long axis of the table; pull gently on the patient's legs or under the patient's arms to straighten the patient.
- Position the patient's hands comfortably on the upper chest or radiographic table *(Figure 10–55)*.

Central Ray

- Direct the central ray perpendicular to the film through the L4–5 interspace (14 × 17-in. cassette) or L3 (11 × 14-in. cassette). L4–5 is at the level of the iliac crests; L3 is approximately 1 to 1.5 in. above the crests.
- Center the cassette to the central ray.

Breathing Instructions

- Instruct the patient to take a breath in, blow it out, and hold it out during the exposure.

Image Evaluation

- The vertebral bodies of T12 through S2 should be included in the collimated area.
- Bony trabeculae should be seen within the vertebral bodies.
- The fourth (14 × 17-in. cassette) or third (11 × 14-in. cassette) lumbar vertebral body should be centered to the film.
- The iliac crests should be symmetrical.
- Spinous processes should be seen at the midline of the vertebrae and in the middle of the film.
- The intervertebral disk spaces should be clearly demonstrated *(Figure 10–56)*.

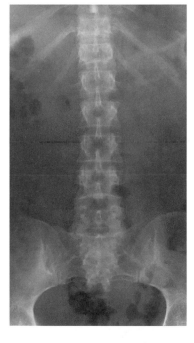

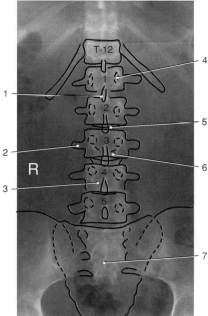

1. Spinous process
2. Transverse process
3. Vertebral body
4. Pedicle
5. Intervertebral disk space
6. Lamina
7. Sacrum

Figure 10–56. AP lumbar spine.

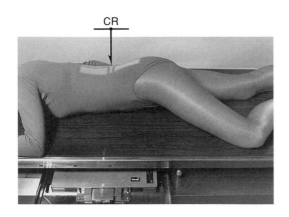

Figure 10–57. RAO lumbar spine to demonstrate the left zygapophyseal joints.

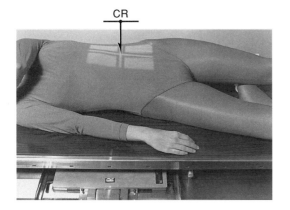

Figure 10–58. RPO lumbar spine.

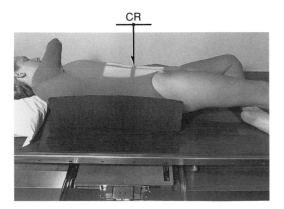

Figure 10–59. LPO lumbar spine.

▶ AP OBLIQUE LUMBAR SPINE

Technical Considerations

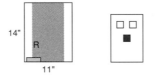

- Film size: 11 × 14 in. lengthwise.
- Grid required.
- 70–80 kVp.
- Collimate to the spine crosswise and to film size lengthwise.

Shielding

- Gonadal shielding should be used on male patients, especially children and adults of reproductive age.

Patient Positioning

- Assist the patient to the supine position on the radiographic table; the patient's spine should remain parallel with the long axis of the table.

Part Positioning

- Keeping the patient supine, off-center the patient approximately 3 to 4 in. toward the left side of the table (for the RPO position); both obliques are obtained for comparison. **Note:** The zygapophyseal joints can also be demonstrated with the patient in the anterior or PA oblique (RAO and LAO) position. When doing so, the joints farthest from the film will be demonstrated *(Figure 10–57)*.
- Rotate the patient 45° toward the right side (left side up); the arm of the elevated side should be brought across the patient's chest to prevent twisting or unequal rotation of the spine.
- Position a lumbar sponge behind the patient to support the shoulder and hip; the hip and shoulder should be in the same plane.
- Flex the knee of the dependent side for support and extend the leg of the elevated side and position so the foot points upward.
- Center the plane passing 2 in. medial to the elevated ASIS to the midline of the table; check for uniform rotation of the hips and shoulders from the head or foot of the table.
- Adjust the long axis of the patient to lie parallel with the long axis of the table.
- The opposite oblique should be obtained in a similar manner for comparison *(Figures 10–58, 10–59)*.

Central Ray

- Direct the central ray perpendicular to the film through L3, located approximately 1 to 1.5 in. above the iliac crests.
- Center the cassette to the central ray.

Breathing Instructions

- Instruct the patient to take a breath in, blow it out, and hold it out during the exposure.

Image Evaluation

- The vertebral bodies of T12 through S2 should be included in the collimated area.
- Bony trabeculae should be seen within the vertebral bodies.
- The third lumbar vertebral body should be in the middle of the film.
- When the RPO and LPO projections are compared, the ilia should be symmetrical.
- The right (RPO) or left (LPO) zygapophyseal joints should be clearly demonstrated.

- When the patient is crrectly rotated, the pedicles will be demonstrated in the middle of the vertebral body; anterior or posterior placement indicates less than or greater than 45° rotation, respectively.
- The zygapophyseal joints should be adequately exposed and clearly demonstrated.
- The superior and inferior articular processes, transverse process, pedicle, lamina, and pars interarticularis will be demonstrated as parts of a "Scotty dog" when the patient is correctly positioned *(Figures 10–60, 10–61)*.

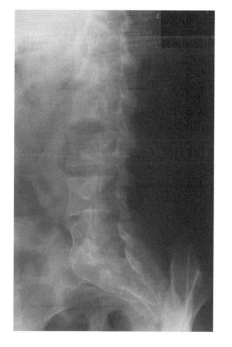
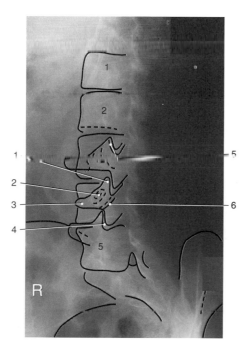

Figure 10–60. RPO lumbar spine.

1. Superior articular process, right	3. Transverse process, right	5. Zygapophyseal joint, right
2. Pedicle, right	4. Inferior articular process, right	6. Pars interarticularis, right

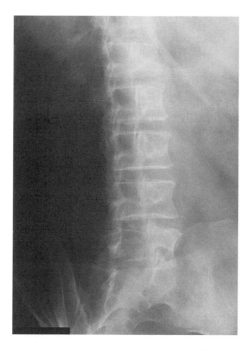
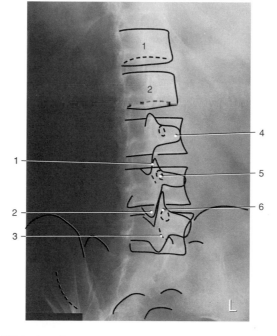

Figure 10–61. LPO lumbar spine.

1. Zygapophyseal joint, left	3. Pars interarticularis, left	5. Pedicle, left
2. Inferior articular process, left	4. Transverse process, left	6. Superior articular process, left

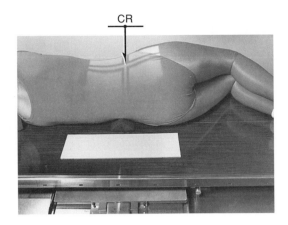

Figure 10–62. Lateral lumbar spine.

► LATERAL LUMBAR SPINE

Technical Considerations

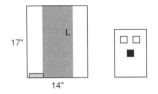

- Film size: 14 × 17 in. or 11 × 14 in. lengthwise.
- Grid required.
- 80–90 kVp.
- Collimate to the spine crosswise and to film size lengthwise.

Shielding

- Gonadal shielding should be used on male patients, especially children and adults of reproductive age.

Patient Positioning

- Assist the patient to the left lateral position on the radiographic table; the patient may flex the knees and hips for comfort and balance. **Note:** This projection can also be obtained with the patient erect.

Part Positioning

- Center the midaxillary plane to the midline of the table; position the arms at a right angle with the body.
- Adjust the long axis of the spine to lie parallel with the long axis of the table. The right leg should be directly over the left leg; a small sandbag between the knees will help prevent rotation.
- Position a firm pillow under the head and radiolucent supports under the waist and lower thoracic area so the spine is parallel with the tabletop.
- Adjust the body so a line through the shoulders and another through the hips are perpendicular to the film plane; looking down from above the patient or head of the table will help detect any patient rotation.
- Place a sheet of leaded rubber on the table behind the patient to reduce the amount of scatter reaching the film and improve radiographic quality *(Figure 10–62)*.

Positioning Tip. Men with broad shoulders and narrow hips may need an additional support under the hips; women with wide hips and narrow shoulders will need support under the shoulders. Look at and feel the spinous processes to determine the need for supports.

Central Ray

- Direct the central ray perpendicular to the film through the L4–5 interspace (14 × 17-in. cassette) or L3 (11 × 14-in. cassette). L4 is at the level of the iliac crests; L3 is approximately 1 to 1.5 in. above the crests. **Note:** If radiolucent supports are not used to place the spine parallel with the film plane, a 5° to 8° caudal central ray angle may be required to demonstrate the intervertebral disk spaces.
- Center the cassette to the central ray.

Breathing Instructions

- Instruct the patient to take a breath in, blow it out, and hold it out during the exposure.

Image Evaluation

- The vertebral bodies of T12 through S2 should be well visualized within the collimated area.
- Bony trabeculae should be seen within the vertebral bodies.
- The fourth (14 × 17-in. cassette) or third (11 × 14-in. cassette) lumbar vertebral body should be in the middle of the film.
- The first through fifth lumbar bodies should be adequately penetrated.
- The vertebral bodies should appear boxlike; posterior ribs of T12 should be superimposed.
- The spine should be parallel to the transverse axis of the film.
- The intervertebral disk spaces and pedicles should be clearly demonstrated *(Figure 10–63)*.

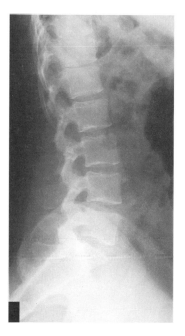 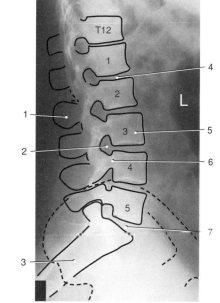

Figure 10–63. Lateral lumbar spine.

1. Spinous process	3. Sacrum	6. Pedicles, superimposed
2. Intervertebral foramina, super-imposed	4. Intervertebral disk space	7. Lumbosacral junction
	5. Vertebral body	

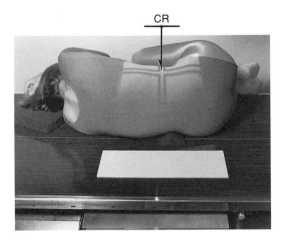

Figure 10–64. Hyperflexion lateral lumbar spine.

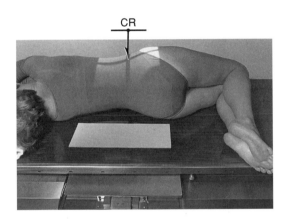

Figure 10–65. Hyperextension lateral lumbar spine.

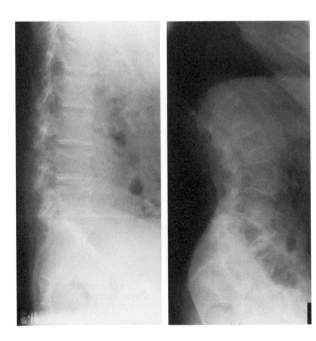

Figure 10–66. and Figure 10–67. Hyperflexion lateral lumbar spine **(left)** Hyperextension lumbar spine **(right);** note the calcified aorta on the hyperextension projection.

► HYPERFLEXION/HYPEREXTENSION LATERAL LUMBAR SPINE

Technical Considerations

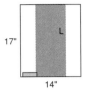

- Film size: 14 × 17 in. lengthwise.
- Grid required.
- 80–90 kVp.
- Collimate to the spine crosswise and to film size lengthwise.

Shielding

- Gonadal shielding should be used on male patients, especially children and adults of reproductive age.

Patient Positioning

- Assist the patient to the left lateral position on the radiographic table; the patient may flex the knees and hips for comfort and balance. **Note:** This projection can also be obtained with the patient erect.

Part Positioning

- Instruct the patient either to bend forward at the waist, bringing the knees upward and the shoulders downward (hyperflexion), or to bend backward, arching the back and bringing the shoulders and legs backward (hyperextension).
- Center the midaxillary plane to the midline of the table.
- Adjust the long axis of the spine to lie near parallel with the long axis of the table; the right leg should be directly over the left leg.
- Position a firm pillow under the head and radiolucent supports under the waist and lower thoracic area so the spine is parallel with the tabletop.
- Adjust the body so a line through the shoulders and another through the hips are perpendicular to the film plane; looking down from above the patient or head of the table will help detect any patient rotation.
- Place a sheet of leaded rubber on the table behind the patient to reduce the amount of scatter reaching the film and improve radiographic quality *(Figures 10–64, 10–65).*

Central Ray

- Direct the central ray perpendicular to the area of the spinal fusion, if known, or L3, approximately 1 to 1.5 in. above the iliac crests.
- Center the cassette to the central ray.

Breathing Instructions

- Instruct the patient to take a breath in, blow it out, and hold it out during the exposure.

Image Evaluation

- The vertebral bodies of T12 through S1 should be well visualized within the collimated area.
- Bony trabeculae should be seen within the vertebral bodies.
- The third lumbar vertebral body should be in the middle of the film.
- The first through fifth lumbar bodies should be adequately penetrated.
- The vertebral bodies should appear boxlike; posterior ribs of T12 should be superimposed.
- The intervertebral disk spaces and pedicles should be clearly demonstrated.
- The spinous processes will be separated on the hyperflexion projection and closer together on the hyperextension view, whereas the anterior aspect of the disk spaces will be narrower on the hyperflexion but wider on the hyperextension projection *(Figures 10–66, 10–67).*

► AP AXIAL LUMBOSACRAL JUNCTION

Technical Considerations

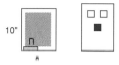

- Film size: 8 × 10 in. or 10 × 12 in. lengthwise or 9 × 9 in.
- Grid required.
- 70–80 kVp.
- Collimate to a 5 × 5-in. field size.

Shielding

- Gonadal shielding should be used on male patients, especially children and adults of reproductive age, as long as it does not compromise the examination.

Patient Positioning

- Assist the patient to the supine position on the radiographic table; the patient's legs should be extended.
  Note: This projection can also be obtained with the patient prone, directing the central ray caudad.

Part Positioning

- Center the midsagittal plane of the patient to the midline of the table; check for rotation of the head and shoulders.
- Adjust the long axis of the patient to lie parallel with the long axis of the table; pull gently on the patient's legs or under the patient's arms to straighten the patient.
- Position the patient's arms comfortably on the radiographic table *(Figure 10–68).*

Central Ray

- Direct the central ray 30° or 35° cephalad (males or females, respectively) to the level of the ASISs.
- Center the cassette to the central ray.

Breathing Instructions

- Instruct the patient to take a breath in, blow it out, and hold it out during the exposure.

Image Evaluation

- The vertebral bodies of L5 through S1 should be included in the collimated area.
- Bony trabeculae should be seen within the vertebral bodies.
- The iliac crests should be symmetrical.
- Spinous processes should be seen at the midline of the vertebrae and in the middle of the film.
- The L5–S1 intervertebral disk space should be clearly demonstrated in the middle of the film *(Figure 10–69).*
  Note: This projection also demonstrates the sacroiliac joints, as described in Chapter 9.

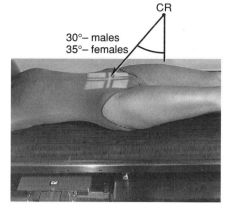

Figure 10–68. AP axial lumbosacral junction.

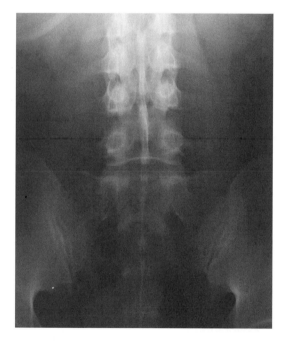

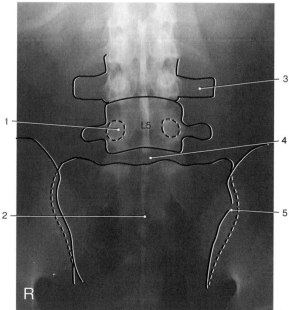

Figure 10–69. AP axial lumbosacral junction.

1. Pedicle
2. Sacrum
3. Transverse process
4. Lumbosacral junction (L5–S1 intervertebral disk space)
5. Sacroiliac joint, left

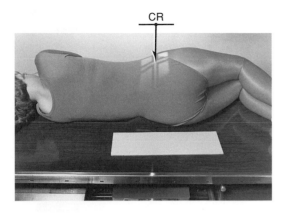

Figure 10–70. Lateral lumbosacral junction.

► LATERAL LUMBOSACRAL JUNCTION

Technical Considerations

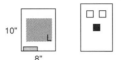

- Film size: 8 × 10 in. lengthwise or 9 × 9 in.
- Grid required.
- 85–100 kVp.
- Collimate to a 5 × 5 in. field size.

Shielding

- Gonadal shielding should be used on all patients, especially children and adults of reproductive age as long as it does not compromise the examination.

Patient Positioning

- Assist the patient to the left lateral position on the radiographic table; the patient may flex the knees and hips for comfort and balance. **Note:** This projection can also be obtained with the patient erect.

Part Positioning

- Center the coronal plane passing 1.5 in. posterior to the midaxillary plane to the midline of the table; position the arms at a right angle with the body.
- Adjust the long axis of the spine to lie parallel with the long axis of the table. The right leg should be directly over the left leg; a small sandbag between the knees will help prevent rotation.
- Position a firm pillow under the head and radiolucent supports under the waist and lower thoracic area so the spine is parallel with the tabletop.
- Adjust the body so a line through the shoulders and another through the hips are perpendicular to the film plane; looking down from above the patient will help detect any patient rotation.
- Place a sheet of leaded rubber on the table behind the patient to reduce the amount of scatter reaching the film and improve radiographic quality *(Figure 10–70)*.

Positioning Tip. When the patient is correctly positioned, the central ray should pass through the two soft tissue depressions (dimples) seen on the backs of most people.

Central Ray

- Draw an imaginary line between the right and left iliac crests. Direct the central ray parallel to that line through the L5–S1 junction; the central ray should enter midway between the level of the iliac crests and ASISs. **Note:** If radiolucent supports are not used to place the spine parallel with the film plane, the central ray is usually directed caudad; palpate the iliac crests to determine the degree of angulation as previously described.
- Center the cassette to the central ray.

Breathing Instructions

- Instruct the patient to take a breath in, blow it out, and hold it out during the exposure.

Image Evaluation

- The vertebral bodies of L5 through S1 should be well visualized within the collimated area.
- Bony trabeculae should be seen within the vertebral bodies.
- The L5–S1 intervertebral disk space should be clearly demonstrated in the middle of the film.
- The first sacral and fifth lumbar bodies should be adequately penetrated.
- The vertebral body of L5 should appear boxlike.
- The spine should be parallel with the longitudinal axis of the film.
- The ASISs should be in the same longitudinal plane (Figure 10–71).

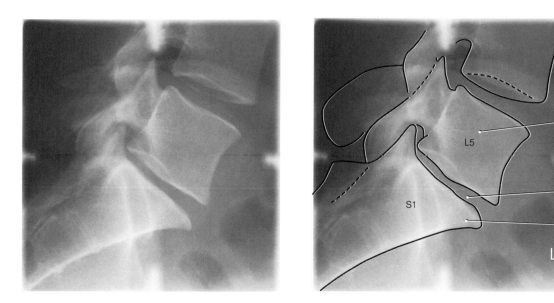

Figure 10–71. Lateral lumbosacral junction.

1. Vertebral body, L5

2. Lumbosacral junction (L5–S1 intervertebral disk space)

3. Sacral promontory

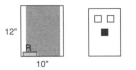

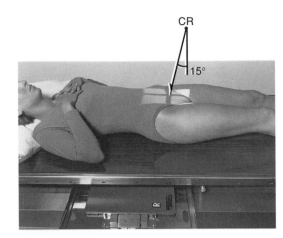

Figure 10–72. AP sacrum.

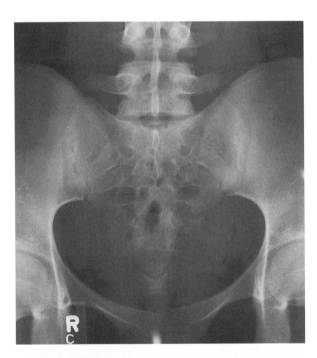

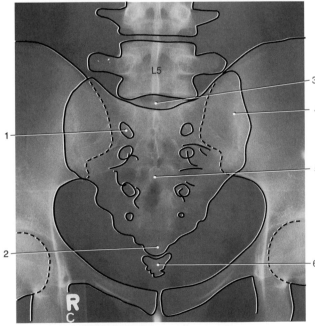

Figure 10–73. AP sacrum.

► AP SACRUM

Technical Considerations

- Film size: 10 × 12 in. lengthwise.
- Grid required.
- 65–75 kVp.
- Collimate to include ASISs crosswise and to film size lengthwise.

Shielding

- Gonadal shielding should be used on male patients, especially children and adults of reproductive age, as long as it does not compromise the examination.

Patient Positioning

- Assist the patient to the supine position on the radiographic table. **Note:** In addition to the aforementioned patient preparation, the patient should empty the bladder prior to radiographic examination to improve image quality. The physician may also need to order a cleansing enema to remove fecal material from the sigmoid colon and rectum; fecal material often makes evaluation of the sacrum difficult.

Part Positioning

- Center the midsagittal plane of the patient to the midline of the table.
- Adjust the long axis of the patient to lie parallel with the long axis of the table; pull gently on the patient's legs or under the patient's arms to straighten the patient.
- Adjust the pelvis to true anatomical position.
- Check for rotation of the pelvis by measuring the distance from the ASISs to the table; to maintain equal distances, small sponges may be needed to support one or both sides of the pelvis.
- Position the patient's hands comfortably on the upper chest or radiographic table (*Figure 10–72*).

Central Ray

- Direct the central ray 15° cephalad to a point approximately 2 in. superior to the symphysis pubis.
- Center the cassette to the central ray.

Breathing Instructions

- Instruct the patient to take a breath in, blow it out, and hold it out during the exposure.

Image Evaluation

- The L5–S1 intervertebral disk space and superior rami of the pubic bones should be included in the collimated area.
- Bony trabeculae should be seen within the sacrum.
- The sacrum should be demonstrated in the middle of the film.
- The alae of the sacrum should be symmetrical.
- The sacrum should be demonstrated without unnecessary distortion superior to the pubic bone (*Figure 10–73*).

1. Sacral foramina
2. Apex
3. Lumbosacral junction
4. Ala
5. Sacral body
6. Coccyx

▶ LATERAL SACRUM

Technical Considerations

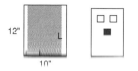

- Film size: 10 × 12 in. lengthwise.
- Grid required.
- 70–85 kVp.
- Collimate to an 8 × 10-in. field size.

Shielding

- Gonadal shielding should be used on all patients, especially children and adults of reproductive age, as long as it does not compromise the examination.

Patient Positioning

- Assist the patient to the left lateral position on the radiographic table; the patient may flex the knees and hips for comfort and balance.

Part Positioning

- Center the coronal plane passing 3 in. posterior to the midaxillary plane to the midline of the table; position the arms at a right angle with the body.
- Adjust the long axis of the spine to lie parallel with the long axis of the table. The right leg should be directly over the left leg; a small sandbag between the knees will help prevent rotation.
- Position a firm pillow under the head and radiolucent supports under the waist and lower thoracic area so the spine is parallel with the tabletop.
- Adjust the body so a line through the shoulders and another through the hips are perpendicular to the film plane; looking down from above the patient will help detect any patient rotation.
- Place a sheet of leaded rubber on the table behind the patient to reduce the amount of scatter reaching the film and improve radiographic quality (Figure 10–74).

Central Ray

- Direct the central ray perpendicular to the level of the ASISs.
- Center the cassette to the central ray.

Breathing Instructions

- Instruct the patient to take a breath in, blow it out, and hold it out during the exposure.

Image Evaluation

- The L5–S1 intervertebral disk space, S1, and the entire sacrum, including the promontory, should be well visualized within the collimated area.
- Bony trabeculae should be seen within the sacrum.
- The sacrum should be clearly demonstrated in the middle of the film.
- The entire sacrum should be adequately penetrated without overpenetration of the distal segments.
- The femoral heads should be nearly superimposed.
- The sacrum should be parallel with the longitudinal axis of the film (Figure 10–75).

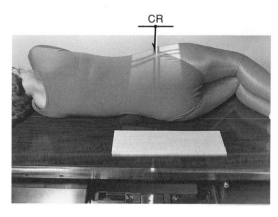

Figure 10–74. Lateral sacrum.

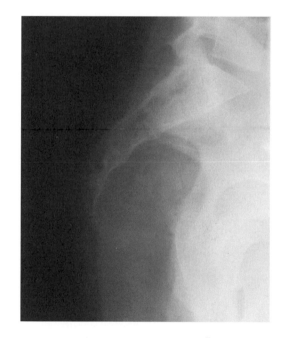

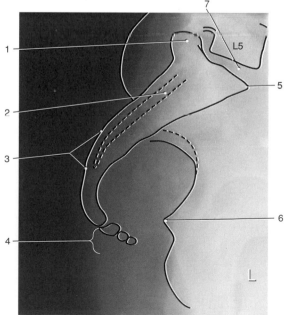

Figure 10–75. Lateral sacrum.

1. Superior articular processes, superimposed
2. Sacral canal
3. Median sacral crest
4. Coccyx
5. Promontory
6. Ischial spines, superimposed
7. Lumbosacral junction

311

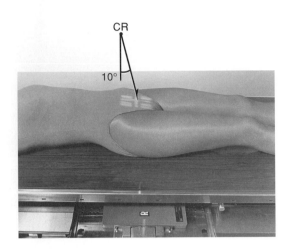

Figure 10–76. AP coccyx.

► AP COCCYX

Technical Considerations

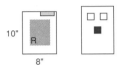

- Film size: 8 × 10 in. lengthwise or 9 × 9 in.
- Grid required.
- 60–70 kVp.
- Collimate to a 4 × 5-in. field size.

Shielding

- Gonadal shielding should be used on male patients, especially children and adults of reproductive age, as long as it does not compromise the examination.

Patient Positioning

- Assist the patient to the supine position on the radiographic table. **Note:** In addition to the aforementioned patient preparation, the patient should empty the bladder prior to radiographic examination to improve image quality. The physician may also have to order a cleansing enema to remove fecal material from the sigmoid colon and rectum; fecal material often makes evaluation of the coccyx nearly impossible.

Part Positioning

- Center the midsagittal plane of the patient to the midline of the table; check for rotation of the head and shoulders.
- Adjust the long axis of the patient to lie parallel with the long axis of the table; pull gently on the patient's legs or under the patient's arms to straighten the patient.
- Adjust the pelvis to true anatomic position.
- Check for rotation of the pelvis by measuring the distance from the ASISs to the table; to maintain equal distances, a small sponge may be needed to support one or both sides of the pelvis.
- Position the patient's hands comfortably on the upper chest or radiographic table *(Figure 10–76)*.

Central Ray

- Direct the central ray 10° caudad to a point approximately 2 in. superior to the symphysis pubis.
- Center the cassette to the central ray.

Breathing Instructions

- Instruct the patient to take a breath in, blow it out, and hold it out during the exposure.

Image Evaluation

- The coccyx and distal one third of the sacrum should be included in the collimated area.
- The coccyx should be clearly demonstrated in the middle of the film.
- The coccyx should be adequately penetrated using an appropriately low kVp to produce a high-contrast image (see Note above).
- The coccyx should be directly above the symphysis pubis *(Figure 10–77)*.

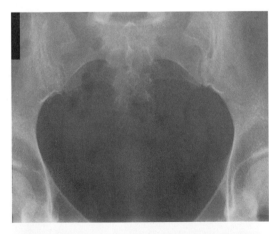

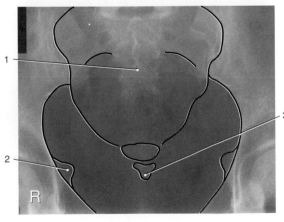

Figure 10–77. AP coccyx.

1. Sacrum   2. Ischial spine   3. Coccyx

► LATERAL COCCYX

Technical Considerations

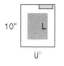

- Film size: 8 × 10 in. lengthwise or 9 × 9 in.
- Grid required.
- 65–75 kVp.
- Collimate to the 4 × 4-in. field size.

Shielding

- Gonadal shielding should be used on male patients, especially children and adults of reproductive age, as long as it does not compromise the examination.

Patient Positioning

- Assist the patient to the left lateral position on the radiographic table; the patient may flex the knees and hips for comfort and balance.

Part Positioning

- Center the coronal plane passing 5 in. posterior to the midaxillary plane to the midline of the table; position the arms at a right angle with the body.
- Adjust the long axis of the spine to lie parallel with the long axis of the table. The right leg should be directly over the left leg; a small sandbag between the knees will help prevent rotation.
- Position a firm pillow under the head and radiolucent supports under the waist and lower thoracic area so the spine is parallel with the tabletop.
- Adjust the body so a line through the shoulders and another through the hips are perpendicular to the film plane; looking down from above the patient or head of the table will help detect any patient rotation.
- Place a sheet of leaded rubber on the table behind the patient to reduce the amount of scatter reaching the film and improve radiographic quality *(Figure 10–78)*.

Central Ray

- Direct the central ray perpendicular to the coccyx; the coccyx can be palpated at the base of the spine.
- Center the cassette to the central ray.

Breathing Instructions

- Instruct the patient to take a breath in, blow it out, and hold it out.

Image Evaluation

- The coccyx and distal third of the sacrum should be well visualized within the collimated area.
- The coccyx should be clearly demonstrated in the middle of the film.
- The coccyx should be adequately penetrated using a low enough kVp to produce a high-contrast image.
- The posterior ilia and ischia should be nearly superimposed.
- The sacrum should be parallel with the longitudinal axis of the film *(Figure 10–79)*.

1. Sacrum   2. Cornua, coccyx   3. Coccyx

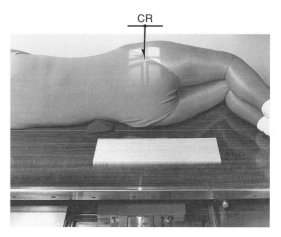

Figure 10–78. Lateral coccyx.

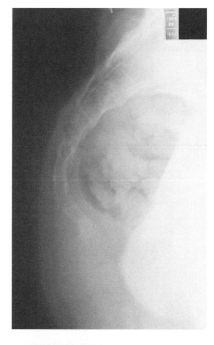

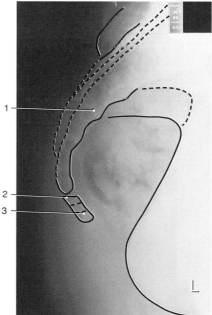

Figure 10–79. Lateral coccyx.

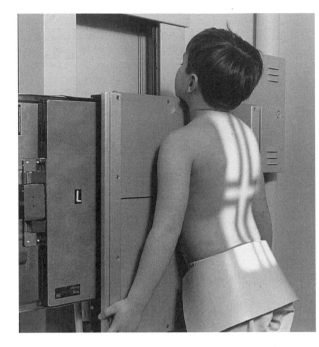

Figure 10–80. PA scoliosis.

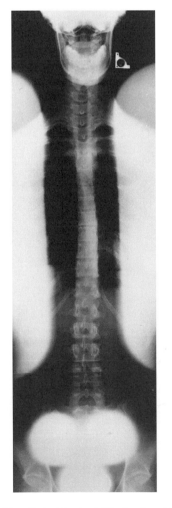

Figure 10–81. PA scoliosis. (*Courtesy of Nuclear Associates, Carle, NY.*)

► PA SCOLIOSIS

Technical Considerations

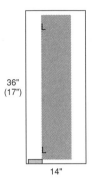

- Film size: 14 × 36 in. or two 14 × 17 in. lengthwise.
- Grid required.
- 75–90 kVp.
- Collimate to the spine crosswise and from the hips to the level of ASIS lengthwise.

Shielding

- Gonadal shielding should be used on all patients; breast shields should also be used for female patients.

Patient Positioning

- Assist the patient to the erect position facing an upright grid device; weight should be equally distributed on both feet. **Note:** An AP projection may also be performed; however, the dose to the radiosensitive breasts is significantly greater.

Part Positioning

- Adjust the patient's body so there is no rotation; the patient's head should be directed forward and the arms can hang comfortably at the sides. **Note:** Compression bands or other supports should not be used for immobilization.
- Center the midsagittal plane to the midline of the grid *(Figure 10–80)*.

Central Ray

14 × 36-in. Cassette
- Direct the central ray perpendicular to the level of T10, using a 72-in. SID; center the cassette to the central ray and position lead shielding and compensating filter appropriately. **Note:** If two different intensifying screen speeds are used, the faster-speed screen should be at the level of the abdomen.

14 × 17-in. Cassette
- Center the cassette so the bottom edge is at the level of the ASIS; approximately 1 in. of the iliac crests should be included on the radiograph.
- Direct the central ray perpendicular to the middle of the cassette, using a 72-in. SID; position lead shielding and compensating filter appropriately.

Breathing Instructions

- Instruct the patient to stop breathing during the exposure.

Image Evaluation

- The vertebral bodies of C1 through S2 should be included in the collimated area.
- The vertebral column should be centered crosswise with the film.
- Appropriate collimation and shielding should be evident on the radiograph *(Figure 10–81)*.

► LATERAL SCOLIOSIS

Technical Considerations

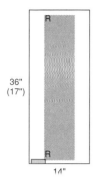

- Film size: 14 × 36 in. or two 14 × 17 in. lengthwise.
- Grid required.
- 85–100 kVp.
- Collimate to the spine crosswise and from the lips to the level of ASIS lengthwise.

Shielding

- Gonadal shielding should be used on all patients; breast shields should also be used for female patients.

Patient Positioning

- Assist the patient to the erect lateral position adjacent to an upright grid device; weight should be equally distributed on both feet.

Part Positioning

- Adjust the patient's body so there is no rotation; the patient's head should be directed forward and the arms should be elevated as for the lateral chest projection.
- Center the midaxillary plane to the midline of the grid *(Figure 10–82)*.

Central Ray

14 × 36-in. Cassette
- Direct the central ray perpendicular to the level of T10, using a 72-in. SID; center the cassette to the central ray and position lead shielding and compensating filter appropriately. **Note:** If two different intensifying screen speeds are used, the faster-speed screen should be at the level of the abdomen.

14 × 17-in. Cassette
- Center the cassette so the bottom edge is at the level of the ASIS.
- Direct the central ray perpendicular to the middle of the cassette, using a 72-in. SID; position lead shielding and compensating filter appropriately.

Breathing Instructions

- Instruct the patient to stop breathing during the exposure.

Image Evaluation

- The vertebral bodies of C1 through S2 should be included in the collimated area.
- The vertebral column should be centered crosswise with the film.
- Appropriate collimation and shielding should be evident on the radiograph *(Figure 10–83)*.

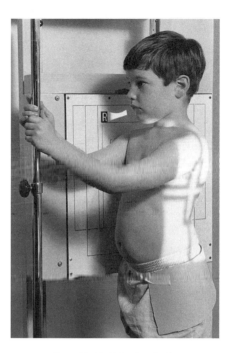

Figure 10–82. Lateral scoliosis.

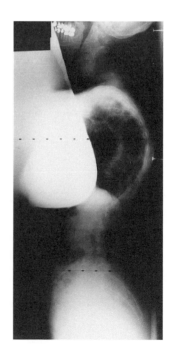

Figure 10–83. Lateral scoliosis. (*Courtesy of Nuclear Associates, Carle, NY.*)

$\mathcal{S}$UMMARY

▶ All radiographic examinations of the vertebral column include AP and lateral projections; oblique projections may be required or optional.

▶ The spine should be parallel with the long axis of the cassette for most projections.

▶ Instability of the injured cervical spine is a significant factor with respect to patient care and patient positioning.

▶ The cross-table lateral cervical spine is the initial projection obtained following trauma.

▶ Hyperflexion/hyperextension studies of the cervical and lumbar spine may be performed to evaluate anteroposterior mobility or potential instability as a result of injury, surgery, or disease.

▶ A scoliosis series is performed to evaluate lateral curvature of the vertebral column; the PA projection is preferred to the AP projection to minimize the dose to the breast.

▶ To minimize magnification, a 72-in. SID should be used for lateral and oblique cervical spine and scoliosis films.

▶ Although breathing instructions vary according to the area of interest, in general, the lateral cervical and all lumbar spine projections are obtained during suspended expiration; the thoracic projections may be obtained during shallow breathing.

▶ The kVp used for the vertebral column ranges from 60 to 100, depending on the area of interest and patient position.

▶ Although all other projections of the vertebral column should be obtained using a grid, the oblique and lateral cervical spine projections may be obtained without a grid.

▶ The anode–heel effect and compensating filters may be used to produce a more uniform density for thoracic spine and scoliosis studies.

$\mathcal{Q}$UESTIONS FOR CRITICAL THINKING & APPLICATION

1. How does poor posture adversely affect the vertebral column? What conditions are most likely to result in an individual who is constantly round-shouldered or one who wears shoes with very high heels?

2. Differentiate between the vertebral and intervertebral foramina with respect to location and function.

3. What region of the vertebral column is affected by a whiplash injury? Specifically, what structures are involved in such an injury? Describe how this can be a potentially fatal injury.

4. Which joints permit you to nod your head "yes" or turn your head from side to side to indicate "no"? Identify the classification and type of movement permitted by each joint. How is it possible to bend forward at the waist if there are no hinge joints in the vertebral column?

5. What effect would the absence of intervertebral disks have on the vertebral column?

6. List the questions that might be asked when obtaining a patient history for someone scheduled for radiographic examination of the vertebral column.

7. A patient admitted through the emergency room is brought to the radiology department for radiographic examination of the cervical spine, humerus, and femur. Identify the first projection you would obtain and describe how you would produce an acceptable radiograph.

8. The patient described in Question 7 is experiencing some paralysis and the radiologist has requested oblique cervical spine projections. Describe how you would obtain these radiographs. Discuss patient care, including patient movement and communication, for someone who has experienced severe spinal injury.

9. With radiography of the thoracic spine, obtaining a uniform density can be a challenge. Describe technical adjustments that you, as the radiographer, can make to produce a more uniform density on both the AP and lateral projections of the thoracic spine.

10. Preoperative scoliosis films have been requested. Identify the projections that might be included in this examination and describe the appropriate patient positioning for these projections.

FILM CRITIQUE

Describe the positioning accuracy of the AP atlas and axis projection shown *(Figure 10–84)*.

Is the part correctly positioned?

What criteria did you use to evaluate positioning accuracy?

How would you correct any positioning errors?

Was the part correctly centered to the film and the central ray correctly centered to the part and film?

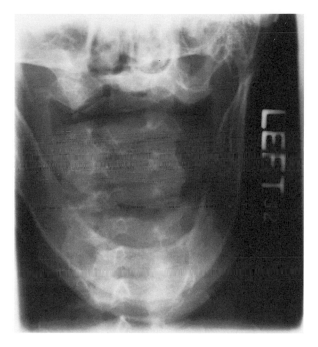

Figure 10–84

Evaluate the positioning accuracy of this lateral thoracic spine radiograph *(Figure 10–85)*.

Was the patient correctly positioned?

Why or why not?

State the criteria you used to make this evaluation.

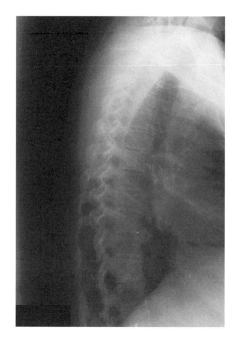

Figure 10–85

SKULL

► OBJECTIVES

Following the completion of this chapter the student will be able to:

- Given diagrams, radiographs, or dry bones, name and describe the bones of the skull.

- Using a lab partner or a drawing of the head, identify the localizing lines and planes used for radiographic positioning of the skull.

- Classify the articulations of the skull according to structure and function.

- Differentiate between the three shape classifications of the skull, and discuss their implications on positioning of the petrous portions.

- State the criteria used to determine positioning accuracy on radiographs of the skull, petrous portions, and mastoids and evaluate radiographs of the skull in terms of positioning, centering, image quality, radiographic anatomy, and pathology.

- Describe positioning modifications that might be necessary depending on a patient's bodily habitus.

- Define terminology associated with the skull, to include anatomy, procedures, and pathology.

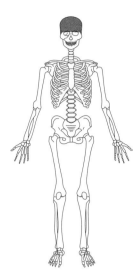

Figure 11–1. The cranium.

► ANATOMY OF THE SKULL

The skull is located superiorly to the vertebral column and, in fact, rests on the first vertebra *(Figure 11–1)*. It is a very complex structure composed of 22 bones plus 6 auditory ossicles. It can be separated into 8 cranial *(Table 11–1)* and 14 facial bones. The 8 cranial bones are discussed in this chapter; the facial bones are covered in depth in Chapter 12 *(Figure 11–2)*.

The bones of the cranium (KRA-ne-um) unite to form the **cranial vault.** This vault can be compared with a bony helmet that encloses and protects the brain, blood vessels, and nerves of the head. It is sometimes referred to as the "brainbox" because the brain actually resides inside the cranium in the cranial cavity or fossa. The outer surface of the cranium serves as the site of muscle attachments that allow for the movement of the head. The cranium can be divided into the calvarium (kal-VA-re-um) and the floor. The **calvarium,** or skull cap, consists of four bones that are classified as flat bones even though their outer surface is curved. These bones are thin, but their curved shape makes them strong. They are constructed of a layer of cancellous bone known as diploe (DIP-lō-e) sandwiched between inner and outer tables of compact bone. The **floor of the cranium** is also formed by four bones; however, these bones are irregular in shape. *Table 11–2* identifies the bones in the calvarium and cranial floor.

Each of the bones of the cranium is unique and has numerous surface markings. For this reason, the bones are discussed individually.

Table 11–1. Summary of the Skull

Bones of the Skull	Description

Frontal (1)	• Forehead, orbital roof, cranial floor
	• Squamous portion
	   Frontal tuberosity, glabella
	   Superciliary arch
	   Frontal sinuses
	   Supraorbital margin and foramen
	• Orbital portion
	   Orbital plates
	   Ethmoidal notch

Parietal (2)	• Lateral walls and roof • Parietal eminence • Superior and inferior temporal lines

Occipital (1)	• Posteroinferior wall and floor
	• Squamous portion
	   Foramen magnum
	   External occipital protuberance
	   Superior and inferior nuchal lines
	• Two lateral portions
	   Occipital condyles
	• Basilar portion
	   Clivus

Ethmoid (1)	• Horizontal portion (cribriform plate)
	   Crista galli
	• Vertical portion (perpendicular plate)
	• Two lateral masses (labyrinths)
	   Superior and middle nasal conchae (turbinates)

Sphenoid (1)	• Body
	   Sella turcica, dorsum sellae, posterior clinoid processes
	• Lesser wings
	   Anterior clinoid processes
	• Greater wings
	   Numerous foramina

Temporal (2)	• Squamous portion
	   Zygomatic process
	   Mandibular fossa
	• Tympanic portion
	   Styloid process
	• Mastoid portion
	   Air cells
	• Petrous portion
	   Organs of hearing and balance

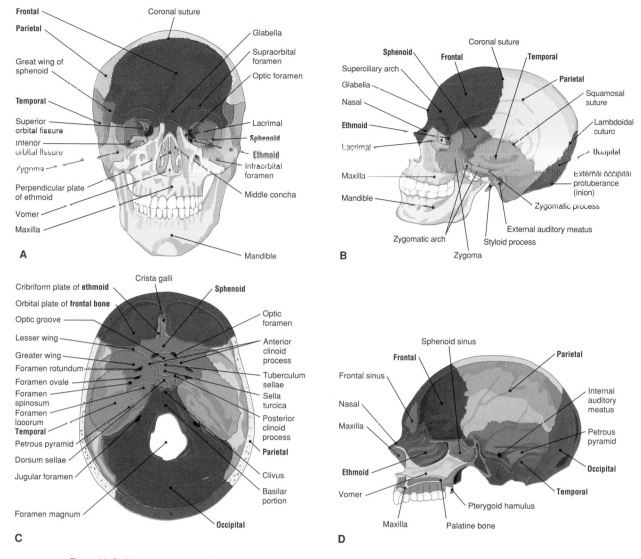

Figure 11–2. Bones of the cranium: **(A)** frontal aspect, **(B)** lateral aspect, **(C)** superior aspect of cranial floor, **(D)** lateral section of cranial vault.

FRONTAL BONE

The frontal bone is located on the anterior aspect of the cranium. It forms the forehead, superior wall (roof) of each orbit, and anterior portion of the cranial floor. The single frontal bone actually develops from two ossification centers. At birth, the bone is divided in two halves. The halves unite shortly after birth and are completely fused by age 6. The frontal bone has two main parts: a squamous (SKWA-mus) portion and an orbital portion.

The **squamous portion** (*squama* = "platelike") of the frontal bone is also known as the **vertical portion.** This part of the bone articulates with both parietal bones at the coronal suture, from which point it extends forward to form the forehead. This area of the frontal bone is fairly thick. A rounded projection

Table 11–2. Bones of the Calvarium and Cranial Floor

Calvarium	Floor
Frontal	Ethmoid
Right parietal	Sphenoid
Left parietal	Right temporal
Occipital	Left temporal

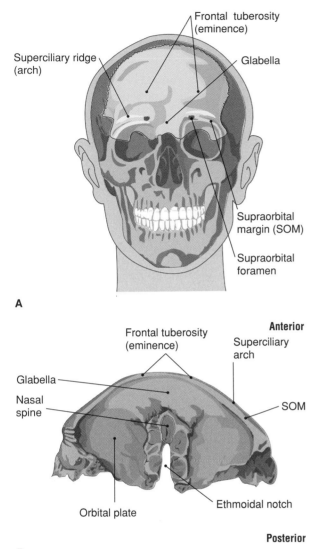

A

B

Figure 11–3. Frontal bone: **(A)** anterior view demonstrating the squamous portion, **(B)** inferior view demonstrating orbital portion.

known as the **frontal tuberosity** or **eminence** can be palpated on either side of the upper forehead. The **superciliary** (soo-per-SIL-e-er-e) **ridge** or **arch** is a curved ridge of bone located beneath each eyebrow. The **glabella** (glah-BEL-ah) is the smooth area between the eyebrows just above the articulation of the frontal bone with the nasal bones. The **frontal sinuses** are paired cavities situated between the inner and outer tables of the frontal bone behind the glabella. The **supraorbital margin** is the thick, upper rim of each orbit. This area is located just below the superciliary arch. There is a hole or notch just medial to the midpoint of each supraorbital margin called the **supraorbital foramen,** through which the supraorbital nerve and artery pass.

The **orbital** or **horizontal portion** of the frontal bone is formed by two flat plates of bone known as the **orbital plates.** Each orbital plate forms the roof of an orbit and the anterior aspect of the floor of the cranial fossa. The **ethmoidal notch** is a somewhat horseshoe-shaped opening located between the two orbital plates. The cribriform plate of the ethmoid bone (bone of cranial floor) fits perfectly in this gap. A spike of bone positioned at the anterior end of the ethmoidal notch on the frontal bone is called the **nasal spine.** This structure forms a very small portion of the upper nasal septum. The posterior aspect of the orbital portion of the frontal bone articulates with the lesser wings of the sphenoid bone *(Figure 11–3).*

PARIETAL BONES

The two parietal (pah-RI-e-tal) bones (*paries* = "wall") form the lateral walls and roof of the skull. Each bone is roughly square in shape, with a convex outer surface and concave inner surface. The **parietal eminence** is a rounded tuberosity located on the lateral surface of the bone. The skull is measured between the two parietal eminences to find its widest dimension. There is a pair of slight ridges called the **superior** and **inferior temporal lines** that run horizontally across the bone. They serve as the attachment points for the muscles that close the mouth. The inner surface of the parietal bone has many depressions, which are the impressions of the veins and arteries supplying the brain. The parietal bones articulate with each other at the sagittal suture on the midline of the skull. Each one also articulates anteriorly with the frontal bone, posteriorly with the occipital, inferiorly with the temporal, and inferiorly and anteriorly with a small part of the greater wing of the sphenoid *(Figure 11–4).*

OCCIPITAL BONE

The single occipital (ok-SIP-i-tal) bone forms the posteroinferior wall and floor of the cranium. In fact, the term *occiput* (OK-si-put) refers to the back of the head. The occipital bone can be divided into four parts: squamous, right and left lateral, and basilar.

The **squamous portion** of the occipital bone is the largest segment. It curves upward from the foramen magnum to form the posterior wall and articulates with both parietal and temporal bones. The **fora-**

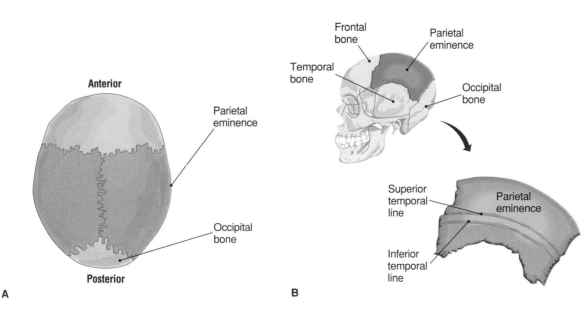

A

B

Figure 11–4. Parietal bones: **(A)** superior aspect, **(B)** lateral aspect.

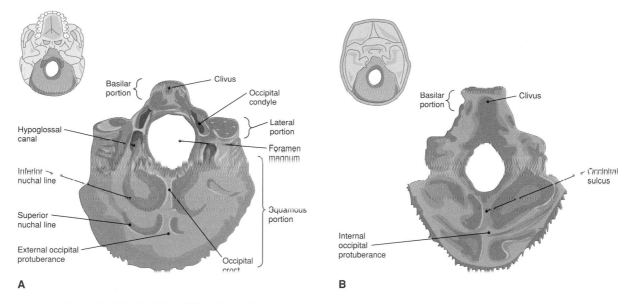

Figure 11–5. Occipital bone: **(A)** inferior view demonstrating the outer aspect, **(B)** superior view demonstrating the inner aspect.

men magnum is a large hole through which the spinal cord passes downward from the medulla oblongata of the brain. The **occipital crest** is a small bony ridge that extends from the foramen magnum to the **external occipital protuberance** or **inion** (IN-ē-on), which is a palpable bump located on the midline of the squamous portion. Two parallel ridges called the **superior** and **inferior nuchal** (NOO-kal) **lines** run horizontally through the occipital crest. These bony landmarks serve as the attachment sites for muscles and ligaments that provide support and balance to the right and left occipitoatlantal joints. On the inner surface of the occipital bone, there is a bump called the **internal occipital protuberance** that corresponds in location to its external counterpart. There are also grooves or **sulci** (SUL-kī) (singular, sulcus) that accommodate the venous (dural) sinuses of the brain.

The two **lateral portions** of the occipital bone are situated between the squamous and basilar portions. They lie to either side of the foramen magnum. Each lateral portion has a convex, rockerlike **occipital condyle** on which it articulates with the corresponding articular surface on the first cervical vertebra. There is also a **hypoglossal canal** located at the superior end of the condyle through which the 12th cranial or **hypoglossal nerve** is transmitted to the brain.

The **basilar** (BAS-i-lar) **portion** forms part of the base of the skull. It is located in front of the foramen magnum and extends anteriorly and superiorly to articulate with the body of the sphenoid bone. As this area of bone slopes forward to meet the sphenoid, it is known as the **clivus** (KLĪ-vus) *(Figure 11–5).*

ETHMOID BONE

The ethmoid (ETH-moid) bone is a small, complex-shaped bone located on the midline of the skull between the orbits. Situated anteriorly to the sphenoid bone and posteriorly to the nasal bones, it forms the anterior part of the cranial floor, medial wall of each orbit, lateral walls of the nasal cavity, and upper part of the nasal septum. The ethmoid bone consists of four parts: a horizontal portion, vertical portion, and two lateral masses. The **horizontal portion** is known as the **cribriform** (KRIB-ri-form) **plate** (*cribrum* = "sieve"). It fits snugly in the ethmoidal notch of the frontal bone to form the anterior portion of the cranial floor, as well as the roof of the nasal cavity. It has numerous tiny perforations for passage of the olfactory (smell) nerves, which account for the sievelike appearance. The **crista galli** (KRIS-tah GAH-le) is a triangular process that projects upward from the cribriform plate to extend up through the ethmoidal notch of the frontal bone. The name actually means "rooster's comb" and accurately describes its appearance. The projection serves as an attachment point for the membranes that cover and secure the brain in the cranial fossa.

The **vertical portion** is called the **perpendicular plate.** It projects inferiorly from the bottom of the cribriform plate to form the superior portion of the bony nasal septum. Together, the horizontal and vertical portions assume the shape of a cross.

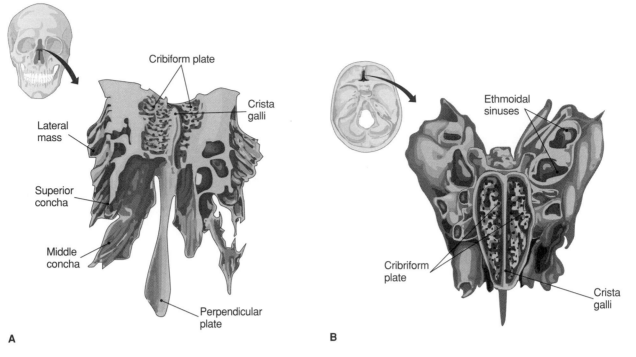

Figure 11–6. Ethmoid bone: **(A)** anterosuperior aspect, **(B)** superior aspect.

The right and left **lateral masses** or **labyrinths** are thin-walled, spongelike structures that hang from the underside of the cribriform plate on either side of the perpendicular plate. Each of these structures has a spongy or honeycomb appearance because it contains anywhere from 3 to 18 air cells which form the ethmoid sinuses. The lateral surface of the labyrinth forms the medial wall of an orbit; the medial surface forms the lateral wall of the nasal cavity. Two thin, scroll-shaped structures project into the nasal cavity from the medial wall. They are known as the **superior nasal concha** (KONG-kah) or **turbinate** and the **middle nasal concha** or **turbinate.** These shelflike projections filter, warm, and moisten inhaled air before it passes to the lungs. A third turbinate, the inferior nasal concha, is a facial bone and is discussed in Chapter 12 *(Figure 11–6).*

SPHENOID BONE

The single sphenoid (SFE-noid) bone is located on the midline of the cranial floor. It acts as an anchor or keystone to hold the eight cranial bones together, as it articulates with each of the other seven bones. Although it can be described as an irregular, wedge-shaped bone, the sphenoid actually has the appearance of a bat with outstretched wings and dangling legs. It forms the base of the skull and a small portion of each lateral wall, as well as part of the posterior wall of each orbit. It consists of a body, paired lesser wings, greater wings, and pterygoid processes *(Figure 11–7).*

The **body** forms the central portion of the bone. It is located between the ethmoid and occipital bones, and its anterior surface forms the posterior wall of the nasal cavity. The body is a hollow, cube-shaped area that encloses the air-filled sphenoid sinuses. The **sella turcica** (SEL-ah TUR-si-kah) *(sella turcica* — "Turkish saddle"), a saddle-shaped depression on the superior surface of the body, houses the pituitary gland. Because the pituitary gland is also called the hypophysis (hī-POF-i-sis), the deep central cavity of the sella turcica may be referred to as the **hypophyseal** (hī-pō-FE-sē-al) **fossa.** Situated on the midline of the skull, the sella turcica can be localized for radiographic examination by centering ¾ in. anterior and ¾ in. superior to the external acoustic meatus on the lateral projection *(Figure 11–8).* The **dorsum sellae** (DOR-sum SEL-ē) is the posterior border of the sella turcica. Two small, rounded projections known as the **posterior clinoid** (KLĪ-noid) **processes** extend superiorly from the upper, lateral margins of the dorsum sellae. A lateral projection of the skull demonstrates the sella turcica, as well as the underlying sphenoid sinuses. The sella turcica is bordered anteriorly by the **tuberculum sellae** (too-BER-ku-lum SEL-e), which is a small tubercle or eminence. The **optic** or **chiasmatic** (ki-az-MAT-ic) **groove** is a depression that runs horizontally across the body anterior to the sella turcica. The optic chiasm, formed by the crossing of the

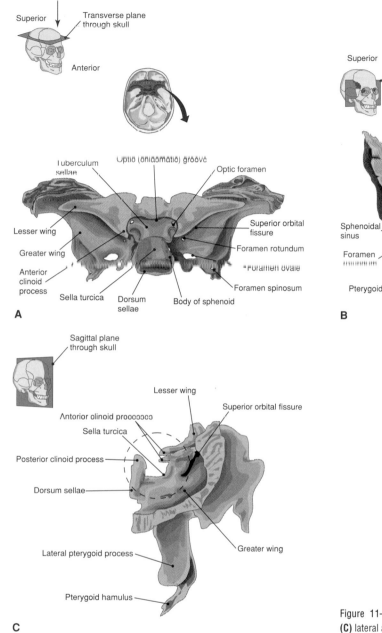

Superior

Transverse plane through skull

Anterior

Tuberculum sellae

Optic (chiasmatic) groove

Optic foramen

Lesser wing

Superior orbital fissure

Greater wing

Foramen rotundum

Anterior clinoid process

*Foramen ovale

Sella turcica

Dorsum sellae

Body of sphenoid

Foramen spinosum

A

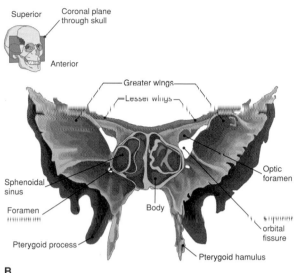

Superior

Coronal plane through skull

Anterior

Greater wings

Lesser wings

Sphenoidal sinus

Optic foramen

Foramen rotundum

Body

Superior orbital fissure

Pterygoid process

Pterygoid hamulus

B

Sagittal plane through skull

Lesser wing

Anterior clinoid processes

Superior orbital fissure

Sella turcica

Posterior clinoid process

Dorsum sellae

Lateral pterygoid process

Greater wing

Pterygoid hamulus

C

Figure 11–7. Sphenoid bone: **(A)** superior aspect, **(B)** anterior aspect, **(C)** lateral aspect.

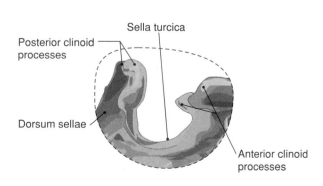

Posterior clinoid processes

Sella turcica

Dorsum sellae

Anterior clinoid processes

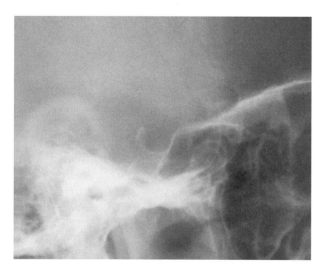

Figure 11–8. Closeup of sella turcica on a lateral projection.

Table 11-3. Summary of the Openings of the Sphenoid Bone

Openings of the Sphenoid Bone	Primary Structures Transmitted
Foramen lacerum	Internal carotid artery; small nerves and blood vessels
Foramen ovale	Meningeal branch of the fifth cranial nerve (sensation to mandible)
Foramen rotundum	Maxillary branch of the fifth cranial nerve (sensation to face)
Foramen spinosum	Meningeal vessels
Optic canal	Optic nerve, ophthalmic artery
Superior orbital fissure	Ophthalmic vein, third to sixth cranial nerves

optic nerves, is situated in this groove. The optic groove ends on each side at the **optic canal.** This short passageway between the body and each lesser wing transmits the optic nerve and blood vessels to the orbit. The circular terminal opening of the optic canal into the bony orbit is called the optic foramen and is discussed more fully in Chapter 12.

Two **lesser wings** extend laterally and horizontally from the anterosuperior aspect of the body. Their junction at the midline is called the **sphenoid ridge.** The triangular lesser wings articulate anteriorly with the orbital plate of the frontal bone. A portion of both lesser wings is demonstrated on an AP or PA projection of the skull, as these structures form the posteromedial segment of the orbital roofs. A small projection known as the **anterior clinoid process** extends from the posterior margin of each lesser wing to project posteriorly and laterally to the opening of the optic canal.

The paired **greater wings** of the sphenoid bone are posterior to the lesser wings. They arise from the lateral surfaces of the body to extend outward. Each greater wing forms part of the posterolateral wall of the orbit, a small portion of the lateral cranial wall, and fossa of the cranial cavity. It also forms the lower margin of the superior orbital fissure. Numerous openings on each greater wing serve as passageways for the nerves and blood vessels supplying the orbits and face. The **superior orbital fissure** is a split in the sphenoid bone between each greater wing and the inferior margin of a lesser wing. It can be seen within the orbit on a frontal drawing or a radiograph obtained with an appropriately angled central ray. The **foramen rotundum** (ro-TUN-dum) is a small, round opening situated close to the body in the anteromedial aspect of the greater wing. As the name implies, the **foramen ovale** (ov-A-le) is an oval opening somewhat larger than the foramen rotundum, to which it is located laterally and posteriorly. The **foramen spinosum** (spi-NO-sum) is a small hole positioned laterally and posteriorly to the foramen ovale in the posterior corner of the greater wing. The **foramen lacerum** (LA-se-rum) is a somewhat jagged opening at the junction of the sphenoid bone, temporal bone, and basilar portion of the occipital bone. It allows for the passage of several blood vessels and nerves, including the internal carotid artery. *Table 11-3* summarizes the structures that pass through the openings of the greater and lesser wings of the sphenoid bone.

The right and left **pterygoid** (TER-i-goid) **processes** (*pterygoid* = "winglike") are extensions of bone that hang from the underside of the sphenoid bone at the junction of the body and greater wings. They are approximately 1 in. long and serve as attachment sites for some of the muscles that move the mandible. They articulate anteriorly with the palatine bones and vomer. Each pterygoid process comprises two plates of bone that are fused together at their upper, anterior surfaces. The medial plate, which is also known as the **pterygoid hamulus** (HAM-u-lus), is longer and more narrow than the lateral plate with a small hook-like process on its distal end.

TEMPORAL BONES

The two irregularly shaped temporal (TEM-po-ral) bones form part of the base and the sides of the cranium. They are named for their location in the region of the temples (*temporo* = "time"). As a person ages, the hair at the temples turns gray, which indicates the passage of time. Each temporal bone is located directly below a parietal bone and also articulates with the greater wing of the sphenoid and occipital bones. It has four regions—squamous, tympanic, mastoid, and petrous—which are illustrated in *Figure 11-9*.

The **squamous portion** is the flaring, upper part of the temporal bone. As the thinnest and flattest portion, it forms the inferior aspect of the cranial wall above the ear. Two structures of importance are the zygomatic process and the mandibular fossa. The **zygomatic** (ZI-go-mat-ik) **process** is a slender bar of bone that extends anteriorly to articulate with a similar process on the zygomatic bone. Together, the zygomatic process of the temporal bone and the temporal process of the zygomatic bone form the **zygomatic arch,** which a person can palpate on the lateral aspect of the cheek. The **mandibular fossa** is a small de-

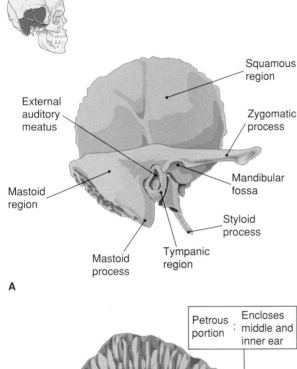

A

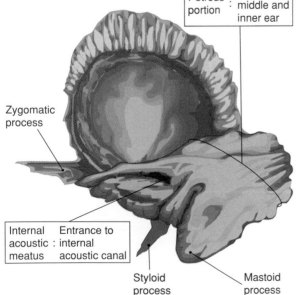

B

Figure 11-9. Temporal bone: **(A)** lateral aspect, and **(B)** medial aspect illustrating the four regions.

Table 11–4. Openings of the Temporal Bone

Openings of the Temporal Bone	Primary Structures Transmitted
External acoustic meatus	Sound waves into the external acoustic canal
Internal acoustic meatus	Blood vessels and nerves to inner ear
Foramen lacerum	Internal carotid artery; small nerves and blood vessels
Jugular foramen	Internal jugular vein; several cranial nerves

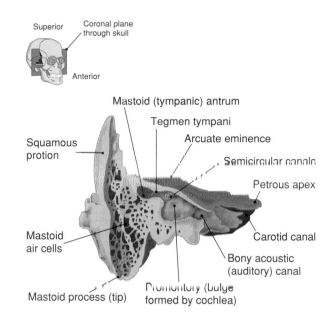

Figure 11–10. Temporal bone: coronal section through mastoid and petrous portions.

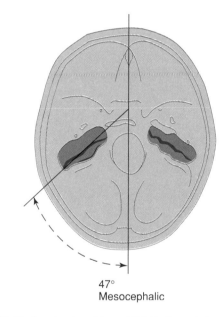

Figure 11–11. Superior view of the cranial floor demonstrating the petrous ridges at a 47° angle to the midsagittal plane.

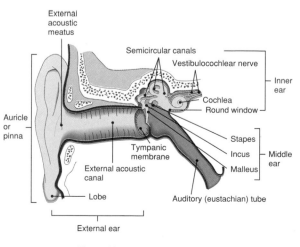

Figure 11–12. Anatomy of the ear.

pression situated below the zygomatic process just anterior to the ear. The condyle of the mandible fits in the fossa to form the movable temporomandibular joint. A small, rounded prominence at the anterior end of the fossa is known as the **articular tubercle.** It serves to keep the mandibular condyle from dislocating anteriorly out of the fossa.

The **tympanic** (tim-PAN-ik) **portion** of the temporal bone is located below the squamous portion and anterior to both the petrous and mastoid portions. This curved plate of bone forms the inferior, anterior, and part of the posterior walls of the external auditory meatus. A slender spike of bone called the **styloid** (STI-loid) **process** projects downward from the temporal bone between the mandible and external auditory meatus. It allows for the attachment of muscles and ligaments of the neck and tongue.

The **mastoid** (MAS-toid) **portion** is that part of the temporal bone that is posterior and inferior to the external auditory meatus. The **mastoid process** is a rounded bump (*mastoid* = "breast-shaped") that can be palpated just behind the ear. It serves as an attachment site for several neck muscles. Beginning early in life and concluding at puberty, a network of air cells develops in the mastoid region of the temporal bone, particularly in the mastoid process. The largest air cell is known as the **mastoid antrum.** Located at the upper, anterior aspect of the mastoid process, the antrum communicates with the tympanic cavity of the middle ear. The size of the mastoid process is variable depending on the number of air cells that develop. Mastoiditis is a condition in which the mastoid air cells become inflamed. It usually results from a middle ear infection, as the communication between the middle ear and mastoid antrum allows for the spread of infection. Although the condition is treatable with antibiotics, it can have serious consequences as the mastoid air cells are separated from the brain by only a thin wall of bone called the *tegman tympani* (TEG-men TIM-pah-ne) and encephalitis can ensue if the infection spreads.

The organs of hearing and balance are sheltered in the **petrous** (PET-rus) **portion.** It is not only the densest part of the temporal bone (*petrous* = "rocky"), but the densest portion of the cranium. Located in the floor of the skull, it is the most inferior segment of the temporal bone. It extends medially and anteriorly from the squamous portion of the temporal bone to articulate with the basilar portion of the occipital bone. Its anterior margin articulates with the greater wing of the sphenoid bone. Because it is roughly pyramid-shaped, it is also referred to as the *petrous pyramid* or *pars petrosa.* The upper border of the petrous portion is a sharp crest called the **petrous ridge,** which corresponds with the level of the infraorbitomeatal line. The **arcuate eminence** is a noticeable arch on the petrous ridge. The semicircular canals of the inner ear are directly below this point *(Figure 11–10).* A superior view of the cranial floor, as seen in *Figure 11–11,* demonstrates each petrous ridge at a 47° angle to the midsagittal plane on the average-shaped head. An opening at the medial end, or apex, of the petrous ridge is known as the **internal acoustic meatus.** It is the entrance into the **internal acoustic canal,** which transmits blood vessels and nerves to the inner ear. Several other openings are present in the petrous portion of the temporal bone. The **jugular foramen** is located between the temporal and occipital bones. It serves as the passageway for the internal jugular vein and several cranial nerves. Immediately anterior to it is the **carotid canal,** which conveys most of the blood supply to the cerebral hemispheres of the brain via the internal carotid artery. The carotid canal opens into the foramen lacerum between the sphenoid, temporal, and occipital bones. The openings of the temporal bone are summarized in *Table 11–4.*

EAR

The ear has a dual function as it controls both hearing and balance. The organs and sensory receptors for hearing and equilibrium are housed within the petrous portion of each temporal bone. The ear is divided into three main divisions: external, middle, and inner *(Figure 11–12).*

The **external ear** is the outer portion and comprises an auricle and an acoustic meatus. The **auricle** or **pinna** is the shell-shaped, cartilaginous structure that directs the sound waves into the external acoustic canal. The rim of the auricle is known as the **helix;** the earlobe is the **lobule.** The **tragus** is a small, liplike

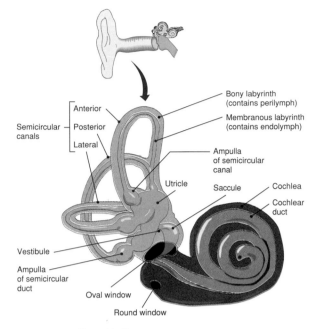

Figure 11–13. Structures of the inner ear.

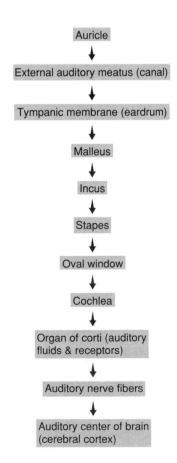

Figure 11–14. Path of sound waves during the hearing process. *(Adapted from Chabner DE. The Language of Medicine. 4th ed. Philadelphia: WB Saunders, 1991, with permission.)*

projection that partially covers and protects the **external acoustic meatus** (EAM), which is the opening to the canal. The **external acoustic (auditory) canal** is a slightly curved, sound-conducting tube that leads toward the middle ear. It is approximately 1 in. (2.5 cm) long and ends at the eardrum. The outer one third of the canal is cartilaginous, whereas the inner two thirds is bony. Although the EAM is located on the tympanic portion, most of the external acoustic canal is situated within the petrous portion of the temporal bone. The external ear ends at the eardrum.

The middle ear is an air-filled chamber that is also known as the **tympanic cavity.** It begins with the eardrum, which is a thin, semitransparent structure called the **tympanic membrane** (*tympanum* = "drum") and ends at a thin, bony wall that contains two small openings or windows. Three tiny bones called **auditory ossicles** (OS-i-kuhlz) are present on the medial side of the eardrum within the tympanic cavity. They are named for their shape: **malleus** (hammer), **incus** (anvil), and **stapes** (stirrup). The handle of the malleus is attached to the tympanic membrane, whereas the base or footplate of the stapes fits into the **oval** or **vestibular window** that opens into the inner ear. When sound waves pass through the external acoustic canal, they strike the tympanic membrane causing it to vibrate, which in turn sets the ossicles in motion. The other opening in the bony partition between the middle and inner ear is the **round** or **cochlear window,** which is covered by a secondary tympanic membrane. The middle ear has two additional openings or communications. The **tympanic opening** of the **auditory** or **eustachian tube** is on the anterior wall of the middle ear. This canal leads directly from the middle ear to the pharynx and is often the passageway for infectious organisms between the throat and ear. The auditory tube serves to equalize the pressure between the external and middle portions of the ear, thus preventing damage to the eardrum. The **aditus** is an opening on the posterior wall of the middle ear into the mastoid antrum. As discussed previously, infection can be spread via this communication resulting in mastoiditis. Because the middle ear is air-filled, it can be evaluated radiographically when the petrous portion of the temporal bone is examined.

The inner ear is also referred to as the *labyrinth* because it has a complicated, mazelike structure deep within the temporal bone. It has two basic divisions: the bony (osseous) labyrinth and the membranous labyrinth. The **bony labyrinth** comprises a vestibule, a cochlea, and three semicircular canals. It is filled with an auditory fluid called **perilymph**. The **membranous labyrinth** is a series of intercommunicating sacs and ducts that basically correspond in shape to the bony labyrinth. It is suspended in the perilymph and is filled with an auditory fluid called **endolymph** *(Figure 11–13).*

The **vestibule** is a centrally located cavity concerned with equilibrium. Its membranous components are the **saccule** (SAK-yool) and the **utricle** (U-tri-kul), which house receptors that are sensitive to movements of the head.

The **cochlea** is located anteriorly to the vestibule. This spiral or snail-shaped bony structure houses the receptors for the sense of hearing. The membranous portion is a coiled tube consisting of the **scala vestibuli** (vestibular duct), **scala tympani** (tympanic duct), and **cochlear duct.** The oval window of the middle ear communicates with the scala vestibuli; the round window is adjacent to the scala tympani. Both the oval and round windows have membranous coverings that separate the fluids of the inner ear from the air in the middle ear. Therefore, the fluid fluctuates within a closed system. Sound waves are conducted to the oval window by ossicular movements. When the vibratory motion of the ossicles is transmitted through the oval window, wavelike movements are induced in the fluid of the inner ear, which, in turn, stimulate the sensory receptors in the cochlear duct, specifically in the **organ of Corti.** Impulses in the receptors or nerve fibers are transmitted to the brain via the **vestibulocochlear** (eighth cranial) **nerve.** *Figure 11–14* diagrams the path that sound waves follow during the process of hearing.

The **anterior, posterior,** and **lateral semicircular canals** are positioned at right angles to each other and are named according to their location. Receptors in the fluid-filled, expanded **ampulla** (am-PUL-ah) of each canal detect head movements in all directions. The information is transmitted to the brain where it is disseminated to the muscles of the body to help maintain equilibrium.

ARTHROLOGY

The bones of the skull are securely joined together to form a fairly solid, protective enclosure for the brain. The joints formed between cranial bones are known as **sutures** (SOO-churz). Most of the cranial bones have irregular edges that interlock like the pieces of a jigsaw puzzle to strengthen the skull. Short pieces of fibrous connective tissue hold the bones tightly together. Structurally, sutures are fibrous joints that are classified as synarthrodial because they do not permit movement. During adulthood, usually between the ages of 20 and 30, the bones fuse together as the fibrous tissue becomes ossified. At this point, the sutures are more accurately described as synostoses *(Figure 11–15).*

Each parietal bone is involved in the formation of four major sutures. The **coronal** (ko-RO-nal) **suture** (*corona* = "crown") is located between the frontal and both parietal bones, in much the same location where the front of a crown would rest on the head. The **sagittal** (SAJ-i-tal) **suture** (*sagitta* = "arrow") is located on the midsagittal plane of the body between the right and left parietal bones. On the newborn

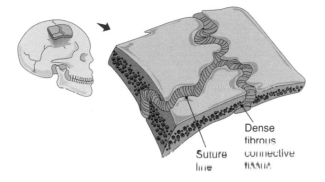

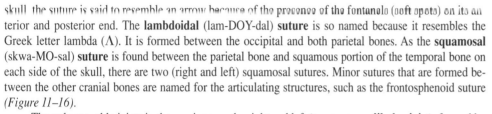

Figure 11–15. Closeup view of a suture demonstrating fibrous tissue between the irregular edges of bone.

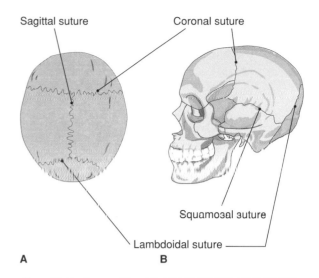

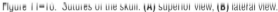

Figure 11–16. Sutures of the skull. (A) superior view, (B) lateral view.

skull, the suture is said to resemble an arrow because of the presence of the fontanels (soft spots) on its anterior and posterior end. The **lambdoidal** (lam-DOY-dal) **suture** is so named because it resembles the Greek letter lambda (Λ). It is formed between the occipital and both parietal bones. As the **squamosal** (skwa-MO-sal) **suture** is found between the parietal bone and squamous portion of the temporal bone on each side of the skull, there are two (right and left) squamosal sutures. Minor sutures that are formed between the other cranial bones are named for the articulating structures, such as the frontosphenoid suture *(Figure 11–16)*.

The only movable joints in the cranium are the right and left **temporomandibular joints** formed by the mandibular fossa of each temporal bone with the corresponding condyle of the mandible. These joints are classified as diarthrodial. They are synovial in structure, allowing both hinge and gliding movements *(Figure 11–17)*.

At birth, the skull is proportionately larger than the remainder of the skeleton. Several of the cranial bones, such as the frontal bone, consist of more than one piece. During fetal development, the frontal bone is divided into two halves by the **metopic** (me-TOP-ik) **suture.** This suture runs down the midsagittal plane on the squamous portion of the bone (*metopic* = "pertaining to the forehead"). The halves unite shortly after birth and are completely fused by the age of 6, with the suture usually undetectable radiographically by the age of 8. Therefore, the frontal bone is considered to be a single structure. Unossified fibrous connective membrane is present at birth in areas where three or more bones adjoin. Known as **fontanels** (fon-ta-NELZ), these "soft spots" allow for modification of the size and shape of the skull as it passes through the birth canal. Another function is to permit rapid growth of the brain to take place during infancy. Although there are six fontanels, the most prominent are the **anterior** and **posterior fontanels,** which are located at the anterior and posterior ends of the sagittal suture, respectively. *Figure 11–18* illustrates the location of the fontanels on the skull. Through the process of intramembranous ossification, the membranous tissue is eventually replaced by bone. This occurs in the posterior fontanel about 2 months af-

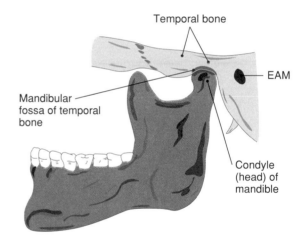

Figure 11–17. Temporomandibular joint.

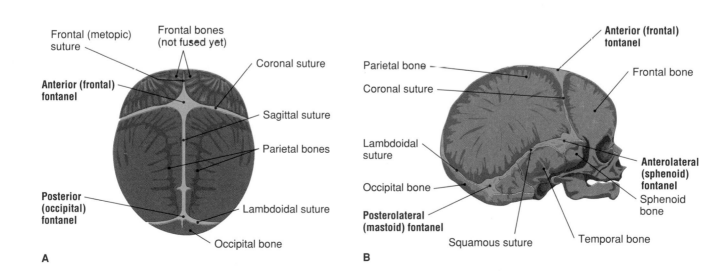

Figure 11–18. Fontanels of the newborn skull: **(A)** superior view, **(B)** lateral view.

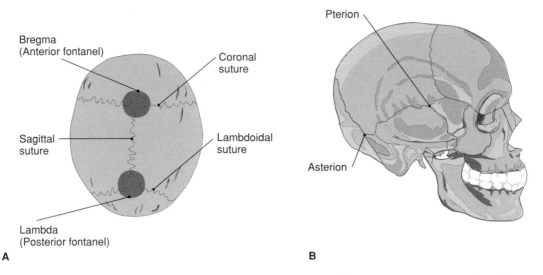

Figure 11–19. **(A)** Superior view of the skull demonstrates the bregma and lambda. **(B)** Lateral view demonstrates pterion and as-terion.

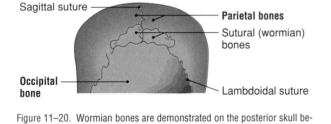

Figure 11–20. Wormian bones are demonstrated on the posterior skull between the sagittal and lambdoidal sutures.

ter birth. As the anterior fontanel is larger, it generally does not ossify or close until the child is 18 to 24 months. In the adult, the point of articulation between the frontal and both parietal bones at the anterior end of the sagittal suture is called the **bregma** (BREG-mah); the similar point between the occipital and both parietal bones at the posterior end is called the **lambda** (LAM-dah). The smaller **anterolateral** (sphenoid) and **posterolateral** (mastoid) **fontanels** are known as the **pterion** (TER-re-on) and **asterion** (as-TE-re-on), respectively, in the adult *(Figure 11–19)*.

  Wormian or **sutural bones** are small, oddly shaped bones that often develop between the sutures of the cranial bones, particularly in the lambdoidal suture. They vary in number (average is 3–4) and actual position from person to person *(Figure 11–20)*.

► PROCEDURAL CONSIDERATIONS

Although CT and MRI have replaced much of the routine radiography of the skull, radiographic examination of the skull is still performed when the more expensive CT and MRI examinations are not warranted. Because these procedures are not requested as frequently today, the radiographer should review skull positioning periodically to remain current.

PATIENT PREPARATION

After being correctly identified, the patient should be instructed to remove all metallic objects, eyeglasses, and dental appliances (eg, dentures, retainers) from the head and neck area. Care should be taken to remove all hairpins, barrettes, and elastic bands from the hair. Buttons or zippers on the shirt collar should also be moved away from the head and neck area.

  Because it is necessary for the patient to place his or her face against the radiographic table or upright grid device, all pertinent surfaces should be cleaned with appropriate solutions. It is recommended that this be done either in front of the patient or immediately prior to the patient entering the room so the surface smells freshly cleaned; the bottle of cleaning solution can also be kept in a spot visible to the patient. In addition, the radiographer's hands must be thoroughly washed immediately prior to touching the patient's head; disposable gloves should be worn, if warranted.

POSITIONING CONSIDERATIONS

Because of the many positioning lines, planes, and central ray angles to remember, skull positioning produces a high level of anxiety in most student radiographers. In addition, the infrequency of skull examinations performed today limits opportunities for observation and practice in the clinical setting. An important

Table 11–5. Routine/Optional Projections: Skull and Petrous Portions

Skull	Mastoids[a]
AP/PA axial	AP/PA axial (collimated)
PA/AP	PA (collimated)
Lateral	Modified lateral (Law)
Submentovertical (SMV)[a]	Axiolateral oblique (Mayer)
Internal auditory canals/petrous portions[a]	Sella turcica
AP/PA axial (collimated)	Lateral
PA (collimated)	AP/PA axial
Posterior/anterior profile	

Note. The routine examination of the petrous portions can include any of a broad variety of projections. This table includes several of the common projections, as well as the traditional projections for the routine skull examination.
[a]Optional projections/examinations that may be routine in some departments.

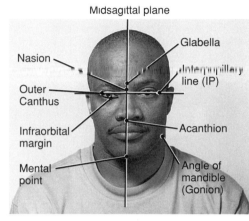

fact to remember is that several of the basic projections discussed in this chapter, with slight modifications for centering, are also included in various examinations of the facial bones and sinuses that are discussed in the next chapter. A thorough knowledge of the basic projections included in this chapter, therefore, will facilitate the learning of many other projections.

Although department protocols vary, radiographic examination of the skull typically includes the AP axial (Grashey/Towne), PA, and lateral projections *(Table 11–5)*. When the patient is unable to lie prone, the AP projection provides an acceptable alternative to the PA. It is important, however, to remember that the AP projection also results in magnification of the orbits and a significant increase in radiation exposure to the lens of the eye (entrance dose is significantly greater than exit dose). Depending on available equipment, patient condition, and radiologist/technologist preference, any of the skull projections can be obtained with the patient either recumbent or erect; the erect position may be more comfortable for the patient.

Accurate positioning of the head is accomplished through the use of specific landmarks, positioning lines, and planes *(Tables 11–6 and 11–7, Figure 11–21)*. Incorrect positioning of the midsagittal plane could result in improper rotation or tilt of the head. Incorrect head flexion is related to inaccurate use of the positioning lines. Topographical, or surface, landmarks, such as the nasion and acanthion, are used for localizing specific structures and for accurate centering. Although patient comfort is important when positioning any body part, it is critical for skull positioning. Unnecessary stress on the muscles can prevent the patient from focusing on maintaining the correct position. Many of the skull positions will be difficult for the patient to maintain; taking the time to ensure the patient is as comfortable as possible will contribute to

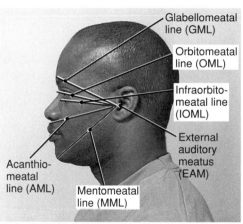

Table 11–6. Topographical Landmarks

Acanthion (ah-KAN-the-on): midline junction of the upper lip and nose

Auricle (pinna): large flap of cartilage commonly referred to as the "ear"

Base of the orbit: bony rim surrounding each eye

External acoustic (auditory) meatus (me-A- tus) (EAM): external opening into the ear canal

Glabella (glah-BEL-ah): smooth, triangular area superior to the bridge of the nose and between the eyebrows

Gonion (GO-ne-on): lower, posterior angle seen on each side of the jaw or mandible

Infraorbital margin (IOM): inferior rim of the orbital base

Inion (IN-e-on): prominent bump, midline at the back of the head; external occipital protuberance

Inner canthus (KAN-thus); (plural, *KAN-thi):* junction of the upper and lower eyelids, near the nose

Mental point: midpoint of the chin; center of a flat, triangular region known as the *mentum*

Midlateral orbital margin: rim of bone near the outer corner of the eye

Nasion (NA-ze-on): slight depression at the bridge of the nose; marks the junction of the frontal and nasal bones

Superciliary ridge (arch): ridge of bone found over each eye and under each eyebrow

Supraorbital groove (SOG): small depression directly above each superciliary arch; corresponds with the highest level of the facial bones and the floor of the anterior fossa of the cranium

Supraorbital margin (SOM): superior rim of the orbital base

Top of ear attachment (TEA): junction of the most superior portion of the ear and the scalp; corresponds with the level of the petrous ridges

Tragus (TRA-gus): small flap of cartilage projecting over the external acoustic meatus

Outer canthus: lateral junction of the upper and lower eyelids

Vertex (VER-tex): most superior point of the head

Note. Topographical, or surface, landmarks can be either seen or palpated and are used for centering, localization of internal structures, and the formation of specific positioning lines.

Figure 11–21. Positioning landmarks, planes, and lines: **(A)** frontal view, **(B)** and **(C)** lateral view.

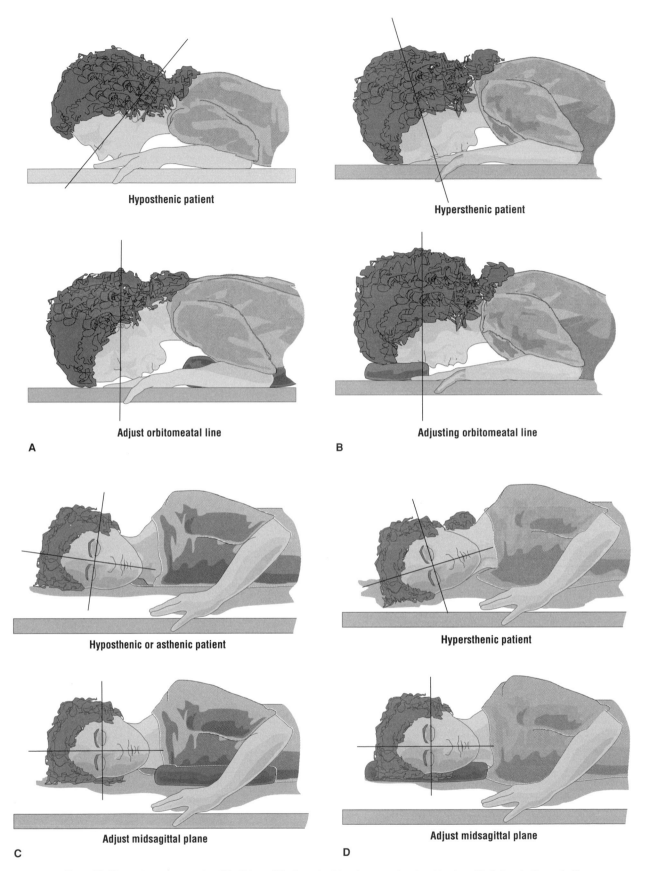

Figure 11–22. The hyposthenic patient **(A)** will have difficulty maintaining the correct head position for a PA skull projection and will benefit by having a radiolucent support placed under the upper thorax. Conversely, the hypersthenic patient **(B)** may be unable to extend the head as necessary and may need a small support under the forehead. The lateral position is often difficult for asthenic **(C)** and hypersthenic **(D)** patients to maintain and may require supports strategically placed as illustrated.

(continued)

Table 11-7. Positioning Lines and Planes

Acanthiomeatal Line (AML): extends from the EAM to the acanthion	**Mentomeatal line** (MML): extends from EAM to mental point
Glabelloalveolar line: connects glabella to anterior part of the alveolar process of maxilla at the midline; used for the tangential projection of the nasal bones	**Midsagittal, median sagittal, or median plane:** plane dividing the head (and body) into equal right and left halves; this plane is either perpendicular to or parallel with the film plane for AP/PA and lateral projections, respectively
Glabellomeatal line: extends from EAM to glabella	
Infraorbitomeatal line (IOML): extends from EAM to infraorbital margin; there is an approximate 7° angle between OML and IOML	**Orbitomeatal line** (OML): extends from EAM to outer canthus of eye; there is an 8° difference between the glabellomeatal and orbitomeatal lines
Interpupillary line (IPL) **or interorbital line:** line connecting the two pupils or outer canthi of the eyes	

Note. Positioning lines are used to achieve the correct head flexion. Planes are used for accurate head rotation. Errors in the use of these lines and planes will result in poor patient positioning and may require repeat radiographs.

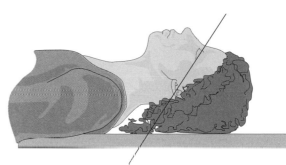

Hypersthenic or round-shouldered patient

better-quality radiographs. Differences in body habitus can also make accurate skull positioning a challenge *(Figure 11–22)*. Although asthenic or hyposthenic patients may require supports under the upper thorax when positioned for the PA skull projection, it may be almost impossible for the hypersthenic patient to depress the chin enough for an acceptable AP axial projection. In this situation, a comparable view can be obtained by positioning the patient prone, as for the PA projection, and directing the central ray cephalad instead of caudad for a PA axial (Haas) projection. To ensure that the part is straight on the film, care should be taken to place the long axis of the patient's body parallel with the long axis of the table or upright grid device.

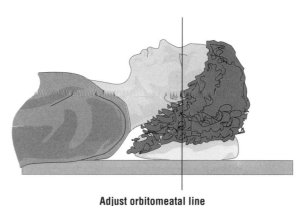

Adjust orbitomeatal line

E

Figure 11–22 *(continued).* The hypersthenic or round-shouldered **(E)** patient may require a radiolucent support to place the orbitomeatal line perpendicular to the film plane.

Skull Morphology

Because the size and shape of most skulls are the same, internal structures can be precisely located. Even though most heads are similar in size and shape, however, assessment of the external features of the patient's head is important. Patients may have features (eg, mandible, orbits, ears) that are asymmetric in size, shape, or location. A patient's features, therefore, can affect part centering, patient positioning, and central ray angle. The typical or average-shaped head is termed *mesocephalic*. In the mesocephalic skull, the petrous portions lie at a 47° angle with the midsagittal plane. Although most individuals have a normally shaped head, others may have either a short, broad, and shallow head, termed *brachycephalic*, or a long, narrow, and deep head, called *dolichocephalic*. In the brachycephalic head, the petrous ridges form a 54° angle with the midsagittal plane, whereas the petrous portions in the dolichocephalic head form a 40° angle *(Figure 11–23)*. Although these differences require negligible adjustments in patient positioning or central ray angle for routine skull examinations, they affect patient positioning for the petrous portions. For projections in which the petrous portions must be parallel to the film (eg, anterior and posterior profile [Arcelin/Stenvers] projections), the brachycephalic head will be rotated less than 45° (approximately 36°); the dolichocephalic head must be rotated approximately 50°. To place the petrous portion perpendicular to the film, as for the axiolateral oblique (Mayer) projection, the brachycephalic head must be rotated approximately 54° and the dolichocephalic head about 40°. Picturing the petrous portions within the head will help the radiographer determine the amount and direction of rotation needed for the projection.

TRAUMA CONSIDERATIONS

Because traumatic lesions, such as brain hemorrhage and edema, may be present without an associated skull fracture, CT is frequently performed on patients with a suspected head injury. For a variety of reasons, however, routine skull films are often obtained prior to CT or as a screening examination for patients with minimal injury. The routine skull projections—AP axial, PA, and both laterals—are often obtained with the patient supine, because of the patient's condition. Note that the AP projection *(Figure 11–24A,B)*, or reverse PA, is performed when the patient cannot or should not be moved. Any central ray angles routinely used on a PA projection are reversed. **Because cervical spine injuries are often associated with head injuries, it is vitally important that cervical spine fractures and dislocations be ruled out prior to moving or manipulating the head.** In the case of a cervical spine fracture or dislocation, the central ray may need to be angled to compensate for the inability of the patient to flex the neck. A horizontal beam used for the cross-table lateral projections will assist in the identification of fluid in the sphenoid sinuses *(Figure 11–25)*.

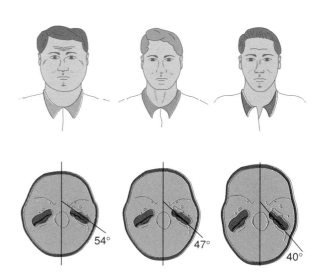

Figure 11–23. The orientation of the petrous ridges within the skull correlates with the general shape of the skull. *(Adapted from Cullinan AM.* Optimizing Radiographic Positioning. *Philadelphia: JB Lippincott, 1992:101.)*

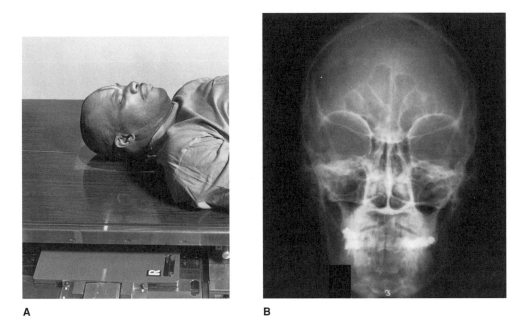

A   **B**

Figure 11–24. AP skull, trauma.

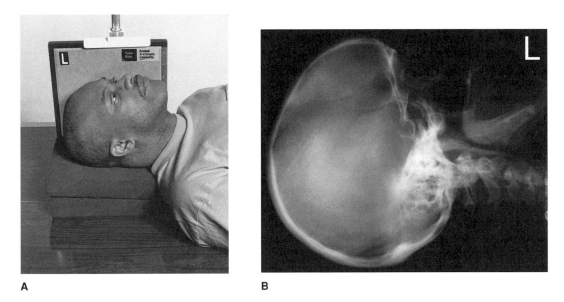

A   **B**

Figure 11–25. If a cervical spine fracture has been ruled out, a support may be used to elevate the head to obtain a lateral projection of the entire skull.

ALTERNATE PROJECTIONS

Although included as part of the routine series in some departments, the submentovertical (full basal) projection is generally obtained only by request. It can be used to demonstrate the petrous portions and various foramina seen in the base of the skull. The key to accurate positioning for this projection is to position the patient so the infraorbitomeatal line (IOML) is as nearly parallel to the film plane as possible; then direct the central ray perpendicular to the IOML *(Figure 11–26)*. The submentovertical (SMV) projection can also be used to evaluate certain facial bones and paranasal sinuses and, therefore, is discussed again in the next chapter.

If the patient is unable to assume the SMV position, the reverse position, the verticosubmental position, can be performed. The patient is positioned prone with the head hyperextended. Although the central ray can be directed perpendicular to the IOML, the IOML cannot be positioned parallel to the film plane, producing increased distortion and decreased sharpness of the mid- and posterior basilar structures.

Table 11–8. Average Skull Measurements by Projection

AP/PA axial	21 cm
PA/AP	19 cm
Lateral	16 cm
SMV/VSM	23 cm

Note. Caliper measurements should coincide with the path of the central ray. Consequently, the AP axial measurement is obtained by measuring the distance from the inferior occipital area to the region of the hairline, the lateral measurement is taken from parietal eminence to parietal eminence, the PA is from the inion to the glabella, and the SMV is from the vertex to the region below the chin.

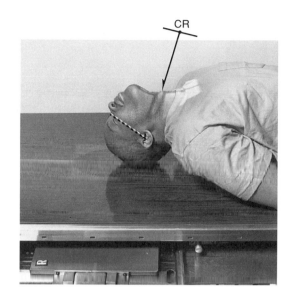

Figure 11–26. If the patient cannot be positioned so the IOML is parallel with the film, the central ray must be angled appropriately so it is perpendicular to the IOML.

Although they are demonstrated primarily by CT today, the pars petrosae can also be evaluated on routine radiographs. Radiographic examination of the mastoids, or petrous portions, can vary significantly from one department to another. AP axial and PA skull projections, collimated to the petrous portion, are often included as part of the series. Additional projections may include the modified lateral (Law) and axiolateral oblique (Mayer), obtained bilaterally for comparison. Either the anterior or posterior profile (Arcelin/Stenvers) projections may also be performed to examine the internal auditory canals and mastoid processes; again, both sides are evaluated. Because these examinations are seldom performed today, many radiographers must consult the department's procedure manual and a positioning atlas prior to beginning the examination.

BREATHING INSTRUCTIONS

Because skull positioning must be precise, any movement prior to or during the exposure could result in an unacceptable radiograph. To minimize the possibility of voluntary or involuntary motion and alert the patient that the exposure is going to be made, the patient should be instructed to suspend respiration for all projections of the skull and petrous portions.

EXPOSURE FACTORS

The kVp for skull projections generally ranges from 65 to 85. Although the lateral skull projections may require only 65 to 70 kVp, the AP/PA axial and basilar projections generally require 80 to 85 kVp. Because the tissue measurement for most adults is fairly standard for each projection *(Table 11–8)*, the mAs required depends on the type of equipment generator, film/screen speed, type of grid, and pathologic conditions present; a small focal spot should be used, when possible. Close collimation and/or the use of a cylinder cone also improves radiographic quality. Because lead right or left markers displayed outside of the anatomy can be overexposed or "burned out," a small, thin piece of aluminum can be placed under the marker during the exposure; the aluminum acts as a filter, allowing visualization of the lead marker.

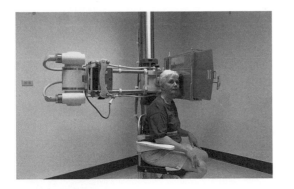

Figure 11–27. Franklin head unit. By moving the grid and film to the side, the radiographer can look through a plexiglass "window" to evaluate patient centering and positioning.

EQUIPMENT CONSIDERATIONS

Because of the density of the skull, a grid should be used for all projections. The patient may be positioned recumbent on a radiographic table or erect in front of a vertical grid device or dedicated head unit. Although head units are not as common as they once were, they offer the advantage of being able to view the patient's position from the perspective of the film, allowing for more accurate centering and positioning *(Figure 11–27)*. In addition, two projections, such as the bilateral modified lateral (Law) projections, can be easily imaged on one film.

A cassette holder is needed for cross-table lateral skull projections. Head clamps may be used to prevent rotation of the head *(Figure 11–28)*. In addition, adhesive tape may be carefully positioned across the chin to immobilize the head for the AP axial projection; sponges may be used to support the head and/or chin for the lateral projections and positioned under the thorax for the PA projection (thin patients). A special protractor *(Figure 11–29)* can be used for accurate positioning of the skull. In lieu of this device, cardboard angles can be made inexpensively and kept for this purpose.

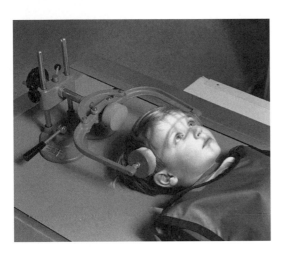

Figure 11–28. Head clamps can be used for immobilization.

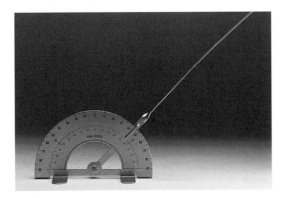

Figure 11–29. Positioning protractor.

RADIOGRAPHIC POSITIONING OF THE SKULL

- ► AP AXIAL (GRASHEY/TOWNE) SKULL

- ► PA AXIAL (HAAS) SKULL

- ► PA (CALDWELL) SKULL

- ► LATERAL SKULL

- ► SUBMENTOVERTICAL (FULL BASAL) SKULL

- ► VERTICOSUBMENTAL SKULL (VSM)

- ► MODIFIED LATERAL (LAW) SKULL FOR PETROUS PORTIONS

- ► AXIOLATERAL OBLIQUE (MAYER) SKULL FOR PETROUS PORTIONS

- ► POSTERIOR PROFILE (STENVERS) SKULL FOR PETROUS PORTIONS

- ► ANTERIOR PROFILE (ARCELIN) SKULL FOR PETROUS PORTIONS

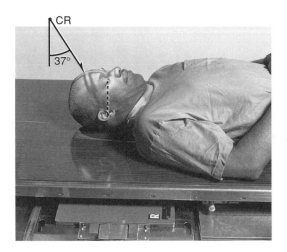

Figure 11-30. AP axial (Grashey/Towne) skull, using infraorbitomeatal line.

► AP AXIAL (GRASHEY/TOWNE) SKULL

Technical Considerations

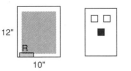

- Film size: 10 × 12 in. lengthwise.
- Grid required.
- 80–85 kVp.
- Collimate to include the top of the head and ears.

Caution: Fracture or dislocation of the cervical vertebrae should be ruled out before moving the head.

Shielding

- Gonadal shielding should be used on all patients, especially children and adults of reproductive age.

Patient Positioning

- Set the technical factors; the position may be difficult for the patient to maintain.
- Assist the patient to the supine position on the table or seated position with back to an upright grid device; the upright position is more comfortable for the hypersthenic patient and facilitates patient positioning without increasing part–film distance.
- Position the patient so the midsagittal plane is centered to and parallel with the long axis of the table or upright grid device; position the arms comfortably at the sides.

Part Positioning

- Position the patient's head so the midsagittal plane is perpendicular to the film plane.
- Depress the patient's chin so the orbitomeatal line is perpendicular to the film plane; if this is not possible, adjust the head so the infraorbitomeatal line is perpendicular.
- Center the cassette so the top edge is just above the top of the head.
- Recheck the head position from the head of the table *(Figure 11–30).*

Central Ray

- Direct the central ray so it enters at a point approximately 2.5 in. above the level of the superciliary arches and exits through the foramen magnum: 30° caudad to the orbitomeatal line or 37° caudad to the infraorbitomeatal line.

Breathing Instructions

- Instruct the patient to stop breathing during the exposure.

Image Evaluation

- The entire cranium and petrous portions should be included within the collimated area.
- The occipital bone and foramen magnum should be adequately penetrated and projected onto the lower half of the film.
- The petrous portions should be symmetrical.
- The dorsum sellae and posterior clinoid processes should be demonstrated within the shadow of the foramen magnum *(Figure 11–31).*

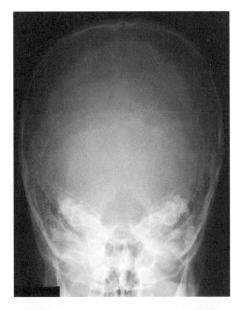

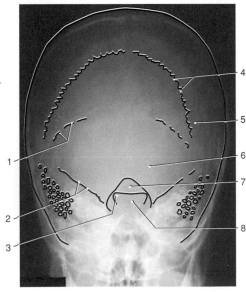

Figure 11-31. AP axial (Grashey/Towne) skull.

1. Coronal suture	4. Lambdoidal suture	7. Foramen magnum
2. Petrous ridge	5. Parietal bone	8. Dorsum sellae
3. Posterior clinoid process	6. Occipital bone	

► PA AXIAL (HAAS) SKULL

Technical Considerations

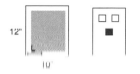

- Film size: 10 × 12 in. lengthwise.
- Grid required.
- 80–85 kVp.
- Collimate to include the top of the head and ears.

Note: This position produces a reverse AP axial projection and may be easier for hypersthenic patients to attain.

Caution: Fracture or dislocation of the cervical vertebrae should be ruled out before moving the head or turning the patient prone.

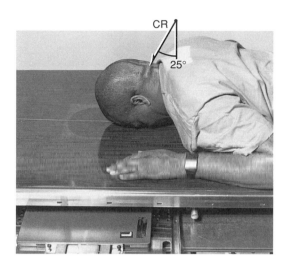

Figure 11–32. PA axial (Haas) skull.

Shielding

- Gonadal shielding should be used on all patients, especially children and adults of reproductive age.

Patient Positioning

- Set the technical factors; the position may be difficult for the patient to maintain.
- Assist the patient to the prone position on the table or seated position facing an upright grid device; the upright position is more comfortable for the hypersthenic patient and facilitates patient positioning without increasing part–film distance.
- Position the patient so the midsagittal plane is centered to and parallel with the long axis of the table or upright grid device; position the arms comfortably with hands near shoulders (on table) or at sides (upright).

Part Positioning

- With the patient's forehead resting on the table or upright grid device, position the head so the midsagittal plane is perpendicular to the film plane.
- Adjust the head so the orbitomeatal line is perpendicular to the film plane; thin patients may require a radiolucent support under the thorax to facilitate positioning and make them more comfortable.
- Recheck the head position from the head of the table; immobilize *(Figure 11–32)*.

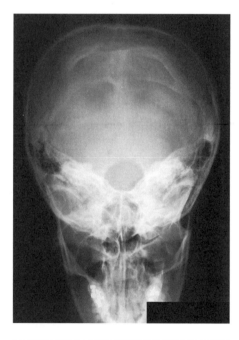

Central Ray

- Direct the central ray 25° cephalad, entering at a point approximately 1.5 in. inferior to the inion and exiting approximately 1.5 in. above the nasion.
- Center the cassette to the central ray.

Breathing Instructions

- Instruct the patient to stop breathing during the exposure.

Image Evaluation

- The entire cranium and petrous portions should be included within the collimated area.
- The occipital bone and foramen magnum should be adequately penetrated and projected onto the lower half of the film.
- The petrous portions should be symmetrical.
- The dorsum sellae and posterior clinoid processes should be demonstrated within the shadow of the foramen magnum *(Figure 11–33)*.

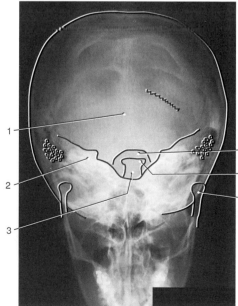

1. Occipital bone	3. Dorsum sellae	5. Posterior clinoid process
2. Petrous ridge	4. Foramen magnum	6. Mandibular condyle

Figure 11–33. PA axial (Haas) skull.

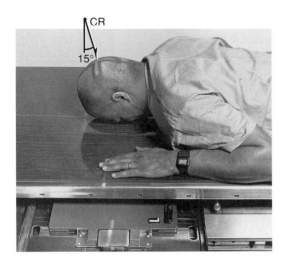

Figure 11–34. PA (Caldwell) skull.

▶ PA (CALDWELL) SKULL

Technical Considerations

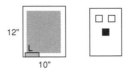

- Film size: 10 × 12 in. lengthwise.
- Grid required.
- 70–80 kVp.
- Collimate to include the top of the head and ears.

Shielding

- Gonadal shielding should be used on all patients, especially children and adults of reproductive age.

Patient Positioning

- Set the technical factors; the position may be difficult for the patient to maintain.
- Assist the patient to the prone position on the table or seated facing an upright grid device. The upright position may be more comfortable for the asthenic or hyposthenic patient. (**Note:** This AP projection may also be obtained with the patient supine when the patient is unable to lie prone or sit erect; however, this projection results in magnification of the orbits and an increased radiation dose to the lens of the patient's eyes.)
- Position the patient so the midsagittal plane is centered to and parallel with the long axis of the table or upright grid device; position the arms comfortably with hands near shoulders (on table) or at sides (upright).

Part Positioning

- With the patient's forehead resting on the table or upright grid device, position the head so the midsagittal plane is perpendicular to the film plane.
- Adjust the head so the orbitomeatal line is perpendicular to the film plane; thin patients may require a radiolucent support under the thorax to facilitate positioning and make them more comfortable.
- Recheck the head position from the head of the table; immobilize as necessary *(Figure 11–34)*.

Central Ray

- Direct the central ray to exit at the nasion; the central ray should be angled according to department routine or structure(s) of interest:

  frontal bone   0° angle
  general survey (Caldwell method)   15° caudad
- Center the cassette to the central ray.

Breathing Instructions

- Instruct the patient to stop breathing during the exposure.

Image Evaluation

- The entire cranium from the vertex through the petrous portions should be included within the collimated area.
- The frontal bone should be adequately penetrated without overexposure of the lateral margins of the skull.
- The petrous portions should fill the entire orbits when 0° angle is used or the lower third of the orbits when a 15° angle is used.
- The distances between the outer margins of the orbits and lateral margins of the skull should be equal.
- The petrous portions should be symmetrical *(Figures 11–35, 11–36)*.

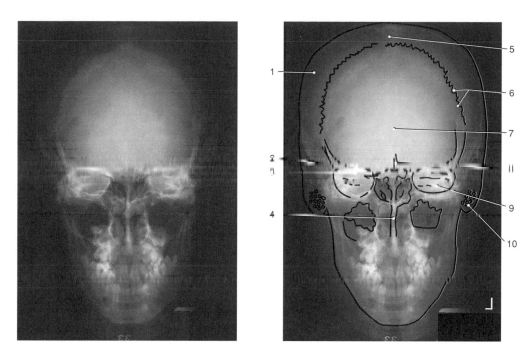

Figure 11-35. PA (Caldwell) skull, 0° central ray angle.

1. Parietal bone
2. Supraorbital rim
3. Petrous ridge
4. Bony nasal septum

5. Sagittal suture
6. Coronal suture
7. Frontal bone
8. Crista galli, ethmoid bone

9. Internal acoustic canal
10. Mastoid process, temporal bone

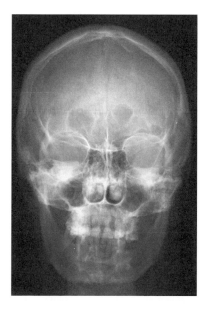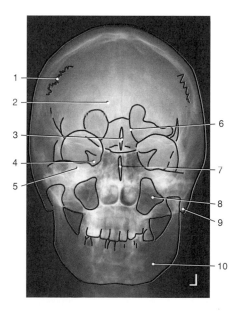

Figure 11-36. PA (Caldwell) skull, 15° caudal central ray angle.

1. Coronal suture
2. Frontal bone
3. Crista galli, ethmoid bone

4. Superior orbital fissure, sphenoid bone
5. Petrous ridge
6. Frontal sinuses

7. Bony nasal septum
8. Maxillary sinuses
9. Mastoid process
10. Mandible

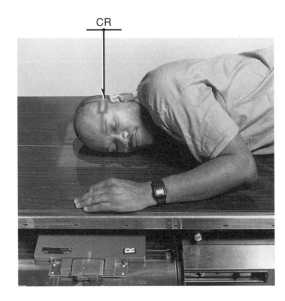

Figure 11–37. Lateral skull.

► LATERAL SKULL

Technical Considerations

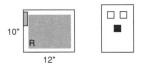

- Film size: 10 × 12 in. crosswise.
- Grid required.
- 65–70 kVp.
- Collimate to include the vertex, C1, inion, and glabella.

Shielding

- Gonadal shielding should be used on all patients, especially children and adults of reproductive age.

Patient Positioning

- Set the technical factors; the position may be difficult for the patient to maintain.
- Assist the patient to the semiprone position on the table or seated facing an upright grid device; the upright position may be more comfortable for the patient; when the patient is recumbent, the arm and leg of the elevated side should be positioned to provide support.
- Position the patient so the ear is centered to the midline of the table or upright grid device.

Part Positioning

- Adjust the head so the midsagittal plane is parallel with the film plane; the patient's body should be rotated to provide support when the patient is recumbent.
- Flex the neck and head so the infraorbitomeatal line is parallel with the transverse axis of the film.
- Adjust the head so the interpupillary line is perpendicular to the film plane. Radiolucent supports may be needed to elevate the thorax of very thin patients; the head of hypersthenic patients may require elevation.
- From the head of the table, recheck the head for rotation; immobilize the head *(Figure 11–37)*.

Central Ray

- Direct the central ray perpendicular to a point midway between the inion and the glabella, approximately 2 in. above the EAM.
- Center the cassette to the central ray. **Note:** If the sella turcica is the primary area of interest, the central ray should be directed perpendicular to a point ¾ in. anterior and ¾ in. superior to the external acoustic meatus.

Breathing Instructions

- Instruct the patient to stop breathing during the exposure.

Image Evaluation

- The vertex, inion, glabella, and C1 should be included within the collimated area.
- The parietal bones should be adequately penetrated without overexposure of the frontal bone.
- The skull should be in the center of the film.
- The temporomandibular joints should be superimposed; the orbital roofs (plates) should also be super-imposed.
- The infraorbitomeatal line and floor of the maxillary sinus should be parallel with the transverse axis of the film (*Figure 11–38*).

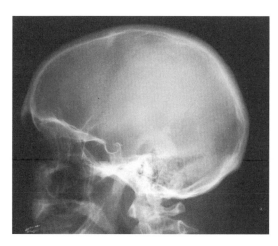 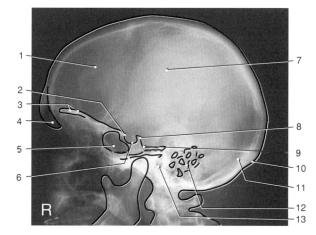

Figure 11–38. Lateral skull.

1. Frontal bone
2. Anterior clinoid processes
3. Orbital roofs
4. Frontal sinuses
5. Sphenoid sinuses

6. Sella turcica, sphenoid bone
7. Parietal bones
8. Dorsum sellae
9. Clivus
10. Inion

11. Occipital bone
12. Mastoid air cells, temporal bone
13. External acoustic meatus (EAM)

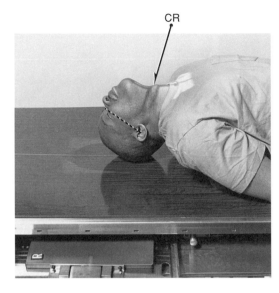

Figure 11–39. Submentovertical skull, recumbent.

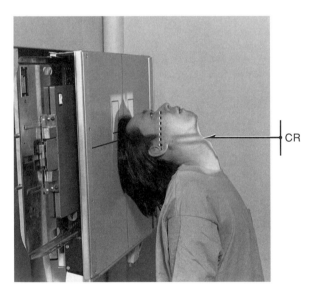

Figure 11–40. Submentovertical skull, erect.

► SUBMENTOVERTICAL (FULL BASAL) SKULL

Technical Considerations

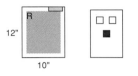

- Film size: 10 × 12 in. lengthwise.
- Grid required.
- 80–85 kVp.
- Collimate to include the nose, ears, and posterior skull.

Caution: Do not hyperextend the neck until a fracture or dislocation of the cervical vertebrae has been ruled out.

Shielding

- Gonadal shielding should be used on all patients, especially children and adults of reproductive age.

Patient Positioning

- Set the technical factors; the position will be difficult for the patient to maintain.
- Assist the patient to the AP seated position in front of the upright grid device; the projection may also be obtained with the patient supine and the torso elevated on radiolucent supports *(Figure 11–39)*.
- Position the patient so the midsagittal plane is centered to the midline of the grid device.

Part Positioning

- Move the cassette approximately to the level of the gonia and direct the central ray horizontally to the midpoint of the cassette; this centering may need to be adjusted after the patient is positioned.
- Hyperextend the patient's neck and head so the infraorbitomeatal line is parallel or nearly parallel with the film plane; rest the vertex against the grid device *(Figure 11–40)*.

Central Ray

- Direct the central ray perpendicular to the infraorbitomeatal line to a point midway between the gonia; if the infraorbitomeatal line is not parallel with the film, the central ray will need to be directed cephalad.
- Center the cassette to the central ray.

Breathing Instructions

• Instruct the patient to stop breathing during the exposure.

Image Evaluation

• The nose, mandible, and lateral and posterior margins of the skull should be included within the collimated area.
• The basilar structures of the cranium should be adequately penetrated and exposed.
• The mandibular condyles should be projected anterior to the petrous portions.
• The distances between the mandibular condyles and the lateral margins of the skull should be equal.
• The petrous portions should be symmetrical (*Figure 11–41*).

Note: When the exposure factors are decreased, this projection can also be used to demonstrate the zygomatic arches; the exact centering is described in Chapter 12.

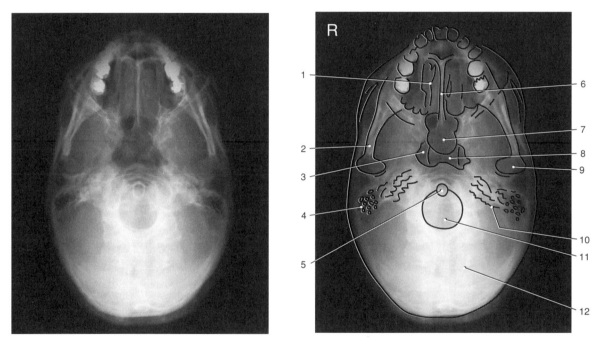

Figure 11–41. Submentovertical skull.

1. Ethmoid sinuses	6. Vomer	10. Petrous pyramid, temporal bone
2. Mandibular ramus	7. Sphenoid sinuses	11. Foramen magnum
3. Pharynx	8. Clivus	12. Occipital bone
4. Mastoid air cells, temporal bone	9. Mandibular condyle	
5. Dens, C1		

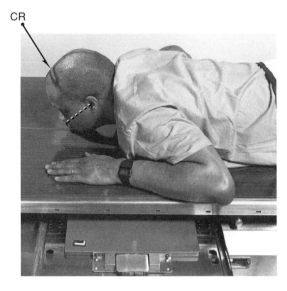

CR

Figure 11–42. Verticosubmental skull.

► VERTICOSUBMENTAL SKULL (VSM)

Technical Considerations

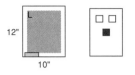

- Film size: 10 × 12 in. lengthwise.
- Grid required.
- 80–85 kVp.
- Collimate to include the nose, ears, and posterior skull.

Caution: Do not hyperextend the neck until a fracture or dislocation of the cervical vertebrae has been ruled out.

Shielding

- Gonadal shielding should be used on all patients, especially children and adults of reproductive age.

Patient Positioning

- Set the technical factors; the position will be difficult for the patient to maintain.
- Assist the patient to the prone position on the radiographic table.
- Position the patient so the midsagittal plane is centered to the midline of the grid device.
- Place the patient's arms in a comfortable position with the hands resting on the table at the level of the neck.

Part Positioning

- Hyperextend the patient's neck and head; rest the patient's head on the chin.
- Adjust the head so the midsagittal plane is perpendicular to the film plane; head clamps can be used for immobilization *(Figure 11–42)*.

Central Ray

- Direct the central ray perpendicular to the infraorbitomeatal line through a plane passing ¾ in. anterior to the EAM; the central ray should pass through the sella turcica. **Note:** This position is a reverse submentovertical projection. Because of the necessary angle of the central ray and the OID of the posterior skull, however, the middle and posterior basilar structures are distorted and exhibit decreased sharpness.
- Center the cassette to the central ray.

Breathing Instructions

- Instruct the patient to stop breathing during the exposure.

Image Evaluation

- The nose, mandible, and lateral margins of the skull should be included within the collimated area.
- The anterior basilar structures of the cranium should be adequately penetrated and exposed.
- The mandibular condyles should be projected anterior to the petrous portions.
- The distance between the mandibular condyles and the lateral margins of the skull should be equal.
- The petrous portions should be symmetrical *(Figure 11–43).*

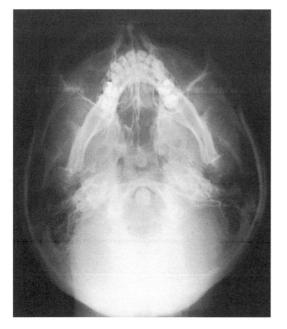
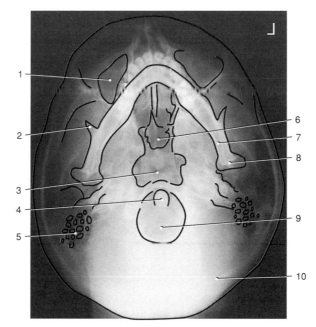

Figure 11–43. Verticosubmental skull.

1. Maxillary sinuses
2. Mandibular coronoid process
3. Pharynx
4. Dens, C2

5. Mastoid air cells, temporal bone
6. Sphenoid sinuses
7. Mandibular ramus

8. Mandibular condyle
9. Foramen magnum
10. Occipital bone

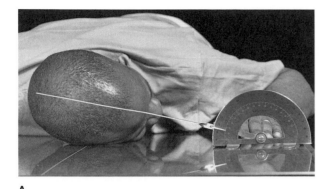

A

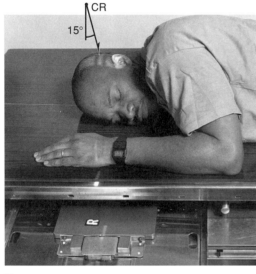

B

Figure 11–44. Modified lateral (Law) for petrous portions.

► MODIFIED LATERAL (LAW) SKULL FOR PETROUS PORTIONS

Technical Considerations

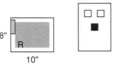

- Film size: 8 × 10 in. crosswise.
- Grid required.
- 65–75 kVp.
- Collimate to a 5 × 6-in. field.

Shielding

- Gonadal shielding should be used on all patients, especially children and adults of reproductive age.

Patient Positioning

- Set the technical factors; the position may be difficult for the patient to maintain.
- Assist the patient to the semiprone position on the table or seated facing an upright grid device with the side of interest nearest the grid device; both sides should be examined for comparison.
- Folding the auricle of the side being examined forward, position the patient so the folded ear is resting against the midline of the table or upright grid device.

Part Positioning

- Rotate the head to place the nose closer to the table; the midsagittal plane should be rotated 15° from a true lateral position. The patient's body should be appropriately rotated to provide support when the patient is recumbent.
- Adjust the head so the interpupillary line is perpendicular with the film plane and the infraorbitomeatal line is parallel with the transverse axis of the film.
- Center the point 1 in. posterior to the EAM of the dependent side to the midline of the table or upright grid device *(Figure 11–44)*.

Central Ray

- Direct the central ray 15° caudad to a point approximately 1 in. posterior and 2 in. superior to the EAM furthest from the film. The central ray should exit at the level of the EAM.
- Center the cassette to the central ray.

Breathing Instructions

- Instruct the patient to stop breathing during the exposure.

Image Evaluation

- The temporomandibular joint and mastoid air cells of the side nearest the film must be included within the collimated area.
- The temporal bone should be adequately penetrated without overexposure of the mastoid air cells.
- The mastoid air cells nearest the table should be in the center of the film.
- The internal and external acoustic (auditory) meatuses should be superimposed *(Figure 11–45)*.

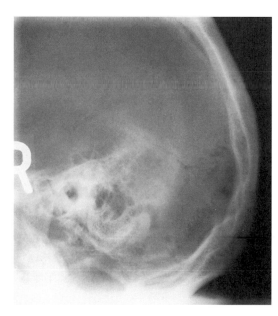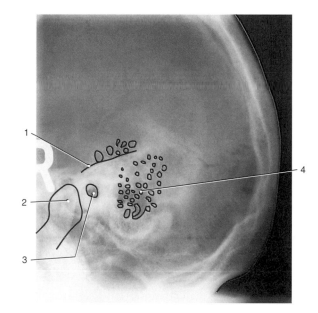

Figure 11–45. Modified lateral (Law) projection.

1. Tegman tympani
2. Mandibular condyle, right
3. External and internal acoustic meati superimposed
4. Mastoid air cells, temporal bone

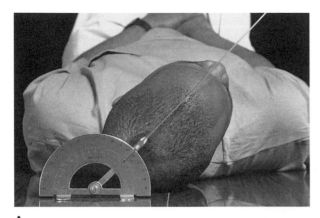

A

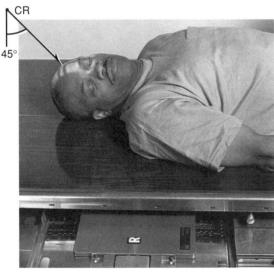

B

Figure 11–46. Axiolateral oblique (Mayer) for petrous portions.

▶ AXIOLATERAL OBLIQUE (MAYER) SKULL FOR PETROUS PORTIONS

Technical Considerations

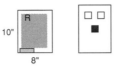

- Film size: 8 × 10 in. lengthwise.
- Grid required.
- 70–80 kVp.
- Collimate to a 5 × 8-in. field size.

Shielding

- Gonadal shielding should be used on all patients, especially children and adults of reproductive age.

Patient Positioning

- Assist the patient to the supine position on the table or seated position with back to an upright grid device; the upright position is more comfortable for the hypersthenic patient.
- Set the technical factors; the position may be difficult for the patient to maintain.

Part Positioning

- Fold the auricles forward and carefully tape to immobilize in this position.
- Rotate the patient's head toward the side of interest until the midsagittal plane forms a 45° angle with the film plane; both sides should be examined for comparison.
- Center the point directly behind the EAM at the junction of the auricle and head to the midline of the grid device.
- Adjust the flexion of the head and neck so the infraorbitomeatal line is parallel with the transverse axis of the film *(Figure 11–46)*.

Central Ray

- Direct the central ray 45° caudad through the EAM nearest the film plane.
- Center the cassette to the central ray.

Breathing Instructions

- Instruct the patient to stop breathing during the exposure.

Image Evaluation

- The temporomandibular joint and mastoid air cells of the side of interest should be included within the collimated area.
- The bony labyrinth should be appropriately penetrated without overexposure of the mastoid air cells.
- The mastoid air cells of the side examined should be in the middle of the collimated area.
- The petrous portion should be perpendicular to the film plane.
- The dependent temporomandibular joint should be seen anterior to the EAM *(Figure 11–47)*.

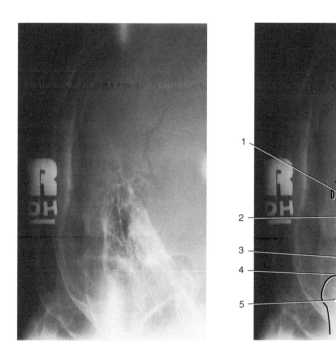

Figure 11–47. Axiolateral oblique (Mayer) projection.

1. Mastoid air cells
2. Mastoid antrum
3. Bony labyrinth
4. External acoustic canal
5. Mandibular condyle

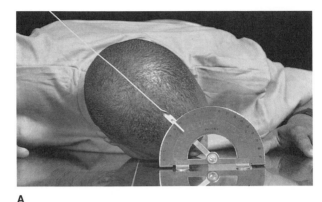

A

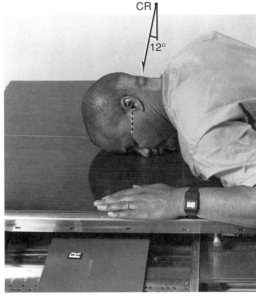

B

Figure 11–48. Posterior profile (Stenvers) for petrous portions.

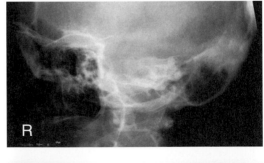

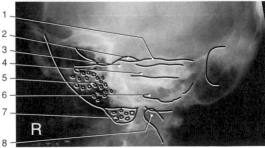

Figure 11–49. Posterior profile (Stenvers) projection.

▶ POSTERIOR PROFILE (STENVERS) SKULL FOR PETROUS PORTIONS

Technical Considerations

- Film size: 8 × 10 in. crosswise.
- Grid required.
- 70–80 kVp.
- Collimate to a 5 × 7-in. field size.

Shielding

- Gonadal shielding should be used on all patients, especially children and adults of reproductive age.

Patient Positioning

- Set the technical factors; the position may be difficult for the patient to maintain.
- Assist the patient to the prone position on the table or seated facing an upright grid device; for patients unable to sit or lie prone, the reverse projection (Arcelin) may be performed as described next.
- Position the patient so the midsagittal plane is centered to and parallel with the long axis of the table or upright grid device; position the arms comfortably with hands near shoulders (on table) or at sides (upright).

Part Positioning

- Position the patient's head on the forehead, nose, and right cheek ("three-point landing"); both sides should be done for comparison.
- Adjust the rotation of the head so the midsagittal plane forms a 45° angle with the film plane; a protractor can be used for accuracy. **Note:** As discussed earlier, the brachycephalic head needs to be rotated slightly less than 45° (more AP) and the dolichocephalic head needs to be rotated more than 45° (more lateral).
- Adjust the head flexion so the infraorbitomeatal line is parallel with the transverse axis of the film.
- Center the point 1 in. directly anterior to the EAM nearest the film to the midpoint of the cassette; immobilize as necessary *(Figure 11–48)*.

Central Ray

- Direct the central ray 12° cephalad, exiting at the point 1 in. anterior to the EAM nearest the film; center the cassette to the central ray.

Breathing Instructions

- Instruct the patient to stop breathing during the exposure.

Image Evaluation

- The mastoid air cells, mastoid process, and lateral margin of the orbit should be included within the collimated area.
- The petrous pyramid should be adequately penetrated without overexposure of the mastoid air cells.
- The mastoid process should be demonstrated in profile, away from the bony structures of the skull and cervical spine.
- The tip of the petrous pyramid should be near the lateral margin of the orbit.
- The petrous ridge should be parallel with the transverse axis of the film *(Figure 11–49)*.

1. Petrous ridge
2. Arcuate eminence
3. Bony labyrinth
4. Internal acoustic canal

5. Mastoid air cells
6. External acoustic meatus and canal

7. Mastoid process
8. Mandibular condyle

▶ ANTERIOR PROFILE (ARCELIN) SKULL FOR PETROUS PORTIONS

Technical Considerations

- Film size: 8 × 10 in. crosswise.
- Grid required.
- 70–80 kVp.
- Collimate to a 5 × 7-in. field size.

Shielding

- Gonadal shielding should be used on all patients, especially children and adults of reproductive age.

Patient Positioning

- Set the technical factors; the position may be difficult for the patient to maintain.
- Assist the patient to the supine position on the table or seated facing an upright grid device.
- Position the patient so the midsagittal plane is centered to and parallel with the long axis of the table or upright grid device; position the arms comfortably at the sides.

Part Positioning

- Rotate the patient's head toward the left side; both sides should be done for comparison.
- Adjust the rotation of the head so the midsagittal plane forms a 45° angle with the film plane; a protractor can be used for accuracy. **Note:** As discussed previously, the brachycephalic head needs to be rotated slightly less than 45° (more AP) and the dolichocephalic head needs to be rotated more than 45° (more lateral).
- Center the point 1-in. directly anterior to the EAM furthest from the film to the midpoint of the cassette.
- Adjust the head flexion so the infraorbitomeatal line is parallel with the transverse axis of the film; immobilize as necessary *(Figure 11–50)*.

Central Ray

- Direct the central ray 10° caudad, entering at the point approximately 1 in. anterior to and 0.75 in. superior to the EAM furthest from the film.
- Center the cassette to the central ray.

Breathing Instructions

- Instruct the patient to stop breathing during the exposure.

Image Evaluation

- The mastoid air cells, mastoid process, and lateral margin of the orbit should be included within the collimated area.
- The petrous pyramid should be adequately penetrated without overexposure of the mastoid air cells.
- The mastoid process should be demonstrated in profile, away from the bony structures of the skull and cervical spine.
- The tip of the petrous pyramid should be near the lateral margin of the orbit.
- The petrous ridge should be parallel with the transverse axis of the film *(Figure 11–51)*.

1. Arcuate eminence
2. Internal acoustic canal
3. Mastoid air cells
4. External acoustic meatus and canal
5. Mastoid process
6. Mandibular condyle

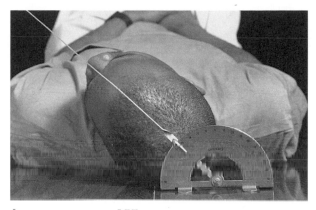

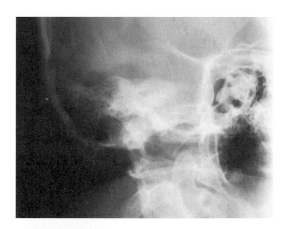

B

Figure 11–50. Anterior profile (Arcelin) for petrous portions.

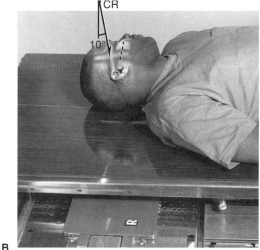

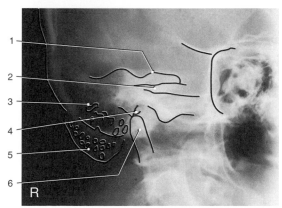

Figure 11–51. Anterior profile (Arcelin) projection.

SUMMARY

▶ Although radiographic examinations may be performed with the patient recumbent or erect using a dedicated head unit or other vertical grid device, the upright position may be more comfortable for the patient.

▶ The routine examination of the skull typically includes the AP axial, PA, and lateral projections.

▶ Specific positioning lines and planes should be used for accurate patient positioning.

▶ An individual's head may be described as mesocephalic, brachycephalic, or dolichocephalic, depending on the shape; the average-shaped head is called mesocephalic.

▶ An adjustment in routine patient positioning may be required for those patients with a brachycephalic or dolichocephalic head shape.

▶ Cervical spine fractures or dislocations must be ruled out before moving or manipulating the head.

▶ A cross-table lateral skull projection, using a horizontal beam, can be used to detect fluid in the sphenoid sinus.

▶ The verticosubmental or submentovertical projection can be used to demonstrate the pars petrosae and other basilar skull structures.

▶ Although CT is usually requested for examination of the mastoids, traditional radiography of the mastoids is still occasionally requested.

▶ To minimize the possibility of motion, patients should be instructed to stop breathing for all examinations of the skull.

▶ Because the skull is relatively dense, a moderate kVp, 65 to 85, is recommended.

▶ A grid is recommended for all skull radiography.

QUESTIONS FOR CRITICAL THINKING & APPLICATION

1. Which of the senses would be impaired if a person had no holes in the cribriform plate of the ethmoid bone? Explain your answer.

2. When reading a skull series, the radiologist noticed an irregularity of the sella turcica. Discuss the implications of this abnormality, to include the important structure(s) affected.

3. What role does the ethmoid bone play in the structural formation of the nasal cavity?

4. Suppose the temporal bones were not fully developed in a person. What possible problems might result from this defect?

5. A patient stated that he was changing a fuse in his basement when he stumbled in the dark and struck the side of his head against a metal support column. On radiographic examination, he was told that he had a small depressed skull fracture. What role does diploe play in a such a fracture? Given the patient's history, which bone was most likely injured?

6. When evaluating an AP axial skull radiograph, you are unable to see the dorsum sellae, and the foramen magnum is obscured by the sinuses. Describe your positioning error.

7. Your patient is suffering from an uncontrollable, severe nosebleed. Describe the best way to obtain the routine skull radiographs.

8. Having been involved in a car accident, your patient has sustained trauma to the forehead and neck. The patient is lying on a stretcher with sandbags on either side of the head when she arrives in the radiology department. Because the clinical neurologic examination suggests a possible cervical spine fracture, you are instructed to obtain all films without moving the patient. Describe the projections you would obtain for a skull series, including patient positioning and central ray angles, if appropriate.

9. The radiologist has requested just one radiograph of the internal acoustic canals. If given a choice, which projection would you obtain to best demonstrate this structure? Justify your answer.

10. When assessing your patient prior to radiographing the mastoids, you determine that the head has a dolichocephalic shape. Describe how you would modify the head positioning for the axiolateral oblique and posterior profile projections.

FILM CRITIQUE

Evaluate the positioning accuracy of this lateral skull radiograph *(Figure 11–52)*.

How did you determine accuracy or error?

Which positioning lines or planes should be used?

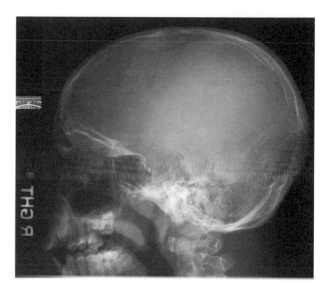

Figure 11–52.

12

FACIAL BONES & PARANASAL SINUSES

► OBJECTIVES

Following the completion of this chapter the student will be able to:

- Given diagrams, radiographs, or dry bones, name and describe the bones of the face.

- Discuss the location and structural makeup of the four groups of paranasal sinuses.

- Describe the bony construction of the orbits, to include a discussion of their shape and placement within the cranium, as well as their openings.

- Classify the articulations between the facial bones according to structure and identify their type of movement, if applicable.

- Explain the rationale for performing a radiographic examination of the paranasal sinuses using the upright position and a horizontal beam.

- Describe procedural modifications that might be helpful when radiographing the facial bones in a trauma situation and when specific pathology is suspected.

- Discuss the positioning modifications necessary to demonstrate either the ramus or the body of the mandible.

- State the criteria used to determine positioning accuracy on radiographs of the facial bones, paranasal sinuses, and optic foramina and evaluate radiographs of the facial bones, paranasal sinuses, and optic foramina in terms of positioning, centering, image quality, radiographic anatomy, and pathology.

- Define terminology associated with the facial bones, paranasal sinuses, and optic foramina, to include anatomy, procedures, and pathology.

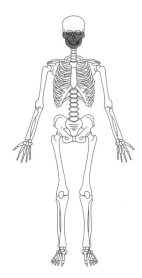

Figure 12–1. The facial bones.

► ANATOMY OF THE FACIAL BONES

The facial bones form in the fetus through the process of intramembranous ossification. They continue to grow after birth and reach full maturity around age 16. The facial bones form the structural frame of the face, which, to some extent, defines a person's facial appearance *(Figure 12–1)*. For example, the facial structure of a female is generally more rounded and less angular than that of a male.

There are a total of 14 facial bones, which include 6 paired bones (maxillae, zygomatic bones, nasal bones, lacrimal bones, palatine bones, inferior nasal conchae) and two single bones (vomer and mandible) *(Table 12–1)*. In addition to assisting in the formation of mouth, nasal cavity, and orbits, the facial bones serve to protect those structures housed within them, such as the eyes and the entrances to the digestive and respiratory tracts. They are irregularly shaped bones that provide attachment sites for the muscles which allow a person to smile, frown, squint, and make many other facial expressions ranging from happiness to anger *(Figure 12–2)*.

MAXILLA

The paired maxillae (mak-SIL-e) (singular, maxilla) or maxillary bones are the largest immovable bones of the face. Like the sphenoid of the cranial bones, the maxillae form the anchor or keystone of the facial skeleton as they articulate with every facial bone except the mandible. They assist in the formation of the floor of each orbit, lateral wall and floor of the nasal cavity, and majority of the roof of the mouth. Each maxilla consists of a body and four processes: frontal, zygomatic, alveolar, and palatine *(Figure 12–3)*.

The **body** of each maxilla is a boxlike area in the central portion of the bone. Situated laterally to the nose, it forms a portion of the cheek. It contains a large air-filled cavity above the teeth, the **maxillary sinus,** which communicates with the nasal cavity. The **infraorbital foramen** is a small hole located just below the infraorbital margin. It allows for the passage of the infraorbital nerve and artery to the face. The **inferior orbital fissure** is an elongated opening located within the floor of the orbit. It is formed between the maxilla, zygoma, and the greater wing of the sphenoid. The zygomatic nerve and blood vessels are trans-

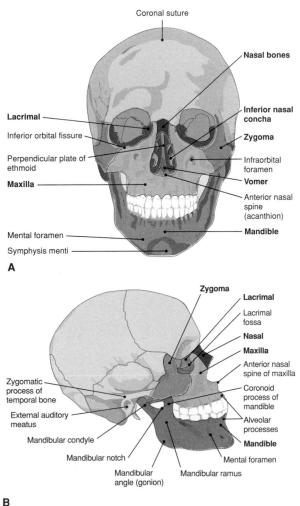

A

B

Figure 12–2. Facial bone mass: **(A)** anterior aspect, **(B)** lateral aspect.

Table 12–1. Summary of the Facial Skeleton

Facial Bones	Description
Maxilla (2)	• Anchor bone of facial skeleton • Maxillary sinus • Four processes: frontal, zygomatic, alveolar, palatine • Anterior nasal spine = acanthion
Palatine (2)	• Horizontal and vertical plates • Hard palate • Lateral walls of nasal cavity
Zygomatic (2)	• Malar bone • Cheekbone • Three processes: frontal, maxillary, temporal • Forms part of zygomatic arch
Lacrimal (2)	• Medial orbital wall • Lacrimal fossa/tear duct
Nasal (2)	• Bridge of nose • Frontonasal suture = nasion
Inferior nasal concha (2)	• Turbinate • Scroll-shaped shelf projecting into nasal cavity
Vomer (1)	• Plow-shaped • Part of bony nasal septum

Mandible (1)	• Lower jawbone
	• Horseshoe-shaped
	• Body
	    Alveolar process
	    Mental protuberance/mental point
	• Two rami
	    Coronoid process
	    Condyloid process (head)
	    Mandibular notch

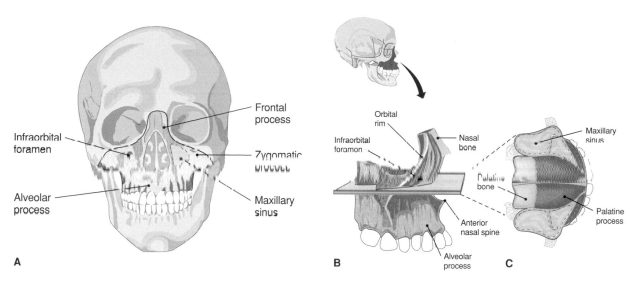

Figure 12–3. Maxillae: **(A)** frontal aspect, **(B)** lateral aspect, **(C)** cross-sectional aspect.

mitted to the maxillary and zygomatic area of the face via this opening. The bodies of the maxillae meet at the midsagittal plane and fuse solidly together early in life. At the upper border of their junction, a small, pointed structure known as the **anterior nasal spine** is formed. It can be palpated just at the base of the nasal septum.

The **frontal process** of the maxilla projects upward from the body to lie between the medial margin of the orbit and the lateral margin of the nose. It articulates with the frontal, nasal, and lacrimal bones. The **zygomatic process** extends laterally from the body of the maxilla to articulate with the zygomatic bone, where it forms part of the prominence of the cheek. The **alveolar** (al-VE-o-lar) **process** is a thick, spongy area on the inferior aspect of the body. Together, the two alveolar processes form the horseshoe-shaped upper jawbone in which the upper teeth are embedded. The **palatal** or **palatine process** extends horizontally and medially from the lower part of the body. It meets the palatine process of the other maxilla at the midline to form the anterior three fourths of the hard palate or roof of the mouth, which separates the nasal and oral cavities. The fusion of these processes usually takes place prior to birth. If this does not happen, a congenital defect known as **cleft palate** occurs in which there is an opening between the palatine processes of the maxillae, occasionally involving the palatine bones, and the lip. The condition is surgically repaired before the child begins to talk around the age of 1 or 2.

PALATINE BONES

Each of the paired palatine (PAL-ah-tin) bones is L-shaped to include a vertical plate and a horizontal plate. The **horizontal plate** is the lower foot of the "L" and extends medially from the vertical plate. It articulates at the midline with its counterpart on the other palatine bone and anteriorly with the palatine process of the maxilla to form the posterior one fourth of the hard palate. The **vertical plate** is the upward projection of the "L." It extends between the maxilla and the pterygoid plate of the sphenoid to form the posterior part of the lateral walls of the nasal cavity and a very small portion of the orbital floor *(Figure 12–4)*.

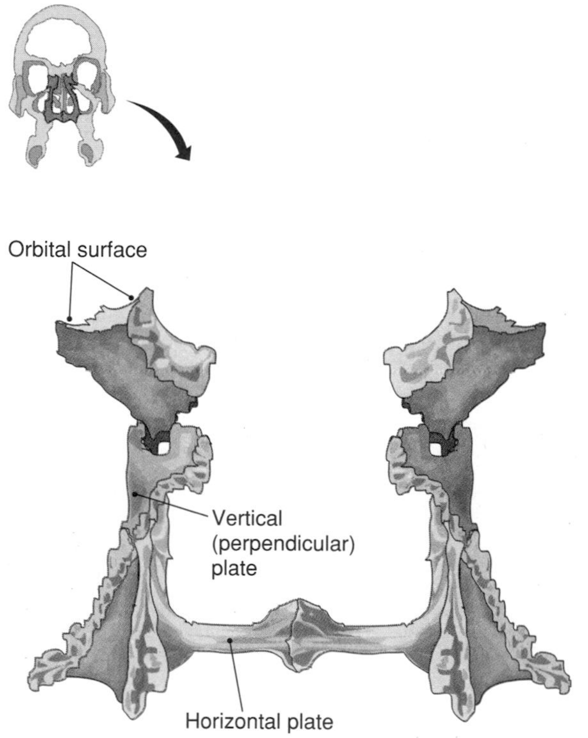

ZYGOMATIC BONES

The zygomatic (ZI-go-mat-ik) or malar (MA-lar) bones are typically called the cheekbones. Each zygomatic bone is an irregularly shaped bone that is roughly four-sided. In addition to forming the prominence of the cheek, it makes up the inferolateral wall and floor of the orbit. It consists of three processes, which are named according to the bone with which they articulate. The **frontal process** articulates with the frontal bone at the upper, lateral margin of the orbit. The **maxillary process** at the lower, medial portion of the bone joins the zygomatic process of the maxilla. The **temporal process** projects posteriorly to articu-

Figure 12–4. Palatine bones: posterior aspect of both palatine bones demonstrating their "L" shape.

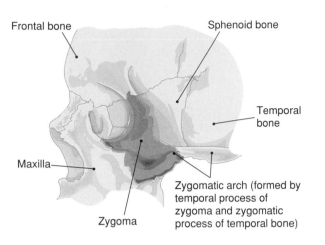

Figure 12–5. Articulations of the zygomatic (malar) bone are demonstrated on a lateral view.

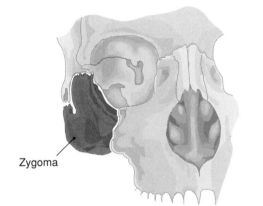

A

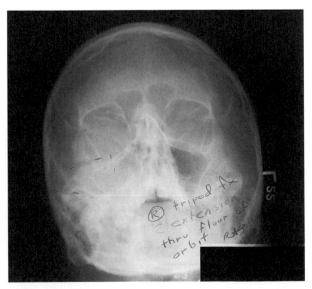

B

Figure 12–6. "Tripod" fracture affects the zygomatic bone at its attachment points as illustrated on **(A)** an anterior view and **(B)** parietoacanthial projection.

late with the zygomatic process of the temporal bone to form the delicate zygomatic arch. The zygomatic bone also articulates posteriorly with the sphenoid bone *(Figure 12–5)*. A blow aimed directly at the cheek can result in a depressed fracture of the zygomatic arch or cause the zygomatic bone to become severed from its attachments with the frontal, maxilla, and temporal bones, or "free-floating." This is known as a **tripod fracture** *(Figure 12–6)*.

LACRIMAL BONES

The lacrimal (LAK-ri-mal) bones (*lacrima* = "tears") are the smallest of the facial bones. They are delicate, flat bones that roughly approximate a fingernail in shape and size. Each lacrimal bone is located in the anterior part of the medial orbital wall between the maxilla anteriorly, ethmoid posteriorly, and frontal bone superiorly. The **lacrimal fossa** is a cavity on the bone's anterior surface that houses the lacrimal sac. A groove between the anterior portion of the lacrimal bone and the maxilla serves as a passageway for the nasolacrimal duct through which tears drain into the nasal cavity *(Figure 12–7)*.

NASAL BONES

The right and left nasal (NA-zal) bones lie side-by-side and articulate at the midsagittal plane to form the upper portion of the bridge of the nose. Each of the paired nasal bones is small, rectangular, and flat. There is a great deal of variation in size between individuals. The nasal bone lies medial to and articulates with the frontal process of the maxilla. It is located just inferior to the frontal bone. The articulation of the two nasal bones with the frontal bone is called the **frontonasal suture** and is the location of the **nasion,** a positioning landmark. Both nasal bones also join the perpendicular plate of the ethmoid bone posteriorly inside the skull. They attach inferiorly to cartilage which forms the distal structure of the nose. The bony nasal septum lies posteriorly to the junction of the two nasal bones on the midline *(Figure 12–8)*.

INFERIOR NASAL CONCHAE

The right and left inferior nasal conchae (KONG-ke) (singular, choncha) or turbinates are similar to the superior and middle nasal conchae of the ethmoid bone, but are larger and separate from those structures. They are readily visible on an AP or PA projection of the skull. Each inferior nasal concha (*concha* = "shell") is a thin, curved bone with a scroll-like appearance. Like a shelf, it extends medially into the nasal cavity from the lower third of the lateral wall formed by the maxilla. The **lacrimal** and **ethmoid processes** are located on the superior border of each inferior nasal concha. The lacrimal process attaches to the lacrimal bone and assists in the formation of the bony lacrimal canal. The ethmoid process joins the ethmoid bone superiorly. The inferior nasal conchae serve the same function as the superior and middle nasal conchae—to warm, moisten, and filter the inspired air before it reaches the lungs. Together, the superior, middle, and inferior nasal conchae divide the nasal cavity into compartments. The space or area between the nasal septum and the conchae is called the **common nasal meatus** *(Figure 12–9)*.

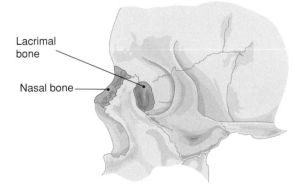

Figure 12–7. Lacrimal and nasal bones.

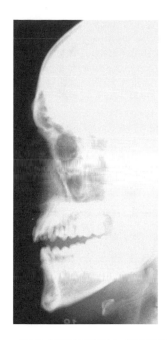

Figure 12–8. Lateral projection demonstrates the superimposed nasal bones, frontonasal suture, and superimposed anterior nasal spines of the maxillae.

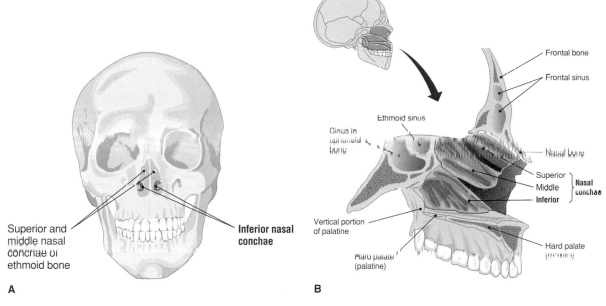

A

B

Figure 12–9. Inferior nasal conchae: **(A)** anterior aspect, **(B)** sagittal section.

VOMER

The single vomer (VO-mer) is a thin, somewhat plow-shaped bone (*vomer* = "plowshare") which is roughly triangular with three borders: anterior, posterior, and inferior. It is oriented vertically in the nasal cavity and forms the inferior and posterior portions of the bony nasal septum. The superior portion of the posterior border of the vomer articulates with the sphenoid bone, whereas the superior portion of its anterior border articulates with the perpendicular plate of the ethmoid bone. From this point, the anterior border of the vomer slants inferiorly and anteriorly so that the inferior border rests on the upper surface of the hard palate, where it articulates with parts of the maxillary and palatine bones.

The **nasal septum** is a partition that divides the nasal cavity into right and left sides. It consists of a bony portion and a cartilaginous portion. The bony portion comprises the perpendicular plate of the ethmoid bone superiorly and the vomer inferiorly and posteriorly. Septal cartilage articulates with the bony portion anteriorly. When the nasal septum is deviated or moved out of place as a result of injury, one side of the nasal cavity becomes smaller than the other. The nasal passageways may become blocked, resulting in the person having difficulty breathing through the nose. Oftentimes, this problem contributes to sleep disorders *(Figure 12–10)*.

MANDIBLE

The mandible (MAN-di-b'l) is the single U-shaped bone that forms the lower jawbone. Not only is it the largest and strongest bone in the face, it is the only movable bone. It consists of three main parts: a body and two rami.

The **body** is the horizontal portion of the mandible. During fetal development and early infancy, the mandible is actually separated into two equal halves joined at the midline by a fibrous joint. The halves are solidly united when the joint ossifies completely by the age of 1. The only remnant of the fusion is a small, vertical ridge on the midline called the **symphysis menti,** which terminates at the flat, triangular surface on the chin known as the **mentum** (*mentum* = "chin") or **mental protuberance.** The midpoint of this area is a positioning landmark known as the **mental point.** The superior border of the body, the **alveolar process,** is a spongy ridge in which the lower teeth are embedded. The **mental foramina** are located at the lateral aspects of the body under the alveolar process. Blood vessels and nerves are transmitted through these openings to the chin.

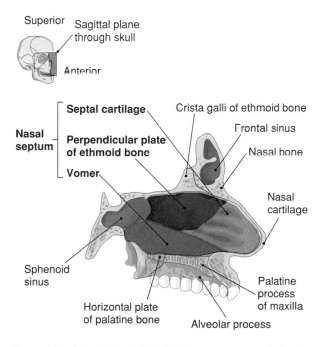

Figure 12–10. Sagittal section of the facial bone mass demonstrating the nasal septum and surrounding structures.

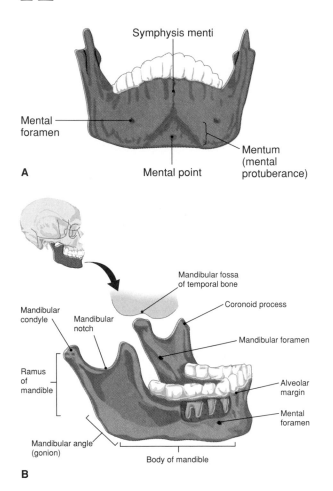

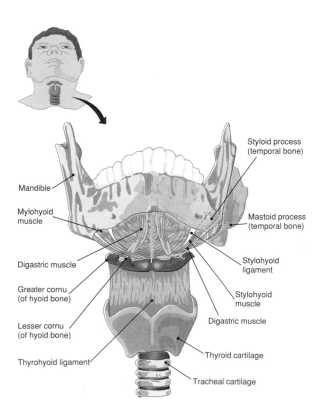

Figure 12–12. Hyoid bone is located between the mandible and larynx in the anterior portion of the neck.

Figure 12–11. Mandible: **(A)** frontal view, **(B)** oblique view.

The **rami** (RA-mi) (singular, ramus) are the two ascending or vertical portions of the mandible. Each ramus meets the body at the **mandibular angle** or **gonion** (GO-ne-on). The superior part of the ramus consists of two processes separated by a concave, half-moon-shaped **mandibular notch.** The anterior process is known as the **coronoid process.** Thin and tapered in structure, it serves as the attachment point for the temporalis muscle, which moves the mandible and opens the mouth. The posterior **condyloid process** comprises a rounded head called the **condyle** and a more inferior constricted **neck.** The head of the condyle is that portion of the mandible that articulates with the mandibular fossa of the temporal bone to form the temporomandibular joint. A **mandibular foramen** is located on the inner surface of the lower half of each ramus. It is the origin of the mandibular canal, which passes anteriorly below the roots of the teeth to terminate at the mental foramen. Blood vessels and nerves are transmitted through the canal to the lower teeth. Prior to working on the lower teeth, dentists often anesthetize the nerves in this area *(Figure 12–11).*

HYOID BONE

The hyoid (HI-oid) bone is a small bone situated at the base of the tongue. Although it is a component of the axial skeleton, it is not actually part of the vertebral column, skull, or facial bone mass. It does not articulate with any other bone in the skeleton and is quite mobile. Located between the mandible and the larynx in the anterior portion of the neck, the hyoid bone is suspended from the styloid process of each temporal bone *(Figure 12–12).* It comprises a curved, anterior body, two greater cornua or horns *(cornua =* "horns"), which extend posteriorly from the body, and two small lesser cornua or horns, which extend from the greater cornua *(Figure 12–13).* Muscles and ligaments attach to the hyoid bone to allow the larynx to move during speech and deglutition (swallowing). The hyoid bone is demonstrated radiographically on a lateral soft tissue neck or cervical spine projection.

ORBITS

The orbits are bony cavities in the skull that house the organs of vision, as well as the lacrimal glands and muscles that move the eyeball. Each orbit is cone-shaped with a base and apex. The outer rim of the orbit, encompassing the frontal, maxilla, and zygomatic bone, forms the **base.** As the base is closer in shape to a square than a circle, the orbit structurally has a roof, floor, and medial and lateral walls. A total of seven cranial and facial bones contribute to the composition of each orbit. The roof of the orbit is formed by the frontal and sphenoid bones. The floor is formed by the maxilla, zygomatic, and palatine bones. The medial wall is formed by the sphenoid bone, ethmoid bone, maxilla, and lacrimal bone. The lateral wall is formed by the sphenoid and zygomatic bones. *Table 12–2* summarizes the locations of the bones forming the orbit.

From the base, the bony orbit projects 30° superiorly and 37° medially into the skull to its posterior end, or **apex.** The **optic foramen** is the circular opening to the optic canal seen at the apex of the orbit *(Figure 12–14).* Two other openings seen within each orbit are the superior orbital fissure and the inferior orbital fissure. The **superior orbital fissure** is a split on the sphenoid bone between the greater and lesser wings. It lies laterally to and is separated from the optic foramen by a small piece of bone called the **sphenoid strut.** The **inferior orbital fissure** is formed between the greater wing of the sphenoid bone, maxilla, and zygomatic bone at the point where the floor and lateral wall meet. *Figure 12–15* illustrates the position of each of the seven bones in the formation of the orbit.

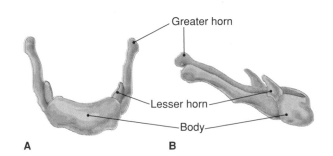

Figure 12–13. Hyoid bone: **(A)** anterior aspect, **(B)** lateral aspect.

Table 12–2. Bony Composition of the Orbit

Roof	Floor	Medial Wall	Lateral Wall
	Maxilla	Sphenoid	
Frontal	Zygoma	Ethmoid	Sphenoid
Sphenoid	Palatine	Maxilla	Zygomatic
		Lacrimal	

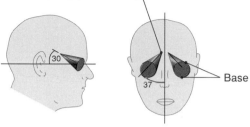

Figure 12–14. Orientation of the cone-shaped orbits.

Blunt trauma to the face directly over the orbit pushes the fluid-filled eyeball downward where it can break through the maxilla in the floor of the orbit. Directly below the site of the fracture, the maxillary sinus fills with blood from the injury. This type of fracture, known as a **blow-out fracture,** generally occurs from a solid punch to the eye or contact with a baseball. It is demonstrated radiographically on a modified parietoacanthial (Waters) projection, with the affected sinus exhibiting a cloudy, opaque appearance *(Figure 12–16).*

ARTHROLOGY

With the exception of the mandible, the facial bones articulate with one another and the cranial bones to form synarthrodial joints called *sutures.* As described in Chapter 11, these are fibrous, immovable joints named for the articulating bones, such as the frontonasal and maxillopalatine sutures *(Figure 12–17).*

Gomphoses are synarthrodial joints formed by the articulation of the teeth with the mandible and maxillae. The roots of the teeth are embedded in bony sockets and held in place by fibrous ligaments. Thus, they are immovable, fibrous joints *(Figure 12–18).*

The mandible forms the only two movable joints in the cranium as its condyles articulate with the mandibular fossae of the temporal bones to form the right and left **temporomandibular joints.** These joints are classified as diarthrodial. They are synovial in structure, allowing both hinge and gliding movements *(Figure 12–19). Table 12–3* summarizes the joints involving the bones of the facial skeleton.

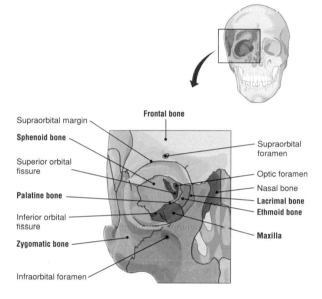

Figure 12–15. Bony composition of an orbit.

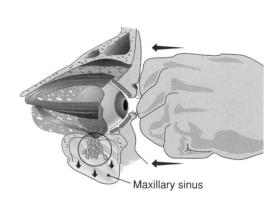

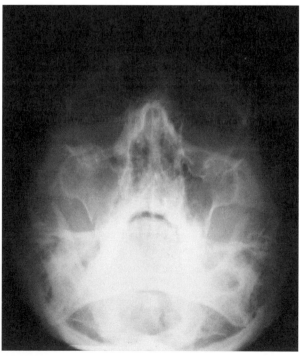

Figure 12–16. Effect of a "blow-out" fracture on the orbit. **(A)** A lateral view demonstrates mechanism of injury. **(B)** Fracture is demonstrated on the right orbit on a parietoacanthial projection.

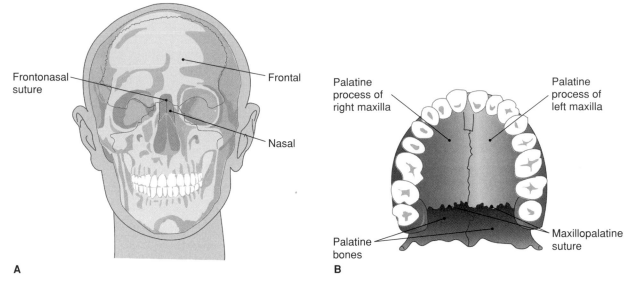

Figure 12–17. Examples of synarthrodial joints formed by the facial bones are the **(A)** frontonasal and **(B)** maxillopalatine sutures.

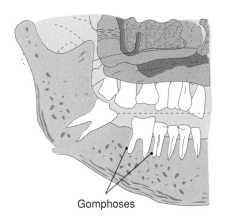

Figure 12–18. Gomphoses formed by the articulation of the teeth with the maxillae and mandible.

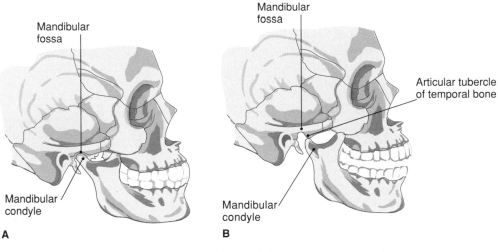

Figure 12–19. Temporomandibular joints allow both hinge and gliding movements. **(A)** Closed mouth. **(B)** Open mouth.

Table 12–3. Summary of Joints Involving the Facial Bones

Name	Classification	Structure	Movement
Sutures	Synarthrodial	Fibrous	Immovable
Gomphoses	Synarthrodial	Fibrous	Immovable
Temporomandibular	Diarthrodial	Synovial	Hinge/gliding

▶ ANATOMY OF THE PARANASAL SINUSES

The paranasal (*para* = "beside") sinuses are air-filled cavities in the frontal, sphenoid, ethmoid, and maxillary bones of the skull and face as illustrated in *Figure 12–20*. These mucus-lined chambers begin to form during fetal development as small sacs that grow and gradually encroach on the diploe in the bone so that cavities are formed between the inner and outer tables. All of the paranasal sinuses are adjacent to and communicate with the nasal cavity. Therefore, the mucosal lining is continuous in each of the sinuses and with the nasal cavity. The sinuses serve to lighten the total weight of the skull, warm and humidify air before it passes to the lungs, and intensify the resonance of the voice.

The paired **frontal sinuses** are located behind the glabella in the squamosal portion of the frontal bone. Although they can be described as being somewhat pyramidal in shape, their size and shape vary greatly so that they are generally not symmetric. Multiple septa may divide them into smaller subcompartments. In some cases, the frontal sinuses may be absent altogether.

The **ethmoid sinuses** are situated between the nasal cavity and each orbit. If a person pinched the bridge of his or her nose by placing the thumb of one hand in the corner of one orbit and the index finger in the other orbit, the ethmoid sinuses would lie in the area between those digits. The sinuses are located in the lateral masses or labyrinths of the ethmoid bone. Each one consists of three groups of air cells named according to their position: anterior, middle, and posterior. The number of cells varies per group and also per individual, ranging from 3 to 18. The ethmoid sinuses are also referred to as ethmoidal air cells.

The **sphenoid sinus** may or may not be paired depending on the presence of a thin bony septum dividing the air-filled cavity in the body of the sphenoid bone. This cavity is located directly below the sella turcica and extends from the area of the posterior ethmoid air cells to the dorsum sellae. Because the sphenoid sinus is so close to the base of the skull, blood or cerebrospinal fluid may seep through a basal skull fracture into the sinus. A cross-table lateral projection of the skull will demonstrate an air–fluid level in the sphenoid sinus in this case.

The paired **maxillary sinuses** are located in the body of each maxilla posteriorly to the cheek. They are also known as the **antra of Highmore** or simply **antra** (singular, antrum) (*antro* = "cavity"). Normally symmetrical in shape, they can be described as pyramidal, although they appear somewhat boxlike on a lateral projection. The pointed apices of maxillary sinuses project laterally and inferiorly so that the roots of the upper teeth are in close proximity to the antral floors. As a result, an infection of an upper tooth can spread to the maxillary sinus. Occasionally, the floor of the sinus is disturbed when one of the upper teeth is pulled.

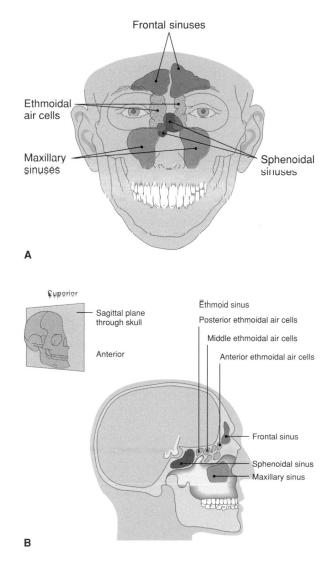

Figure 12–20. Paranasal sinuses: **(A)** frontal aspect, **(B)** sagittal section.

▶ PROCEDURAL CONSIDERATIONS

Although numerous projections can be used to demonstrate the sinuses and facial bones, many are modifications of the basic skull projections discussed in Chapter 11. Sometimes all that is necessary is a change in technical factors, as when the submentovertical projection is used for demonstration of the zygomatic arches. In any case, precise patient positioning is critical for accurate diagnosis.

PATIENT PREPARATION

After being correctly identified, the patient should be instructed to remove all metallic objects, including eyeglasses, jewelry, and dental appliances (eg, dentures, retainers) from the head and neck area. Special care should be taken to ensure that all hairpins, barrettes, and elastic bands are removed from the hair. Buttons or zippers on the shirt collar should be moved away from the head and neck area.

As discussed in Chapter 11, any surface that might be touched by the patient's face should be cleaned with appropriate cleaning/disinfecting solutions. This should be done either in front of the patient or immediately prior to the patient entering the room, so the surface smells freshly cleaned; the bottle of cleaning solution can also be kept in a spot visible to the patient. In addition, the radiographer's hands must be thoroughly washed immediately prior to touching the patient's head; disposable gloves should be worn, if warranted.

As for all radiographic examinations, a pertinent patient history is important for accurate diagnosis. In the case of sinus and facial bone examinations when a single lateral projection is usually obtained, a pertinent patient history helps in determining which lateral to perform.

POSITIONING CONSIDERATIONS

Although patient comfort is important when positioning any body part, it becomes more critical when positioning the head. Unnecessary stress on the muscles can prevent the patient from maintaining the correct position. Taking the time to make sure the patient is as comfortable as possible will contribute to better-quality radiographs. To ensure that the part is straight on the film, care should be taken to place the long axis of the patient's body parallel with the long axis of the table or upright grid device.

Although all radiography of the skull and facial bones can be performed with the patient either erect or recumbent, radiographic examinations of the sinuses should be performed with the patient upright for the demonstration of air–fluid levels. A true horizontal beam is preferred; however, it may not be possible for all projections. The PA projection, for example, requires either a 15° caudal angle or angulation of the cassette in a head unit or other upright grid device. The routine sinus examination generally includes the PA (Caldwell), parietoacanthial (Waters), and single lateral projections; when the lateral projection is obtained, the affected side should be nearest the film. The lateral sinus projection is the only one that demonstrates all paranasal sinuses *(Table 12–4)*. The parietoacanthial projection is frequently performed with the patient's mouth open to demonstrate the sphenoid sinuses through the open mouth. The submentovertical (SMV) projection can also be obtained to demonstrate the sphenoid sinuses.

The projections included in the facial bone series can vary tremendously, but the routine series frequently includes the parietoacanthial (Waters), PA (Caldwell), and single lateral projections; again, the side of interest is nearest the film for the lateral projection. This series may also include the SMV projection and various other projections for evaluation of specific facial bones (see *Table 12–4*).

For accurate diagnosis of fractures or other pathology related to the orbits, the superior and inferior orbital fissures, optic foramina, wings of the sphenoid, and ethmoidal air cells must be clearly demonstrated. When the orbits are radiographed, a modified parietoacanthial projection, achieved by adjusting the head flexion so the orbitomeatal line forms a 37° to 55° angle with the film, is often substituted for the standard Waters projection to better demonstrate the orbital floors. Bilateral parieto-orbital oblique (Rhese) projections may also be obtained as part of the routine series. For this projection, the central ray should be collimated to include both orbits. When using a "hot light," the radiologist can evaluate the orbital rim of the orbit furthest from the film, as well as the opposite orbit. Although the parieto-orbital oblique (Rhese) projection was originally developed for demonstration of the optic foramina, it is seldom performed for this purpose today; CT and MRI are far superior for evaluation of the optic nerves and canals.

Prior to MRI examination of the head, an orbital series is often obtained to rule out a foreign body. When a foreign body is suspected in the eye, the patient should be instructed to close the eyes and hold them in a fixed position during the exposure. As an alternative to traditional radiographic approaches to the localization of foreign objects in the eye, ultrasound and CT are frequently used. MRI, however, is contraindicated because of the strong magnetic fields and the potential for further damage.

Radiographic examination of the mandible can be quite challenging for the radiographer. Numerous positioning techniques can be used to obtain comparable images; no single technique is necessarily better than another. The position and method used often depend on the condition of the patient and available equip-

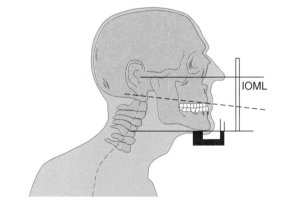

Figure 12–21. Axiolateral oblique mandible obtained with the patient supine.

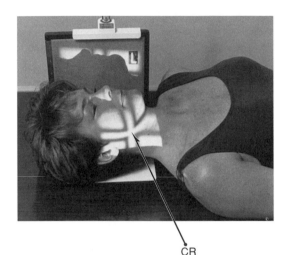

A

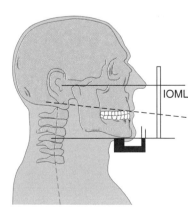

B

Figure 12–22. Careful patient positioning is required when obtaining panoramic radiographs of the mandible. Incorrect **(A)** and correct **(B)** patient positions.

Table 12–4. Routine/Optional Projections: Sinuses and Facial Bones

Sinuses	Orbits
PA/AP erect	Parietoacanthial (Waters)
Lateral erect	Lateral
Parietoacanthial (Waters) erect	Parieto-orbital oblique (Rhese)[a]
Submentovertical[a] erect	PA (25° caudal angle)[a]
Facial Bones	Optic Foramina[a]
PA/AP	Parieto-orbital oblique (Rhese)
Lateral	Mandible
Parietoacanthial (Waters)	PA
Submentovertical[a]	Axiolateral oblique
Zygomatic Arches	PA/AP axial[a]
Submentovertical or tangential	Submentovertical[a]
Parietoacanthial (Waters)	Panorex[a]
Superoinferior (Titterington)[a]	Temporomandibular Joints
AP axial (Grashey/Towne)[a]	Axiolateral or axiolateral oblique (open/closed)
Nasal Bones	PA/AP axial (exaggerated)[a]
Parietoacanthial (Waters)	Panorex[a]
Lateral(s)	Tomography[a]
PA (Caldwell)[a]	

Note. Although there are many modifications of these projections that can be used, this table lists most of the basic ones used for the sinuses and facial bones.

[a]Optional projections/examinations that may be routine in some departments.

ment. Although a head unit or upright cassette holder capable of angulation is often the easiest method, the condition of the patient and/or availability of the equipment often preclude this method. The standard "text-book" method is also frequently contraindicated because of patient condition. Patients unable to sit or turn from the supine position must be radiographed using a cross-table technique *(Figure 12–21)*.

Radiographic examination of the temporomandibular joints is performed bilaterally with the mouth open and closed (four exposures). The films must be clearly marked with right or left and open or closed markers. For consistent patient positioning a sterilized bite block can be placed between the patient's teeth for the open-mouth projections. CT may be performed as an alternative to this traditional method.

TRAUMA CONSIDERATIONS

Facial fractures can be the result of motor vehicle accidents or localized trauma, such as impact by a hard object or fist. The swelling and/or hemorrhage that accompany facial fractures can make imaging difficult. In addition, associated skull or spinal injury may prohibit moving the head into the necessary positions. In severe cases, anteroposterior and cross-table projections have to be substituted for the routine posteroanterior and lateral projections. Because trauma to the mandible, especially a displaced fracture, often results in a second fracture of the mandible or dislocation of the temporomandibular joint (TMJ), imaging of the entire mandible, including both TMJs, is necessary for a thorough diagnosis. Traditional tomography or CT may be necessary to evaluate the TMJs or orbital fractures.

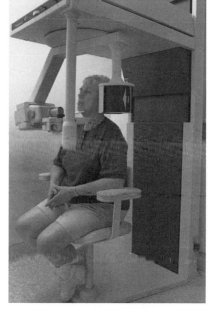

Figure 12–23. Panelipse unit.

ALTERNATE PROJECTIONS

The **panorex** or **panolipse,** a type of tomographic unit, employs a special technique to tomograph curved surfaces, like the mandible. A dedicated radiographic unit is required and may be one of two types. In one type, the patient and film rotate before a stationary x-ray tube. In the second type, the patient is stationary, and the x-ray tube and film rotate around the patient. The x-ray beam is tightly collimated by a leaded slit diaphragm at the tube aperture and another between the patient and film to prevent overlap and fogging of the film and to minimize patient exposure.

When positioning a patient for a panographic view of the mandible, the patient's spine must be straight, with the hips slightly forward; the head should not lean forward. The patient should rest the chin on the chin rest. The height of the chin rest must then be adjusted so the infraorbitomeatal line is parallel with the floor; the occlusal plane will slant 10° from posterior to anterior *(Figures 12–22, 12–23)*. Exposure time varies from 10 to 20 seconds and the kVp ranges from 70 to 80. The patient should be instructed to close the mouth, bite on a spacer, and hold the tongue against the roof of the mouth during the exposure.

In evaluation of the finished radiograph, the entire mandible, both TMJs, and the inferior portions of the nasal fossae and maxillary sinuses should be demonstrated with the upper and lower teeth slightly separated. The density should be uniform across the entire mandible, with no density loss near the mentum *(Figure 12–24)*. Because it cannot be used to describe the position of fracture fragments, this projection is generally used to supplement traditional radiography of the mandible and TMJs, but may also be used for a general survey of dental abnormalities.

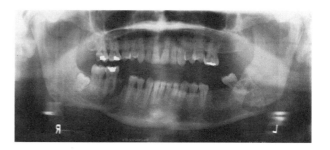

Figure 12–24. Panoramic tomogram.

BREATHING INSTRUCTIONS

Because positioning for the sinuses and facial bones must be accurate, any movement prior to or during the exposure could result in an unacceptable radiograph. To minimize the possibility of voluntary or involuntary motion and alert the patient that the exposure is going to be made, the patient should be instructed to suspend respiration for all projections of the sinuses and facial bones.

EXPOSURE FACTORS

As several facial bone projections can be performed without a grid, the kVp for facial bones and sinuses can vary from 50 to 85. Generally, 50 to 60 kVp penetrates the zygomatic arches (SMV and tangential), nasal bones (lateral), and mandible (axiolateral oblique) when these projections are obtained without a grid. The use of a grid for sinus and facial bone projections requires 65 to 85 kVp. Because the tissue measurement for most adults is fairly standard for each projection, the mAs required depends on the type of equipment generator, film/screen speed, type of grid, and pathologic conditions present. A small focal spot size should be selected to enhance bony detail. Close collimation and/or the use of a cylinder cone also improves radiographic quality. Because lead right or left markers displayed outside of the anatomy can be overexposed or "burned out," a small, thin piece of aluminum can be placed under the marker during the exposure; the aluminum acts as a filter, allowing visualization of the lead marker.

Automatic exposure control (AEC) is not recommended for radiography of the paranasal sinuses. Because the AEC averages the radiation passing through both air and bone, the bones appear too dark and the sinuses are too dark to evaluate air–fluid levels. For similar reasons, AEC is also not recommended for several routine facial bone projections.

EQUIPMENT CONSIDERATIONS

Any projection in which the central ray must penetrate most or all of the skull (eg, PA, SMV) requires a grid. A vertical grid device or dedicated head unit must be used for adequate demonstration of air–fluid levels in the sinuses; facial bone projections may be performed using either the radiographic table or vertical grid device. Because some of the facial bones are fairly small, a grid is not required for the SMV or tangential zygomatic arches, lateral nasal bone, or axiolateral mandible projections. In addition, detail cassettes can be used for the lateral projection of the nasal bones.

A cassette holder is needed for cross-table lateral projections that might be necessary for trauma patients. Head clamps, or other immobilization devices, should be used to prevent rotation of the head. Tape, if used, should be used carefully. Sponges may be used to support the head or torso, facilitating patient positioning and improving patient comfort. A special protractor, or other suitable device, should be used to ensure accurate positioning. A special "bite" block can be used to immobilize the mandible for the open-mouth TMJ projections *(Figure 12–25)*.

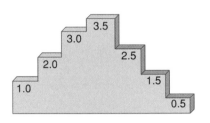

Figure 12–25. Bite block.

RADIOGRAPHIC POSITIONING OF THE PARANASAL SINUSES & FACIAL BONES

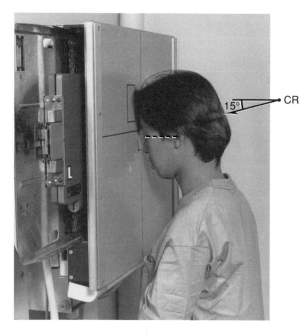

Figure 12–26. PA (Caldwell) paranasal sinuses with 15° caudal central ray angle.

▶ PA (CALDWELL) PARANASAL SINUSES

Technical Considerations

- Film size: 8 × 10 in. lengthwise or 9 × 9 in.
- Grid required.
- 70–80 kVp.
- Collimate to a 6 × 6-in. field size.

Shielding

- Gonadal shielding should be used on all patients, especially children and adults of reproductive age.

Patient Positioning

- Set the technical factors; the position may be difficult to maintain.
- Assist the patient to the seated position facing an upright grid device.
- Position the patient so the midsagittal plane is centered to and parallel with the long axis of the upright grid device; position the arms comfortably at the sides.

Part Positioning

- With the patient's forehead resting against the upright grid device, adjust the head so the midsagittal plane is perpendicular to the film plane.
- Adjust the head flexion so the orbitomeatal line is perpendicular to the film plane; immobilize as necessary (Figure 12–26).

Central Ray

- Direct the central ray 15° caudad to exit at the nasion. **Note:** If a dedicated head unit or other upright grid device capable of angulation is used, the film can be angled and the central ray directed horizontally; this method is actually better for demonstrating a sharp air–fluid level.
- Center the cassette to the central ray.

Breathing Instructions

- Instruct the patient to stop breathing during the exposure.

Image Evaluation

- The frontal sinuses, lateral margins of the orbits, and maxillary sinuses should be included within the collimated area.
- The orbits should be adequately penetrated without over- or underexposure.
- The frontal and ethmoidal sinuses should be seen in the middle of the collimated area.
- The petrous portions should fill the lower third of the orbits; the anterior ethmoidal sinuses should be seen above the petrous ridges.
- The distances between the outer margin of the orbits and lateral margins of the skull should be equal.
- The petrous ridges should be symmetrical *(Figure 12–27)*.

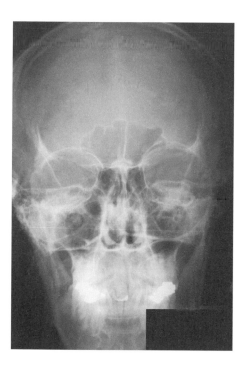 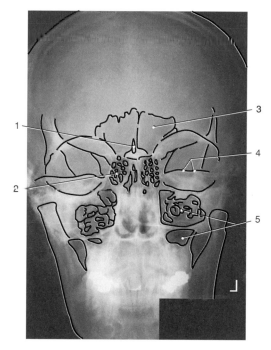

Figure 12–27. PA (Caldwell) paranasal sinuses; the petrous ridges should fill the lower one third of the orbits.

1. Crista galli, ethmoid bone
2. Ethmoid sinuses
3. Frontal sinuses
4. Petrous ridges, temporal bone
5. Maxillary sinuses

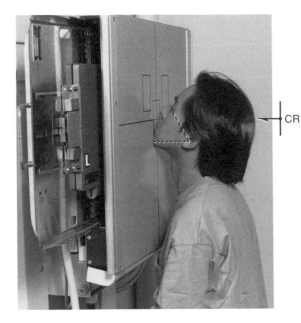
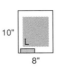

Figure 12–28. Parietoacanthial (Waters) paranasal sinuses.

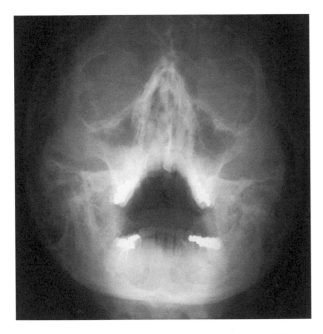

Figure 12–29. Parietoacanthial, open-mouthed (Waters) paranasal sinuses.

► PARIETOACANTHIAL (WATERS) PARANASAL SINUSES

Technical Considerations

- Film size: 8 × 10 in. lengthwise or 9 × 9 in.
- Grid required.
- 70–80 kVp.
- Collimate to a 6 × 6-in. field size.

Shielding

- Gonadal shielding should be used on all patients, especially children and adults of reproductive age.

Patient Positioning

- Set the technical factors; the position may be difficult to maintain.
- Assist the patient to the seated position facing an upright grid device.
- Position the patient so the midsagittal plane is centered to and parallel with the long axis of the upright grid device; position the arms comfortably at the sides.

Part Positioning

- With the patient's chin resting against the upright grid device, adjust the head so the midsagittal plane is perpendicular to the film plane.
- Adjust the head so the orbitomeatal line forms a 37° angle with the film plane and immobilize; the mentomeatal line will be perpendicular to the film plane on the average patient *(Figure 12–28)*.

Central Ray

- Direct the central ray perpendicular to the film, exiting at the acanthion.
- Center the cassette to the central ray.

Breathing Instructions

- Instruct the patient to stop breathing during the exposure. **Note:** For department routines that require it, the patient's mouth is opened prior to the exposure to demonstrate the sphenoid sinuses through the open mouth *(Figure 12–29)*.

Image Evaluation

- The frontal sinuses, orbits, and maxillary sinuses should be included within the collimated area.
- The orbits should be adequately penetrated without over- or underexposure.
- The lower margins of the orbit should be seen in the middle of the collimated area lengthwise, and the bony nasal septum should be in the middle crosswise.
- The petrous ridges will be projected just below the maxillary sinuses when the head flexion is correct.
- The distances between the outer margins of the orbits and lateral margins of the skull should be equal.
- The petrous ridges should be symmetrical *(Figure 12–30)*.

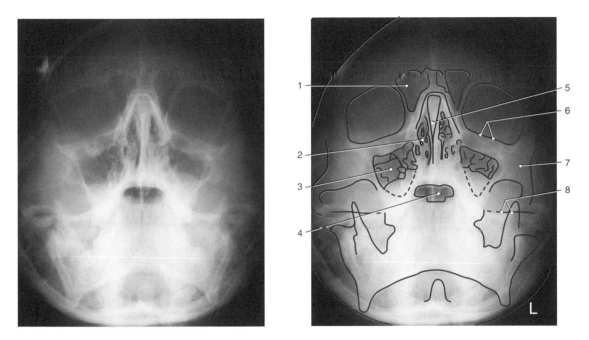

Figure 12–30. Parietoacanthial (Waters) paranasal sinuses; the petrous ridges should be projected just below the maxillary sinuses.

1. Frontal sinuses
2. Ethmoid sinuses
3. Maxillary sinuses
4. Sphenoid sinuses
5. Bony nasal septum
6. Inferior orbital margin
7. Zygomatic bone
8. Petrous ridge, temporal bone

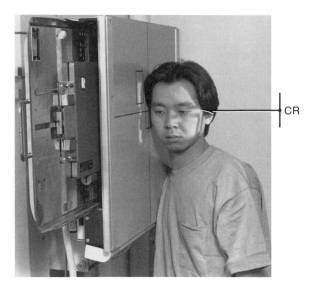

Figure 12–31. Lateral paranasal sinuses.

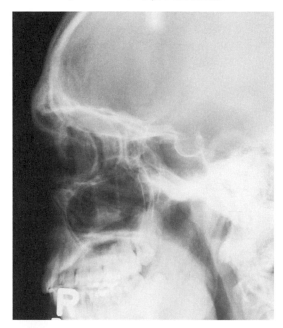

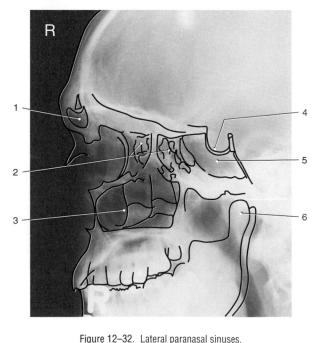

Figure 12–32. Lateral paranasal sinuses.

► LATERAL PARANASAL SINUSES

Technical Considerations

- Film size: 8 × 10 in. lengthwise or 9 × 9 in.
- Grid required.
- 60–70 kVp.
- Collimate to include TMJ, nose, maxilla, and forehead.

Shielding

- Gonadal shielding should be used on all patients, especially children and adults of reproductive age.

Patient Positioning

- Set the technical factors; the position may be difficult to maintain.
- Assist the patient to the seated position facing an upright grid device.

Part Positioning

- Rotate the patient and head to place the affected side against the upright grid device in a true lateral position.
- Center the point approximately 0.5 to 1 in. posterior to the outer canthus of the eye to the midline of the grid.
- Adjust the head so the midsagittal plane is parallel with and the interpupillary line is perpendicular to the film.
- Flex the neck and head so the infraorbitomeatal line is parallel with the transverse axis of the film (*Figure 12–31*).

Central Ray

- Direct the central ray horizontally to a point approximately 0.5 to 1 in. posterior to the outer canthus of the eye. **Note:** For accurate preoperative measurement, precise positioning and a 72-in. SID are required.
- Center the cassette to the central ray.

Breathing Instructions

- Instruct the patient to stop breathing during the exposure.

Image Evaluation

- The frontal, ethmoid, sphenoid, and maxillary sinuses should be included within the collimated area.
- The paranasal sinuses should be adequately penetrated without over- or underexposure.
- The paranasal sinuses should be in the center of the collimation field.
- The orbital roofs should be superimposed; the mandibular rami should also be superimposed.
- The floor of the maxillary antra should be parallel with the transverse axis of the film (*Figure 12–32*).

1. Frontal sinuses
2. Ethmoid sinuses
3. Maxillary sinuses

4. Sella turcica, sphenoid bone
5. Sphenoid sinuses

6. Mandibular condyles, superimposed

► SUBMENTOVERTICAL PARANASAL SINUSES (SMV)

Technical Considerations

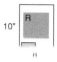

- Film size: 8 × 10 in. lengthwise or 9 × 9 in.
- Grid required.
- 70–80 kVp.
- Collimate to include nose and EAMs; an approximate 5 × 6-in. field size.

Shielding

- Gonadal shielding should be used on all patients, especially children and adults of reproductive age.

Patient Positioning

- Set the technical factors; the position will be difficult to maintain.
- Assist the patient to the seated position with the back toward an upright grid device; the chair should be approximately 6 in. from the grid unit.
- Position the patient so the midsagittal plane is centered to the midline of the grid device.

Part Positioning

- Center the cassette to the level of the gonia and direct the central ray horizontally to the midpoint of the cassette; this centering may need to be adjusted after the patient is positioned.
- Hyperextend the patient's neck and head to place the infraorbitomeatal line parallel or nearly parallel with the film plane; rest the vertex against the grid device.
- Adjust the head to place the midsagittal plane perpendicular to the film plane and centered to the midline of the grid; immobilize as necessary *(Figure 12–33)*.

Central Ray

- Direct the central ray perpendicular to the infraorbitomeatal line through the coronal plane passing 1 in. anterior to the EAMs; if the infraorbitomeatal line is not parallel with the film, the central ray will need to be directed cephalad.
- Center the cassette to the central ray.

Breathing Instructions

- Instruct the patient to stop breathing during the exposure.

Image Evaluation

- The nose, mandible, and petrous portions should be included within the collimated area.
- The sphenoid sinuses should be adequately penetrated and exposed.
- The mandibular condyles should be projected anterior to the petrous portions.
- The distances between the mandibular condyles and the lateral margins of the skull should be equal.
- The petrous portions should be symmetrical *(Figure 12–34)*.

1. Sphenoid sinuses	3. Ethmoid sinuses	5. Mastoid portion, temporal bone
2. Petrous ridge, temporal bone	4. Mandibular condyle	

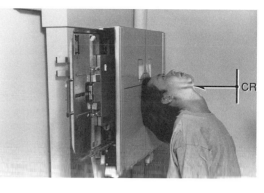

Figure 12–33. Submentovertical paranasal sinuses.

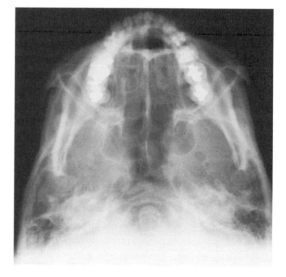

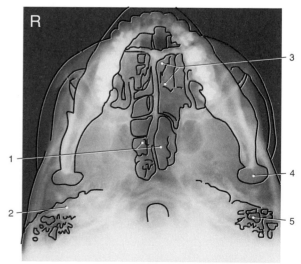

Figure 12–34. Submentovertical paranasal sinuses.

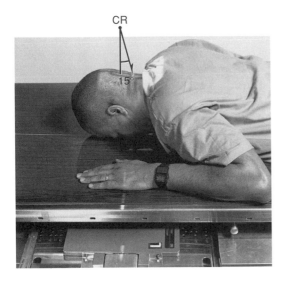

Figure 12–35. PA facial bones.

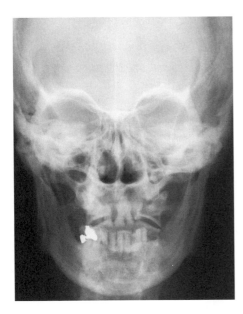

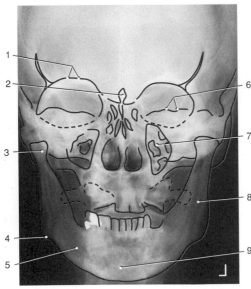

Figure 12–36. PA facial bones, 15° caudad central ray angle.

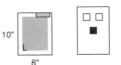

▶ PA FACIAL BONES

Technical Considerations

- Film size: 8 × 10 in. lengthwise or 9 × 9 in.
- Grid required.
- 70–80 kVp.
- Collimate to a 6 × 8-in. field size.

Shielding

- Gonadal shielding should be used on all patients, especially children and adults of reproductive age.

Patient Positioning

- Set the technical factors; the position may be difficult to maintain.
- Assist the patient to the prone position on the radiographic table; this projection may also be obtained with the patient upright.
- Position the patient so the midsagittal plane is centered to the midline and parallel with the long axis of the table.
- Adjust the shoulders so they lie in the same transverse plane; position the arms comfortably with the hands above the shoulders.

Part Positioning

- With the patient's forehead resting against the table, adjust the head so the midsagittal plane is perpendicular to the film plane.
- Adjust the head so the orbitomeatal line is perpendicular to the film plane; immobilize as necessary (Figure 12–35).

Central Ray

- Direct the central ray according to the area of interest:
  - general survey   15° caudad to the acanthion
  - orbits   25° caudad through the orbits
  - mandibular rami   perpendicular to the acanthion
- Center the cassette to the central ray.

Breathing Instructions

- Instruct the patient to stop breathing during the exposure.

1. Supraorbital margin
2. Crista galli, ethmoid bone
3. Mandibular condyle
4. Gonion
5. Mandibular body
6. Petrous ridge
7. Maxillary sinuses
8. Mandibular ramus
9. Mentum

Image Evaluation

- The supraorbital and lateral margins of the orbits and mentum of the mandible should be included within the collimated area.
- The orbits should be adequately penetrated without over- or underexposure.
- The acanthion or orbits should be in the middle of the collimated area (general survey-mandibular rami or orbits, respectively).
- The distances between the outer margins of the orbits and lateral margins of the skull should be equal.
- The petrous ridges should be symmetrical.
- The location of the petrous ridges will vary depending on the central ray angle:

  general survey   will fill the lower third of the orbits

  orbits   will be visualized just inferior to the orbits

  mandibular rami   will fill the orbits (Figures 12–36, 12–37, 12–38).

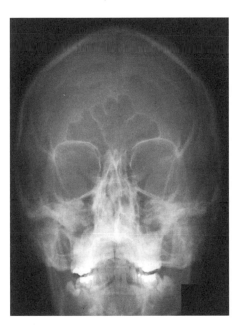

1. Supraorbital margin
2. Floor of orbit
3. Zygomatic bone
4. Petrous ridge, temporal bone
5. Mandibular condyle
6. Frontal sinuses
7. Superior orbital fissure, sphenoid
8. Maxilla
9. Maxillary sinuses

Figure 12–37. PA facial bones, 25° caudad central ray angle.

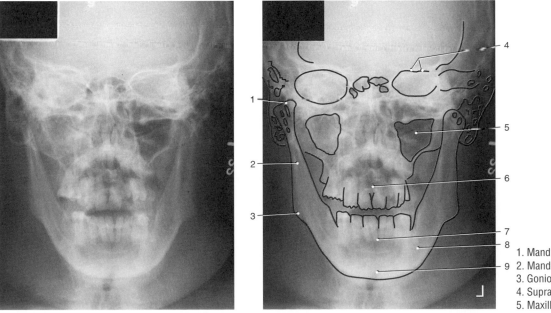

1. Mandibular condyle
2. Mandibular ramus
3. Gonion
4. Supraorbital margin
5. Maxillary sinuses
6. Alveolar process, maxillae
7. Alveolar process, mandible
8. Mandibular body
9. Mentum

Figure 12–38. PA facial bones, 0° caudad central ray angle.

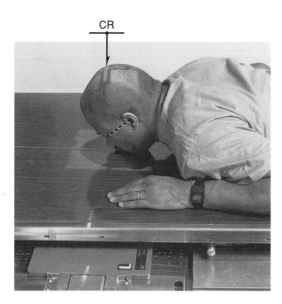

Figure 12–39. Parietoacanthial (Waters) facial bones.

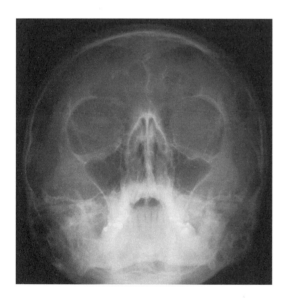

Figure 12–40. Modified parietoacanthial facial bones.

▶ PARIETOACANTHIAL (WATERS) FACIAL BONES

Technical Considerations

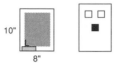

- Film size: 8 × 10 in. lengthwise or 9 × 9 in.
- Grid required.
- 70–80 kVp.
- Collimate to include orbits and mandible.

Shielding

- Gonadal shielding should be used on all patients, especially children and adults of reproductive age.

Patient Positioning

- Set the technical factors; the position may be difficult to maintain.
- Assist the patient to the prone position on the radiographic table; this projection may also be obtained with the patient erect.
- Position the patient so the midsagittal plane is centered to the midline of the table and parallel with the long axis of the table.
- Adjust the shoulders so they lie in the same transverse plane; position the arms comfortably with the hands near the shoulders.

Part Positioning

- With the patient's chin resting against the table, adjust the head so the midsagittal plane is perpendicular to the film plane.
- Tilt the head backward until the orbitomeatal line forms a 37° angle with the film plane and immobilize; the mentomeatal line will be perpendicular to the film plane on the average patient *(Figure 12–39)*.

  Note: When the modified Waters projection is used to demonstrate a blow-out fracture in the floor of the orbit, the orbitomeatal line may form a 55° angle with the film *(Figure 12–40)*.

Central Ray

- Direct the central ray perpendicular to the film, exiting at the acanthion.
- Center the cassette to the central ray.

Breathing Instructions

- Instruct the patient to stop breathing during the exposure.

Image Evaluation

- The orbits, zygomatic arches, and entire mandible should be included within the collimated area.
- The orbits should be adequately penetrated without over- or underexposure.
- The acanthion should be in the middle of the collimated area.
- The petrous ridges will be projected just below the maxillary sinuses when the head flexion is correct; the ridges will be in the lower maxillary sinuses for the modified Waters projection.
- The distances between the outer margins of the orbits and lateral margins of the skull should be equal.
- The petrous ridges should be symmetrical *(Figure 12–41)*.

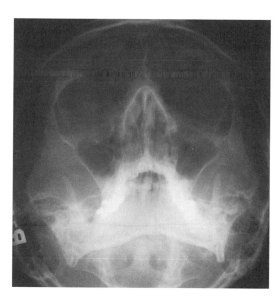 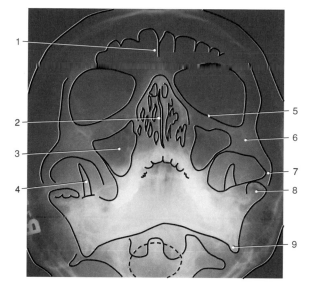

Figure 12–41. Parietoacanthial (Waters) facial bones.

1. Frontal sinuses
2. Bony nasal septum
3. Maxillary sinuses
4. Mandibular coronoid process
5. Infraorbital margin
6. Zygomatic bone
7. Zygomatic arch
8. Mandibular condyle
9. Gonion

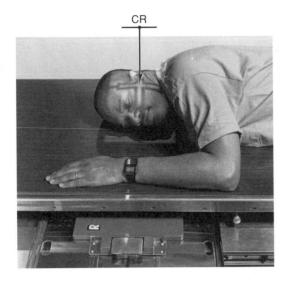

Figure 12–42. Lateral facial bones.

► LATERAL FACIAL BONES

Technical Considerations

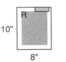

- Film size: 8 × 10 in. lengthwise or 9 × 9 in.
- Grid required.
- 60–70 kVp.
- Collimate to include TMJ, nose, mandible, and orbits.

Shielding

- Gonadal shielding should be used on all patients, especially children and adults of reproductive age.

Patient Positioning

- Set the technical factors; the position may be difficult to maintain.
- Assist the patient to the RAO or LAO position on the radiographic table; the affected side should be nearest the table. **Note:** This projection may also be obtained with the patient erect.

Part Positioning

- Adjust the rotation of the body and head so the midsagittal plane is parallel with and the interpupillary line is perpendicular to the film.
- Position the head so the infraorbitomeatal line is parallel with the transverse axis of the film.
- Center the zygoma to the midline of the grid *(Figure 12–42)*.

Central Ray

- Direct the central ray perpendicular to the cassette through the zygoma.
- Center the cassette to the central ray.

Breathing Instructions

- Instruct the patient to stop breathing during the exposure.

Image Evaluation

- The frontal sinuses, EAM, and entire mandible should be included within the collimated area.
- The mandible and orbital roofs should be adequately penetrated without overexposure.
- The facial bones should be in the center of the collimation field.
- The orbital roofs should be superimposed; the mandibular rami should also be superimposed.
- The floor of the maxillary antra should be parallel with the transverse axis of the film *(Figure 12–43)*.

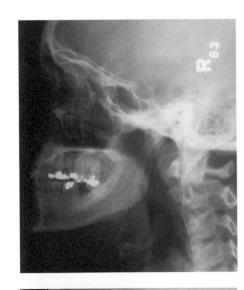

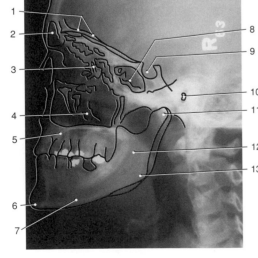

Figure 12–43. Lateral facial bones.

1. Orbital roofs
2. Frontal sinuses
3. Ethmoid sinuses
4. Maxillary sinuses
5. Maxillae, superimposed
6. Mentum
7. Mandibular body
8. Sphenoid sinuses
9. Sella turcica
10. External acoustic meatus (EAM)
11. Mandibular condyles, superimposed
12. Mandibular rami, superimposed
13. Gonia, superimposed

► PARIETO-ORBITAL OBLIQUE (RHESE) OPTIC CANAL/FORAMEN

Technical Considerations

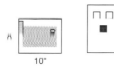

- Film size: 8 × 10 in. crosswise or 9 × 9 in.; may be masked crosswise for single orbit.
- Grid required. • 70–80 kVp. • Collimate to include both orbits.

Shielding

- Gonadal shielding should be used on all patients, especially children and adults of reproductive age.

Patient Positioning

- Set the technical factors; the position may be difficult to maintain.
- Assist the patient to the prone position on the radiographic table; this projection may also be obtained with the patient erect.
- Position the patient so the midsagittal plane is centered to the midline of the table and parallel with the long axis of the table.
- Adjust the shoulders so they lie in the same transverse plane; position the arms comfortably with the hands near the shoulders.

Part Positioning

- Position the patient's head so the nose, chin, and right cheek are resting on the table; both obliques are obtained for comparison.
- Center the orbit nearest the film to the midline of the grid.
- Flex the head and neck so the acanthiomeatal line is parallel with the transverse axis of the film.
- Rotate the head until the midsagittal plane forms a 53° angle with the film plane; a protractor or other device should be used to ensure accurate positioning *(Figure 12–44)*.
- Immobilize the head by using headclamps, tape, sponges, or sandbags.

Central Ray

- Direct the central ray perpendicular to the level of the outer canthus nearest the film. **Note:** If this projection is used as a survey for all the facial bones, the central ray should be perpendicular to the level of the infraorbital margin; collimation should include the orbits and mandible.
- Center the cassette to the central ray.

Breathing Instructions

- Instruct the patient to stop breathing during the exposure.

Image Evaluation

- The optic canal should be centered within the collimated area; both orbits should be included when imaging the orbits.
- The orbit nearest the film should be adequately penetrated; the elevated orbit will be dark but can be seen with a "hot light."
- The orbit nearest the film should be in the center of the collimation field.
- The petrous ridges should be level with or slightly above the level of the infraorbital margin.
- The optic canal of the side nearest the film should be demonstrated in the lower, outer quadrant of the orbit; lateral deviation indicates incorrect head rotation and longitudinal displacement indicates an error in head flexion.
- The optic foramen should normally appear round *(Figure 12–45)*.

1. Superior orbital margin   3. Optic canal/foramen   4. Sphenoid strut
2. Lateral orbital margin

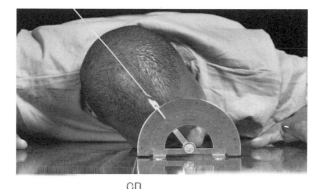

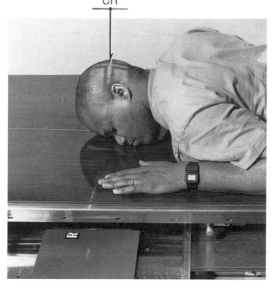

Figure 12–44. Parieto-orbital oblique (Rhese) projection right optic canal.

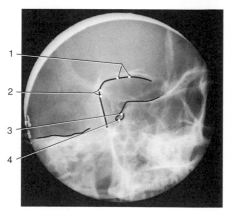

Figure 12–45. Parieto-orbital oblique for optic foramen, obtained using a Franklin head unit; field size was limited to one orbit.

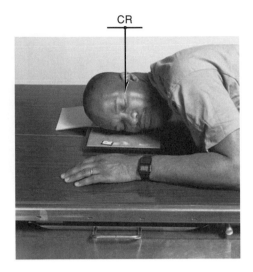

Figure 12–46. Right lateral nasal bones.

► LATERAL NASAL BONES

Technical Considerations

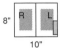

- Film size: 8 × 10 in. masked in half crosswise.
- Nongrid; detail cassette optional.
- 50–60 kVp.
- Collimate to include the nasion, acanthion, and soft tissue nose.

Shielding

- Gonadal shielding should be used on all patients, especially children and adults of reproductive age.

Patient Positioning

- Set the technical factors; the position may be difficult to maintain.
- Assist the patient to the RAO or LAO position on the radiographic table; both laterals will be obtained using one cassette.

Part Positioning

- Adjust the rotation of the body and head so the midsagittal plane is parallel with and the interpupillary line is perpendicular to the film.
- Position the head so the infraorbitomeatal line is parallel with the transverse axis of the film.
- Center the point approximately ¾ in. distal to the nasion to the unmasked half of the cassette *(Figure 12–46)*.

Central Ray

- Direct the central ray perpendicular to the cassette through the point ¾ in. inferior to the nasion.

Breathing Instructions

- Instruct the patient to stop breathing during the exposure.

Image Evaluation

- The frontonasal suture, soft tissue structures of the nose, and anterior nasal spine of the maxilla should be included within the collimated area.
- The frontonasal junction and anterior nasal spine should be adequately penetrated.
- The nasal bones and anterior nasal spine should be demonstrated in profile without rotation *(Figure 12–47)*.

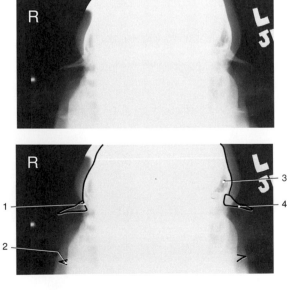

Figure 12–47. Right and left lateral nasal bones.

1. Frontonasal suture
2. Anterior nasal spine, maxillae
3. Frontal sinuses
4. Nasal bones, superimposed

► SUBMENTOVERTICAL ZYGOMATIC ARCHES (SMV)

Technical Considerations

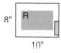

- Film size: 8 × 10 in. crosswise or 9 × 9 in.
- Nongrid or grid.
- 55–60 kVp.
- Collimate to include the nose and EAMs; an approximate 8 × 4-in. field size.

Shielding

- Gonadal shielding should be used on all patients, especially children and adults of reproductive age.

Patient Positioning

- Set the technical factors; the position will be difficult to maintain.
- Assist the patient to the seated position with the back facing an upright cassette holder; the chair should be approximately 6 in. from the cassette or grid unit. **Note:** This projection may also be obtained with the patient recumbent on the radiographic table.
- Position the patient so the midsagittal plane is centered to the midline of the cassette; adjust the shoulders so they lie in the same plane, parallel with the film plane.

Part Positioning

- Center the cassette to the level of the cheek (zygoma) and direct the central ray horizontally to the midpoint of the cassette; this centering and/or tube direction may need to be adjusted after the patient is positioned.
- Hyperextend the patient's neck and head to place the infraorbitomeatal line parallel or nearly parallel with the film plane; rest the vertex against the cassette or grid device.
- Adjust the head to place the midsagittal plane perpendicular to the film plane and centered to the midline of the cassette or grid; immobilize as necessary *(Figure 12–48)*.

Central Ray

- Direct the central ray perpendicular to the infraorbitomeatal line to a point midway between the gonia at the level of the zygomatic arches.
- Center the cassette to the central ray.

Breathing Instructions

- Instruct the patient to stop breathing during the exposure.

Image Evaluation

- Both zygomatic arches should be included within the collimated area.
- The zygomatic arches should be adequately penetrated and demonstrated in their entirety.
- The zygomatic arches should be demonstrated symmetrically *(Figure 12–49)*.

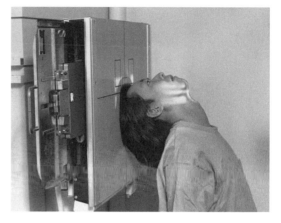

Figure 12–48. Submentovertical zygomatic arches, erect.

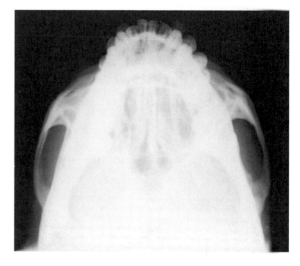

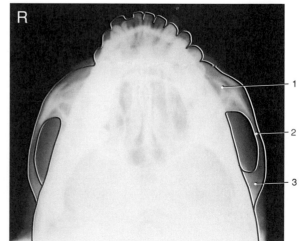

1. Zygomatic bone   2. Zygomatic arch   3. Temporal bone

Figure 12–49. Submentovertical zygomatic arches.

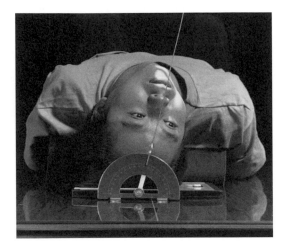

Figure 12–50. Tangential zygomatic arches, recumbent.

► TANGENTIAL ZYGOMATIC ARCHES

Technical Considerations

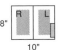

- Film size: 8 × 10 in. crosswise or 9 × 9 in.; may be masked in half, if performed nongrid.
- Nongrid or grid.
- 55–65 kVp.
- Collimate to include the zygoma and EAM; an approximate 3 × 4-in. field size.

Note: Depressed fractures or "flat" cheekbones usually are best demonstrated with this projection.

Shielding

- Gonadal shielding should be used on all patients, especially children and adults of reproductive age.

Patient Positioning

- Set the technical factors; the position will be difficult to maintain.
- Assist the patient to the seated position with the back facing an upright cassette holder; the chair should be approximately 6 in. from the cassette or grid unit. **Note:** This projection may also be obtained with the patient recumbent on the radiographic table *(Figure 12–50)*.
- Position the patient so the midsagittal plane is centered to the midline of the cassette or grid; adjust the shoulders so they lie in the same plane, parallel with the film plane.

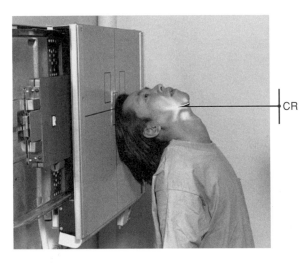

Figure 12–51. Tangential zygomatic arches, erect.

Part Positioning

- Center the cassette to the level of the cheek (zygoma) and direct the central ray horizontally to the midpoint of the cassette; this centering and/or tube direction may need to be adjusted after the patient is positioned.
- Hyperextend the patient's neck and head to place the infraorbitomeatal line parallel or nearly parallel with the film plane; rest the vertex against the grid device.
- Rotate the head 15° toward the side of interest; the midsagittal plane will be rotated 15°.
- Center the zygomatic arch of interest to the cassette; immobilize as necessary. Both sides are usually obtained for comparison *(Figure 12–51)*.

Central Ray

- Direct the central ray perpendicular to the infraorbitomeatal line, through the zygomatic arch of interest.

Breathing Instructions

- Instruct the patient to stop breathing during the exposure.

Image Evaluation

- The zygomatic arch should be demonstrated in the middle of the collimated area.
- The zygomatic arch should be adequately penetrated at both the anterior and posterior ends.
- The zygomatic arch should be demonstrated free of superimposition by adjacent structures (Figure 12–52).

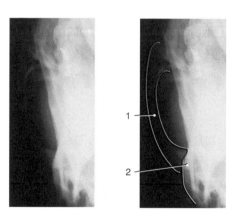

Figure 12–52. Tangential right zygomatic arch.

1. Zygomatic arch   2. Temporal bone

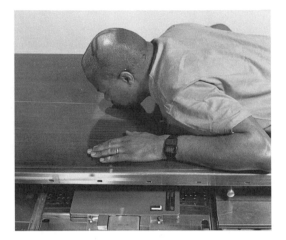

Figure 12–53. Superoinferior (Titterington) zygomatic arches.

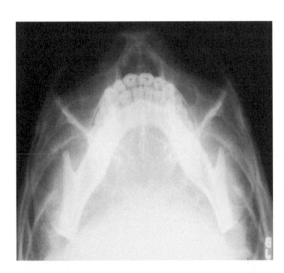

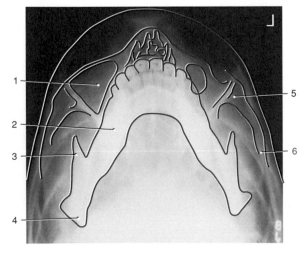

Figure 12–54. Superoinferior (Titterington) zygomatic arches, 38° angulation.

► SUPEROINFERIOR (TITTERINGTON) ZYGOMATIC ARCHES

Technical Considerations

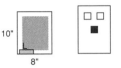

- Film size: 8 × 10 in. lengthwise or 9 × 9 in.
- Grid required.
- 70–80 kVp.
- Collimate to include the orbits and mandible.

Shielding

- Gonadal shielding should be used on all patients, especially children and adults of reproductive age.

Patient Positioning

- Set the technical factors; the position may be difficult to maintain.
- Assist the patient to the prone position on the radiographic table; this projection may also be obtained with the patient erect.
- Position the patient so the midsagittal plane is centered to the midline of the table and parallel with the long axis of the table.
- Adjust the shoulders so they lie in the same transverse plane; position the arms comfortably with the hands near the shoulders.

Part Positioning

- With the patient's chin resting against the table, adjust the head so the midsagittal plane is perpendicular to the film plane.
- Tilt the head backward until the nose is barely touching the table or upright grid device; immobilize as appropriate (Figure 12–53).

Central Ray

- Direct the central ray 23° to 38° caudad through a line passing through the zygomatic arches, exiting approximately at the mental point of the chin; the amount of angulation may depend on department protocol (a 23° angle will produce a projection similar to the Waters).
- Center the cassette to the central ray.

Breathing Instructions

- Instruct the patient to stop breathing during the exposure.

Image Evaluation

- The orbits, zygomatic arches, and entire mandible should be included within the collimated area.
- The orbits should be adequately penetrated without over- or underexposure.
- The petrous ridges will be projected below the level of the zygomatic arches.
- The distances between the outer margins of the orbits and lateral margins of the skull should be equal.
- The zygomatic arches should be symmetrical (Figure 12–54).

1. Maxillary sinus	3. Mandibular coronoid process
2. Mandibular body	4. Mandibular condyle
5. Zygomatic bone	6. Zygomatic arch

▶ PA AXIAL MANDIBULAR CONDYLES

Technical Considerations

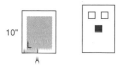

- Film size: 8 × 10 in. lengthwise or 9 × 9 in.
- Grid required.
- 70–80 kVp.
- Collimate to a 6 × 8-in. field size.

Shielding

- Gonadal shielding should be used on all patients, especially children and adults of reproductive age.

Patient Positioning

- Set the technical factors; the position may be difficult to maintain.
- Assist the patient to the prone position on the radiographic table; this projection may also be obtained with the patient upright.
- Position the patient so the midsagittal plane is centered to the midline and parallel with the long axis of the table.
- Adjust the shoulders so they lie in the same transverse plane; position the arms comfortably with the hands near the shoulders.

Part Positioning

- With the patient's forehead resting against the table, adjust the head so the midsagittal plane is perpendicular to the film plane.
- Adjust the head so the orbitomeatal line is perpendicular to the film plane; immobilize as necessary (Figure 12–55).

Central Ray

- Direct the central ray 20° to 25° cephalad, exiting through the glabella.
- Center the cassette to the central ray.

Breathing Instructions

- Instruct the patient to stop breathing during the exposure.

Image Evaluation

- The mandibular condyles and rami should be included within the collimated area.
- The condyles and rami of the mandible should be adequately penetrated without over- or underexposure.
- The acanthion should be in the middle of the collimated area.
- The mandibular rami should be symmetrical.
- The dorsum sellae should be seen within the shadow of the foramen magnum (Figure 12–56).

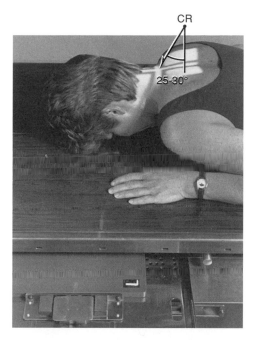

Figure 12–55. PA axial mandibular condyles.

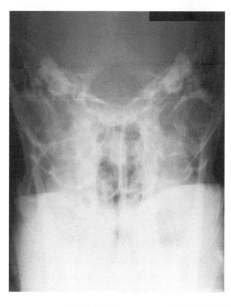

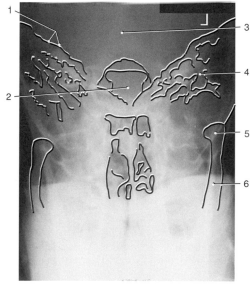

Figure 12–56. PA axial mandibular condyles.

1. Petrous ridge
2. Dorsum sellae, sphenoid bone
3. Occipital bone
4. Mastoid air cells, temporal bone
5. Mandibular condyle
6. Mandibular ramus

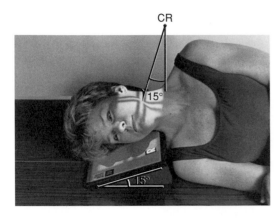

Figure 12–57. Axiolateral oblique mandible, ramus.

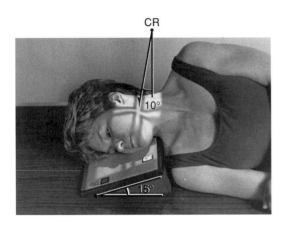

Figure 12–58. Axiolateral oblique mandible, body.

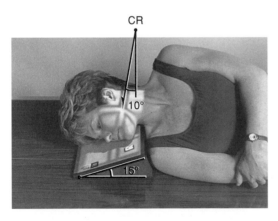

Figure 12–59. Axiolateral oblique mandible, mentum.

▶ AXIOLATERAL OBLIQUE MANDIBLE

Technical Considerations

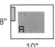

- Film size: 8 × 10 in. crosswise.
- Nongrid.
- 50–60 kVp.
- Collimate to include the entire mandible.

Shielding

- Gonadal shielding should be used on all patients, especially children and adults of reproductive age.

Patient Positioning

- Set the technical factors; the position may be difficult to maintain.
- Assist the patient to the semisupine position on the radiographic table; both obliques will be obtained for a complete examination. **Note:** This projection may also be obtained with the patient erect, using a vertical cassette holder or head unit.

Part Positioning

- Adjust the rotation of the body so the head can be placed in a lateral position with the patient's cheek on a 10° to 15° inclined cassette; the elevated side of the cassette should be adjacent to the shoulder.
- Position the head so the infraorbitomeatal line is parallel with the transverse axis of the film and the interpupillary line is perpendicular to the film plane.
- Adjust the rotation of the head so the part of the mandible of greatest interest is parallel to the film plane:

ramus	head is in a true lateral position *(Figure 12–57)*
body	head is rotated approximately 30° toward the film *(Figure 12–58)*
mentum	head is rotated approximately 45° toward the film *(Figure 12–59)*

Central Ray

- Direct the central ray approximately 10° to 15° cephalad to a point approximately 2 in. inferior to the gonion furthest from the film; the central ray should be angled just enough to separate the two halves of the mandible and will depend on the angulation of the sponge and patient position (greater angle for the ramus than for the body).
- Adjust the cassette position to coincide with the central ray.

Breathing Instructions

- Instruct the patient to stop breathing during the exposure; the mouth should be closed and the teeth together, if possible.

Image Evaluation

- The condyle, gonion, body, and mentum of the side nearest the film should be included within the collimated area.
- The condyle should be adequately penetrated without overexposure of the mandibular body.
- The ramus and gonion should be demonstrated anterior to the cervical vertebrae (ramus).
- The opposite side of the mandible should not be superimposed over the side of interest.
- The area of interest should be demonstrated without distortion *(Figures 12–60, 12–61)*.

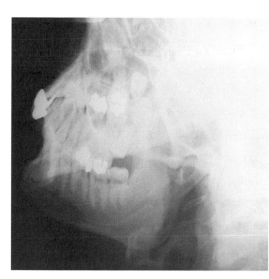

1. Mentum
2. Mental foramen
3. Mandibular body
4. Mandibular coronoid process
5. Mandibular condyle
6. Mandibular notch
7. Mandibular ramus
8. Gonion

Figure 12–60. Axiolateral oblique mandible, ramus.

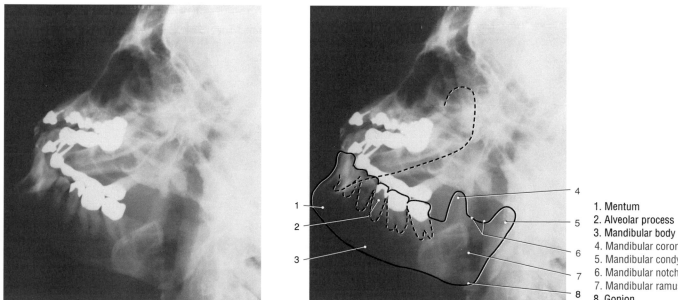

1. Mentum
2. Alveolar process
3. Mandibular body
4. Mandibular coronoid process
5. Mandibular condyle
6. Mandibular notch
7. Mandibular ramus
8. Gonion

Figure 12–61. Axiolateral oblique mandible, body.

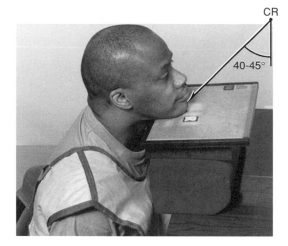

Figure 12–62. AP axial extraoral mandibular symphysis.

► AP AXIAL EXTRAORAL MANDIBULAR SYMPHYSIS

Technical Considerations

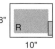

- Film size: 8 × 10 in. crosswise or occlusal film.
- Nongrid.
- 55–65 kVp.
- Collimate to include the mental symphysis.

Shielding

- Gonadal shielding should be used on all patients, especially children and adults of reproductive age.

Patient Positioning

- Assist the patient to a chair at the end of the table. **Note:** This projection can also be obtained with the patient supine, the film holder supported vertically below the chin, and the central ray directed caudally through the mental symphysis.
- Elevate the cassette or occlusal film on sponges, sandbags, or other support; the film holder should be elevated to the level of the patient's chin.

Part Positioning

- Instruct the patient to rest the chin on the distal end of the film holder; the inferior surface of the chin should be in close contact with the film holder.
- Adjust the head so the midsagittal plane is perpendicular to the film plane and centered to the film crosswise (*Figure 12–62*).

Central Ray

- Direct the central ray 40° to 45° toward the patient through the mandibular symphysis, midway between the lower lip and chin; align the film to the central ray.

Breathing Instructions

- Instruct the patient to stop breathing during the exposure.

Image Evaluation

- The entire mentum should be included within the collimated area.
- The two halves of the mandible should be symmetrical.
- The mental symphysis should be in the middle of the collimated area *(Figure 12–63)*.

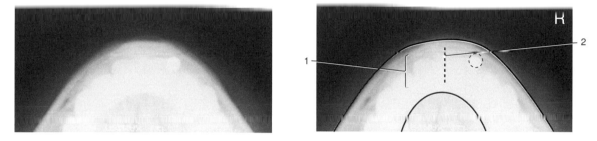

Figure 12–63. AP axial external mandibular symphysis; note the presence of the BB to the right of the symphysis.

1. Mentum

2. Mandibular symphysis

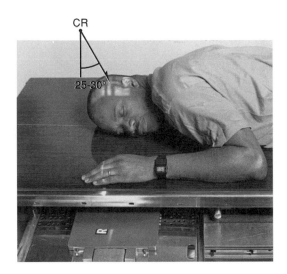

Figure 12–64. Axiolateral (Schüller) temporomandibular joint, closed mouth.

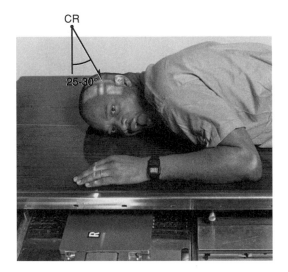

Figure 12–65. Axiolateral (Schüller) temporomandibular joint, open mouth.

► AXIOLATERAL (SCHÜLLER) TEMPOROMANDIBULAR JOINTS

Technical Considerations

- Film size: 8 × 10 in. crosswise.
- Grid required.
- 65–75 kVp.
- Collimate to a 5 × 5-in. field size.

Shielding

- Gonadal shielding should be used on all patients, especially children and adults of reproductive age.

Patient Positioning

- Set the technical factors; the position may be difficult to maintain.
- Assist the patient to the RAO or LAO position on the radiographic table or seated facing an upright grid device; the side nearest the table will be demonstrated. **Note:** Both sides are examined with open and closed mouth for comparison (four exposures).

Part Positioning

- Adjust the rotation of the body and head so the midsagittal plane is parallel with and the interpupillary line is perpendicular to the film; the head should be in true lateral position.
- Position the head so the infraorbitomeatal line is parallel with the transverse axis of the film.
- Center the TMJ to the midline of the grid; immobilize the head as necessary *(Figures 12–64, 12–65)*.

Central Ray

- Direct the central ray 25° to 30° caudad to the cassette, exiting through the TMJ nearest the film.
- Center the cassette to the central ray.

Breathing Instructions

- Instruct the patient to stop breathing during the exposure; two exposures will be obtained of each TMJ—one with the mouth closed and teeth together, the other with the mouth open as wide as possible (a bite block may be used for immobilization). Remember to change or move the cassette between exposures!

Image Evaluation

- The entire TMJ nearest the film should be included within the collimated area.
- The mandibular condyle and mandibular fossa should be adequately penetrated.
- The TMJ should be in the center of the collimation field.
- The TMJ furthest from the film should be approximately 2.5 to 3 in. below the TMJ being examined on the radiograph *(Figures 12–66, 12–67).*

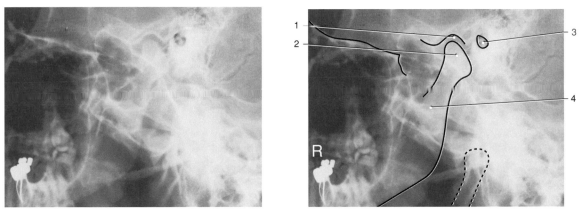

1. Mandibular fossa, temporal bone
2. Mandibular condyle
3. External acoustic meatus (EAM)
4. Mandibular ramus

Figure 12–66. Axiolateral (Schüller) temporomandibular joint, closed mouth.

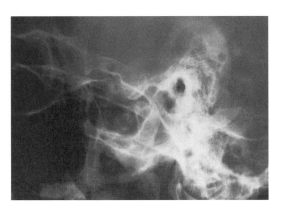

1. Mandibular fossa, temporal bone
2. Articular tubercle
3. Mandibular condyle
4. External acoustic meatus (EAM)

Figure 12–67. Axiolateral (Schüller) temporomandibular joint, open mouth.

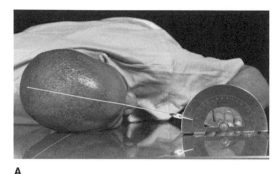

A

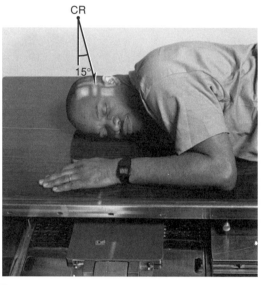

B

Figure 12–68. Axiolateral oblique temporomandibular joint, closed mouth.

► AXIOLATERAL OBLIQUE TEMPOROMANDIBULAR JOINTS

Technical Considerations

- Film size: 8 × 10 in. crosswise.
- Grid required.
- 65–75 kVp.
- Collimate to a 5 × 5-in. field size.

Shielding

- Gonadal shielding should be used on all patients, especially children and adults of reproductive age.

Patient Positioning

- Set the technical factors; the position may be difficult to maintain.
- Assist the patient to the RAO or LAO position on the radiographic table or seated facing an upright grid device; the side nearest the table will be demonstrated. **Note:** Both sides will be examined with open and closed mouth for comparison (four exposures).

Part Positioning

- With the head resting comfortably on the cheek, center the point 0.5 in. anterior to the EAM nearest the table to the midline of the grid.
- From a true lateral position, rotate the head so the midsagittal plane is directed 15° toward the film. **Note:** With exception of the acanthiomeatal line and the centering point, the head should be positioned as for the modified lateral (Law) method for demonstration of the mastoids.
- Position the head so the acanthiomeatal line is parallel with the transverse axis of the film; immobilize as necessary *(Figures 12–68, 12–69)*.

Central Ray

- Direct the central ray 15° caudad to the cassette, exiting through the TMJ nearest the film.
- Center the cassette to the central ray.

Breathing Instructions

- Instruct the patient to stop breathing during the exposure; two exposures will be obtained of each TMJ— one with the mouth closed and teeth together, the other with the mouth open as wide as possible (a bite block may be used for immobilization). Remember to change or move the cassette between exposures!

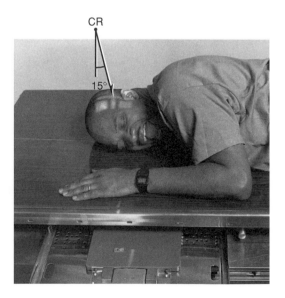

Figure 12–69. Axiolateral oblique temporomandibular joint, open mouth.

Image Evaluation

- The entire TMJ nearest the film should be included within the collimated area.
- The mandibular condyle and mandibular fossa should be adequately penetrated.
- The TMJ nearest the film should be in the center of the collimation field.
- The TMJ furthest from the film should be approximately 1.5 in. anterior and inferior to TMJ being examined (*Figures 12–70, 12–71*).

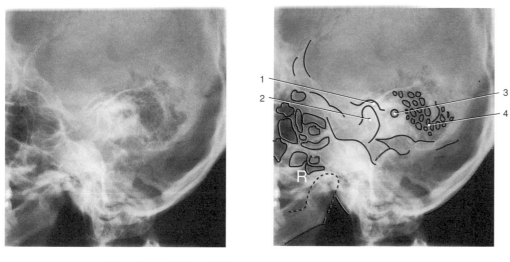

1. Mandibular fossa, temporal bone
2. Mandibular condyle
3. External acoustic meatus (EAM)
4. Mastoid air cells

Figure 12–70. Axiolateral oblique temporomandibular joint, closed mouth.

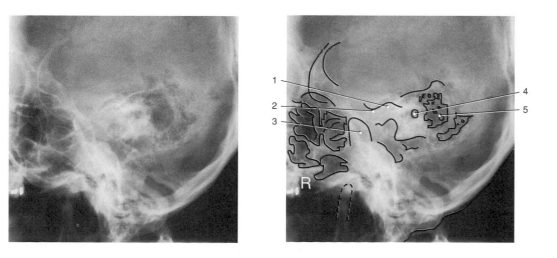

1. Mandibular fossa, temporal bone
2. Articular tubercle
3. Mandibular condyle
4. External acoustic meatus (EAM)
5. Mastoid air cells

Figure 12–71. Axiolateral oblique temporomandibular joint, open mouth.

$\mathcal{S}$UMMARY

▸ To demonstrate air–fluid levels, radiographic examinations of the sinuses must be performed using a horizontal beam.

▸ The routine sinus examination generally includes the PA (modified Caldwell), parietoacanthial (Waters), and lateral (affected side nearest the film) projections; the routine facial bone examination often includes these same projections.

▸ Because patient positioning may be difficult to maintain, technical factors and preliminary cassette and central ray centering should be set before placing the head in position.

▸ Traumatic injury of the skull and spine may prohibit movement of the patient and require modifications of the standard projections.

▸ The panorex, a special type of tomographic unit, can be used to radiograph the mandible, temporomandibular joints, and various dental abnormalities.

▸ To minimize the possibility of motion, patients should be instructed to stop breathing for all examinations of the sinuses and facial bones.

▸ Facial bone projections obtained without the use of a grid require only 50 to 60 kVp; projections requiring a grid need 65 to 85 kVp.

$\mathcal{Q}$UESTIONS FOR CRITICAL THINKING & APPLICATION

1. A baseball player was hit in the face by a fly ball. On radiographic examination, he was told that he had a "deviated septum." Explain what is meant and which structures are involved in this condition.

2. How do the paranasal sinuses act as "resonating chambers" for the voice when a person sings or talks? Why does the voice become muffled when a person has a sinus infection?

3. Why is "cleft palate" considered to be a congenital condition? What bone(s) is/are generally affected? Could any other structures be involved?

4. In old age, the facial skeleton seems to shrink, leaving an older person with the appearance of a small face. Explain this phenomenon of aging as it relates to the structure of the mandible.

5. The emergency department sent a patient to the radiology department but had not yet entered the order for the examination into the computer. As the radiographer on duty, you began an initial assessment of the patient and noticed that her mouth was continually open. She indicated in writing to you that she yawned and felt a popping sensation that left her jaw "stuck" in an open position. What do you suppose is the problem? What examination will most likely be ordered by the emergency department physician? What structures are involved? Discuss the movement that normally occurs when a person opens and closes her mouth.

6. A quadriplegic patient who is unable to sit has been scheduled for radiographic examination of the sinuses. Describe how you would obtain diagnostic films for this study.

7. Describe the projections you would obtain to demonstrate the zygomatic arches on a patient with fairly "flat" cheekbones.

8. The victim of a car accident has sustained a fracture of the cervical vertebrae and severe trauma to the face. Describe how you would obtain the necessary radiographs to demonstrate any possible facial bone fractures. Justify your methods.

9. Radiographic examination of the facial bones can be completed with the patient erect or recumbent. List advantages and disadvantages of each general patient position.

10. A patient with a severe nosebleed is waiting for radiographic examination of the nasal bones. Describe how you would obtain the necessary films.

FILM CRITIQUE

Evaluate this parietoacanthial projection that was taken as part of a facial bone examination *(Figure 12–72)*.

Was the patient accurately positioned?

Why or why not?

What criteria did you use to determine positioning accuracy?

Were proper exposure factors used?

How can you tell?

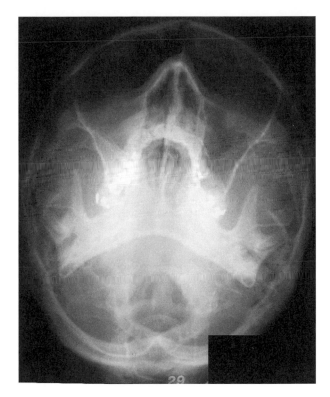

Figure 12–72.

13

INTRODUCTION TO CONTRAST STUDIES

▶ OBJECTIVES

Following the completion of this chapter the student will be able to:

- Discuss the term *contrast medium,* to include its definition, purpose, and use in radiography.

- Identify specific materials that are used as contrast agents, including the chemical, physical, and radiographic characteristics of each.

- Differentiate between positive and negative contrast media.

- Identify the routes of administration of contrast media for various radiographic examinations.

- Compare and contrast the use of ionic and nonionic iodinated contrast media.

- Identify contraindications to the administration of a contrast medium and possible complications resulting from its use.

- Describe possible reactions to contrast media and categorize them according to severity.

- Describe the radiographer's responsibilities with regard to contrast examinations.

- Discuss recommended sequencing of various diagnostic examinations and provide a rationale for this sequencing.

- Discuss terminology related to the use of contrast media.

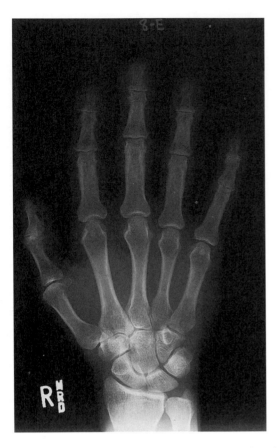

Figure 13–1. Calcium in bones has a higher atomic number than skin. Therefore, the bones appear more radiopaque on this PA projection of the hand.

Contrast studies are those examinations in which contrast media are used to enhance visualization of specific body structures. Because of the low subject contrast of the abdomen, contrast media are used to demonstrate the anatomic structures of the urinary, digestive, and biliary systems. Contrast media are also used to evaluate other areas of the body, such as the spinal canal, female reproductive system, and vasculature. The radiographer must understand the composition of contrast media, the effects they can have on the body, and how they are used. *Table 13–1* provides an overview of the contrast media used in diagnostic radiography.

► BASIC PRINCIPLES OF CONTRAST MEDIA

Many structures and organs within the body have similarly low tissue densities. This is determined by their atomic number, which is the number of protons (positive charges) in the nuclei of their atoms. When the x-ray beam is directed at a specific structure during a radiographic examination, some of the x-rays pass through, and others are absorbed (attenuated) by the structure. More x-rays are absorbed by structures having a high atomic number, resulting in less radiation reaching the film, whereas fewer x-rays are absorbed by structures having a low atomic number. This accounts for the visible difference in densities on a radiograph. For example, the calcium in bone has a higher atomic number than skin or muscle tissue; therefore, the bone appears light on a radiograph and the soft tissue appears dark *(Figure 13–1)*. Many organs, such as those of the digestive, urinary, biliary, and cardiovascular systems, are about the same density as soft tissue, which has an atomic number of approximately 7.4. For this reason, they absorb nearly the same amount of x-radiation and appear relatively similar on a radiograph. In other words, they have low contrast because there is little difference in the attenuation of the x-ray beam by the structures and they may not be distinguishable from one another on a radiograph. To make these structures more visible for diagnostic purposes, a contrast medium or agent must be used.

A *contrast medium* is a pharmaceutical agent that is administered to a patient for a radiographic examination to enhance the contrast of a particular structure. Its use allows for differentiation between a structure and surrounding tissues by altering the density of the structure, which in turn alters the absorption of x-rays. The type of contrast medium (negative or positive) affects the amount of radiation reaching the film, and produces a visible change in the radiographic appearance of the structure *(Figure 13–2)*.

Table 13–1. Summary of Contrast Media Used in Radiography

Negative contrast agents	• Radiolucent • Low atomic number • Gases • Appear dark on the radiograph • Used singly or combined with positive contrast agents
Positive contrast agents	• Radiopaque • High atomic number • Liquid, powder, tablet, or granule form • Appear light on the radiograph
• Barium sulfate	• Inert compound • Atomic number 56 • Used in alimentary canal • Administered orally or rectally
• Iodinated compounds	• Organic iodine compounds • Atomic number 54
—Oil-based	• Fatty acid base • Insoluble in water • Slowly absorbed • Used primarily in lymphangiography
—Water-soluble	• Triiodobenzoic acid base • Ionic—dissociates into (+) and (−) particles; high osmolality • Nonionic—does not dissociate; low osmolality • Administered orally, rectally, intravascularly, or directly • Used in examinations of the cardiovascular, urinary, biliary, and digestive systems

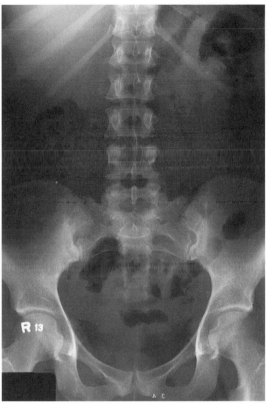

A

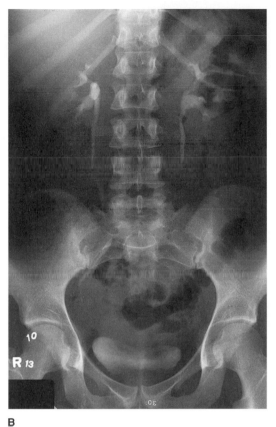

B

Figure 13–2. The kidneys and urinary bladder are not well demonstrated on a routine KUB **(A),** but are visualized after the administration of contrast medium **(B).**

The study and use of contrast agents date back to 1896 when researchers administered compounds of lead, potassium, or bismuth to animals to study gastric motility. Follow-up studies disclosed problems with toxicity with the original contrast media; however, contrast agents have been continually refined over the years and a wide variety of products are available from several pharmaceutical companies.

► TYPES OF CONTRAST MEDIA

The two basic classifications of contrast media are negative contrast agents and positive contrast agents *(Figure 13–3).*

A **negative contrast agent** is radiolucent, has a low atomic number, and allows x-rays to pass through quite easily. As more x-radiation reaches the film, the structure that is filled with a negative contrast agent appears dark (black) on a radiograph. Gases, such as oxygen, carbon dioxide, and nitrous oxide, may be used as negative contrast media, although room air is the most common agent. For example, the air in the lungs serves as a negative contrast medium on a chest radiograph *(Figure 13–4).* A negative contrast medium may be used alone, as in the case of an air arthrogram. It can also be combined with a positive contrast agent to produce a double-contrast effect, such as a barium enema examination with air *(Figure 13–5).* As a second contrast agent for upper gastrointestinal examinations, a negative contrast medium is generally administered as an effervescent agent in powder, granule, or tablet form which forms carbon dioxide (CO_2) when mixed with water *(Figure 13–6).* The uses of negative contrast media are limited, however, as they may not provide sufficient contrast of a structure when used singly. Also, they must never be injected intravenously; doing so will have serious, if not fatal, consequences.

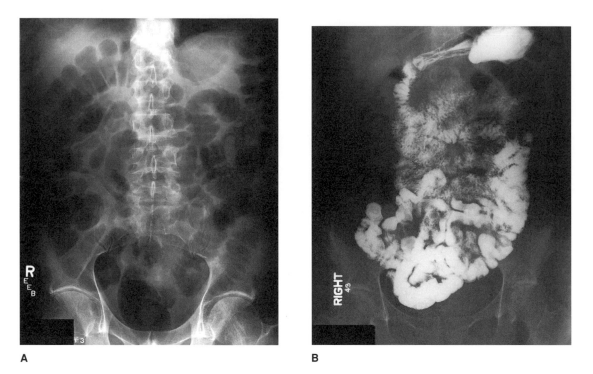

A   B

Figure 13–3. Air in the small intestine is a negative contrast medium on radiograph **(A)**. Barium sulfate, a positive contrast medium, is present in the small intestine on radiograph **(B)**.

A **positive contrast agent** is radiopaque and has a high atomic number. As it absorbs approximately three times more x-rays than bone and five times as many x-rays as soft tissue, an organ filled with a positive contrast agent appears light on the resulting radiograph. Barium sulfate ($BaSO_4$) and iodinated compounds are positive contrast media used in radiography to enhance the visibility of particular structures. As demonstrated on the Periodic Table of the Elements *(Figure 13–7)*, the elements iodine (53) and barium (56) have high atomic numbers compared with that of oxygen (8). Gadolinium, a positive contrast medium used in magnetic resonance imaging, also has a high atomic number (64). As it is not used in diagnostic radiography, gadolinium is not included in this discussion of positive contrast media.

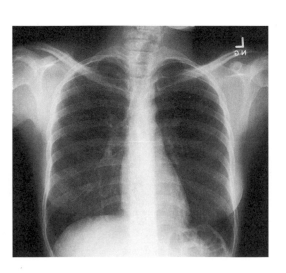

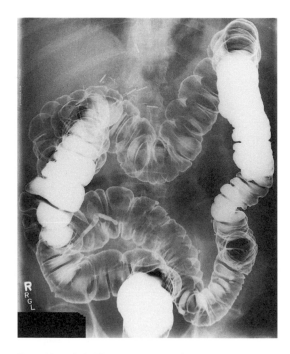

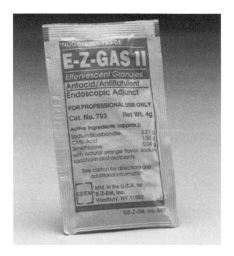

Figure 13–4. Air acts as a negative contrast agent on this PA chest radiograph.

Figure 13–5. A double-contrast examination of the large intestine requires the administration of barium sulfate and air.

Figure 13–6. This effervescent product is a negative contrast agent.

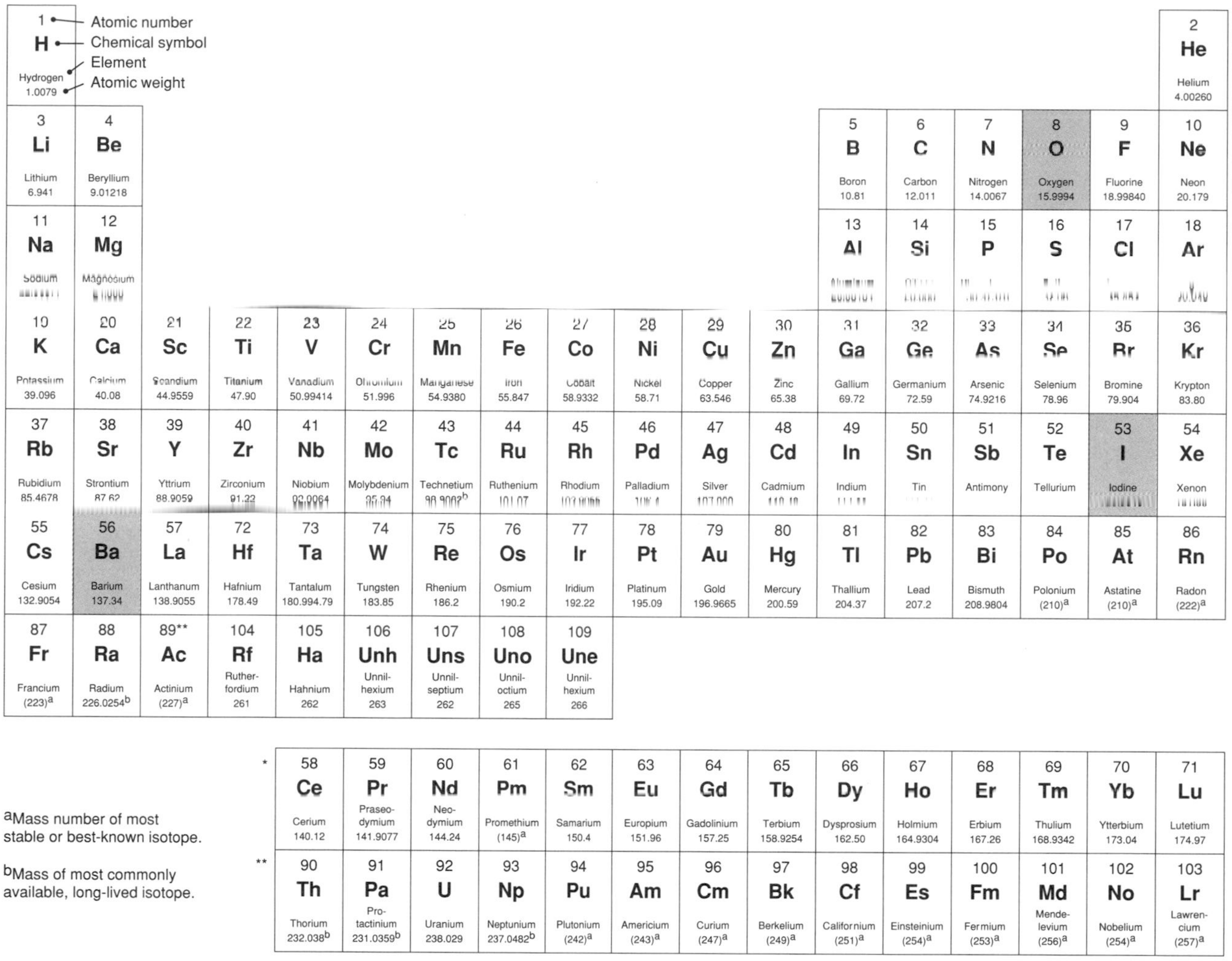

Legend:
- 1 — Atomic number
- H — Chemical symbol
- Element
- Hydrogen 1.0079 — Atomic weight

1 H Hydrogen 1.0079																	2 He Helium 4.00260
3 Li Lithium 6.941	4 Be Beryllium 9.01218										5 B Boron 10.81	6 C Carbon 12.011	7 N Nitrogen 14.0067	8 O Oxygen 15.9994	9 F Fluorine 18.99840	10 Ne Neon 20.179	
11 Na Sodium	12 Mg Magnesium										13 Al Aluminum	14 Si Silicon	15 P Phosphorus	16 S Sulfur	17 Cl Chlorine	18 Ar Argon	
19 K Potassium 39.096	20 Ca Calcium 40.08	21 Sc Scandium 44.9559	22 Ti Titanium 47.90	23 V Vanadium 50.99414	24 Cr Chromium 51.996	25 Mn Manganese 54.9380	26 Fe Iron 55.847	27 Co Cobalt 58.9332	28 Ni Nickel 58.71	29 Cu Copper 63.546	30 Zn Zinc 65.38	31 Ga Gallium 69.72	32 Ge Germanium 72.59	33 As Arsenic 74.9216	34 Se Selenium 78.96	35 Br Bromine 79.904	36 Kr Krypton 83.80
37 Rb Rubidium 85.4678	38 Sr Strontium 87.62	39 Y Yttrium 88.9059	40 Zr Zirconium 91.22	41 Nb Niobium 92.9064	42 Mo Molybdenum 95.94	43 Tc Technetium 98.9062	44 Ru Ruthenium 101.07	45 Rh Rhodium 102.9055	46 Pd Palladium 106.4	47 Ag Silver 107.868	48 Cd Cadmium 112.40	49 In Indium 114.82	50 Sn Tin	51 Sb Antimony	52 Te Tellurium	53 I Iodine 126.9045	54 Xe Xenon 131.30
55 Cs Cesium 132.9054	56 Ba Barium 137.34	57 La Lanthanum 138.9055	72 Hf Hafnium 178.49	73 Ta Tantalum 180.9479	74 W Tungsten 183.85	75 Re Rhenium 186.2	76 Os Osmium 190.2	77 Ir Iridium 192.22	78 Pt Platinum 195.09	79 Au Gold 196.9665	80 Hg Mercury 200.59	81 Tl Thallium 204.37	82 Pb Lead 207.2	83 Bi Bismuth 208.9804	84 Po Polonium (210)a	85 At Astatine (210)a	86 Rn Radon (222)a
87 Fr Francium (223)a	88 Ra Radium 226.0254b	89** Ac Actinium (227)a	104 Rf Rutherfordium 261	105 Ha Hahnium 262	106 Unh Unnilhexium 263	107 Uns Unnilseptium 262	108 Uno Unniloctium 265	109 Une Unnilhexium 266									

*	58 Ce Cerium 140.12	59 Pr Praseodymium 141.9077	60 Nd Neodymium 144.24	61 Pm Promethium (145)a	62 Sm Samarium 150.4	63 Eu Europium 151.96	64 Gd Gadolinium 157.25	65 Tb Terbium 158.9254	66 Dy Dysprosium 162.50	67 Ho Holmium 164.9304	68 Er Erbium 167.26	69 Tm Thulium 168.9342	70 Yb Ytterbium 173.04	71 Lu Lutetium 174.97
**	90 Th Thorium 232.038b	91 Pa Protactinium 231.0359b	92 U Uranium 238.029	93 Np Neptunium 237.0482b	94 Pu Plutonium (242)a	95 Am Americium (243)a	96 Cm Curium (247)a	97 Bk Berkelium (249)a	98 Cf Californium (251)a	99 Es Einsteinium (254)a	100 Fm Fermium (253)a	101 Md Mendelevium (256)a	102 No Nobelium (254)a	103 Lr Lawrencium (257)a

aMass number of most stable or best-known isotope.

bMass of most commonly available, long-lived isotope.

Figure 13–7. Periodic table of the elements.

BARIUM SULFATE

Properties

Barium is a heavy metal having an atomic number of 56. It is combined with oxygen and sulfate to form the inert compound barium sulfate ($BaSO_4$). Barium sulfate is a white, crystalline powder that is insoluble in water. For use in radiography, it is mixed with water and stabilizing agents to form a suspension. Often, artificial flavors and colors are added to the suspension used for upper gastrointestinal radiography to make the barium sulfate more palatable to the patient.

Barium sulfate is used for examination of the entire alimentary canal. Ideally, the suspension should be dense to coat the mucosa and outline the visceral walls, yet it must have the ability to flow smoothly through the alimentary canal. Barium sulfate products can be procured in a variety of concentrations depending on the type of examination and specific anatomy of interest. The products are available commercially in paste, liquid, powder, and tablet form *(Figure 13–8)*. Paste, having a viscosity approximate to that of honey, may be recommended for an esophagram. As it will not pass down the esophagus as swiftly as a thinner suspension, the radiologist and/or radiographer have more time to take radiographs of the contrast-filled esophagus. A liquid barium sulfate suspension can also be used for radiographic examination of the esophagus, as well as the stomach and both small and large intestines. It can be purchased in premixed liquid form or in powder form, which must be mixed with water prior to use. In either case, it should be shaken or stirred immediately before administration, as suspensions tend to settle. Barium sulfate tablets are helpful in evaluating foreign objects or strictures in the esophagus. They dissolve in either the esophagus or stomach when mixed with water.

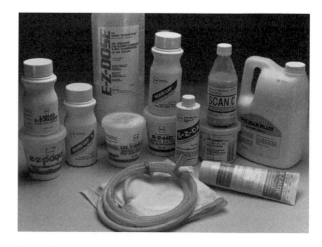

Figure 13–8. Barium sulfate products are available in a variety of forms.

Contraindications

Because of its inability to be absorbed by the body, barium sulfate cannot be used intravascularly or intrathecally. Also, its use is contraindicated in the case of a suspected perforation in the alimentary canal, as it may leak into the peritoneal cavity, causing avascular adhesions and peritonitis. For this reason, it is also contraindicated in cases of recent or impending abdominal surgery.

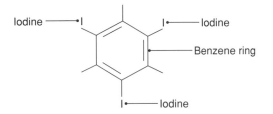

Figure 13–9. The benzene ring forms the base of iodinated contrast media.

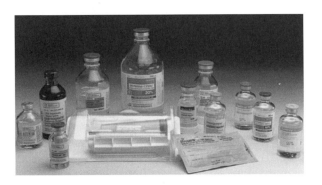

Figure 13–10. Examples of iodinated contrast agents.

IODINATED COMPOUNDS

Properties

With an atomic number of 53, the element iodine is almost as radiopaque as barium sulfate. A triiodinated benzene ring containing three atoms of iodine per molecule forms the base of iodinated contrast media *(Figure 13–9)*. Iodine is the element of choice for use as a contrast agent, as it forms stable compounds and does not break down in the body. Like barium sulfate, it has a relatively low toxicity and high atomic number. Unlike barium sulfate, it is generally absorbed by the body and excreted by the kidneys within 24 hours of intravascular administration. As iodinated contrast media have a tendency to break down in the light, they should be shielded from bright light. The viscosity, or thickness, of the contrast medium is greatly determined by the size and concentration of the molecules in the solution. It is recommended that liquid iodinated contrast media be prewarmed to body temperature prior to use. Doing so reduces their viscosity, allowing for easier administration and lessening the possibility of adverse reactions.

Iodinated contrast agents are administered for a variety of radiographic examinations. From the many products available commercially, the radiology department or physician selects a particular contrast agent according to the area of interest and type of examination *(Figure 13–10)*. As pharmaceutical products, iodinated contrast media are referred to by their generic name, chemical name, or trade name, which is the manufacturer's brand name for the product. For example, Reno-60 is a trade name, whereas diatrizoate meglumine 60% is the generic name for the same product. The opacity of an iodinated contrast agent is determined by its iodine content; therefore, a product containing a high percentage of iodine will characteristically exhibit high opacity and high radiographic contrast. Iodinated contrast agents often have a number or percentage after their names representing the weight-to-volume ratio or concentration of iodine-containing compounds in the solution. Again, using Reno-60 as an example, this product contains 60 g of iodine-containing salts per 100 mL of solvent, which is equivalent to a 60% concentration. An iodinated contrast agent with a higher concentration is generally used for cardiovascular studies, whereas a lower concentration is used for urography and cholography.

Iodinated contrast media are available as either oil-based or water-soluble agents. Each type of medium is selected for use based on the anatomy to be examined.

Oil-based Iodinated Contrast Media

The use of oil-based iodinated contrast media in radiography is relatively limited. They are used primarily for studies of the lymphatic system (lymphangiography). In the past, they were also used for studies of the female reproductive system (hysterosalpingography), spinal cord (myelography), bronchial tree of the respiratory system (bronchography), salivary glands (sialography), and tear ducts (dacryocystography), but have been replaced by water-soluble iodinated nonionic contrast media. The oil-based iodinated contrast

Table 13–2. Examples of Water-soluble Iodinated Ionic and Nonionic Contrast Media

Trade Name	Generic Name
Ionic Contrast Media	
Reno-60	Diatrizoate meglumine 60%
Conray	Iothalamate meglumine 60%
Hypaque meglumine 60%	Diatrizoate meglumine 60%
Hexabrix	Ioxaglate
Nonionic Contrast Media	
Isovue-300	Iopamidol 61%
Optiray 320	Ioversol 68%
Omnipaque 300	Iohexal 61%
Amipaque	Metrizamide
Ultravist 300	Iopromide 62%

Table 13–3. Advantages of Nonionic Contrast Media Over Ionic Contrast Media

- Well tolerated by the patient
- Less heat and discomfort on injection
- Low osmolality
- Does not dissociate into charged particles
- Low neurotoxicity
- Approximately one-fifth fewer adverse reactions than with the use of ionic contrast media

medium is used in hollow anatomic areas to show by the radiographic contrast in the structure. The oily base of the contrast medium is a fatty acid, which is responsible for making the solution viscous (thick) and insoluble in water and body fluids. Because it is not miscible with blood, it should never be injected intravenously or intraarterially. It should also be noted that the oily medium tends to persist in the area that was examined, as it is very slowly absorbed by the body.

Water-soluble Iodinated Contrast Media

Water-soluble (aqueous) iodinated contrast media are routinely used for radiographic examinations of the urinary, biliary, and cardiovascular systems, as well as the digestive system if barium sulfate is contraindicated. Water-soluble iodinated contrast media are also used in special examinations of the skeletal system, such as myelography and arthrography. They are available in liquid, tablet, or granule form, depending on the intended use. The injectable liquid media can be divided into ionic and nonionic contrast agents *(Figure 13–11).*

An ionic contrast agent is an organic iodine compound that has triiodinated benzoic acid as its base. The compound dissociates or separates in water into two electrically charged particles. One of the particles, called a *cation,* has a positive charge; the other particle, an *anion,* has a negative charge. A nonionic contrast agent also contains iodine and is a derivative of the triiodinated benzoic acid base, but it does not contain an ionizing group. It is more soluble in water and does not dissociate into charged particles; it is said to have a lower osmolality than an ionic contrast agent. *Table 13–2* lists commonly used ionic and nonionic contrast agents.

Osmolality (oz-mō-LAL-i-tē) refers to the concentration or number of particles (cations and anions) in the solution per kilogram of water and is directly related to the occurrence of adverse patient reactions. It is measured in osmoles, which are units of osmotic pressure. A contrast agent with a high osmolality has an increased number of particles and more osmoles in the solution.

Any time a foreign substance is injected into the bloodstream, the homeostasis of the body can be affected. There is less chance of an interruption of homeostasis if the osmolality of the injected contrast agent closely resembles that of blood plasma, which is approximately 300 osmol/kg. On the average, nonionic contrast agents have around 750 osmol/kg, whereas ionic contrast agents range from 1000 to 2400 osmol/kg. Because of their hyperosmolality, ionic contrast agents can cross the blood–brain barrier, which is also a factor in the occurrence of adverse reactions. Nonionic contrast agents have a much lower level of neurotoxicity. Although the osmolality of nonionic contrast agents is still higher than that of blood plasma, it is significantly lower then the osmolality of ionic contrast agents. For this reason, the use of nonionic contrast agents tends to produce fewer physiologic reactions than use of their ionic counterparts. The advantages of nonionic contrast media are summarized in *Table 13–3;* however, there is a disadvantage to the use of nonionic contrast agents, as they are more difficult to produce and expensive, costing about six times the price of ionic agents. It should also be noted that severe adverse reactions to ionic contrast agents are rare, making it difficult to justify exclusive use of nonionic contrast agents. To control costs, many radiology departments may routinely use ionic contrast agents except when patient history and condition warrant the use of nonionic contrast agents. The American College of Radiology (ACR) has identified high-risk patients and criteria for using nonionic contrast agents instead of ionic contrast agents, summarized in *Table 13–4.*

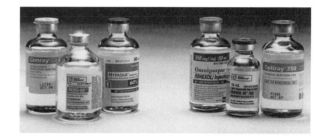

Figure 13–11. Examples of ionic and nonionic iodinated contrast agents.

Table 13–4. Criteria for the Use of Nonionic Contrast Media

- History of previous adverse reaction (except mild reactions of heat, flush, and nausea)
- History of cardiac impairment
- History of allergies and/or asthma
- Generalized debilitation/poor patient condition
- Increased patient anxiety
- Patient request for nonionic contrast medium
- Sickle cell disease
- Other situations in which there is poor communication about history because of patient's condition

Table 13–5. Contraindications to the Intravascular Administration of Water-soluble Contrast Media

- Allergy/hypersensitivity to iodine
- Anuria
- High creatinine level
- Renal disease and other conditions that compromise renal function
  (eg, diabetes mellitus, multiple myeloma, sickle cell anemia, pheochromocytoma)
- Congestive heart failure
- Severe dehydration

Note. Intravascular Injection of water-soluble iodinated contrast media puts
patients with these conditions at a higher risk for adverse reactions.

Contraindications

The most significant contraindication to the use of iodinated contrast media is an allergic history to iodine. In some cases, the patient can be premedicated with steroids and/or antihistamines and the contrast medium can be administered without causing an adverse reaction. Allergic reactions to oil-based iodinated contrast media can occur but are rare. Other contraindications to the intravascular administration of water-soluble iodinated contrast media are identified in *Table 13–5*.

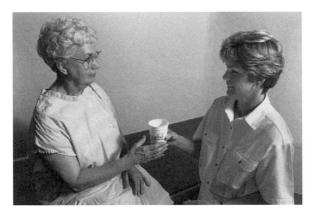

Figure 13–12. Barium sulfate is administered orally for a radiographic examination of the stomach or small intestine.

► ROUTES OF ADMINISTRATION

Contrast media are considered to be pharmaceuticals (drugs), and as such, they must be administered appropriately to achieve the desired effect and to avoid unwanted complications. Radiographers are not licensed to dispense medications on their own; this is the physician's responsibility. As the physician's assistant in radiographic procedures using contrast media, however, the radiographer must be knowledgeable about the safest and most effective methods of administrating contrast agents.

Table 13–6 illustrates the *Five Rights* system, which applies to the administration of all medications, including contrast agents. The patient must be properly identified. The name of the contrast agent should be checked by the radiographer at least three times—at the time of selection, preparation, and just prior to administration. Although many contrast media are packaged in average dosages, the amount may have to be adjusted depending on the patient's age, size, and condition. The radiologist should make the decision to alter the dosage. The contrast medium must be administered by the proper route to be effective and to avoid adverse complications. Contrast media should be administered at the correct time, which is dependent on the type of examination and the radiologist's orders. After a contrast medium is administered, a notation should be made in the patient's chart indicating the name of the contrast medium, dosage, route of administration, and time of administration. Any adverse reaction to the contrast medium should also be documented.

The route of administration depends on the anatomy of interest, type of examination, and particular contrast medium. Contrast media can be administered orally, rectally, or intravascularly, or introduced directly into the intended site.

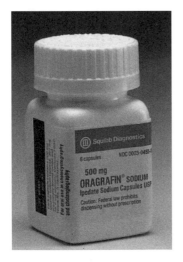

Figure 13–13. This cholecystopaque is administered orally to promote visualization of the gallbladder.

ORAL/RECTAL ROUTE

Barium sulfate products are administered by means of the oral route for examinations of the esophagus, stomach, and small intestine *(Figure 13–12)*. Iodinated contrast agents such as Gastrografin and Hypaque can also be administered orally for these same examinations. Iodinated agents known as **oral cholecystopaques** are administered orally in pill or granule form for visualization of the gallbladder *(Figure 13–13)*.

Table 13–6. The Five Rights of Medicine Administration

- The *right patient* should receive
- The *right medication*
- In the *right amount*
- Via the *right route*
- At the *right time*

A contrast medium is administered rectally as an enema for an examination of the large intestine. Although barium sulfate is the most commonly used contrast medium for this purpose, Hypaque or similar iodinated products may also be used. Guidelines for correct insertion of the enema tip are provided in Chapter 15.

INTRAVASCULAR ROUTE

Only water-soluble iodinated contrast media can be administered intravascularly. Intravascular injection of contrast media includes both intravenous and intraarterial routes.

The **intravenous route** is employed for excretory urography and intravenous cholangiography, as well as for CT and MRI examinations using contrast media. A vein in the antecubital region of the arm or on the dorsum of the hand provides the easiest access site for injection *(Figure 13–14)*. The radiographer or physician performing the venipuncture should follow universal precautions, which include the use of gloves. After visual inspection of the site, it is then thoroughly cleansed by applying a sterile alcohol or antiseptic swab in a circular motion, working outward from the center of the site. The site should be allowed to dry completely. A tourniquet is applied snugly approximately 3 to 4 in. (7 to 10 cm) above the site. A butterfly needle *(Figure 13–15)*, straight needle, or venous catheter is inserted smoothly at a 15° angle to the skin (the bevel of the needle should face upward). Backflow of blood indicates correct placement of the needle in the vein. After the tourniquet is released, the contrast medium can be injected in bolus fashion, infusion, or by means of an automatic injector. At the completion of the injection, a sterile gauze pad is placed over the site, the needle is removed, and pressure is applied for several minutes until the bleeding stops *(Figure 13–16)*. This is a cursory description of venipuncture; a more detailed explanation can be found in a patient care book or phlebotomy handbook. Although it is within the scope of practice for radiographers, some states do not permit radiographers to practice venipuncture. Therefore, the radiographer should be aware of applicable statutes regulating the practice of venipuncture in the state of his or her employment.

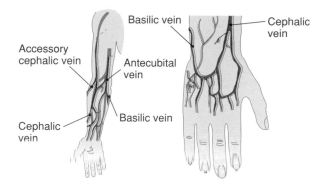

Figure 13–14. A vein in the antecubital region of the arm or on the dorsum of the hand provides the easiest access site for intravenous injection of water-soluble iodinated contrast media.

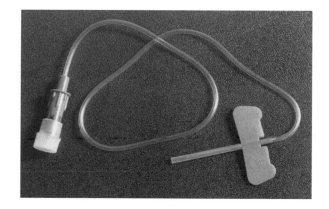

Figure 13–15. A butterfly needle is also called a winged infusion set. The "wings" on the butterfly needle are used to guide the needle into the vein.

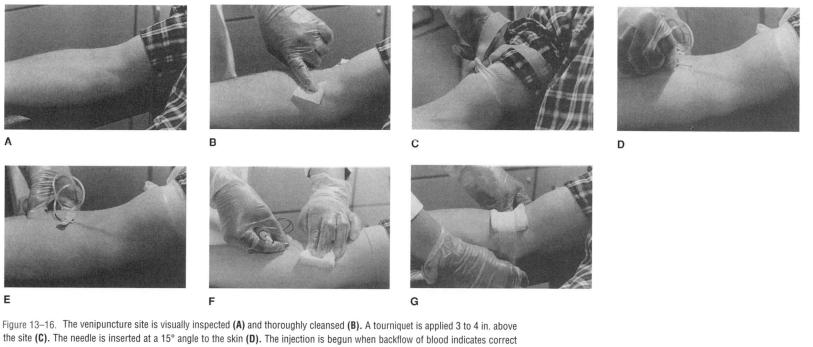

Figure 13–16. The venipuncture site is visually inspected **(A)** and thoroughly cleansed **(B)**. A tourniquet is applied 3 to 4 in. above the site **(C)**. The needle is inserted at a 15° angle to the skin **(D)**. The injection is begun when backflow of blood indicates correct placement of the needle in the vein **(E)**. At the completion of the injection, the needle is removed **(F)** and pressure is applied with a gauze pad until the bleeding stops **(G)**. *(From Garza, D. and Becan-McBride, K. Phlebotomy Handbook, 3rd ed. Norwalk, CT: Appleton & Lange; 1993: 126–128, with permission.)*

The **intraarterial route** is used for special radiographic procedures of the cardiovascular system. Access to the artery is accomplished via the Seldinger technique, which is described in Chapter 18.

In lymphangiography, the contrast medium is injected intravascularly into the lymphatic vessels. This procedure is also described in Chapter 18.

DIRECT ROUTE

Some radiographic examinations require that the contrast medium be introduced directly into the anatomy of interest. This can be achieved by means of a catheter or needle. For example, in a cystogram a catheter is inserted into the urinary bladder and a water-soluble iodinated contrast medium (either ionic or non-ionic) is allowed to flow into the bladder until it is full. During a myelogram, an intrathecal injection is performed by inserting a spinal needle into the subarachnoid space between two vertebrae and injecting a water-soluble iodinated (nonionic) contrast medium into the thecal sac. Examples of other examinations in which contrast media are directly administered include arthrography, hysterosalpingography, sialography, and percutaneous transhepatic cholangiography.

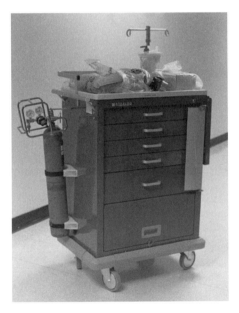

Figure 13–17. A crash cart or emergency drug box should be readily available.

► REACTIONS TO CONTRAST MEDIA

The potential exists for an adverse reaction to occur when a contrast medium is administered to a patient. Although reactions can take place with the use of any contrast agent, they are more likely to occur after intravascular injection. Very few reactions actually occur following administration of barium sulfate or oil-based iodinated contrast agents. The radiographer should be aware of the possibility of adverse reactions and be prepared to handle them according to the institution's protocol. All reactions must be properly documented in the patient's chart. An emergency drug box or crash cart should be in the examination room or readily available *(Figure 13–17)*. It is recommended that the patient's blood pressure, pulse, and respiration be assessed prior to contrast medium administration. This provides baseline information in the event a reaction occurs.

Because it is inert, barium sulfate rarely causes any allergic reactions; however, it does tend to cause constipation as the water is absorbed from the mixture, leaving the solid barium sulfate in the intestines. This is especially true in elderly patients who tend to have decreased bowel motility. Following any examination in which barium sulfate is administered, the patient should be advised to drink plenty of fluids to prevent a bowel obstruction. Care should be taken when a patient feels nauseous or vomits after ingestion of barium sulfate so that the contrast material is not aspirated. Aspiration of barium sulfate into the lungs can result in pneumonia. Occasionally, a condition known as hypervolemia can occur from administration of a barium enema. In this very serious condition, excessive water is absorbed from the large intestine by the circulatory system. Pulmonary edema and/or other complications can result from the fluid overload.

An allergic reaction is possible with the use of any iodinated contrast agent; however, few reactions occur with the use of oil-based iodinated contrast media. The reactions to injectable contrast agents can be described as systemic because the physiologic response of the body's systems is affected when the contrast media are injected into the cardiovascular system. According to the Chemotoxic Theory, hemodynamic changes occur as the body's normal physiologic functions and homeostasis are interrupted. The reactions seem to be directly related to the following factors:

- Degree of chemotoxicity of the contrast medium
- Concentration of iodine in the contrast medium
- Certain properties of the contrast medium, including osmolality, viscosity, and purity of the solution
- Dosage administered
- Pace of the injection
- Physical condition of the patient

An **anaphylactoid** (an-ah-fah-LAK-toid) **reaction** closely resembles a true allergic reaction in which the patient demonstrates hypersensitivity when a foreign substance is injected. Although such a reaction cannot be predicted, certain patients seem to be predisposed to experiencing adverse reactions. It is critical that the radiographer take an accurate patient history prior to the administration of a contrast medium, particularly to determine any allergies and previous reactions to contrast media. Examples of patient histories for particular examinations can be found in the following chapters on the urinary, digestive, and biliary systems.

Table 13–7. Adverse Reactions to Iodinated Contrast Media

System	Reaction	Severity of Reaction		
		Mild	Moderate	Severe
Cardiovascular	Arrhythmia		X	
	Tachycardia or bradycardia		X	
	Extreme hypotension			X
	Cardiac arrest			X
	Hypervolemia			X
Neurologic	Headache		X	May become severe
	Unconsciousness			X
	Coma			X
	Seizures			X
	Aphasia			X
Respiratory	Coughing/sneezing	X		
	Dyspnea			X
	Extreme change (up or down) in rate of respiration			X
	Laryngospasm/laryngeal edema			X
	Cyanosis			X
	Respiratory arrest			X
Urinary	Flank pain		X	
	Hematuria		X	
	Renal impairment/failure			X
Gastrointestinal	Nausea/vomiting	X		
	Uncontrolled vomiting		X	
	Metallic taste	X		
Integumentary	Hot flash/flush	X		
	Mild urticaria	X		
	Excessive urticaria		X	
	Pain or burning sensation from extravasation	X		
	Itching	X		
	Facial edema		X	

A **vasovagal** (vā-sō-VĀ-gal) **reaction** is one that occurs in response to anxiety or fear. It generally involves a vascular as well as a neurogenic response, with the patient experiencing mild symptoms of pallor, dizziness, diaphoresis, nausea, and possibly bradycardia. The radiographer can help alleviate the symptoms by being supportive and reassuring.

Extravasation (eks-trav-ah-ZĀ-shun) occurs during injection if some of the contrast medium seeps out of the vein into the surrounding tissue. This reaction usually involves pain and discoloration at the site of injection. The radiographer should apply a warm, moist compress to the site to decrease pain and aid in the absorption of the extravasated contrast medium.

Adverse reactions are usually acute, with the majority occurring 5 to 20 minutes after injection of the contrast medium. Although delayed reactions are possible, they are rare and typically mild. Reactions are classified as mild, moderate, or severe according to the symptoms experienced by the patient and the treatment needed to alleviate them. **Mild (minor) reactions,** such as a warm flush or metallic taste, generally need little or no treatment and are considered to be self limiting. **Moderate reactions** require the administration of medication to relieve the symptoms. For example, a patient who develops hives on several areas of the body might be given an antihistamine such as Benadryl. **Severe reactions** are considered to be life-threatening. Immediate treatment is necessary to stabilize the patient, beginning with administration of 100% oxygen and accessing a vein to start an intravenous line (5% dextrose in water or normal saline). The patient's blood pressure, pulse, and respiration should be closely monitored. *Table 13–7* summarizes a variety of adverse reactions, the particular body systems affected, and the severity of the reactions.

▶ Related Terminology

bolus injection (BŌ-lus)—injection of a concentrated amount of contrast medium over a short period

diaphoresis (dī-ah-fō-RĒ-sis)—condition in which a person sweats profusely

extravasation (eks-trav-ah-ZĀ-shun)—occurs during injection if some of the contrast medium seeps out of the vein into the surrounding tissue

hemodynamic (he-mo-dī-NAM-ik)—concerning the movement of blood within the circulatory system

homeostasis (hō-mē-ō-STĀ-sis)—maintenance of constant conditions within the body; state of equilibrium of the body's biological systems

hypervolemia (hī-per-vōl-E-mē-ah)—abnormal condition in which there is excess volume of fluid in the circulatory system; this condition can occur with the use of water-soluble iodinated contrast media or barium sulfate

infusion (in-FŪ-shun)—slow intravenous administration of contrast medium diluted with sterile water

miscible (MIS-i-bl)—able to be mixed or combined with other components

pharmaceutical (far-mah-SŪ-ti-kal)—drug; the term also applies to contrast agents used in radiography

toxicity (tok-SIS-i-tē)—refers to the degree that something is poisonous

urticaria (ur-ti-KĀ-rē-ah)—hives or wheals; may occur as a vascular reaction of the skin after injection of iodinated contrast medium

viscosity (vis-KOS-i-tē)—refers to the resistance of a solution to flow; a viscid substance is one that is thick and sticky (eg, honey is more viscid than water)

► PROCEDURAL CONSIDERATIONS

The procedures for completing contrast studies are somewhat different from those for noncontrast studies, with most examinations requiring the use of advanced patient preparation, fluoroscopy, and a higher level of patient care. Because contrast examinations tend to be more lengthy and involved than noncontrast procedures, room preparation, organization, and appropriate patient communication are vital to a safe and successful examination.

RADIOGRAPHER'S RESPONSIBILITIES

Most contrast studies use fluoroscopy and require the expertise of the radiologist or other physician, making them more complex than plain skeletal radiography. In addition to obtaining overhead radiographs, the radiographer is also responsible for preparing the room for fluoroscopy and assisting the physician with the examination.

Although patient education should be provided for all radiographic examinations, it is especially critical for contrast examinations. Because the health care environment often seems impersonal, radiographers must develop their skills relative to compassion, caring, and empathy. Patients preparing for contrast examinations are often anxious because they do not know what to expect and may be very afraid of the outcome of the procedure. A high level of anxiety could ultimately affect the success of the examination. The radiographer must be sensitive to the patient's needs and take the time to explain the entire procedure to the patient, including what will happen, who will be involved in the procedure, any contrast media used and how it will be administered, any side effects that may occur, and the length of the examination. Because patients do not always process information quickly, it is important to speak slowly and provide the patient the opportunity to ask questions at the end of the explanation. As the primary caretaker in the radiology department, it is the radiographer's responsibility to introduce other health care professionals participating in the procedure to the patient.

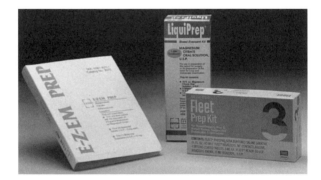

Figure 13-18. Examples of bowel preparation kits.

Patient Preparation

Most radiographic examinations that use contrast media require preparation that must be completed prior to the day of the study. Patient preparation can range from fasting for 8 hours prior to the examination to a restricted diet and thorough cleansing of the bowel, depending on the examination and department protocol *(Figure 13–18)*. It is the radiographer's responsibility to be familiar with the department protocols for examination preparation (please see relevant chapters for generic guidelines).

Because information obtained from a pertinent patient history can assist the radiologist with diagnosis and determination of proper procedure protocol, the radiographer must learn specific patient information relative to the examination. When iodinated contrast is used, an allergy history and information regarding previous examinations using iodinated contrast should be obtained. In addition to the typical questions regarding symptoms and previous history, the patient should also be asked the type of preparation followed prior to the examination. If the patient vomited the pills for a gallbladder study or ate breakfast prior to an upper gastrointestinal examination, the study may have to be rescheduled. Examination-specific patient preparation guidelines and history information are discussed in the chapters that follow.

Room Preparation

The radiographer is responsible for ensuring that all supplies and equipment that may be needed for the examination are available and ready prior to starting the procedure. Although the list of needed supplies varies depending on the procedure to be performed, it generally includes appropriate contrast medium, equipment for administration of contrast, emergency box or crash cart, disposable gloves, emesis basin, towels, and sheets or blankets. Other equipment may also be needed for specific examinations; this will be identified in the relevant chapters.

Before a patient is brought into the radiographic room, the appropriate contrast medium should be prepared according to department protocol or specific patient needs. The equipment should also be thoroughly cleaned using an appropriate disinfectant. Unclean rooms can contribute to nosocomial (hospital-acquired) infections and lead to a lack of patient confidence in the radiographer's competence. Clean linens should be on the table for those examinations performed with the table in the horizontal position.

For upper gastrointestinal studies, the radiographic table is generally turned to the upright position in preparation for fluoroscopy *(Figure 13–19)*. Prior to doing so, the Bucky tray must be moved to the foot of the table. This action must always be done prior to fluoroscopy as it closes the Bucky slot with protective shielding and provides a clear path between the fluoroscopic tube and image intensifier. The footboard

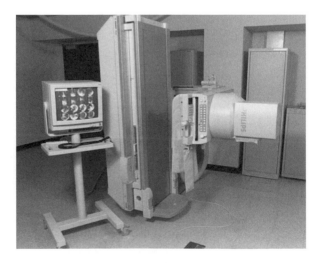

Figure 13-19. The radiographic table is turned 90° upright to start fluoroscopic studies of the upper gastrointestinal tract.

must also be securely attached; force should be applied to the footboard to ensure it is correctly locked into place. When the table is in the upright position, the foot switch should be moved within reach and the lead drape on the image intensifier should be appropriately positioned to protect the fluoroscopist.

Fluoroscopy

Although a radiologist or other trained professional operates the fluoroscope, it is the radiographer's responsibility to ensure it is functioning properly. Some departments may have a phantom that can be imaged. A quality-control check should be performed on a regular basis per department routine. The spot film device or other mechanism for recording images should also be ready for the procedure; cassettes to be used for spot films should be available. Prior to starting the procedure, the radiographer must set the control panel for fluoroscopy, including appropriate technical factors. The fluoroscopic timer should also be set for 5 minutes.

Radiation Protection

Because contrast studies often require the use of fluoroscopy, radiation protection is an important consideration for the patient and radiation workers. It is the radiographer's responsibility to ensure that lead protective aprons and gloves are available for anyone present during the examination; thyroid shields and leaded glasses may also be available. The cardinal rules of time, distance, and shielding are important considerations. Anyone assisting or observing the fluoroscopic examination must wear a lead apron with a minimum 0.5-mm lead equivalent. When not needed to assist the patient or to adjust the flow of barium for a barium enema, the radiographer should maximize the distance from the radiographic table. The fluoroscopist is trained to operate the fluoro using an on–off technique to minimize the amount of time the patient and others in the room are exposed to radiation. To expedite the procedure, the radiographer should assist in turning and holding patients having difficulty moving. When significant patient assistance is anticipated, a lead shield can be placed on the table under the patient's head and shoulders, as long as it does not compromise the procedure. Doing so reduces the radiographer's exposure from scatter coming from the undertable fluoroscopic tube, as well as reduces patient dose.

To minimize the gonadal dose of a pediatric patient during fluoroscopy of the upper gastrointestinal tract, a lead shield can be placed on the table under the patient's buttocks. The use of videotape or digital fluoroscopy can also reduce the amount of fluoro time used.

SEQUENCING OF EXAMINATIONS

Based on the symptoms, patients are often scheduled for multiple diagnostic tests, both in and out of the radiology department. Because contrast media may compromise the success of other diagnostic tests, the radiographer must understand how various procedures should be scheduled so that all studies can be successfully completed in as little time as possible; several studies can often be completed on the same day. Since residual barium can cause unacceptable artifacts, barium studies are generally performed last. The following guidelines should be considered when scheduling patients or communicating with nursing services or a physician's office:

1. All radiographic examinations that do not require contrast media should be performed first.
2. Laboratory studies for thyroid uptake and nuclear medicine thyroid scans should be performed prior to any examination using iodinated contrast media; administration of iodinated contrast could delay a thyroid study for at least 3 weeks.
3. Because iodinated contrast media is less dense than barium and readily excreted, radiographic examinations that use iodinated contrast should be performed before those using barium sulfate.
4. Ultrasound examinations of the abdomen and radioisotope studies of the liver and spleen should be performed before any barium study.
5. Fiberoptic studies of the gastrointestinal tract (eg, gastroscopy, sigmoidoscopy) are usually performed prior to barium studies of the gastrointestinal tract to prevent the possibility of the barium interfering with visual assessment.
6. CT studies of the abdomen should be completed before any other examination using barium sulfate; the barium sulfate used for gastrointestinal studies is much denser than that used for CT examinations and may compromise the results of the CT.
7. Radiographic examinations of the lower gastrointestinal tract (barium enema) are generally performed before upper gastrointestinal studies.

In addition to the above guidelines, examinations that require the patient to fast for 8 or more hours should be scheduled early in the morning. Because diabetic patients may be at risk of an insulin reaction, they should be scheduled first; pediatric and geriatric patients should be scheduled next, as they may have difficulty remaining NPO for lengthy periods. When multiple examinations requiring the intravenous administration of iodinated contrast are scheduled on the same day, care must be taken to ensure that the total dosage of iodine does not exceed the recommended limit.

▶ **Exam Sequence**

- *Noncontrast examinations*

- *Thyroid studies*

- *Iodinated contrast examinations*

- *Abdominal ultrasound examinations*

- *Abdominal CT examinations*

- *Fiberoptic studies of the GI tract*

- *Barium studies of the GI tract*

SUMMARY

▶ Contrast media alter a structure's density, thus affecting its radiographic appearance.

▶ Contrast media can be used to enhance structures that have low subject contrast such as the urinary, digestive, and biliary systems, spinal canal, female reproductive system, and vasculature.

▶ Negative contrast media are radiolucent and appear dark on a radiograph. Room air is a common example of a negative contrast agent.

▶ Positive contrast media are radiopaque and appear light on a radiograph. Iodine and barium sulfate form the bases of positive contrast agents.

▶ Iodinated contrast media that are ionic dissociate into charged particles, whereas nonionic agents do not dissociate.

▶ Contrast media are pharmaceutical agents (drugs) and must be administered appropriately with a physician's order.

▶ Contrast media can be administered orally, rectally, or intravascularly or introduced directly, depending on the type of examination and the type of contrast agent.

▶ An adverse reaction can occur with the use of any contrast medium.

▶ Reactions are classified as mild (minor), moderate, or severe, depending on the symptoms and required treatment.

▶ Most contrast examinations use fluoroscopy and require some type of patient preparation prior to the day of the examination.

▶ The radiographer's responsibilities include patient care and education, patient preparation, preparation of contrast media, room and equipment preparation, and radiation protection.

▶ Although more than one diagnostic test can usually be performed on the same day, care must be taken to ensure that examinations are properly sequenced so all studies can be completed in as little time as possible.

QUESTIONS FOR CRITICAL THINKING & APPLICATION

1. Identify radiographic examinations that require the administration of contrast media for optimum demonstration of the anatomy. Which type of contrast medium is used for each?

2. Explain the correlation between an element's atomic number and its appearance radiographically.

3. Why should a patient be instructed to drink plenty of fluids following the administration of contrast media?

4. Your neighbor tells you that she is scheduled for an excretory urogram. She has concerns about the examination, but has heard that a new "dye" is being used that does not contain iodine. What explanation will you give in the way of "patient education"?

5. What is the relationship between iodinated contrast media and the kidneys? How can excessive administration of iodinated contrast media result in renal failure? What are some of the high-risk factors relating to the urinary system that should be identified prior to contrast media administration?

6. Describe how the radiographer's responsibilities with respect to contrast studies differ from those for noncontrast examinations.

7. A 4-year-old child has been scheduled for an upper gastrointestinal study, which will take approximately 30 minutes. Demonstrate how you would explain this procedure to the patient.

8. Describe the differences in room preparation for noncontrast and contrast examinations.

9. When scheduling contrast studies, diabetic patients should be first on the list. Explain why this is done. In consideration of this, what should the radiographer be aware of with respect to patient care? When scheduling the examination, what information should be given to the patient relative to patient preparation and insulin?

10. A patient must be scheduled for an upper gastrointestinal study, a CT study of the chest, a nuclear medicine thyroid study, and an oral cholecystogram. List the order in which these examinations should be completed. Can any be done on the same day? If so, describe.

FILM CRITIQUE

Describe the type of contrast medium that could be used for this examination *(Figure 13–20)*.

How would the contrast be administered?

What precautions should the radiographer take with respect to patient safety?

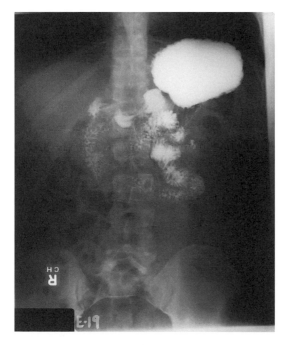

Figure 13–20

14

URINARY SYSTEM

OBJECTIVES

Following the completion of this chapter the student will be able to:

- Given diagrams or radiographs, name and describe the anatomy of the urinary system, to include the kidneys, ureters, urinary bladder, urethra, and vascular structures.

- Discuss the microscopic structure of the kidney and its role in producing urine.

- Discuss the relationship of the adrenal and prostate glands to the urinary system with regard to location.

- Identify the key function of the urinary system and explain why it is vital for a person's health and well-being.

- Define *nephrolith* and *renal calculus* and identify the three constricted areas along the urinary tract where they are most likely to lodge.

- Discuss the use of contrast media in radiographic examinations of the urinary tract, to include type and route of administration.

- Differentiate between functional and nonfunctional radiographic examinations of the urinary tract.

- State the criteria used to determine positioning accuracy on radiographs of the urinary tract and evaluate radiographs of the urinary tract in terms of positioning, centering, image quality, radiographic anatomy, and pathology.

- Define terminology associated with the urinary tract, to include anatomy, procedures, and pathology.

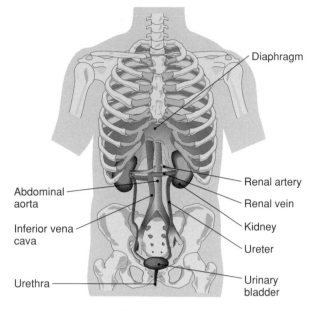

Figure 14–1. The urinary system.

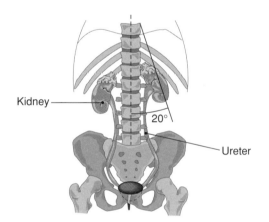

Figure 14–2. Anterior view of the abdomen demonstrating the orientation of the kidneys.

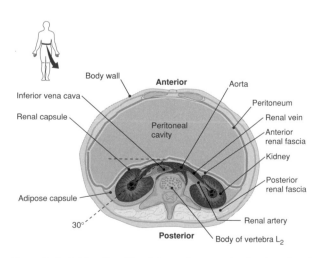

Figure 14–3. Axial section of the abdomen demonstrating the orientation of the kidneys.

► ANATOMY OF THE URINARY SYSTEM

Through the process of metabolism, cells generate excess water and organic waste products, including ammonia, urea, uric acid, carbon dioxide, and bilirubin. The urinary system has the primary responsibility of eliminating these waste materials from the body *(Table 14–1)*. In doing so, it plays a major role in maintaining the homeostasis of the body by regulating the volume, pH, and concentration of the blood, along with controlling blood pressure. The urinary system comprises two kidneys, two ureters, one urinary bladder, and one urethra *(Figure 14–1)*.

KIDNEYS

The paired kidneys (KID-nēz) (singular, kidney) are the organs of the urinary system responsible for producing urine. Their role is so vital to a person's well-being that death will eventually result if renal *(reno = "kidney")* failure occurs as a result of disease or trauma. The kidneys are situated under the diaphragm in the upper, posterior abdominal cavity. Located approximately in the region between the twelfth thoracic and third lumbar vertebrae, they lie behind the parietal peritoneum and are therefore considered to be retroperitoneal structures. The kidneys rest obliquely against the psoas major muscles at an angle of 20°, with the superior portion of each kidney closer to the vertebral column than its inferior portion *(Figure 14–2)*. These muscles also cause the kidneys to tilt posteriorly at a 30° angle to the midsagittal plane *(Figure 14–3)*. The right kidney is displaced somewhat inferiorly as a result of the presence of the liver in the right upper quadrant of the abdomen. The lower posterior ribs afford protection to the kidneys in the case of blunt trauma to the middle back region.

Gross Anatomy

The kidneys are bean-shaped structures. Considering the amount of work they perform daily, they are relatively small, constituting only 1% of the body's mass. *Table 14–2* summarizes the average dimensions of one normal kidney.

The medial border of each kidney is adjacent to the vertebral column. It is concave with a deep cleft or fissure, the **renal hilum** (HĪ-lum), which leads to a cavity within the kidney called the **renal sinus.** The

Table 14–1. Production & Pathway of Urine in the Urinary System

Main Component	Subcomponent	Description
Renal artery ↓		Right and left; branches from abdominal aorta to supply blood to kidney
Kidney ↓		Right and left; under diaphragm in posterior abdomen; produces urine
Cortex →	Nephron (glomerulus and renal tubule) ↓	Filtration Reabsorption Secretion
← ← ← ← ← ← ← ↓		
Medulla →	Renal pyramids (collecting tubules)	8–18 conical structures
Renal pelvis	↓	Branches into major and minor calyces and funnel-shaped cavity
	Minor calyces ↓	7–12; cup-shaped ends
	Major calyces ↓	2 or 3; short and tubelike
	Cavity of renal pelvis ↓	Funnel-shaped cavity; continuous with ureter
← ← ← ← ← ← ← ↓		
Ureter ↓		Right and left; 25 to 30-cm tube; transports urine from kidney to bladder
Urinary bladder ↓		Expandable reservoir that stores urine
Urethra →	External urethral orifice	Tube that transports urine to exterior of body; 4 cm in females, 20 cm in males

Table 14–2. Average Dimensions of the Kidney

Length	10–12 cm	4–5 in.
Width	5–7.5 cm	2–3 in.
Thickness	2.5 cm	1 in.
Weight	150 g	5 oz

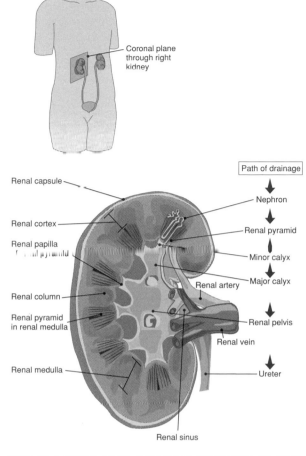

Figure 14–4. Coronal section of the kidney demonstrating the internal structures.

renal blood vessels, lymphatic vessels, nerves, and ureter occupy the renal sinus and are conveyed to and from the kidney via the renal hilum. The kidney is partitioned into an **upper pole** and a **lower pole,** with the hilum being the dividing point.

Each kidney is surrounded by three layers of tissue that safeguard it from injury. The **renal fascia** (RĒ-nal FASH-ē-ah) is the outermost covering. It is a thin layer of dense, fibrous tissue that completely encompasses the kidney and its proximate adrenal gland (part of the endocrine system) and secures them to the abdominal wall and other adjacent structures. The middle layer is the **adipose capsule,** which is also referred to as **perirenal fat.** This fatty cushion surrounds each kidney to protect it from trauma and helps maintain the normal position of the kidney against the psoas major muscle. The innermost layer is the **renal capsule.** This translucent, fibrous covering helps protect the kidney from the spread of infection from other abdominal structures.

The internal anatomy of the kidney can be divided into three definite areas: cortex, medulla, and pelvis. The **cortex** (KOR-teks) is the smooth-textured tissue located just beneath the renal capsule and extending to the bases of the renal pyramids. It also projects into the spaces between the pyramids to extend to the renal sinus, forming the **renal columns.**

The **renal medulla** comprises approximately 8 to 18 **renal pyramids.** These triangular or cone-shaped structures are formed primarily by bundles of collecting tubules, giving the pyramids a striated appearance. Their broad bases are adjacent to the cortex, whereas the more pointed apices, called **papillae** (pah-PIL-ē) (singular, *papilla* = "nipple"), project inward to the renal sinus. The term *parenchyma* (pah-RENG-ki-mah) refers collectively to the cortex and medulla, which constitute the functional tissue of the kidney.

The **renal pelvis** consists of major and minor calyces, as well as a large cavity. The small tubelike **calyces** (KĀ-li-sēz) (singular, calyx) are branches off of the outer margin of the cavity. The cup-shaped ends of approximately 7 to 12 minor calyces enclose the papillae to direct the urine from the collecting tubules toward the renal pelvis. The minor calyces join together to form two or three short major calyces. The major calyces merge at a large, funnel-shaped cavity that lies mostly within the renal sinus. The more medial portion of the renal pelvis is expanded and lies partly outside of the kidney to continue as the ureter *(Figure 14–4).*

Physiology

The **nephron** (NEF-ron) is the physiologic or functional element of the kidney. There are approximately one million microscopic nephrons located within the parenchyma of each kidney. The process of forming urine and regulating the composition of the blood actually takes place in the nephrons as they perform the following three functions: (1) filtration, (2) reabsorption, and (3) secretion.

Structurally, each nephron comprises a glomerulus and a renal tubule. The **glomerulus** (glō-MER-ū-lus) is a ball-like cluster of approximately 50 intertwining capillaries enclosed within a cup-shaped **glomerular (Bowman's) capsule.** The glomerulus and glomerular capsule are often referred to collectively as the **renal corpuscle.** The glomerulus has thin, semipermeable walls that allow nitrogenous wastes, water, sugar, and salts to filter out of the bloodstream *(Figure 14–5).* Larger cells, such as red blood cells, are unable to filter through its membrane. The filtered substances, or filtrate, are collected and absorbed into the glomerular capsule and then passed through a twisted and looped tube known as the **renal tubule.** This portion of the nephron is approximately 3 cm long and consists of a *proximal convoluted tubule, loop of Henle* (HEN-lē), and a *distal convoluted tubule.* Although the majority of the nephron is located within the cortex of the kidney, the loop of Henle penetrates into the medulla *(Figure 14–6).*

The renal tubule is surrounded by a capillary network. It is here that vital salts, nutrients, and water are filtered out of the renal tubule and reabsorbed into the bloodstream. Selective secretion also occurs as substances such as creatinine, potassium, ammonia, and some drugs (eg, penicillin) filter out of the capillaries and are absorbed into the renal tubule. Approximately 99% of the filtrate is reabsorbed. The remaining 1%, constituting the liquid waste product known as urine, moves through the renal tubules and drains into the collecting tubules of the renal pyramids, minor calyces, major calyces, and renal pelvis, respectively. From this point, it is excreted from the kidney via the ureter.

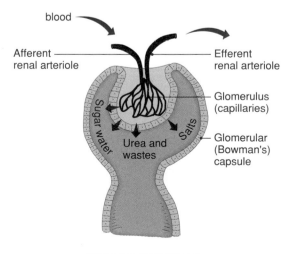

Figure 14–5. Renal corpuscle.

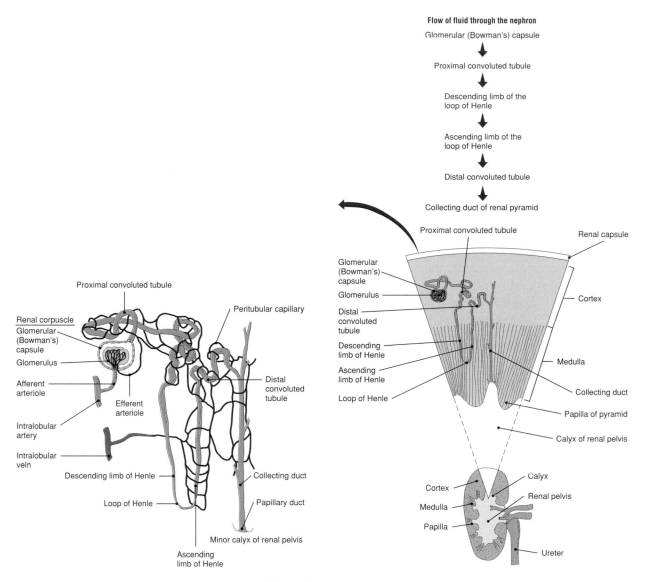

Flow of fluid through the nephron

Glomerular (Bowman's) capsule
↓
Proximal convoluted tubule
↓
Descending limb of the loop of Henle
↓
Ascending limb of the loop of Henle
↓
Distal convoluted tubule
↓
Collecting duct of renal pyramid

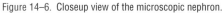

Figure 14–6. Closeup view of the microscopic nephron.

Urine is basically 95% water and 5% solid substances generated through cellular metabolism (ie, urea, creatinine, salts, and acids). It is a transparent, yellow-colored liquid that is slightly acidic in nature with a pH of 5.0 to 7.0. Urine is produced continually, amounting to approximately 1 to 2 qt (1 to 2 L) daily. A person's urinary output is dependent on such factors as diet, blood pressure, and overall general health. Variation in the normal constituents of urine, as revealed through urinalysis, can indicate an abnormal or pathologic condition.

Blood Supply

The kidneys cleanse approximately 1200 mL of blood per minute, regulating the homeostasis of the body. They have a rich blood supply, receiving about 25% of the total cardiac output each minute. The large right and left renal arteries branch off of the abdominal aorta to supply their respective kidney with oxygenated blood. On entering the kidney at the hilum, the renal artery continually divides and subdivides until an expansive capillary network is established *(Figure 14–7)*. The **afferent arteriole** conveys blood into the glomerulus, whereas the **efferent arteriole** transmits blood from the glomerulus and divides to form a network of peritubular capillaries, which surround the renal tubule. The capillaries then unite to form venules, which in turn unite to form the renal vein. Blood leaves the kidney at the hilum via the renal vein.

URETERS

The right and left ureters (Ū-rē-terz or ū-RĒ-terz) (singular, ureter) function to convey urine from the renal pelvis of the kidney to the urinary bladder. They extend inferiorly from the renal pelvis of the kidney; this

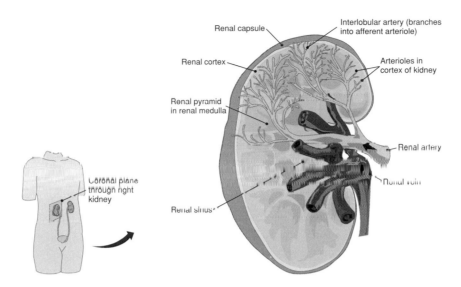

Figure 14–7. Blood supply to the kidney is demonstrated on a coronal section.

area is known as the **ureteropelvic junction** (UPJ). Like the kidneys, the ureters are retroperitoneal structures, passing posteriorly to the peritoneum and anteriorly to the psoas major muscles while following the curve of the vertebral column *(Figure 14–8)*.

Each ureter is a narrow, hollow tube measuring 10 to 12 in. (25 to 30 cm) in length, with the left ureter being slightly longer than the right because of the higher position of the left kidney. It has an average diameter of 0.25 in. (6 mm) and is composed of three layers of tissue: (1) inner mucosa layer, (2) middle muscularis layer, and (3) fibrous adventitia outer layer. The muscular layer allows for rhythmic contraction of the ureters. Urine is transported continually to the urinary bladder via gravity and peristaltic waves occurring every 10 to 30 seconds. The ureter enters the posterolateral aspect of the urinary bladder at the **ureterovesical junction** (UVJ). Renal calculi or kidney stones can obstruct the ureter, preventing the flow of urine and resulting in a great deal of pain. The more constricted areas along the length of the ureter where stones are likely to lodge occur at the ureteropelvic junction, the brim of the pelvis, and the ureterovesical junction *(Figure 14–9)*.

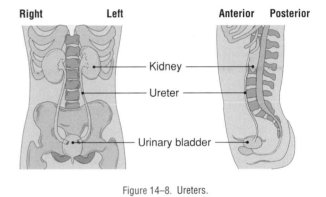

Figure 14–8. Ureters.

URINARY BLADDER

The urinary bladder is an expandable sac located in the pelvic cavity. It is situated directly posterior to the pubic symphysis and under the parietal peritoneum, making it an infraperitoneal structure. In a female, the urinary bladder is anterior to the vagina and anteroinferior to the uterus, whereas it is directly anterior to the rectum in a male. The exact size, shape, and location of the urinary bladder are determined by urine volume. When it is empty, the urinary bladder collapses and its top flattens. As it becomes distended with urine, it assumes a more oval or pear shape and projects upward into the abdominal cavity *(Figure 14–10)*.

The walls of the urinary bladder consist of three layers: (1) inner mucosa, (2) intermediate or middle muscularis, and (3) outer fibrous adventitia. The intermediate muscularis is actually composed of three heavy layers of muscle, which allow the urinary bladder to expand and contract. The inner mucosal lining falls into folds or rugae when it is empty. The **trigone** (TRĪ-gon) is a triangular area in the urinary bladder. It appears smooth because the muscular layer is firmly attached to the floor of the pelvic cavity. The ureters enter the urinary bladder at the upper corners of the trigone, whereas the entrance to the urethra is at the apex or lowest portion of the trigone. A circular muscle known as the **internal urethral sphincter** surrounds the urethral opening in the bladder. Its normal state is one of contraction, which prevents an involuntary, continual flow of urine from the bladder into the urethra. An **external urethral sphincter,** located more inferiorly at the proximal portion of the urethra, can voluntarily contract and relax. *(Figure 14–11)*.

The urinary bladder functions as a reservoir for the storage of urine until it can be conveniently expelled from the body. The average capacity of the bladder is approximately 500 mL (1 pint); however, an individual will get the urge to void when it becomes moderately distended at 250 mL. Pressure in the bladder stimulates the nerves, which transmit impulses to the brain. Both the internal and external sphincters relax and the muscular walls of the bladder contract to expel the urine. The act of voiding or urinating is known as *micturition* (mik-tū-RISH-un). *Incontinence* (in-KON-ti-nens) is involuntary micturition.

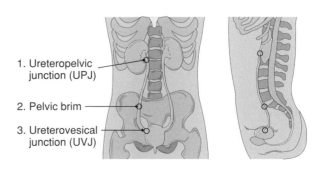

1. Ureteropelvic junction (UPJ)

2. Pelvic brim

3. Ureterovesical junction (UVJ)

Figure 14–9. Renal calculi are likely to lodge at any of the three areas of constriction in the ureters.

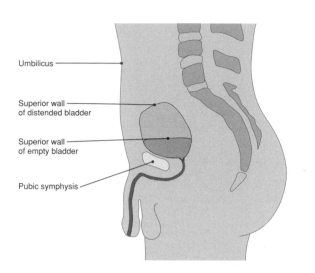

Figure 14–10. Position of an empty urinary bladder relative to a full (distended) urinary bladder.

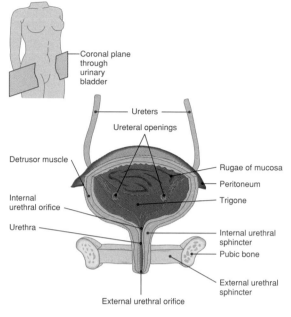

Figure 14–11. Urinary bladder.

URETHRA

The urethra (ū-RĒ-thrah) is a hollow tube leading from the urinary bladder to the exterior of the body. Its function is to transport urine during micturition. The length and exact location of the urethra differ between the sexes *(Figure 4–12)*. The female urethra is approximately 1.5 in. (4 cm) long. It is situated directly posterior to the pubic symphysis and is embedded in the anterior wall of the vagina. The male urethra is approximately 8 in. (20 cm) long because it extends through the prostate gland and the penis. It is subdivided into three regions according to location: (1) prostatic, (2) membranous, and (3) spongy or penile. The male urethra also functions in the reproductive system as it carries semen on ejaculation. The opening of the urethra to the outside of the body is called the **external urethral orifice.**

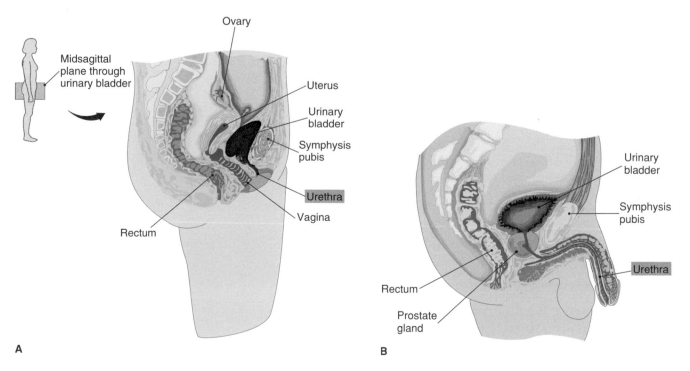

Figure 14–12. Location of the urethra in relation to surrounding structures in a female **(A)** and a male **(B)**.

► PROCEDURAL CONSIDERATIONS

Urography is a general term used to describe radiography of the urinary system and is accomplished by injecting iodinated contrast media into a vein or into a catheter that has been introduced into the structure to be studied. Radiographic examination of the urinary system is performed to evaluate function, location of the various structures, and presence of pathologic conditions such as inflammation, calculi, obstruction, renal hypertension, urinary tract infections, hematuria, tumors, and cysts. Several different procedures can be performed to evaluate the urinary system.

EXCRETORY UROGRAPHY

The *excretory urogram* (ExU), also called *intravenous pyelogram* (IVP) or *intravenous urogram* (IVU), includes a series of radiographs taken at timed intervals following an intravenous injection of contrast medium. Because one of the functions of the kidneys is to filter and excrete waste products, including contrast media from the circulating blood, this examination can be used to evaluate functional disorders, as well as the size, shape, and position of urinary system structures and pathology. The timing of the radiographs may be determined by department protocol or by individual radiologists after evaluating the preceding film(s) and patient history.

Nephrograms are those films that are taken soon after the injection in what is sometimes referred to as the nephron or "blush" phase. At this time, the contrast is seen in the parenchyma of the kidney, but not yet in the calcyces. Because the nephrons are microscopic and exist in the millions, the contrast medium makes them appear as a blush. A nephrogram should be obtained no later than 1 minute after the start of the injection.

Although rarely performed today, the *hypertensive IVP* may be performed on patients with high blood pressure to determine if the kidneys are responsible for the hypertension. Films are obtained at a relatively rapid rate to demonstrate differences in kidney function in smaller time intervals. Although contrast media is normally injected over a 1- to 2-minute period, contrast media for a hypertensive IVP is given as a bolus injection within about 30 seconds. Radiographs of the kidneys are usually obtained at 1, 2, 3, and 5 minutes following the start of injection; additional films may also be obtained per department routine *(Figure 14–13)*. Because films are obtained at such a rapid rate, cassettes with appropriate time markers should be prepared prior to the injection. The time the injection was started should be documented on the patient history form. Right and left renal function is compared; differences in renal function may be a result of renal artery stenosis that can contribute to renal hypertension.

The creatinine and blood urea nitrogen (BUN) levels, as stated on a laboratory report in the patient's chart, are indicators of renal function *(Table 14–3)*. Abnormally high levels might indicate impaired renal function, which could contraindicate excretory urography or delay visualization of contrast media within the kidneys. When a patient has impaired renal function, an infusion urogram may be performed. A large quantity of diluted contrast medium is "infused" at a rapid rate into the patient through an intravenous line. Some radiologists prefer the first film to be obtained when half of the bottle has been infused and the second when the bottle is empty; routine kidney, ureter, and bladder (KUB) films are then obtained per routine, considering the time the infusion was started. Because of the length of time it takes for the contrast to be administered, the comparison of right and left renal function may be inaccurate; infusion urograms, therefore, may not provide an accurate assessment of kidney function.

RETROGRADE PYELOGRAPHY

The retrograde pyelogram is frequently performed for identification and removal of urethral calculi and may also be performed as an alternative to the IVP when routine excretory urography is contraindicated.

Table 14–3. Normal Creatinine & Blood Urea Nitrogen (BUN) Levels

Creatinine	
Female adult	0.6–1.5 mg/100 mL
Male adult	0.7–1.6 mg/100 mL
BUN	6–17 g/d

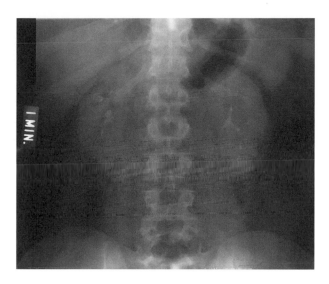

Figure 14–13. AP hypertensive excretory urogram, 1 minute.

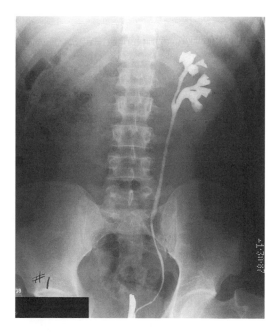

Figure 14–14. Retrograde pyelogram, AP.

This is a nonfunctional examination demonstrating the internal structures of the kidneys and ureters *(Figure 14–14)*. The retrograde pyelogram can be performed in a specialized urologic suite, usually located in surgery. For comfort and compliance, the patient is usually sedated or anesthetized for this examination. Under sterile procedure, the urologist inserts a cystoscope through the urethra and into the bladder, prior to administration of contrast media. The urologist can then examine the inside of the bladder using the cystoscope before inserting a catheter(s) into one or both ureters. The tip of the ureteral catheter is generally placed at the lower level of the renal pelvis. A water-soluble contrast medium is injected into the catheter for evaluation of the renal pelvis, calyces, and ureter. Films are obtained on request by the physician, usually a urologist. Although not technically considered a retrograde pyelogram, a similar procedure is followed for the placement of a stent in the ureter; however, no contrast media is administered.

CYSTOGRAPHY

A **cystogram** is a radiographic examination of the urinary bladder that can demonstrate shape and position of the bladder, as well as possible vesicoureteral reflux of contrast medium and other abnormalities. It involves administration of a urinary retention catheter through the urethra and into the bladder using sterile technique. Approximately 150 to 500 mL (depending on the size of the patient) of diluted contrast media flows into the bladder by gravity until the patient expresses discomfort. Fluoroscopic images may be obtained by the physician; overhead films may also be obtained by the radiographer.

A **voiding cystourethrogram** (VCUG) is a cystogram in which the patient is instructed to "void" or empty the bladder following removal of the urinary retention catheter. This examination is performed primarily on patients suspected of having a lower urinary tract obstruction or vesicoureteral reflux. With the radiographic table either horizontal or tilted so the feet are lower than the head, the patient's bladder and urethra are filmed fluoroscopically while the patient voids. Either strategically positioned towels or a collection bag should be used to collect the eliminated contrast media. Because voiding away from the rest room is usually difficult for adults and children, the sound of running water and/or warm water poured over the perineum may stimulate the urge to void. Although a cystogram may be performed in either a fluoroscopic room in the radiology department or in a surgical urography suite, the VCUG is usually performed in the radiology department.

PATIENT PREPARATION

Time permitting, patient preparation for most urinary radiography begins before the day of the examination. Specific preparation often depends on the examination to be performed.

Preliminary Preparation

Although department protocols vary, the primary goal of patient preparation prior to a urographic study is removal of gas and fecal material from the intestines. To accomplish this, the patient is generally instructed to:
- Eat low-residue foods for 1 to 2 days before the examination
- Eat a light meal the night before the examination
- Take a nongas-producing cathartic to cleanse the bowel the evening prior to the examination
- Remain NPO (except for water) after midnight the day of the examination

Although the intestines should be cleansed, the patient should not be dehydrated for this examination. Pediatric, and some adult, patients may undergo a modified patient preparation; at times, the patient will not have had any preparation (eg, emergency situations).

In preparation for a retrograde pyelogram, a patient may be instructed to drink four to five glassfuls of water to ensure adequate excretion of urine for the study. Because the patient may be sedated or anesthetized for this procedure, however, he or she may be instructed to remain NPO prior to the procedure. Other than voiding, no patient preparation is required for a cystogram. The radiographer should be familiar with specific department protocols.

Examination Preparation

After being correctly identified, an outpatient should be instructed to remove any long necklaces and all clothing except shoes and socks and put on a patient gown. Patients should be checked for any radiopaque objects that might obscure the abdominal anatomy on the radiograph. A pertinent patient history should be

---

► *Renal Calculus*

Along with the term nephrolith, *renal calculus refers to a kidney stone. It can result from a diet high in calcium, lack of fluid intake, or a parathyroid tumor that increases serum calcium levels.*

Although 80% of kidney stones are composed of calcium salts, they may also be formed from crystallized magnesium or uric acid. They can form anywhere in the urinary tract, but are most likely to lodge in a narrow ureter as they attempt to pass to the urinary bladder. This condition causes extreme pain and possibly hydronephrosis if the urine backs up and distends the kidney.

Shock wave lithotripsy is a noninvasive method of treating kidney stones. The patient is immersed in water, and high-intensity sound waves are directed at the stone, causing it to shatter. The small, sandlike particles can easily pass down the ureter without causing an obstruction and are excreted on urination.

History Sheet: Urinary Radiography

Patient Name: _____ Age: _____

Date: _____ X-ray No.: _____ Pregnant? _____

Allergy History (Y/N):   **Medical Problems (Y/N):**

_____ Hayfever/asthma?   _____ Hepatic/renal disease?

_____ Food/medication?   _____ Multiple myeloma?

_____ Hives? Cause: _____   _____ Sickle cell disease?

_____ Previous IVP?   _____ Cardiovascular problems?

_____ Reaction? _____   _____ Bronchial asthma?

_____ Symptoms: _____   _____ Hyperthyroidism?

Symptoms (check all that apply):

_____ Nephrolithiasis   _____ Dysuria

_____ Hematuria   _____ Abdominal pain

_____ Anuria   _____ Incontinence

_____ Oliguria   _____ Unexplained weight loss

_____ Polyuria

Duration of symptoms: _____

Abdominal Surgical History: _____

Procedural Notes:

Patient voided prior to KUB (Y/N)? _____

Type/amount of contrast administered: _____ cc _____ % _____

Time of injection: _____ Injected by: _____

Reactions: _____

Technologist: _____ **Radiologist:** _____

Figure 14–15. History sheet for urinary radiography. *Note:* The acquisition of specific information is imperative for patient safety, as well as accurate diagnosis. Documentation is important for patient records and legal liability.

► RELATED TERMINOLOGY

agenesis (a-JEN-e-sis)—condition in which the kidney or other organ is absent because it failed to develop in the embryo

anuria (an NŪ re an)—abnormal condition in which urine is not being produced by the kidneys

catheterization (kath-e-ter-i-ZĀ-shun)—introduction of a flexible, rubber tube into the urinary bladder via the urethra to remove urine

cystitis (sis-TĪ-tis)—inflammation of the urinary bladder

cystocele (sis-tō-sel)—herniation of the urinary bladder, specifically into the vagina

cystoscope (SIS-tō-skope)—instrument with a light source used to visually examine the inside of the bladder

diuresis (di-ū-RĒ-sis)—increased discharge of urine

dysuria (dis-Ū-rē-ah)—difficult or painful urination, such as from cystitis

gout (gowt)—form of arthritis in which there is an excessive amount of uric acid in the bloodstream; affects the cartilage in the joint and causes inflammation, pain, and swelling, especially in the big toe; long-term effects include renal impairment and/or kidney stones

hematuria (hē-mah-TŪ-rē-ah)—abnormal presence of blood in the urine

hemodialysis (hē-mō-dī-AL-i-sis)—procedure used to artificially clean the blood in an individual with kidney failure; the individual's blood is filtered to remove toxic waste materials and then returned to the bloodstream

horseshoe kidney—congenital condition in which the lower poles of both kidneys are fused together at the midline, forming a horseshoe shape

hydronephrosis (hī-drō-nef-RŌ-sis)—distention of the renal pelvis from a collection of urine due to an obstruction or atrophy

nephrectomy (ne-FREK-tō-mē)—excision of the kidney

nephrolith (nef-RŌ-lith)—kidney stone; also called *renal calculus*

nephrology (nef-ROL-ō-jē)—branch of medicine that studies the function and structure of the kidneys

nephroptosis (nef-rop-TŌ-sis)—condition in which the kidney is prolapsed or displaced downward; also called a *floating kidney*

(continued)

obtained; procedural notes may also be recorded on this form *(Figure 14–15)*. Prior to starting the examination, the radiographer should explain the entire procedure to the patient, including the length of the procedure and what can be expected. To prevent discomfort and dilution of the contrast media in the bladder, the patient should void prior to the start of the examination. When a patient has a urinary catheter, the catheter should be clamped prior to administration of the contrast to ensure adequate filling of the bladder; the clamp should be released following completion of the procedure or prior to the postvoid film.

Because the retrograde pyelogram is routinely performed in a special "cysto" suite in surgery, surgery personnel are responsible for assisting the patient onto a specialized combination cystoscopic–radiographic table. In addition to radiographic capabilities, the table is fitted with stirrups, allowing the patient to be placed in the modified lithotomy position.

► RELATED TERMINOLOGY *(continued)*

nephrostomy (nef-ROS-tō-mē)—permanent opening into the pelvis of the kidney

oliguria (ol-ig-Ū-rē-ah)—scanty urine output

polycystic kidney disease (PKD)—a congenital condition in which there are multiple cysts in the kidney, resulting in loss of functional tissue

pyelonephritis (pī-e-lō-ne-FRĪ-tis)—inflammation of the renal pelvis and the kidney

pyonephritis (pī-ō-ne-FRĪ-tis)—inflammation of the kidney with the presence of pus

pyuria (pī-ū-RĒ-ah)—abnormal condition of pus in the urine

renal ectopia (RĒ-nal ek-TŌ-pē-ah)—malposition of the kidney (eg, pelvic kidneys)

uremia (ū-RĒ-mē-ah)—toxic condition in which there is a buildup of nitrogenous waste materials in the blood, indicative of renal failure; also known as *azotemia*

urinalysis (ū-ri-NAL-i-sis)—laboratory procedure in which the urine is analyzed to aid in the diagnosis of abnormal conditions

Table 14–4. Supplies for Excretory Urography

Contrast medium: correct amount in syringe

Sterile needles: variety to include 19-gauge butterfly and tubing

Alcohol wipes/sponges

Tourniquet

Arm board/towels for support

Emesis basin

Emergency drugs (eg, Benadryl, epinephrine)

Emergency ("crash") cart

Radiolucent pad (if used by department)

Sponges or other supports for under knees

Gonadal shield

Urethral compression device (if used)

Lead markers: right/left, minute, numbers

ROOM PREPARATION

In addition to the usual room preparation, the radiographer must also prepare the contrast medium to be used for the examination, as well as any equipment to be used for its administration *(Table 14–4)*. For verification, the empty bottle of contrast medium should be saved and shown to the individual administering the contrast; it can be discarded when the examination is completed. Because needles can invoke a vasovagal response in many patients, the syringe should be filled out of sight of the patient. For the same reason, the emesis basin should also be placed out of sight, but readily available. An emergency box with medications to be used in case of allergic response, as well as a crash cart, should also be nearby and ready.

When performing a cystourethrogram, diluted contrast media, sterile gloves, sterile water, urinary retention catheter, a lidocaine jelly, towels, and sterile basins are needed. Frequently, a department nurse or representative from nursing services inserts the catheter and provides the necessary equipment for catheter insertion; a trained radiographer may also perform this procedure.

POSITIONING CONSIDERATIONS

Excretory Urogram

A preliminary, or "scout," film should be taken prior to administration of any contrast media. This initial film should be evaluated for proper exposure factors, patient positioning and centering, and presence of radiopaque calculi or any other abnormality that may later be obscured by contrast media. Care must be taken to include both entire kidneys and the superior portion of the symphysis pubis (to ensure the bladder is included). Two films, a 14 × 17-in. lengthwise to include the symphysis and an 11 × 14-in. crosswise centered over the kidneys, may be necessary for tall or hypersthenic patients. Additional evaluation criteria are listed in Figure 3–22 in Chapter 3.

Because it usually takes several minutes for the kidneys to excrete contrast media, a 1- to 2-minute film may include only the kidneys, as little or no contrast media will be seen in the bladder. For radiographs obtained 5 minutes or more after the start of injection, a 14 × 17-in. cassette should be centered to include the kidneys and bladder. Time markers should be placed on all cassettes prior to exposure to indicate the amount of elapsed time since the **start** of injection.

Although most radiographs will be acquired with the patient supine, oblique projections may also be obtained to identify the location of calcifications or to separate gas shadows from the kidneys or ureters. A 30° posterior oblique places the elevated kidney parallel with the film and moves the ureter of the side down away from the spine. Both obliques are usually obtained. The prone position can be used to enhance pelvicalyceal and ureteral filling *(Figure 14–16)*. An upright projection may also be obtained to better visualize the ureters, as well as mobility of the kidneys. Upright bladder films may also be obtained to evaluate a prolapsed bladder or an enlarged prostate. The Trendelenburg position is another method used to enhance the filling of the renal pelvis and calyces for the early films in the series. Quite often, the presence of urinary calculi results in slow filling of the ureter. Delayed films, therefore, may be requested every 1 to 2 hours, per radiologist instructions. Postvoid films are often obtained at the end of the study, after the patient has voided. This projection may be obtained with the patient prone, supine, or erect per radiologist request

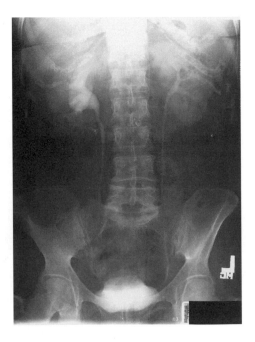

Figure 14–16. Excretory urogram, prone position.

and must include the entire bladder. The postvoid film is generally routine for patients with a history of prostate problems.

To enhance filling of the renal pelves, calyces, and proximal ureters, a ureteral compression device may be used. Prior to administration of contrast, deflated balloons are positioned over each ureter at the level of the pelvic brim; the top edge of the balloon should be at the level of the ASIS. The balloons are held in place by a plastic plate and sponge that are immobilized by a velcro strap or radiolucent compression band *(Figure 14–17)*. The balloons are inflated immediately following the injection of contrast media. Because contrast media cannot reach the bladder when the compression balloons are correctly placed and filled, small films centered over the kidneys may be used. The air in the balloons is usually released approximately 8 to 10 min after injection, with a full film taken immediately after compression has been released; this radiograph should demonstrate both ureters filled with contrast.

Although the ureteral compression device is an excellent tool for enhancing the pelvicalyceal structures, its use is contraindicated when:

1. Ureteral stones may be present (a stone may also restrict passage of contrast).
2. An abdominal mass is suspected.
3. An abdominal aortic aneurysm is present (it may rupture).
4. The patient suffers from severe abdominal pain or acute abdominal trauma.
5. The patient has had recent abdominal surgery.
6. The patient has a pelvic kidney, colostomy, or suprapubic catheter.

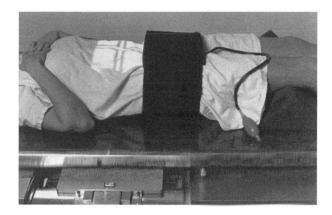

Figure 14–17. Ureteral compression may be used when not contraindicated.

Retrograde Pyelogram

Because the protocol for this procedure is urologist driven, the actual procedure may vary depending on the patient and physician. The scout radiograph may be obtained either before or after the catheter(s) is inserted. Approximately 3 to 5 mL of iodinated contrast media is injected into the catheters prior to making the exposure for the second film, the *pyelogram.* Typically, the third radiograph is obtained after the urologist withdraws the ureteral catheter and simultaneously injects contrast into the ureter(s). This film is referred to as a *ureterogram,* as it is used to visualize the ureters.

Most films are obtained with the patient supine; however, shallow oblique projections may be requested. In addition, the head may be elevated for the ureterogram to help fill the ureters with contrast media remaining in the renal pelvis. If the patient is sleeping, the radiographer should confer with the anesthestist regarding the procedure to be followed to ensure that respiration is suspended for the exposure. Films should be numbered to indicate the correct sequence for later reference.

When the primary purpose is stone retrieval, plain films are taken without contrast media. A catheter with a special mesh "basket" is inserted through the urethra and bladder and into the affected ureter *(Figure 14–18)*. The catheter is advanced to the level of the calculus and the basket is opened adjacent to the stone in hopes of capturing and removing the stone from the ureter. Fluoroscopy or AP radiographs are used to monitor progress.

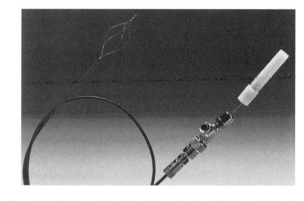

Figure 14–18. A special mesh basket may be placed in the ureter for stone retrieval.

Cystogram

Imaging for a cystogram can include fluoroscopic spots and/or overhead films. If overhead films are obtained, the routine usually includes an AP projection with a 15° caudal angle, to project the symphysis pubis inferior to the bladder and urethra, and both posterior obliques, to demonstrate the ureterovesical junction. A postvoid AP projection may also be requested.

Voiding Cystourethrography

AP and/or right and left posterior oblique radiographs may be obtained prior to voiding to evaluate the ureterovesical junctions and possible reflux of the contrast upward into the ureters. Fluoroscopy is usually used to image the bladder while voiding. Spot films are generally best obtained with the female in the supine or slight oblique position and the male patient in the 30° right posterior oblique position. A postvoid film might be requested.

ALTERNATE PROJECTIONS/PROCEDURES

Because intestinal gas frequently superimposes the kidneys and ureters, tomography is often employed *(Figure 14–19)*. When performed soon after the contrast is injected, these films are called *nephrotomograms,* as they demonstrate the nephron phase of the examination. Tomograms are also performed, however, to better demonstrate calculi, cysts, and tumors. A 10° or smaller angle is used for thick sections and a 30° to 40° angle is used for thinner sections, per radiologist or department protocol. While protocols vary,

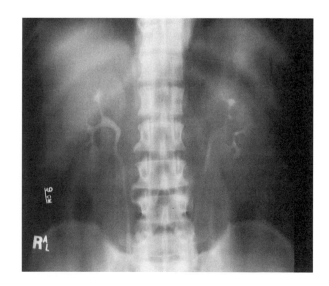

Figure 14–19. Tomogram of the kidneys; obtained as part of an intravenous urogram.

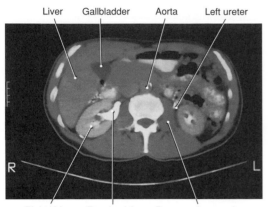

Liver   Gallbladder   Aorta   Left ureter

Right kidney   Renal pelvis   Psoas major muscle

Figure 14–20. Axial CT image obtained at the level of the kidneys.

a scout tomogram is generally obtained after measuring the patient's abdomen and setting the fulcrum level to one third of that measurement. The radiologist specifies which additional sections are needed. Films should be appropriately marked according to fulcrum level and right or left side. A small film size, 11 × 14 in. or 10 × 12 in., is used, permitting appropriate gonadal shielding on all patients.

Although routine excretory or retrograde urography is the first choice for the identification of stones, CT may be preferred for other pathologies *(Figure 14–20)*. Because of its ability to demonstrate very small structures, CT is generally preferred when hematuria is present without obvious cause. Ultrasound is used for differentiation between solid and fluid-filled structures, whereas nuclear medicine can be used to evaluate renal function *(Figure 14–21)*. Renal angiography is performed to diagnose renal artery stenosis that may contribute to renal hypertension *(Figure 14–22)*.

Two procedures rarely performed today should be briefly discussed. The retrograde urethrogram used to be performed on male patients to demonstrate the entire length of the urethra. A special clamp was attached to the distal penis. Contrast was administered retrograde until the urethra was filled; a 30° right posterior oblique was then obtained. The VCUG, as previously described, provides much of the same information and may be performed instead of the retrograde urethrogram.

The metallic bead-chain cystourethrogram is a special type of voiding cystourethrogram that has been performed on females for stress incontinence. Following insertion of a flexible, metallic bead chain into the bladder, contrast media is instilled into the bladder; the catheter is then removed. With the patient erect, two sets of AP and lateral projections are obtained, the first with the patient relaxed and the second with the patient straining (bearing down).

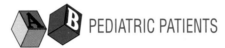 PEDIATRIC PATIENTS

Radiographic examination of the urinary tract may be performed on children to evaluate urinary tract infection (UTI), abdominal masses, childhood polycystic disease, or congenital abnormalities such as renal agenesis, ectopic kidney, and genital abnormalities. Because UTI is a relatively common problem in children, radiographic examination of the urinary system, either excretory urography or cystography, is not unusual. UTIs often occur in children who also have a backward flow of urine from the bladder into the ureter and kidney (vesicoureteral reflux). Reflux is generally the result of an abnormality in the muscular valve located at the junction of the ureter and bladder. This valve normally ensures that urine flows only in one direction—from the ureter to the bladder. When reflux occurs, any bacteria present in the bladder as a result of a UTI are transmitted upward to the kidney, resulting in pyelonephritis. Frequent kidney infections can eventually destroy renal tissue and impair renal function.

For excretory urography, food is usually withheld for 4 hours prior to the examination. Plenty of clear fluids should be encouraged so the patient is hydrated, not dehydrated; fluids should be avoided, however, immediately prior to the examination. There is some evidence that apple juice and milk given prior to the examination may increase the possibility of nausea and vomiting following administration of iodinated contrast media; low-osmolality contrast media decreases this risk. Laxatives are not given to children as they cause unnecessary discomfort; tomography can be performed if stool in the bowel interferes with visualization of the urinary tract.

Fewer films are usually obtained on children than on adults because of the types of diseases and conditions children usually have. Water, apple juice, or ginger ale may be given to the patient after the first postinjection radiograph has been obtained. A carbonated beverage given after injection fills the stomach with gas and pushes the intestines inferiorly, creating a radiolucent window through which the kidneys can be visualized *(Figure 14–23)*. Tomography can be used as an alternative to this procedure.

When an excretory urogram and VCUG are scheduled on the same day, the VCUG is usually performed first. If renal size and morphology are of primary interest, renal ultrasound often replaces the excretory urogram to minimize radiation exposure and may be performed before or after the VCUG.

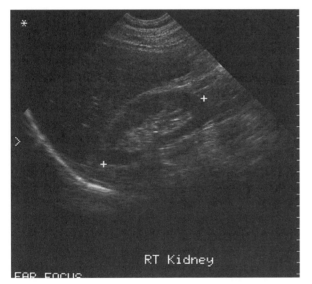

RT Kidney

FAR FOCUS

A

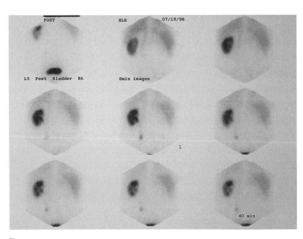

B

Figure 14–21. Ultrasound image **(A)** and nuclear medicine study **(B)** of the kidneys. Note the absence of function in the left kidney in **B**. *(Nuclear medicine scan courtesy of Debbie Kruetzkamp, RT(R) (N).)*

BREATHING INSTRUCTIONS

To elevate the diaphragm to its highest position and prevent compression of the abdominal contents, all radiographs of the urinary system should be obtained during suspended expiration. While preventing abdominal compression, suspended expiration will also reduce the tissue thickness of the patient, thereby requiring less radiation to properly expose the film. For those examinations in which the patient is anesthetized, the anesthetist will have to suspend the patient's respiration for the exposure. This should be coordinated with the urologist prior to administration of the contrast.

EXPOSURE FACTORS

To enhance subject contrast, a moderate kilovoltage of 70 to 75 kVp should be used for adult patients. Technical factors for children should be modified using the guidelines outlined in Chapter 3. Tomographic images should also be obtained using 70 to 75 kVp. The mAs required depends on patient size, type of x-ray generator, film/screen speed, type of grid, and pathologic conditions that may be present.

EQUIPMENT CONSIDERATIONS

A radiographic table with a grid is needed for excretory urography and cystography; fluoroscopic capabilities are preferred for voiding cystourethrography. A vertical grid device should be available for upright films, if needed. Tomography requires a dedicated unit or attachments to the radiographic table. If available, a radiolucent pad can be placed under the patient for comfort; sponges or other supports should be placed under the patient's knees. Other ancillary equipment is listed in *Table 14–4*.

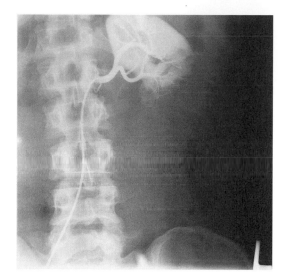

Figure 14–22. Renal arteriogram.

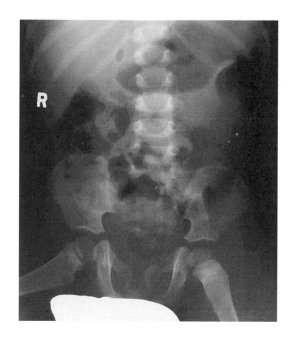

Figure 14–23. Pediatric KUB obtained after ingestion of a carbonated beverage.

RADIOGRAPHIC POSITIONING OF THE URINARY SYSTEM

- ► AP PRE- & POSTCONTRAST URINARY TRACT (EXCRETORY UROGRAM)

- ► AP COLLIMATED RENAL AREA (EXCRETORY UROGRAM)

- ► AP OBLIQUE (RPO & LPO) URINARY TRACT (EXCRETORY UROGRAM)

- ► AP URINARY BLADDER (EXCRETORY UROGRAM OR CYSTOGRAM)

- ► AP OBLIQUE (RPO & LPO) URINARY BLADDER (CYSTOGRAM)

► AP PRE- & POSTCONTRAST URINARY TRACT (EXCRETORY UROGRAM)

Technical Considerations

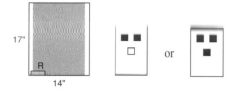

- Film size: Adult: 14 × 17 in. lengthwise. Pediatric: determined by patient size.
- Grid required.
- 70–75 kVp.
- Collimate to the abdominal walls laterally and to film size lengthwise.

Shielding

- Male patients should be shielded according to department policy.

Patient Positioning

- Assist the patient to the supine position on the radiographic table. **Note:** This projection may also be performed with the patient prone or upright.
- Place a pillow under the patient's head and position a small support under the patient's knees for comfort.

Part Positioning

- Center the midsagittal plane of the patient's body to the midline of the table.
- Adjust the long axis of the patient parallel with the long axis of the table; pull gently on patient's legs or under patient's arms to straighten the patient.
- Check for rotation of the pelvis by palpating the ASISs and ensuring they are equidistant from the table; use sponges for support and immobilization, if necessary *(Figure 14–24)*.

Central Ray

- Direct the central ray perpendicular to the level of the iliac crests.
- Center the cassette to the central ray.
- Make any needed adjustment in centering to ensure the symphysis pubis is included on the film; two films may be needed for tall patients.

Breathing Instructions

- Instruct the patient to take in a breath, blow it out, and hold it out during the exposure.

Image Evaluation

- The symphysis pubis, transverse processes of the lumbar spine, hepatic and renal shadows, and lateral margins of the abdomen should be visualized on the radiograph.
- Asymmetry of the iliac crests and ischial spines indicates rotation of the pelvis.
- Unless scoliosis is present, the spine should be straight and centered to the film *(Figure 14–25)*.

1. Upper pole, right kidney
2. Renal cortex
3. Lower pole, right kidney
4. Psoas major muscle

5. Urinary bladder
6. Minor calyx
7. Renal pelvis

8. Major calyx
9. Renal medulla
10. Ureter

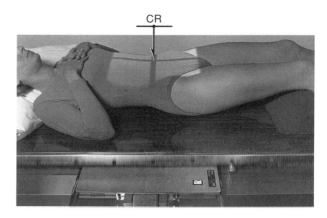

Figure 14–24. AP abdomen for pre- and postcontrast urinary studies.

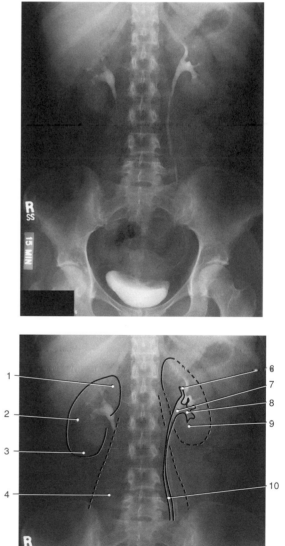

Figure 14–25. AP excretory urogram, 15 minutes postinjection.

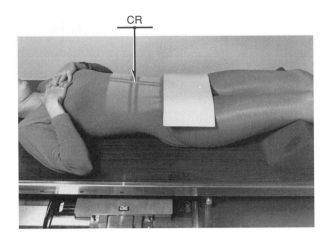

Figure 14–26. Excretory urogram, collimated renal area.

► AP COLLIMATED RENAL AREA (EXCRETORY UROGRAM)

Technical Considerations

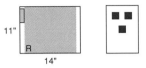

- Film size: 11 × 14 in. or 10 × 12 in. crosswise.
- Grid required.
- 70–75 kVp.
- Collimate to the abdominal walls laterally and to include the iliac crests lengthwise.

Shielding

- Gonadal shielding should be used on all patients, especially children and adults of reproductive age; the top edge of the shield should be at the level of the ASIS.

Patient Positioning

- Assist the patient to the supine position on the radiographic table. **Note:** Ureteral compression or the Trendelenburg position may be used to enhance visualization of the renal pelves and calyces.
- Place a pillow under the patient's head and position a small support under the patient's knees for comfort.

Part Positioning

- Center the midsagittal plane of the patient's body to the midline of the table.
- Adjust the long axis of the patient parallel with the long axis of the table; pull gently on patient's legs or under patient's arms to straighten the patient.
- Check for rotation of the pelvis by palpating the ASISs and ensuring they are equidistant from the table; use sponges for support and immobilization, if necessary *(Figure 14–26)*.

Central Ray

- Direct the central ray perpendicular to the transverse plane passing halfway between the xiphoid process and the iliac crests.
- Center the cassette to the central ray.

Breathing Instructions

- Instruct the patient to take in a breath, blow it out, and hold it out during the exposure.

Image Evaluation

- Thc transverse processes of the lumbar spine, hepatic and renal shadows, and approximately 1 in. of the iliac crest should be visualized on the radiograph.
- Asymmetry of the iliac crests and lower ribs indicates rotation of the patient.
- Unless scoliosis is present, the spine should be straight and centered to the film *(Figure 14–27)*.

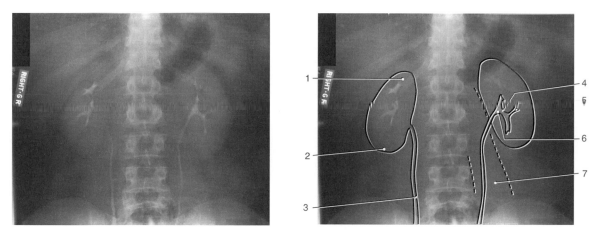

Figure 14–27. AP collimated renal area, 2 minutes postinjection.

1. Upper pole, right kidney	4. Major calyx	6. Renal pelvis
2. Lower pole, right kidney	5. Minor calyx	7. Psoas major muscle
3. Ureter		

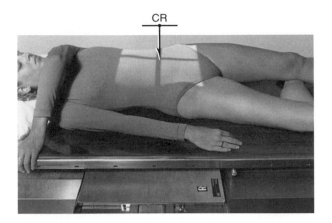

Figure 14–28. Excretory urogram, right posterior oblique.

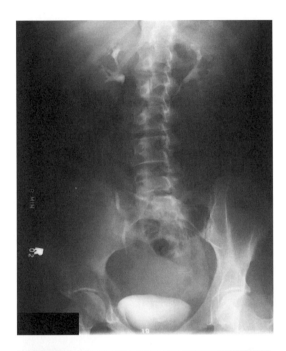

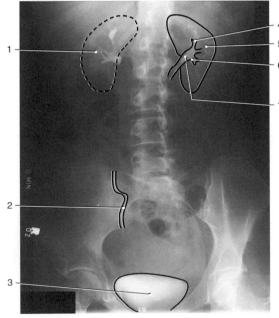

Figure 14–29. Excretory urogram, right posterior oblique; notice that the left kidney appears in profile (parallel with the film plane) whereas the right ureter is projected away from the spine.

► AP OBLIQUE (RPO & LPO) URINARY TRACT (EXCRETORY UROGRAM)

Technical Considerations

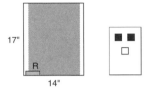

- Film size: Adult: 14 × 17 in. lengthwise. Pediatric: determined by patient size.
- Grid required.
- 70–75 kVp.
- Collimate to the abdominal walls laterally and to film size lengthwise.

Shielding

- Male patients should be shielded according to department policy.

Patient Positioning

- Assist the patient to the supine position on the radiographic table; place a pillow under the patient's head.

Part Positioning

- Rotate the patient 30° toward the one side, bringing the opposite arm across the chest; use a lumbar sponge to support the shoulders and hips. **Note:** Both obliques are usually obtained.
- Center the sagittal plane approximately 3 in. medial to the elevated ASIS to the midline of the table; the vertebral column should be centered to the table.
- Check for rotation to ensure the hips and shoulders are rotated equally; adjust the long axis of the patient to lie parallel with the long axis of the table. **Note:** Flexion of the elevated leg may cause superimposition of the leg over the bladder.
- Examine the opposite side in a similar manner *(Figure 14–28)*.

Central Ray

- Direct the central ray perpendicular to the level of the iliac crests.
- Center the cassette to the central ray.

Breathing Instructions

- Instruct the patient to take in a breath, blow it out, and hold it out during the exposure.

Image Evaluation

- Both kidneys and the symphysis pubis should be visualized on the radiograph.
- The elevated kidney should be seen in profile and the ureter nearest the film should be demonstrated away from the spine.
- The spine should be parallel with and centered to the film *(Figure 14–29)*.

1. Right kidney
2. Right ureter
3. Urinary bladder
4. Minor calyx
5. Left kidney
6. Major calyx
7. Renal pelvis

▶ AP URINARY BLADDER (EXCRETORY UROGRAM OR CYSTOGRAM)

Technical Considerations

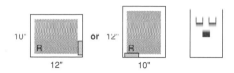

- Film size: 10 × 12 in. crosswise (excretory urogram) or lengthwise (cystogram). **Note:** For the cystogram, lengthwise positioning of the cassette is employed to include the distal ureters for evaluation of ureteral reflux.
- Grid required.
- 70–75 kVp.
- Collimate to the ASISs crosswise and to film size lengthwise.

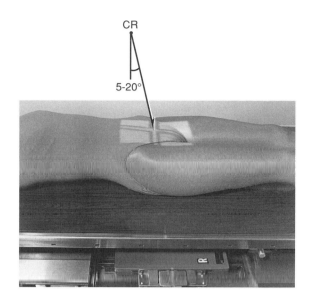

Figure 14–30. AP urinary bladder obtained as part of a cystogram.

Shielding

- Male patients should be shielded according to department policy.

Patient Positioning

- Assist the patient to the supine position on the radiographic table with legs extended. **Note:** This projection may also be performed with the patient prone or upright.

Part Positioning

- Center the midsagittal plane of the patient's body to the midline of the table.
- Adjust the long axis of the patient parallel with the long axis of the table; pull gently on patient's legs or under patient's arms to straighten the patient.
- Check for rotation of the pelvis by palpating the ASISs and ensuring they are equidistant from the table; use sponges for support and immobilization, if necessary *(Figure 14–30)*.

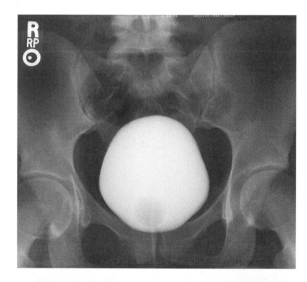

Central Ray

- Direct the central ray 5° to 20° caudad to the point 2 in. directly superior to the symphysis pubis; a greater than 5° angulation may be necessary for patients with a loss of lumbar lordosis.
- Center the cassette to the central ray.

Breathing Instructions

- Instruct the patient to take in a breath, blow it out, and hold it out during the exposure.

Image Evaluation

- The entire bladder and proximal urethra should be visualized above the pubic bones on the radiograph; superimposition indicates insufficient central ray angle.
- The bladder should be appropriately penetrated with short scale contrast.
- Asymmetry of the obturator foramina and ischial spines indicates rotation of the pelvis.
- The sacrum should be straight and centered to the film *(Figure 14–31)*.

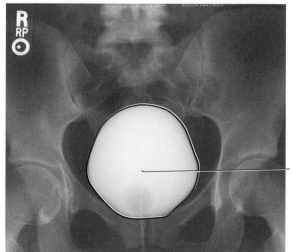

1. Urinary bladder

Figure 14–31. AP urinary bladder.

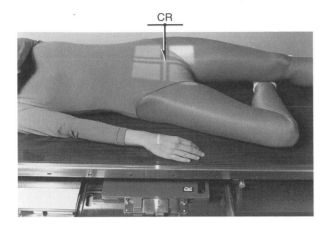

Figure 14–32. Right posterior oblique of the urinary bladder.

▶ AP OBLIQUE (RPO & LPO) URINARY BLADDER (CYSTOGRAM)

Technical Considerations

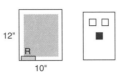

- Film size: 10 × 12 in. crosswise or lengthwise.
- Grid required.
- 70–75 kVp.
- Collimate to include the bladder.

Shielding

- Male patients should be shielded according to department policy.

Patient Positioning

- Assist the patient to the supine position on the radiographic table; place a pillow under the patient's head.

Part Positioning

- Rotate the patient 40° to 60° toward one side, bringing the opposite arm across the chest; use a lumbar sponge to support the shoulders and hips. **Note:** An RPO, LPO, or both obliques are obtained per physician request. A steeper oblique is used to better demonstrate the ureterovesicular region, however, a shallow oblique may be adequate for diffentiation of stones.
- Center the plane passing through the bladder to the midline of the table.
- Check for rotation to ensure the hips and shoulders are rotated equally; adjust the long axis of the patient to lie parallel with the long axis of the table. **Note:** Flexion of the elevated leg may cause superimposition of that leg over the bladder.
- Examine the opposite side in a similar manner *(Figure 14–32)*.

Central Ray

- Direct the central ray perpendicular to a point approximately 2 in. superior to the symphysis pubis and 2 in. medial to a plane passing through the ASIS; the central ray should be directed 10° caudad when the proximal urethra is of interest.
- Center the cassette to the central ray.

Breathing Instructions

- Instruct the patient to take in a breath, blow it out, and hold it out during the exposure.

Image Evaluation

- The urinary bladder and areas of distal ureters and proximal urethra should be visualized above the pubic bones on the radiograph.
- The bladder should be appropriately penetrated with short scale contrast.
- The elevated thigh should not superimpose the bladder.
- The urinary bladder should be centered to the film *(Figure 14–33)*.

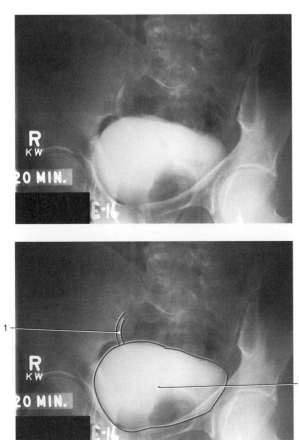

Figure 14–33. **Right posterior oblique of the urinary bladder; a stone is visualized in the right distal ureter.**

1. Right distal ureter   2. Urinary bladder

$\mathscr{S}$UMMARY

▶ Although the retrograde pyelogram and cystogram demonstrate size, shape, and location of various urinary structures, the excretory urogram (intravenous pyelogram) and voiding cystourogram can also be used to evaluate the function of the urinary system.

▶ Radiographs taken when the contrast medium is being filtered from the blood by the nephrons are called nephrograms.

▶ A hypertensive intravenous pyelogram can be used to assist in determining if the cause of hypertension is renal artery stenosis.

▶ Retrograde pyelography is a nonfunctional examination of the ureters, bladder, and pelvicalyceal system that can be performed when routine excretory urography is contraindicated.

▶ Retrograde pyelography, cystography, and voiding cystourethrography are all retrograde procedures performed by introducing contrast media through a catheter that has been introduced into the urethra and urinary bladder under sterile conditions.

▶ Whenever possible, patient preparation for excretory urograms and retrograde pyelograms includes a low-residue diet for 1 to 2 days, a light evening meal the night before the examination, a nongas-producing cathartic, and nothing, other than water, by mouth after midnight; the patient should void prior to the start of the examination.

▶ The acquisition and documentation of a pertinent patient history are important for diagnosis and patient safety and should include information relative to an allergy history and medical problems that might contraindicate the use of iodinated contrast media.

▶ Room preparation includes preparation of contrast media and acquisition of necessary supplies and equipment.

▶ To demonstrate renal shadows, possible calculi, and abnormal lesions, a scout film is taken prior to administration of contrast media for any examination of the urinary tract.

▶ Although most radiographs are obtained with the patient supine, the patient may also be positioned obliquely, prone, upright, or Trendelenburg; delayed films may be necessary when calculi inhibit filling of the ureters.

▶ A ureteral compression device can be used to restrict the flow of contrast media from the kidneys to the bladder, thereby enhancing the renal pelves and calyces.

▶ Tomography is used to eliminate overlying bowel patterns to better evaluate the kidneys in the nephron phase, as well as possible calculi, cysts, and tumors.

▶ CT, ultrasonography, MRI, and nuclear medicine scans are also used to evaluate the structures of the urinary system.

▶ All radiographs of the urinary system should be obtained during suspended expiration.

▶ Urographic imaging of the pediatric patient differs from that of the adult in terms of patient preparation and number of radiographs obtained.

▶ To produce the highest-quality radiographs without excessively high patient exposure, 70 to 75 kVp is recommended for all adult radiography of the urinary system.

▶ A grid device is required for all radiography of the urinary system.

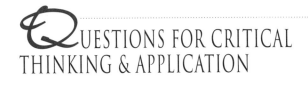

QUESTIONS FOR CRITICAL THINKING & APPLICATION

1. Explain why the kidneys can be referred to as "homeostatic organs."

2. Why would an individual suffering from nephroptosis be susceptible to obstructions caused by tortuous ureters?

3. During an excretory urogram, contrast medum is injected into the median cubital vein in the patient's arm. Trace the path the contrast medum will take in route to the urinary bladder. Your discussion should include vascular structures as well as the structures of the urinary system.

4. What role does the glomerulus play in regulating a person's blood pressure?

5. Why must a person have one working kidney? What are the consequences of renal failure? Describe the process of hemodialysis.

6. List at least four positions or techniques that can be used to enhance filling of the pelvicalyceal structures and/or the ureters.

7. Patient education and communication are important for any examination. Demonstrate your knowledge of excretory urography by explaining to a "patient" what will happen before, during, and after the procedure.

8. A patient with a history of renal cysts has been scheduled for an excretory urogram. After the radiographer obtains a relevant patient history, however, the radiologist feels this examination is contraindicated. What other examination(s) can be done to rule out a cyst without using intravenous contrast media?

9. An excretory urogram has been ordered on the victim of a car accident. The patient has multiple injuries, is unconscious, and has been catheterized; the urine in the output bag is "pink." Describe the procedure you would follow to complete the examination. What are your limitations and concerns?

10. A morbidly obese patient has a creatinine level of 2.0. What might the concerns be relative to performing an excretory urogram? What techniques or procedures could be followed to address those concerns?

FILM CRITIQUE

Looking at this oblique abdominal projection *(Figure 14–34)* that was obtained as part of an excretory urogram, describe the patient positioning.

Was the patient correctly positioned?

What criteria did you use to determine positioning accuracy?

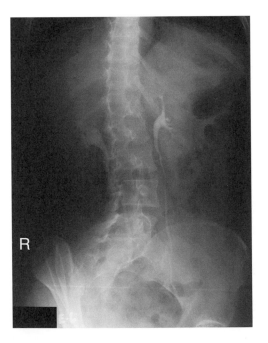

Figure 14–34.

15
DIGESTIVE SYSTEM

► OBJECTIVES:

Following the completion of this chapter the student will be able to:

- Given diagrams or radiographs, name and describe the anatomy of the digestive system, to include the pharynx, esophagus, stomach, small intestine, and large intestine.

- Discuss the orientation of the stomach according to body habitus, physical position, and respiration.

- Identify the functions of each of the structures in the digestive system, outlining the physiologic activities of digestion as they relate to each of the digestive organs.

- Describe room preparation and identify supplies needed for examinations of the digestive system.

- Discuss the use of contrast media in radiographic examinations of the digestive system, to include preferred type and route of administration.

- Identify alternative methods for evaluating the digestive system.

- State the criteria used to determine positioning accuracy on radiographs of the digestive system and evaluate radiographs of the digestive system in terms of positioning, centering, image quality, radiographic anatomy, and pathology.

- Define terminology associated with the digestive system, to include anatomy, procedures, and pathology.

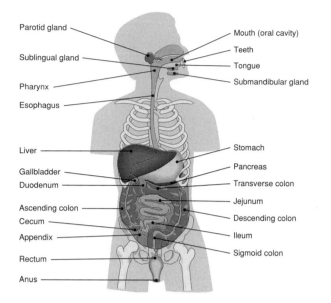

Figure 15–1. Overview of the digestive system.

► ANATOMY OF THE DIGESTIVE SYSTEM

The body needs energy to perform functions that are essential to life. It is the function of the digestive system to take in food and break it down so that it can be converted into energy to keep the body going *(Table 15–1)*. A person's well-being is dependent on a healthy and well-functioning digestive system *(Figure 15–1)*.

The digestive system can be divided into the alimentary (al-i-MEN-tar-ē) canal, also known as the gastrointestinal (GI) tract, and accessory organs *(Figure 15–2)*. The components of each division are identified in *Table 15–2*.

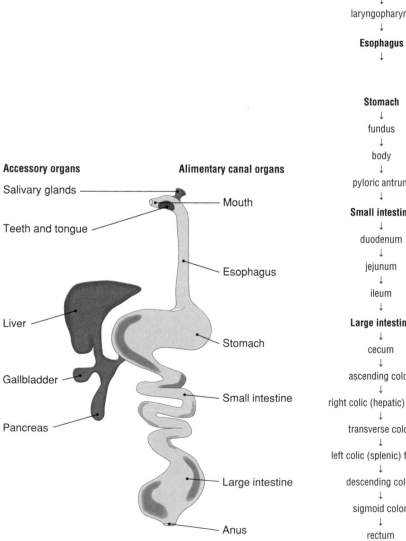

Accessory organs

Salivary glands

Teeth and tongue

Liver

Gallbladder

Pancreas

Alimentary canal organs

Mouth

Esophagus

Stomach

Small intestine

Large intestine

Anus

Figure 15–2. Schematic view of the relationship between the alimentary canal and accessory digestive organs.

Table 15–1. Primary Organs of the Digestive System

Mouth	• Oral/buccal cavity
↓	• Teeth and tongue help direct and move food
Pharynx	• Functions in both respiratory and digestive systems
↓	• Three divisions (nasopharynx does not play a role in digestion)
oropharynx	• 5 in. long
↓	
laryngopharynx	
↓	
Esophagus	• Gullet
↓	• 10 in. long
	• Collapslble
	• Cardiac antrum = abdominal esophagus
Stomach	• Storage chamber
↓	• Rugae = wrinkles in mucosal lining
fundus	• Cardiac and pyloric orifices/sphincters
↓	• Variable size
body	• Greater and lesser curvatures
↓	• Angular and cardiac notches
pyloric antrum	
↓	
Small intestine	• 20 ft long with three segments
↓	• Centrally located in abdomen
duodenum	• Head of pancreas lies in C-loop of duodenum
↓	• Center of most digestive activities
jejunum	• Plicae circularis = circular folds
↓	• Villi on mucosal membrane
ileum	
↓	
Large intestine	
↓	• 5 ft long
cecum	• Arch-shaped
↓	• Peripherally located in abdominopelvic cavity
ascending colon	• Appendix/vermiform process
↓	• Teniae coli = longitudinal bands of muscle
right colic (hepatic) flexure	• Haustra
↓	• Internal and external anal sphincters
transverse colon	
↓	
left colic (splenic) flexure	
↓	
descending colon	
↓	
sigmoid colon	
↓	
rectum	
↓	
anus	

Table 15–2. Components of the Digestive System

Alimentary Canal	Accessory Organs
Mouth	Teeth
Pharynx	Tongue
Esophagus	Salivary glands
Stomach	Liver
Small intestine	Gallbladder
Large intestine	Pancreas

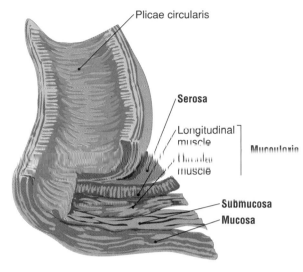

Figure 15–3. Four layers of tissue forming the wall of the alimentary canal are demonstrated on this sectional view of the small intestine.

ALIMENTARY CANAL

The alimentary canal is a long, hollow tube measuring slightly less than 30 ft (9 m) in length. It extends from the mouth to the anus, passing through both the thoracic and abdominopelvic cavities. It is open on both ends, with the inside channel called the **lumen** (LŪ-men).

With some regional modifications, there are generally four layers of tissue forming the walls of the alimentary canal *(Figure 15–3)*. From deep to superficial, the first layer is the **mucosa** (mū-KŌ-sah), which is a mucous membrane forming the inner lining of the canal. In other words, it is adjacent to the lumen of the canal. The second layer is the **submucosa.** Blood vessels supplying the alimentary canal are located in this layer of connective tissue. The third layer, the **muscularis** (mus-kū-LĀ-ris), actually consists of an inner coat of circular muscle tissue and an outer coat of longitudinal muscle tissue. The mouth, pharynx, upper esophagus, and anal sphincter are characterized by skeletal muscle tissue which allows for voluntary movement; the muscle tissue in the remainder of the alimentary canal is typically smooth and involuntary. The **serosa** (se-RŌ-sah) is the fourth and most superficial layer. This serous membrane is the visceral portion of the peritoneum and is found only on those components of the alimentary canal situated in the abdominopelvic cavity: the stomach, small intestine, and large intestine. Recall from Chapter 3 that the peritoneum is a double-walled membrane lining the abdominopelvic cavity. The visceral portion of the peritoneum encloses the organs of the abdomen, whereas the parietal peritoneum lines the walls of the abdominopelvic cavity.

MOUTH

The mouth is also known as the **oral** or **buccal** (BUK-al) **cavity.** The lips or **labia** (LĀ-bē-ah) surround the oral orifice, which is the opening into the mouth. The roof of the cavity is formed by the hard and soft palates; the lateral walls are formed by the cheeks. The **hard palate** is formed by the horizontal portions of both maxillae and palatine bones (facial bones). The movable **soft palate** is a musculomembranous fold of tissue at the posterior portion of the roof that acts as a partition between the mouth and pharynx. The muscular **tongue** lies on the floor of the mouth. Its upper surface is slightly bumpy from the presence of taste buds. The tongue is considered to be an accessory organ of digestion because it moves and directs food inside the mouth. Although it is very mobile, the movement of the tongue posteriorly is limited by the **lingual frenulum** (LING-gwal FREN-ū-lum), a fold of mucous membrane on the underside of the tongue that secures it to the floor of the mouth. The paired **palatine arches** are folds of tissue on each side of the mouth that affix the soft palate anteriorly and posteriorly to the base of the tongue. Respectively, these arches are known as the **palatoglossal** (pal-ah-tō-GLOS-al) (*glosso* = "tongue") and the **palatopharyngeal** (pal-ah-tō-fah-RIN-jē-al) **arches.** The **fauces** (FAW-sēz) is the opening between the oral cavity and the oropharynx bounded by the soft palate, palatoglossal and palatopharyngeal arches, and tongue *(Figure 15–4)*.

Other accessory structures of the digestive system associated with the mouth include the teeth and salivary glands. There are 32 teeth in a full set of permanent teeth. They are positioned in an arched arrangement in the alveolar processes of the maxillae and mandible (facial bones). As accessory structures of digestion, their function is *mastication* (mas-ti-KĀ-shun), which is the process of chewing. They are able to tear and grind food into smaller pieces so that it can mix more readily with saliva *(Figure 15–5)*.

The three pairs of salivary glands are not located within the mouth, but instead empty into it via ducts *(Figure 15–6)*. The **parotid** (pa-ROT-id) **glands** are the largest of the glands. Located in the cheeks, they lie just anterior and inferior to the external ears (*para* = "near," *oto* = "ear") and posterior to the mandibular rami. The **parotid (Stensen's) ducts** are about 2 in. (5 cm) long and empty into the mouth in the area of the second upper molars. The **submandibular glands** are approximately the size of walnuts.

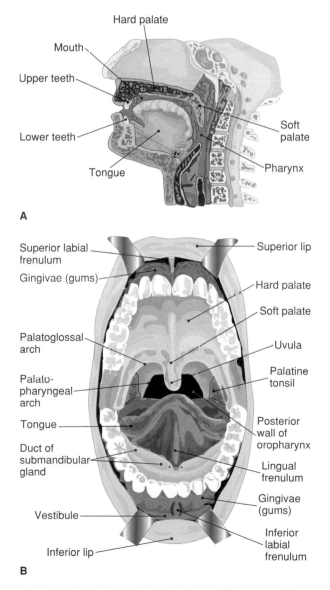

Figure 15–4. Oral cavity: **(A)** sagittal section, and **(B)** open-mouth view.

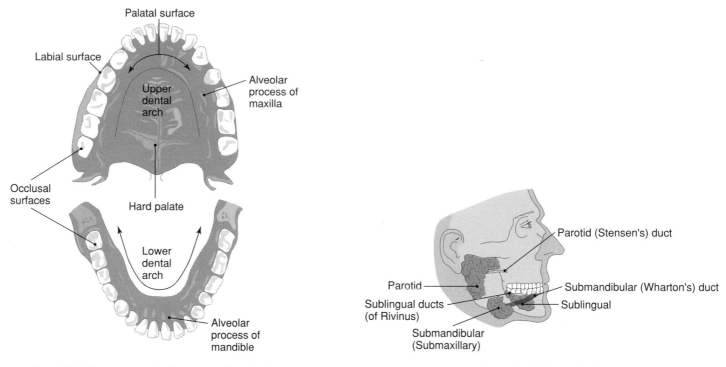

Figure 15–5. Arch arrangement of the upper and lower teeth.

Figure 15–6. Salivary glands.

They are situated under the floor of the mouth between the base of the tongue and the right and left sides of the body of the mandible and are also known as the **submaxillary glands.** The **submandibular (Wharton's) ducts** empty into the oral cavity just lateral to the lingual frenulum. The smallest salivary glands, the **sublingual glands,** are situated anterior to the submandibular glands under the tongue. Approximately 8 to 20 small **sublingual ducts (ducts of Rivinus)** drain into the floor of the mouth. The salivary glands produce approximately 1 to 1.5 quarts (1000–1500 mL) of saliva daily. This slightly acidic fluid is 99.5% water and 0.5% electrolytes, enzymes, proteins, and metabolic waste products. It mixes with food, helping it form into a bolus (small mass) so that it can be easily swallowed. It also serves to initiate digestion of carbohydrates and lubricate the oral cavity.

PHARYNX

The pharynx (FAR-ingks) is often referred to as the throat. It is approximately 5 in. or 12.5 cm in length and is located posteriorly to the mouth, beginning at the fauces. It comprises three divisions which are named according to their location: the nasopharynx, oropharynx, and laryngopharynx are adjacent to the nasal cavity, mouth, and larynx, respectively *(Figure 15–7)*. The anatomy of each division was addressed in Chapter 2, as the pharynx functions in both the respiratory and digestive systems to convey air to the lungs and food/fluids to the esophagus. The nasopharynx does not play any role in the digestive process. During *deglutition* (deg-loo-TISH-un), or swallowing, it is closed off from the rest of the pharynx by the soft palate to prevent the passage of food into the nasal cavities. The oropharynx and laryngopharynx facilitate the propulsion of food and fluids from the mouth to the stomach. The **palatine tonsils** of the lymphatic system lie in the oropharynx between the palatine arches. The **uvula** (Ū-vū-lah) is a small piece of tissue suspended in the oropharynx from the posterior margin of the soft palate. When a person swallows, the uvula moves superiorly with the soft palate so that the swallowed material cannot pass into the nasopharynx. To prevent food from entering the larynx during deglutition, the glottis covers the opening and food passes posteriorly down the laryngopharynx and into the esophagus.

ESOPHAGUS

The esophagus (e-SOF-ah-gus), or gullet, is a hollow, muscular tube that is approximately 10 in. (25 cm) long, beginning approximately at the level of C6 and terminating about T11. Its name translates literally to "carry food," which is an accurate description of its function. The only role of the esophagus in the diges-

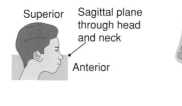

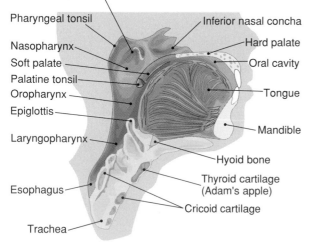

Figure 15–7. Three divisions of the pharynx are demonstrated on a sagittal view.

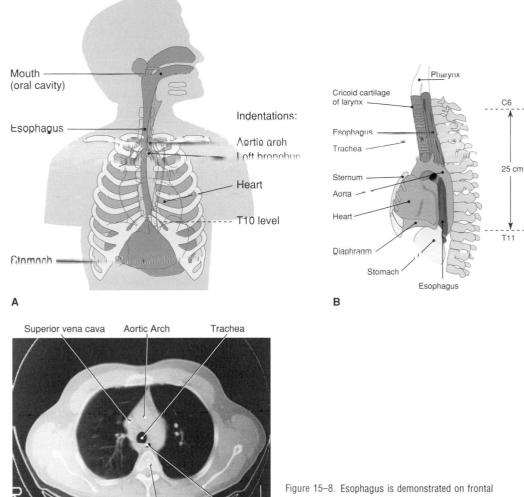

Figure 15–8. Esophagus is demonstrated on frontal **(A)** and lateral **(B)** views. An axial CT image **(C)** through the thorax demonstrates the relative position of the esophagus in the mediastinum.

tive system is to transport food and fluids from the pharynx to the stomach. Its diameter is approximately 0.75 in. (2 cm); however, when it is empty, it collapses and its mucosal lining falls into numerous longitudinal folds. The muscular layer of the upper third of the esophagus is skeletal muscle, allowing for voluntary movement. The middle third is comprised of both skeletal and smooth muscle, and the lower third is just smooth muscle (involuntary movement). As it passes through the mediastinum of the thorax, it is positioned posteriorly to the trachea and heart and anteriorly to the vertebral column *(Figure 15–8)*. The esophagus normally demonstrates two indentations caused by the proximity of the aortic arch and the left bronchus *(Figure 15–9)*. At its distal end, the esophagus veers slightly to the left of the body's midline and passes through an opening in the diaphragm at the level of T10 called the **esophageal hiatus** (e-sof-a-JĒ-al hī-Ā-tus). The abdominal esophagus is less than 1 in. (1 to 2 cm) in length, and may be referred to as the **cardiac antrum** as it is situated near the heart. The esophagus merges with the stomach at the esophagogastric (gastroesophageal) junction, which is located approximately at the level of T11. A condition in which the upper portion of the stomach protrudes up through the esophageal hiatus is known as a *hiatal* (hī-Ā-tal) or diaphragmatic *hernia (Figure 15–10)*.

STOMACH

The stomach (STUM-ak) is located predominately to the left of the midline in the left upper quadrant of the abdomen or, more specifically, in the epigastric, umbilical, and left hypochondriac regions. Because the organ is J-shaped, it crosses the midline into the right side of the abdomen.

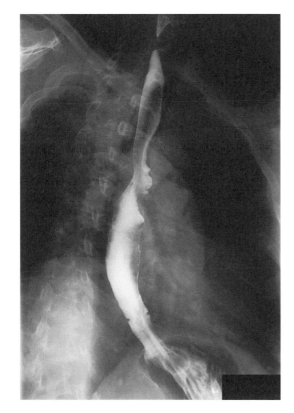

Figure 15–9. Because the esophagus overlies the thoracic vertebrae, it is better seen on an oblique (RAO) projection. Note the indentations caused by the proximity of the aortic arch and left main bronchus.

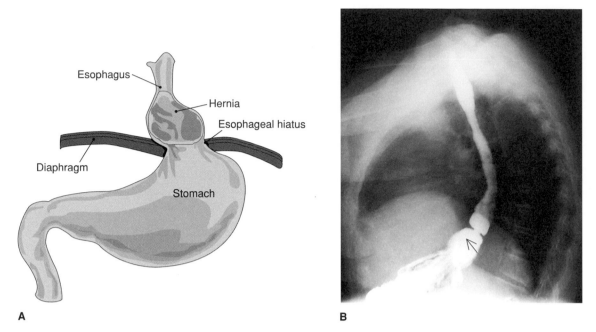

A   **B**

Figure 15–10. **(A)** A hiatal hernia occurs when a portion of the stomach slips up through the esophageal hiatus. **(B)** A hiatal hernia is demonstrated on the lateral esophagram.

Extending between the esophagus and small intestine, the stomach is the most expanded portion of the alimentary canal. When it is empty, its mucosal lining falls into longitudinal ridges and folds called *rugae* (ROO-gē or ROO-guy) (*rugae* = "wrinkles"). Although the average stomach measures about 10 in. (25 cm) in length, the size of the stomach is quite variable as it is capable of distending when eating a large meal. Its volume ranges from 1.7 oz (50 mL) when almost empty to 1.5 qt (1.5 L) when distended. It acts as a holding chamber so that a great volume of food is not passed directly from the esophagus into the small intestine. It is during this holding time that the digestion of proteins is initiated and the food particles are mixed into *chyme* (kīm), a semifluid substance with the consistency of paste.

The esophagus enters the stomach through an opening called the **cardiac orifice.** The opening is guarded by the **cardiac sphincter,** which helps to regulate the movement of food into the stomach. The small area surrounding the cardiac orifice is known as the **cardia** (KAR-dē-ah) because of its proximity to the heart. The three main portions of the stomach are the fundus (FUN-dus), body, and pyloric (pī-LOR-ik) antrum *(Figure 15–11).*

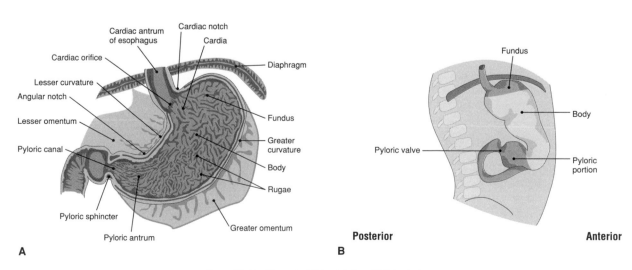

A   **B**   **Posterior**   **Anterior**

Figure 15–11. Stomach: **(A)** frontal view, **(B)** lateral view.

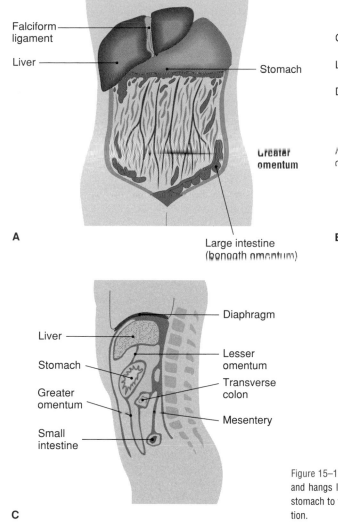
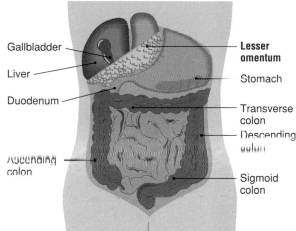

Figure 15–12. **(A)** The greater omentum attaches to the greater curvature of the stomach and hangs like an apron over the small intestine. **(B)** The lesser omentum attaches the stomach to the liver. **(C)** The relative positions of both omenta are seen on a sagittal section.

The **fundus** is the rounded, upper portion of the stomach located laterally to the cardiac orifice. Its upper margin extends above the cardiac orifice to reside just under the left hemidiaphragm. It is the most posterior portion of the stomach. A gas bubble is usually present in the fundus and is often demonstrated on upright projections of the chest. The **body** is the large, central area of the stomach. It is the most anterior portion of the stomach. The **pyloric antrum** is the funnel-shaped area located inferiorly to the body and in the curve of the stomach. The terms *pyloric portion* and *pylorus* are often used interchangeably to refer to this region of the stomach. The pyloric antrum narrows into the **pyloric canal** as it joins the duodenum of the small intestine at the **pyloric orifice.** The **pyloric sphincter** acts as a valve at the orifice to adjust the flow of chyme into the duodenum.

Because of its characteristic J-shape, the stomach has two curved margins and two notches on it. The lateral margin on the left side of the stomach is long and convex. It is known as the **greater curvature.** The medial margin on the stomach's right side is shorter, concave, and called the **lesser curvature.** On the average-sized stomach, the greater curvature is approximately 16 in. (40 cm) long, whereas the lesser curvature is about 4 in. (10 cm) long. The position of the stomach is somewhat secured in the abdomen by two folds of peritoneum called *omenta.* The **greater omentum** extends from the greater curvature to the transverse colon, where it then hangs down like an apron, covering the small intestine in the abdominopelvic cavity. The **lesser omentum** attaches to the lesser curvature of the stomach and stretches to the liver *(Figure 15–12).*

The **angular notch** (incisura angularis) is located on the lesser curvature where the stomach curves to the right side of the abdomen. It marks the transition between the body of the stomach and the pyloric antrum. The **cardiac notch** (incisura cardiaca) is located on the superior aspect of the stomach between the cardiac antrum of the esophagus and the greater curvature.

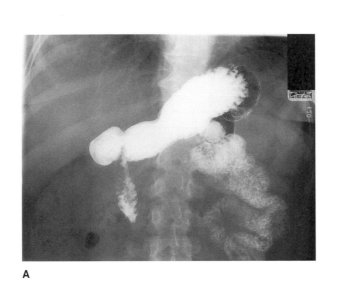

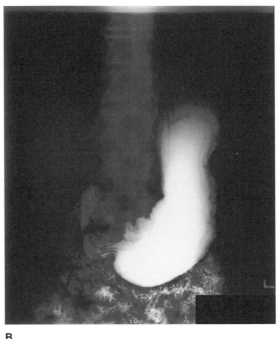

A   **B**

Figure 15–13. The shape and location of the stomach vary with body habitus. **(A)** PA projection of the stomach on a hypersthenic patient. **(B)** PA projection on a hyposthenic/asthenic patient.

The position and shape of the stomach are affected by body habitus, physical position, and respiration. The stomach tends to lie higher and more transverse in the hypersthenic patient, but is situated lower and closer to the spine and appears more elongated in the asthenic patient *(Figure 15–13)*. The stomach is higher when a person is in a supine position and lower when a person is lying in the prone position. Respiration also affects the position of the stomach as the diaphragm pushes the stomach inferiorly on inspiration. The stomach moves upward with the diaphragm on expiration.

SMALL INTESTINE

The majority of the digestive and absorptive processes take place in the small intestine. Also referred to as the small bowel, this is the longest portion of the alimentary canal with an average length of 20 ft (6 m). It is tightly coiled to lie in the central and lower regions of the abdomen *(Figure 15–14)*.

The small intestine consists of three segments: duodenum, jejunum, and ileum. The **duodenum** (dū-ō-DĒ-num) is the first of the segments and is also the shortest. Measuring approximately 10 in. (25 cm) in length, it is usually C-shaped with the head of the pancreas lying in the C-loop. It is arbitrarily divided into four parts. As chyme passes through the sphincter, it enters the **duodenal bulb** or **cap.** This is the expanded initial portion of the **superior duodenum** located approximately at the level of L2. The superior portion projects downward to become the **descending duodenum.** The common bile duct and main pancreatic duct enter on the posterior aspect of the descending portion of the duodenum. The **horizontal duodenum** extends from the descending part to pass across the midline. It continues as the **ascending duodenum,** which passes upward to join the jejunum in the upper left quadrant of the abdomen. The junction between the duodenum and jejunum is a rather sharp bend called the **duodenojejunal flexure** or **angle of Treitz** (trētz). It is the most fixed area of the small intestine as it is held in place by the ligament of Treitz *(Figure 15–15)*.

The **jejunum** (je-JOO-num) is the second segment of the small intestine. It measures approximately 8 ft (2.5 m), constituting two fifths of the remainder of the small intestine. This region of the alimentary canal is relatively mobile, but is generally located in the left upper and lower quadrants of the abdomen. It merges with the **ileum** (IL-ē-um), which forms the last segment and remaining three fifths of the small intestine. The ileum measures in as the longest segment at approximately 11 ft (3.3 m). It is situated primarily in the middle and right regions of the abdomen. The last portion or terminal ileum connects to the large intestine at the **ileocecal valve** located in the right lower quadrant of the abdomen. The muscular **ileocecal**

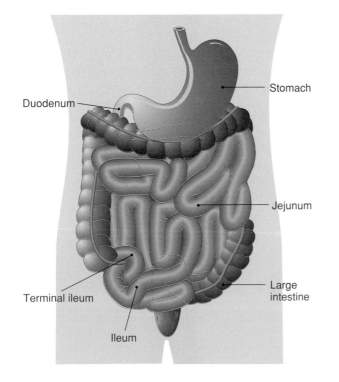

Figure 15–14. Small intestine.

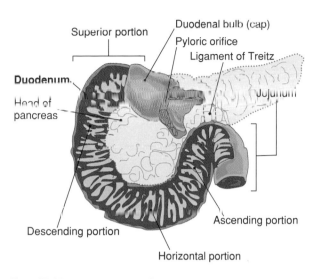

Figure 15–15. The duodenum is a C-shaped structure. The head of the pancreas is situated within the C-loop.

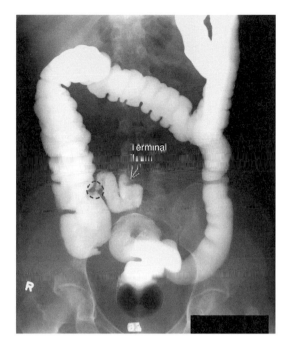

Figure 15–16. The terminal ileum is well demonstrated on this PA projection of the large intestine, as contrast medium has refluxed through the ileocecal valve.

sphincter is present at the valve to prevent reflux of material from the large intestine into the ileum, although some generally occurs during a barium enema examination *(Figure 15–16)*.

The duodenum is a retroperitoneal structure, whereas the jejunum and ileum are intraperitoneal structures. The jejunum and ileum are suspended from the posterior wall of the abdomen by the mesentery. Recall from Chapter 3 that the mesentery is an extension of the parietal peritoneum, which functions to support and secure abdominal organs in place. Blood vessels, nerves, and lymphatic vessels are transported to the small intestine via the mesentery.

The diameter of the small intestine is greatest at the duodenum and becomes progressively smaller through the jejunum and ileum, averaging approximately 1 in. (2.5 cm). Chyme moves through the small intestine in a spiral fashion because of small circular folds in the mucous membrane called **plicae circularis** (PLĪ-kē ser-kū-LAR-ēs) *(Figure 15–17)*. There are about 800 of these folds along the length of the small intestine, with the most prominent number found in the jejunum. The number and size of the folds gradually diminish as the jejunum merges with the ileum. Their presence affects the radiographic appearance of the small intestine, causing it to resemble a coiled wire or spring (like the Slinky® toy) when air is present. After the administration of positive contrast medium, the jejunum normally resembles sponge painting, appearing rather light and feathery. Because the plicae circularis are not as predominant in the ileum, this part of the small intestine appears much smoother *(Figure 15–18)*.

Glands in the mucous membrane of the small intestine secrete intestinal juice that contains digestive enzymes. Another characteristic of the small intestine is the presence of tiny **villi** (VIL-lī) *(S. villus)*. These fingerlike protrusions of the mucosal membrane range from 0.02 to 0.04 in. (0.5 to 1 mm) and serve to increase the absorptive area in contact with the chyme passing through the small intestine.

LARGE INTESTINE

The large intestine extends from the ileum of the small intestine to the anus and has three segments: cecum, colon, and rectum. This arch-shaped structure averages 5 ft (1.5 m) in length and is generally positioned around the periphery of the abdominopelvic cavity *(Figure 15–19)*. Its diameter is larger than that of the small intestine, averaging 2.5 in. (6.5 cm). The large intestine functions to manufacture particular vitamins; to absorb water, which allows feces to form and compact; and to expel the feces from the body.

Chyme moves from the small intestine through the ileocecal valve into the **cecum** (SĒ-kum). This rounded sac or pouch is 2 to 3 in. (5 to 8 cm) long and is actually located inferiorly to the ileocecal valve in the right iliac region or right lower quadrant of the abdomen. The **appendix,** or **vermiform process** (*vermiform* = "wormlike"), is a narrow pocket hanging from the posteromedial surface of the cecum.

Cross section of a circular fold of a small intestine

Circular fold of mucosa or plica circularis

Villi on a circular fold

Plicae circularis

Submucosa
Muscular layers
Serous layer (peritoneum)

Longitudinal section

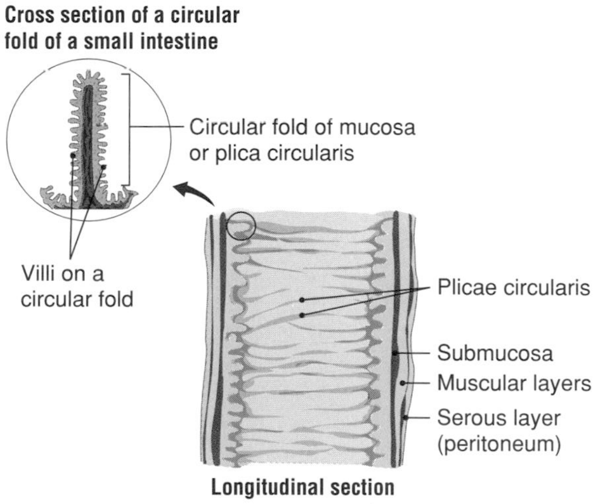

Figure 15–17. Longitudinal section of the jejunum demonstrates the plicae circularis and the location of the villi.

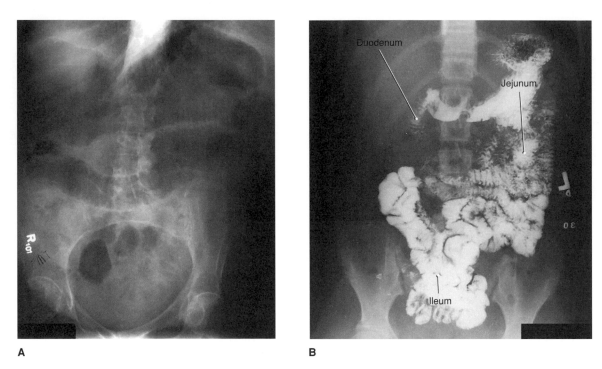

Figure 15–18. (A) When the small intestine is distended with gas, it has the appearance of a spring or coiled wire. **(B)** After the administration of barium sulfate, the jejunum appears light and feathery while the ileum is much smoother.

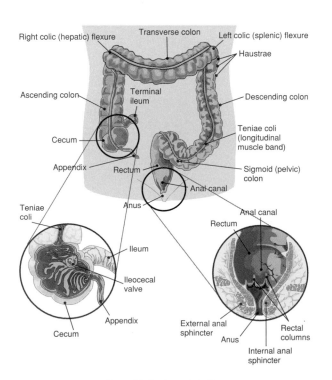

Figure 15–19. Large intestine.

Ranging in length from 2 to 6 in. (5 to 15 cm), its walls contain lymphatic tissue. Feces move freely in and out of the appendix; however, in some cases, the appendix becomes obstructed and inflamed, resulting in appendicitis (ah-pen-di-SĪ-tis).

The second segment of the large intestine called the **colon** (KŌ-lon) is a long tube that continues from the cecum to the rectum. It can be subdivided into four parts:

1. The **ascending colon** is directed superiorly from the cecum to the right upper quadrant, where it bends medially and anteriorly at the **right colic flexure.** This bend is also known as the **hepatic flexure** as it is located under the liver.
2. The **transverse colon** is the longest part of the colon. It crosses the upper anterior abdomen from the right to left sides, where it bends inferiorly and posteriorly under the spleen to form the **left colic** or **splenic flexure.**
3. The **descending colon** is located on the left side of the abdomen and extends inferiorly from the splenic flexure into the pelvis, where it becomes the sigmoid colon.
4. The name **sigmoid** (SIG-moid) **colon** has a Greek origin meaning S-shaped. It is aptly named, as it is an S-shaped loop of the colon extending approximately from the level of the iliac crest or pelvic brim inferiorly to the third segment of the sacrum. At this point, it connects to the rectum. Because of its location, the sigmoid colon is sometimes referred to as the **pelvic colon.**

The transverse colon and sigmoid colon are intraperitoneal structures, but the ascending and descending colon are retroperitoneal, as they are located behind the peritoneum.

The **rectum** (REK-tum) is the last segment of the large intestine, measuring approximately 6 in. (15 cm) in length. It is a retroperitoneal structure, extending inferiorly and posteriorly from the sigmoid colon around the level of S-3 and following the curve of the sacrum. Just anterior to the coccyx, the rectum curves inferiorly and anteriorly and expands into the **rectal ampulla.** Directly below this area, the rectum once again changes directions and extends inferiorly and posteriorly. The anatomic contours of the rectum must be considered when inserting an enema tip so as not to perforate the rectal wall. The last 1 in. (2 to 3 cm) of the rectum is a more constricted area called the **anal canal.** Numerous arteries and veins are present in small longitudinal folds of the mucous membrane known as **rectal columns.** Dilations of these veins are known as *hemorrhoids* (HEM-o-roids). The external opening of the rectum is the **anus** (Ā-nus). Two muscular sphincters are present at the anus. The **internal anal sphincter** comprises smooth muscle and is involuntary, whereas the **external anal sphincter,** composed of skeletal muscle, is voluntary. The anus is typically in a closed state except during defecation *(Figure 15–20).*

In most of the large intestine, the muscularis layer is different than seen elsewhere in the alimentary canal. The longitudinal muscle consists of three bands called **teniae coli** (TĒ-nē-ē KŌ-lī). Because these bands are shorter than the other muscle fibers, they produce a puckering effect in the large intestine much like elastic in the waist of pants. Sacs or pouches called **haustra** (HAUS-tra) are formed as a result of the puckering and are demonstrated along the length of the large intestine, except at the rectum.

Portions of the large intestine are movable, although the **mesocolon,** a double layer of peritoneum, secures it to the posterior abdominal wall. The transverse colon has the ability to move superiorly and inferiorly, whereas the cecum and sigmoid colon are quite mobile and variable in position. Like that of the stomach, the position of the large intestine is affected by body habitus. In the extremely thin (asthenic) patient, the large intestine may be very low in the abdomen, possibly in the pelvis. Conversely, the bowel may be very widespread on the hypersthenic patient, with the flexures extending high in the abdominopelvic cavity (particularly the left colic [splenic] flexure).

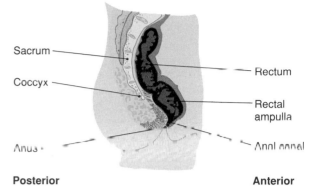

Figure 15–20. Rectum is seen in profile on a lateral view.

DIMENSIONAL ANATOMY

The radiographer should think three-dimensionally about the relative shape or position of the digestive organ. An AP or PA projection of the abdomen demonstrates two dimensions (length and width) of an organ; however, the stomach, small intestine, and large intestine do not lie in a flat plane within the abdomen. The depth, or anteroposterior dimension, should also be considered, as some structures of an organ are situated more anteriorly or posteriorly than others. This is especially relevant for contrast studies of the alimentary canal because a contrast medium will seek its own level depending on the patient's position. Therefore, AP and PA projections of the stomach or large intestine will demonstrate the contrast medium in different regions *(Figure 15–21). Table 15–3* summarizes the anteroposterior position of the particular structure on a digestive organ.

ACCESSORY ORGANS OF DIGESTION

As noted previously, the teeth, tongue, salivary glands, liver, gallbladder, and pancreas are considered to be accessory organs of digestion *(Figure 15–22).* The teeth, tongue, and salivary glands were addressed in the discussion of the mouth.

The **liver** (LIV-er) is a large solid organ of the biliary system. It is situated in the right upper quadrant of the abdomen just inferior to the right hemidiaphragm. Its main contribution to the digestive process is the manufacture of bile. The hepatocytes in the liver manufacture approximately 1 qt (1 L) of bile per

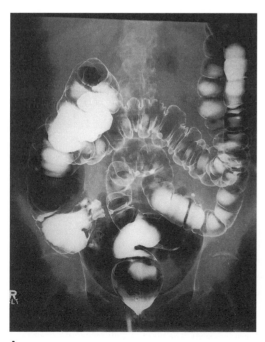

A

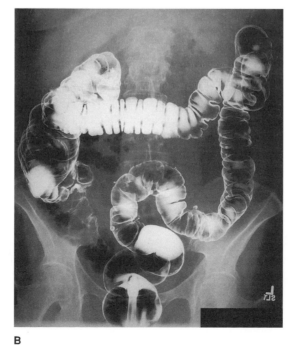

B

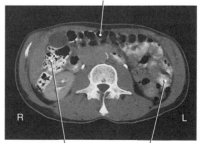

C

Figure 15–21. Transverse colon and sigmoid colon are filled with air on an AP projection because they are located anteriorly **(A)** and contrast-filled on a PA projection **(B)**. Axial CT image demonstrates the relative position of the large intestine in the abdomen **(C)**.

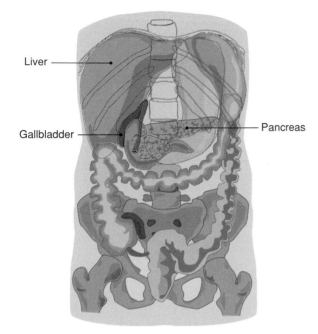

Figure 15–22. Liver, gallbladder, and pancreas are accessory organs of digestion.

Table 15–3. Anterior or Posterior Position of Structures in the Alimentary Canal[a]

	Anterior	Posterior
Stomach		
Fundus		X
Body	X	
Pyloric antrum		(not quite as posterior as fundus)
Small intestine		
Duodenal bulb		X
Jejunum	X	
Ileum	X	
Large intestine		
Cecum	X	
Ascending colon		X
Transverse colon	X	
Descending colon		X
Sigmoid colon	X	
Rectum		X

[a]For example, when a patient is in a supine position, contrast medium fills the fundus of the stomach, duodenal bulb, ascending and descending colons, and rectum.

day. Bile is a liquid substance composed mainly of bile salts, bile pigments, cholesterol, and water. The bile pigments are responsible for its characteristic yellowish color. This fluid plays an important role in the emulsification, absorption, and digestion of ingested fats.

Located on the inferior aspect of the liver, the **gallbladder** is also an organ of the biliary system. It functions to store and concentrate the bile produced by the liver. When stimulated, the gallbladder contracts, releasing the stored bile which is then conveyed by ducts to the duodenum.

The **pancreas** (PAN-krē-as) is an organ of the endocrine system. It spans the right and left upper quadrants of the abdomen. Its large head is situated in the C-loop or curve of the duodenum, whereas the body and tail taper toward the spleen. The pancreas aids in digestion by producing pancreatic juice which contains digestive enzymes. These enzymes break down proteins, carbohydrates, and fats in food. The pancreatic juice is conveyed to the duodenum via the main pancreatic duct. It generally merges with the common bile duct of the biliary system before entering the descending portion of the duodenum.

The anatomy and functions of the liver, gallbladder, and pancreas are covered more extensively in Chapter 16.

PHYSIOLOGY

A mixture of proteins, carbohydrates, lipids (fats), water, vitamins, and electrolytes (eg, sodium, potassium, etc.) are ingested as food. To be used as fuel by the body, most of the materials must be broken down and converted into a usable state, which is one capable of being absorbed by the capillaries of the circulatory system. Some of the substances, such as water, vitamins, and electrolytes, can be absorbed "as is." The process of digestion is twofold. The *mechanical component* is physical in nature, and includes breaking the food into smaller pieces, churning (mixing) it, moving it along the alimentary canal via peristalsis and segmentation, and expelling it as waste material. The *chemical component* consists of changing the chemical composition of the food. Organic catalysts called *enzymes* (EN-zīms) are proteins that expedite chemical reactions when they are mixed with food. *Hydrolysis* (hī-DROL-i-sis) is a process that takes place in the digestive system as compounds in food are mixed with water, acted on by enzymes, and broken down into simpler molecules.

When food is ingested, it is taken into the mouth where mechanical and chemical digestion begin. Through *mastication,* the food is broken into smaller pieces. It is then mixed with saliva, which lubricates it, forms it into a bolus, and begins to break down the carbohydrates. At this point, *deglutition* occurs and propels the food from the mouth. There are three stages of deglutition: buccal, pharyngeal, and esophageal. The *buccal stage* is the only voluntary phase of deglutition. The food is manipulated by the tongue and compressed against the hard palate, whereas the soft palate moves superiorly to close off the nasopharynx. Deglutition continues involuntarily after this point. The *pharyngeal stage* is initiated as food moves through the palatine arches and back against the pharyngeal wall. The epiglottis closes off the trachea as the bolus of food passes through the laryngopharynx. At this time, respiration is temporarily suspended for approximately 1 to 3 seconds. The *esophageal stage* begins as the bolus enters the esophagus. It is moved down the length of the esophagus and through the cardiac sphincter into the stomach by a series of wavelike movements called *peristalsis* (per-i-STAL-sis). It usually takes about 9 seconds for a bolus of food to travel down the esophagus; however, liquids can flow down within a few seconds with the aid of gravity (*Figure 15–23*).

Both mechanical and chemical processes occur in the stomach. Once the bolus enters the stomach, gastric contractions begin that result in mixing waves. Every 20 seconds, the mixing waves cause the bolus to be churned with fluids in the stomach, including gastric secretions, to form *chyme*. This process can continue anywhere from 2 to 6 hours depending on the amount and type of food consumed. The digestion of carbohydrates begun in the mouth continues in the stomach, whereas the digestion of proteins and some lipids is initiated. Alcohol and some drugs (ie, antibiotics and analgesics) may be absorbed from the stomach. Because the duodenum is much smaller than the stomach, the amount of chyme passing from the stomach is limited. A peristaltic wave occurs about every 20 seconds, propelling 2 to 4 teaspoons (10 to 15 mL) of chyme through the pyloric orifice into the duodenal bulb.

The majority of the digestive and absorptive processes take place in the small intestine. The chyme that passes through the pyloric sphincter into the small intestine contains partially digested carbohydrates, proteins, and lipids. Intestinal juice is secreted by glands in the intestinal lining, while bile and pancreatic juice drain into the duodenum. These fluids thoroughly mix with the chyme in a type of movement called *segmentation* (seg-men-TĀ-shun). Muscle contractions occur in separate segments of the small bowel about 12 to 16 times per minute to churn the chyme in a spiral fashion. The food particles are in contact with the mucosa on a large surface area of the small intestine which allows for better absorption. The digestion of carbohydrates, proteins, and lipids is completed in the small intestine, and nutrients (ie, digested food, water, vitamins, and electrolytes) are absorbed by the capillaries through the mucosa of the bowel. The unabsorbed material advances through the small intestine at a very slow rate (less than 0.5 in. [1 cm] per minute) because peristalsis is weaker in this region of the alimentary canal. On average, it takes 3 to 5 hours for chyme to pass completely through the small intestine.

The undigested and unabsorbed chyme moves through the ileocecal valve into the large intestine. At this point, most of the digestion and absorption has taken place. The chyme moves even slower through the large intestine than it did the small intestine. A very slow segmental movement termed *haustral churning* occurs about every 30 minutes. When one area of haustra becomes distended with chyme, the muscles contract and push the chyme into the next region of haustra. Peristalsis also moves the chyme along at a rate of 3 to 12 contractions per minute. Mass movements (mass peristalsis) occur on the average of one to three times per day, moving the food residues from the transverse colon into the sigmoid colon or rectum.

Chyme generally stays in the large intestine from 3 to 10 hours. During this time, a small amount of the residual material is broken down by bacteria naturally present in the large intestine, and amino acids and several vitamins (most notably vitamin K) are produced. Water and some electrolytes, especially sodium chloride, are also absorbed through the mucosa of the large intestine by osmosis, leaving a semisolid material called *feces* (FĒ-sēz). This waste matter is composed of undigested food, mucus, water, bacteria, some salts, and sloughed off cells from the alimentary canal. The feces are eliminated from the large intestine through a process called *defecation* (def-i-KĀ-shun). When the rectum becomes full, pressure increases and its walls distend to start a defecation reflex. When the anal sphincters relax voluntarily, intraabdominal pressure from straining and peristalsis causes the feces to be expelled through the anus. Food or contrast medium ingested orally usually takes about 24 hours to travel through the alimentary canal to the anus.

Mechanical and chemical digestion occurring throughout the alimentary canal is summarized in *Table 15–4* and *Figure 15–24*.

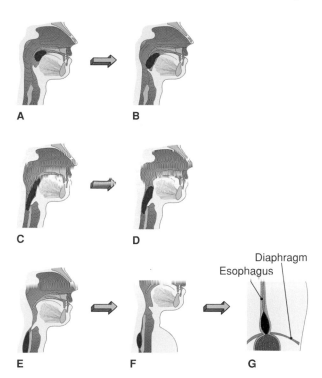

Figure 15–23. This series of illustrations represents the stages of deglutition as seen on an esophagram: buccal (**A, B**); pharyngeal (**C, D**); esophageal (**E–G**).

Table 15–4. Activities of Mechanical and Chemical Digestion in the Alimentary Canal

	Mechanical Activity	Chemical Activity
Mouth	Mastication	Secretion of saliva
	Deglutition	Initial breakdown of carbohydrates
Pharynx	Deglutition	None
Esophagus	Deglutition	None
	Peristalsis	
Stomach	Churning	Secretion of gastric juice
	Peristalsis	Continuation of breakdown of carbohydrates
		Initiates breakdown of proteins and fats
		Absorption of alcohol and certain drugs
Small intestine	Segmentation	Secretion of intestinal juice, which mixes with bile and pancreatic juice
	Peristalsis	Completion of carbohydrate, protein, and fat digestion
		Absorption of nutrients
Large intestine	Haustral churning	Some digestion of residual material
	Peristalsis	Production of amino acids and vitamins from enteric bacteria
	Mass movements	Absorption of water and NaCl
	Defecation	

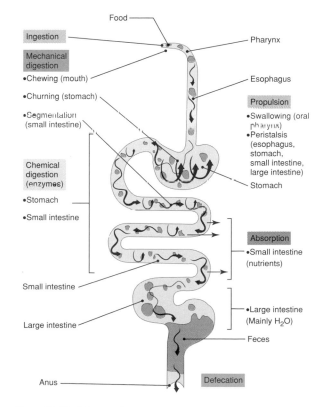

Figure 15–24. Schematic illustration of mechanical and chemical digestion in the alimentary canal.

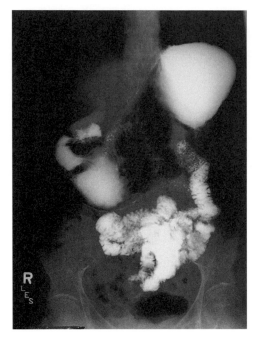

Figure 15–25. Double-contrast AP stomach and duodenum.

► *Water Test*

With the patient in a slight LPO position so the fundus fills with barium, the patient is instructed to swallow a mouthful of water through a straw. The radiologist uses fluoroscopy to monitor the esophagogastric junction for regurgitation of barium from the stomach into the esophagus.

► *Toe-touch Maneuver*

With the radiographic table turned upright, the patient is instructed to bend over and touch the toes. The radiologist uses fluoroscopy to observe the cardiac orifice for possible regurgitation of barium.

► PROCEDURAL CONSIDERATIONS

Radiographic examination of the digestive system includes studies of the primary components of the alimentary canal: esophagus, stomach, and small and large intestines. Although the esophagus, stomach and small intestine are usually examined following the oral ingestion of a contrast medium, the large intestine is evaluated primarily by rectal administration of contrast media.

Esophagram. Radiography of the esophagus, termed an esophagram or barium swallow, is performed to diagnose reflux, inflammation, esophageal varices, diverticula, hiatal hernia, and cancer. With the patient in the upright position, the study begins with a preliminary fluoroscopic examination of the esophagus prior to administration of contrast media. Using fluoroscopy, the radiologist then assesses the esophagus as the patient swallows a barium suspension; thin and/or thick barium may be used. The radiologist typically obtains spot films of the areas of interest at this time. Depending on what the radiologist sees during fluoroscopy, overhead films may or may not be requested. The Trendelenburg position, water test, toe-touch maneuver, or special breathing techniques may be used to diagnose esophageal reflux and/or a diaphragmatic hernia.

Upper GI Series. Radiographic examination of the stomach is generally termed an upper GI (UGI) study as it usually includes a cursory examination of the proximal gastrointestinal tract, including the esophagus and proximal small bowel. It is a fluoroscopic study used primarily to diagnose inflammation, ulcers, and cancer. The examination usually begins with the patient holding a cup of barium in the left hand and standing behind a fluoroscopic tower in the upright position. After the radiologist monitors the path of the initial swallows of barium, the table is lowered to the horizontal position; it is the radiographer's responsibility to hold the cup of barium during this transition and position a pillow behind the patient's head. The radiologist continues to observe the stomach with the patient in various recumbent positions, usually prone, RAO, right lateral, supine, and LPO; fluoroscopic spots may be obtained, as necessary. To perform a double-contrast examination, the patient is instructed to ingest a gas-producing substance or drink a carbonated beverage prior to ingestion of contrast media *(Figure 15–25)*.

Small Bowel Series. A small bowel (small intestine) study, also called a small bowel follow-through (SBFT), may be done to evaluate shape and/or function of the small intestine. An unusual form or shape of the small bowel may indicate the presence of an abdominal cyst, tumor, Crohn's disease, or obstruction; an obstruction may indicate some type of functional disorder. Radiographs are taken at timed intervals following the ingestion of barium. Generally taking 2 hours or less, the examination is complete when barium passes through the ileocecal valve and into the cecum and ascending colon. In most situations, the radiologist obtains fluoroscopic spot films of the ileocecal junction prior to dismissing the patient. Time markers should be included on each film to indicate the amount of time elapsed since ingestion of the barium.

Barium Enema. Radiographic examination of the large intestine is often referred to as a barium enema (BE). A barium enema may be performed to diagnose diverticulitis, colitis, obstruction, volvulus, intussusception, appendicitis, and cancer. Using fluoroscopy, the radiologist monitors the retrograde flow of barium into the patient. When the examination begins, the patient is usually in the supine position, but is rolled to the LPO position after the barium fills the sigmoid colon. As the barium progresses past the splenic flexure, the patient may be asked to turn to the RPO position, to assist with filling of the ascending colon and cecum. During the fluoroscopic portion of this procedure, the radiologist will instruct the radiographer on when to start and stop the flow of barium; barium flow may also be controlled by the fluoroscopist.

Following completion of the fluoroscopy, the radiographer obtains overhead projections per department routine or radiologist's instructions. Once these are completed, the patient may evacuate the barium; the postevacuation film(s) is taken to complete the examination.

Double-contrast barium enemas, also called air-contrast barium enemas, are performed to better evaluate the mucosal lining of the large intestine and are usually preferred for diagnosis of polyps, as heavy barium can flatten the polyps, making them difficult or impossible to see.

PATIENT PREPARATION

Preexamination preparation depends on the procedure, or procedures, to be performed *(Table 15–5)*. For most studies, the preparation begins before the patient comes to the radiology department for the examination.

Table 15–5. Summary of Examination Preparation

Esophagram	No preparation
Upper GI series	NPO after midnight or for at least 8 hours prior to examination; no gum chewing or smoking
Small bowel study	NPO after evening meal; low-residue diet 1–2 days before examination; cleansing enema; empty bladder
Barium enema	Low-residue diet and increased fluid intake for 2–3 days prior to examination; clear liquid diet 24 hours prior to examination; cathartic the afternoon before the examination; cleansing enema morning of examination

Preliminary Preparation

Esophagram. Because any fluids or foods a patient swallows travel through the esophagus rather quickly, there is no advanced preparation for an esophagram; patients can eat and drink normally unless this procedure is combined with another procedure that does require advance preparation.

Upper GI Series. The primary goal of preparation for an upper GI study is an empty stomach. Patients should be instructed to neither eat nor drink anything for at least 8 hours prior to the examination. In addition, the patient should be instructed to refrain from chewing gum or smoking, both of which can stimulate gastric secretions, causing dilution of the contrast which may affect the outcome of the procedure. For similar reasons, medications are usually restricted for 8 hours prior to the examination. To reduce gastric motility and secretions during the procedure, an anticholinergic drug or Glucagon may be administered prior to the start of the examination. **Glucagon should never be administered, however, to a patient who has diabetes mellitus.** When both the esophagram and upper GI have been requested, they may be performed at the same time; the patient must follow the preparation for the upper GI examination.

Small Bowel Series. This examination is frequently combined with the upper GI series and often follows a similar patient preparation. Time permitting, the patient may be instructed to eat a low-residue diet for 1 to 2 days prior to the examination to minimize the amount of stool and gas in the intestines. A cleansing enema may also be ordered to clear the colon of fecal material. Prior to starting the examination, the patient should be instructed to empty the bladder; a full bladder may compress or displace the ileum. At the time of the examination, the patient is asked to drink two large cups of barium sulfate, or approximately twice as much as necessary for the upper GI study.

Barium Enema. Preparation for the barium enema is much more complex and is essential for accurate diagnosis. Although preparation protocols may vary depending on the institution and patient needs, the ultimate goal is a large intestine free of fecal material. The radiographer must be familiar with the department protocol and be able to give outpatients appropriate instructions; nursing staff must also be familiar with these protocols and adequately prepare inpatients.

If time permits, the patient should be instructed to eat a low-residue diet (no fresh fruits or vegetables, fatty or fried foods, whole-grain cereals or breads) for 2 to 3 days prior to the examination. To help clear the large bowel of wastes, the patient should also drink additional fluids during this period. In addition, a clear-liquid diet (coffee or tea without cream or milk, clear gelatin, clear broth, and carbonated beverages) is often prescribed.

A cathartic, or laxative, is often ordered for the afternoon before the examination. It should only be administered with a physician's orders, however, as bowel obstruction, diarrhea, gross bleeding, or patient condition may contraindicate its use. Cleansing enemas may also be ordered for the night before the exam and/or early on the day of the exam.

Examination Preparation

On the day of the examination, an outpatient should be instructed to remove all clothing and any necklaces and put on a patient gown. Patients should be checked for any radiopaque objects that may be superimposed over the anatomy on the radiograph. A pertinent patient history should be obtained at this time *(Figure 15–26)*. Knowledge of previous examinations may provide the radiologist with helpful information regarding the current procedure. The patient's description of the preparation followed may also be important information. For example, if a patient ate breakfast 2 hours before an upper GI examination, the study may

► Related Terminology

appendectomy (ap-en-DEK-to-me)—surgical excision of the appendix

botulism (BOCH-u-lizm)—food poisoning caused by improperly canned foods; characteristic symptoms are abdominal pain, vomiting, headaches, weakness, and diarrhea; may be fatal in severe cases if the respiratory system becomes paralyzed

colectomy (ko-LEK-to-me)—surgical procedure in which all or part of the colon is excised

colitis (ko-LI-tis)—inflammatory condition of the colon

Crohn's disease (kronz)—inflammatory bowel condition usually affecting the terminal ileum segment of the small intestine

diverticulitis (di-ver-tik-u-LI-tis)—inflammation of diverticula, which are sacs or pouches protruding outward from the wall of the alimentary canal

dysentery (DIS-en-ter-e)—condition affecting the intestines, especially the colon, in which an organism such as bacteria, virus, or worms causes diarrhea, abdominal cramps, fever, and weakness

fecalith (FE-kah-lith)—stonelike mass or concretion formed from fecal material

flatus (FLA-tus)—intestinal gas, usually expelled through the anus

gastric ulcer (GAS-trik UL-ser)—type of peptic ulcer; hollow or craterlike lesion on the inner surface of the stomach

gastritis (gas-TRI-tis)—inflammatory condition of the stomach

guaiac test (GWI-ak)—laboratory test that checks for blood in a stool sample

halitosis (hal-i-TO-sis)—condition of malodorous breath; sometimes related to a pathologic condition in the alimentary canal

hemorrhoids (HEM-o-roids)—dilated veins in the rectum, particularly in the anal canal, usually brought on by constipation, hard stools, and continued sitting

(continued)

History Sheet: GI Radiography

Patient Name:_____ Age:_____

Date: _____   X-ray No.:_____   Pregnant?_____

Symptoms (check all that apply):

_____ Nausea   _____ Blood in stool   (color: _____)

_____ Vomiting   _____ Diarrhea

_____ Constipation   _____ Unexplained weight loss/gain

_____ Abdominal pain   _____ General weakness or tiredness

Duration of Symptoms: _____

Abdominal Surgical History: _____

Recent Colonoscopy or Sigmoidoscopy? _____

What Exam Preparation Was Followed? _____

_____

Previous UGI or BE? _____ When/Where?_____

Results (if known): _____

Additional Comments: _____

_____

_____

Technologist: _____   Radiologist: _____

Figure 15–26. History sheet for GI radiography. *Note:* This sample history form includes many of the questions that should be asked prior to radiographic examination of the alimentary canal.

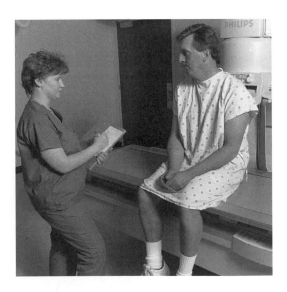

Figure 15–27. A thorough patient history should be obtained before beginning a fluoroscopic procedure.

have to be postponed. In addition, if a sigmoidoscopy, colonoscopy, or colon biopsy was performed prior to a barium enema procedure, the radiologist should be informed to prevent possible perforation of a weakened section of the colon *(Figure 15–27)*.

Radiographic examinations of the digestive system can seem rather foreign to most patients. The radiographer should clearly explain the entire procedure to the patient, including who will perform the procedure, the equipment involved, the instructions to expect during the procedure, contrast media used, how they can expect to feel, and length of examination. Although most examinations of the alimentary canal take no more than 30 to 40 minutes, a small bowel examination may last 2 or more hours.

Barium Enema. To perform the actual examination, an enema tip must be inserted into the patient's rectum. *Table 15–6* provides basic guidelines for tip insertion; the procedure may vary slightly depending on available equipment and department protocol. The enema tip may be a simple, straight type or have a cuff that can be inflated to assist with retention of the barium. After all filled films have been completed, the enema bag can be lowered below the level of the patient to allow the barium to flow back into the bag. When the flow of barium into the bag slows and the patient feels more comfortable, the tip can be removed and the patient can be assisted to the restroom to complete the evacuation of barium. If the cuff has been inflated for the procedure, it must be deflated prior to removing the tip.

Table 15–6. Tips for Tipping

Equipment needed	Enema bag with barium, tubing, clamp, and disposable or sterilized tip IV pole Disposable gloves Water-soluble lubricating gel Towel for wiping excess lubricant Blankets or sheets for under and over the patient
Equipment preparation	1. Prepare the enema bag: clamp tubing about 6 in. from the tip of the tubing and add enough warm water to the barium-filled bag to achieve the desired consistency. Shake the bag to mix thoroughly. Force the bead at the junction of the bag and tubing into the bag. Open the clamp and allow the barium to fill the tubing. 2. Using an IV pole, suspend the enema bag approximately 24–30 in. above the table. 3. Get disposable gloves and towel near the foot end of the table.
Patient preparation	4. When ready, explain the procedure to the patient and instruct the patient to turn to the left Sim's position; cover the patient with a blanket or sheet for warmth and modesty.
Precautions	5. When "tipping" female patients, make sure the catheter enters the anus and not the vagina. 6. If tip insertion is difficult because of extensive hemorrhoids or other pathologic conditions, ask a physician or department nurse for assistance.
Procedure	7. Wearing disposable gloves, cover the tip of the catheter with lubricant. 8. Exposing only the anal area, spread the buttocks with the fingers of your left hand. 9. Ask the patient to take in a breath and blow it out slowly. During exhalation, gently push the lubricated tip through the anus, directing it superiorly and anteriorly into the rectum 2–4 in. Initially, the tip should be pointed in the general direction of the umbilicus. **If resistance is encountered, do NOT apply more force.**

10. Using the towel, wipe away any excess lubricant. Recover and roll the patient to the supine position, positioning the tubing between the patient's legs so it is not compressed. The patient will feel some pressure and should be advised not to bear down.

Note: In some departments, the routine procedure may include inflating the balloon of the rectal retention catheter before the radiologist enters the room to perform the procedure. Once the tip is in place, the rectal retention cuff may be inflated with one squeeze of the bulb. **DO NOT inflate the balloon if it is not the department policy to do so or if it causes patient discomfort.**

Safety Tips for Barium Enema Administration
- Be gentle when inserting an enema tip; using force can lead to a perforated rectum. Tip insertion can be done by the radiologist with fluoroscopic assistance, if necessary.
- Prior to inflating the cuff of a rectal retention catheter, make sure the cuff is inserted beyond the rectal sphincter; inflate with no more than 30 mL (one squeeze) of air unless directed by the radiologist.
- Use water that is neither too cold nor too hot when preparing the contrast; either extreme could cause spasm or injury.
- Unless directed by the radiologist, the height of the enema bag should not exceed 30 in.
- Assist the patient to the rest room following the barium enema; the patient may faint after the procedure.

▶ **Related Terminology** *(continued)*

Hirschbrung's disease (HIRSH-brungz)—megacolon; congenital condition in which the colon and rectum are dilated with loss of muscle function; the absence of peristalsis in the area results in constipation and fecal impaction

imperforate anus (im-PER-fo-rāt)—anus in a neonate is not open because of the presence of an embryonic membrane

intussusception (in-tus-sus-SEP-shun)—condition in which one area of the intestine has telescoped into the lumen of the adjacent area causing an obstruction

microgastria (mī-krō-GAS-trē-ah)—congenital condition in which an individual has an uncommonly small stomach

mumps (mumps)—infectious condition in which one or both of the parotid glands are inflamed; contracted through airborne transmission (droplets); swelling of testes with possible sterility may occur as a complication in the postpubescent male

polyps (POL-ips)—abnormal growth on the mucous membrane of a structure; in the case of the alimentary canal, the growth may extend into the lumen and cause an obstruction; sessile polyps do not have a stem or stalk, whereas pedunculated polyps have a stem

rectocele (REK-tō-sēl)—hernia or prolapse of the rectum; also known as a proctocele

shigellosis (shi-gel-Ō-sis)—bacterial infection caused by bacteria *Shigella* and characterized by abdominal pain, cramps, diarrhea, high fever, and muscle aches; contracted through contaminated food and water or person-to-person contact

-scopy (skō-pē)—examination in which an endoscope is inserted into the area of interest; often biopsies are taken; relevant examinations of the alimentary canal include colonoscopy, esophagoscopy, gastroscopy, proctoscopy, and sigmoidoscopy

-stomy (stō-mē)—surgical opening of a structure to the outside of the body; examples include ileostomy and colostomy in which the particular portion of the intestine is brought through the abdominal wall

volvulus (VOL-vū-lus)—condition in which a loop of the intestine has twisted, resulting in an obstruction

Note: Many terms relevant to the digestive system were defined in Chapter 3.

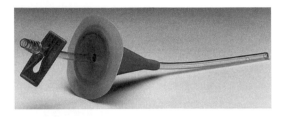

Figure 15–28. Cone-shaped tip for administration of barium through a stoma.

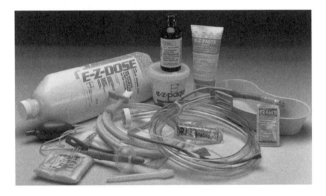

Figure 15–29. Various supplies used for contrast examinations of the GI tract.

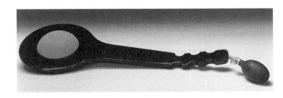

Figure 15–30. Compression paddle used during fluoroscopy.

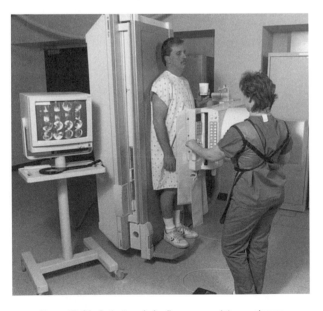

Figure 15–31. Patient ready for fluoroscopy of the esophagus.

Ostomy Patient. As a result of a pathologic condition, such as cancer, diverticulitis, or ulcerative colitis, many patients undergo surgery and receive some type of ostomy as part of their treatment. A *stoma* is an opening created by bringing a loop of bowel to the skin surface of the abdomen. Fecal material passes from the intestine, through the stoma, into a disposable pouch or bag. The area of bowel used to create the stoma gives it its name. When the opening is from the ileum, for example, it is called an **ileostomy,** and when it is from the colon, it is a **colostomy.** Stomas can be located anywhere in the bowel; patients may also have one or two stomas. The bowel distal to the stoma may or may not have been removed.

Because ostomy patients often have a negative body image, the radiographer must be sensitive to the patient's feelings and regard the stoma as nothing unusual or distasteful. Ostomy patients are trained to care for their stoma and often prefer to remove the drainage pouch themselves. The radiographer, however, should be prepared to remove a dressing or drainage pouch; clean gloves should be used and disposed of as contaminated waste. The drainage pouch should be saved and kept clean and dry.

Contrast media may be administered rectally or through the stoma. To administer the barium through a stoma, a special cone-shaped tip *(Figure 15–28)* or a small catheter with an inflatable cuff is used. The tip of the cone or catheter is lubricated prior to insertion. Wearing disposable gloves, the radiologist or radiographer (depending on department protocol) can help the patient insert the tip into the stoma. The radiologist conducts the examination, instilling less barium than for the traditional barium enema. When the procedure is completed, a drainage bag must be attached to the cone or stoma for elimination of the barium. If physical condition permits it, the patient can be assisted to the rest room with the drainage bag in place, allowing the patient to clean the stoma and replace the ostomy pouch; a washcloth, soap, and towel should be made available.

Postexamination Instructions

Because barium sulfate is often constipating, patients receiving it orally or rectally should never be dismissed from the department without receiving appropriate postexamination instructions. If not properly instructed, a patient may ignore symptoms that could lead to fecal impaction and bowel obstruction. In addition, dehydration may occur as a result of the preparation for the procedure. The following information should be included in the radiographer's postexamination instructions to the patient:

1. Until all the barium is expelled, the stools will be white or very lightly colored.
2. Unless contraindicated, increased fluid and fiber in the diet for several days will help with elimination of the barium sulfate.
3. Rest following examination of the large intestines; the preparation for the procedure often weakens patients.
4. Contact his/her personal physician immediately if any of the following conditions or symptoms occur:
   - No bowel movement within 24 hours of the examination
   - Feelings of weakness or faintness
   - Abdominal pain, constipation, or rectal bleeding
   - Failure to pass flatus
   - Abdominal distention

ROOM PREPARATION

Room preparation depends on the specific examination to be performed and includes room setup and contrast media preparation. Fluoroscopy is required for all examinations of the alimentary canal. To remove the Bucky tray from the path of the under-table fluoro beam, the Bucky tray must be moved to the foot of the table; doing so also closes the Bucky slot, providing radiation protection for the fluoroscopist and other personnel. For an upper GI or esophagram, the footboard should be securely attached and the fluoroscopic table should be turned to the upright position. The foot-operated fluoro switch should be accessible and the lead drape on the fluoro tower should be appropriately positioned to provide maximum shielding for the fluoroscopist. Fluoroscopy for small and large intestinal studies is usually performed with the table in the horizontal position.

Supplies must be available for the administration of contrast media, including those supplies needed in case complications arise or the radiologist deviates from the routine procedure *(Figure 15–29)*. Contrast media should be prepared according to radiologist preference. When administering contrast media orally, a straw limits the coating of contrast in the mouth, making ingestion easier and more palatable for most patients. Gas-producing substances should be available for double-contrast studies of the stomach and proximal duodenum, if needed. *Table 15–7* lists miscellaneous supplies needed for radiographic examinations of the alimentary canal. A compression paddle is often used by the radiologist during fluoroscopy *(Figure 15–30)*.

Table 15–7. Supplies for GI Studies

Esophagram
    Contrast media (liquid, paste, pills, capsules)
    Straw and spoon
    Cotton balls or marshmallows
    Emesis basin
Upper GI
    Contrast media
    Straw
    Gas-producing substance (powder,
      pills, crystals, or carbonated
      drink)
    Emesis basin
    Anticholinergic drug or glucagon

Small bowel study
    Contrast media (2 large glasses)
    Straw
    Emesis basin
    Time markers
Barium enema
    Contrast-filled enema bag
    Enema tip
    Lubricant
    Disposable gloves
    Towels
    Sheets/blankets
    Anticholinergic drug or glucagon
    Compression paddle
    Postevacuation marker

Table 15–8. Routine/Optional Projections: Digestive System

Esophagram	Barium enema (colon)	Double-contrast barium enema (colon)
AP or PA	AP and/or PA	AP and/or PA
RAO and/or LAO	RPO/LPO or LAO/RAO	RPO/LPO or LAO/RAO
Right or left lateral	Lateral	Lateral (may be ventral decubitus)
Upper GI (stomach)	AP/PA axial rectosigmoid	AP/PA axial rectosigmoid
PA and/or AP	Postevacuation	Right/left lateral decubitus
RAO and/or LPO		AP upright[a]
Right lateral		RPO/LPO upright[a]
Small bowel series		LPO axial rectosigmoid[a]
PA/AP		

Note. Although department routines for all radiographic examinations can vary, the advent of digital fluoroscopy has significantly changed the routines and reduced the number of overhead projections obtained. The radiographer should be familiar with the department protocol.
[a]Optional projections that may be routine in some departments.

POSITIONING CONSIDERATIONS

All radiographic examinations of the alimentary canal include a fluoroscopic evaluation. Prior to fluoroscopy, however, a preliminary or "scout" radiograph is obtained to assess bowel obstruction, patient preparation, and the presence of radiopaque stones in the biliary or urinary tracts. The films requested after fluoroscopy depend on the specific examination and department protocol. Although digital fluoroscopy has eliminated the need for many overhead radiographs, the basic projections are discussed *(Table 15–8)*.

Esophagram. If a recent PA chest radiograph is not available, one may be requested as a scout film. In preparation for fluoroscopy, the patient is instructed to stand behind the fluoro tower with a cup of barium held in the left hand near the left shoulder *(Figure 15–31)*. Following fluoroscopy, radiographs are obtained per radiologist request. The ultimate objective is to produce radiographs with barium filling the entire esophagus. Typical projections include the AP or PA, RAO, and lateral *(Figure 15–32)*. Although these projections can be obtained with the patient upright or recumbent, the recumbent position minimizes the rate of barium travel through the esophagus.

    Immediately prior to each exposure, two to three spoonfuls of barium paste are administered to the patient, with the last spoonful held in the mouth until ready for the exposure. Within 2 seconds of the patient's swallowing the last spoonful, the exposure should be made; respiration is naturally suspended briefly after deglutition. The patient can also be instructed to continuously drink a barium sulfate suspension through a straw as the exposure is made; the barium sulfate should not be watered down, but thin enough to pass through a straw.

Upper GI Series. Unless contraindicated because of the patient's condition, the fluoroscopic examination begins with the patient upright, holding a cup of barium near the left shoulder. Approximately 12 to 14 oz of barium sulfate is administered to the patient as the radiologist monitors its travel. Additional barium is usually not needed for the overhead films. Although the protocol for overhead radiographs can vary widely from department to department, the standard projections include the AP and/or PA, RAO, and right lateral; the LPO is sometimes included as part of the routine or can be substituted for the RAO when a patient is unable to attain the RAO position. To adequately demonstrate the duodenal bulb, the amount of rotation for the RAO projection must vary depending on body habitus; hypersthenic patients must be rotated more than asthenic patients *(Figure 15–33)*. When the small bowel series is included with an upper GI, the last film is usually an AP or PA taken on a 14 × 17-in. cassette and is considered as the first small bowel film.

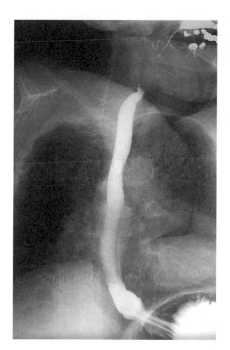

Figure 15–32. Esophagram.

▶ *Positioning Tip*

Body habitus changes the shape and location of the organs of the digestive system. During fluoroscopy the radiographer should observe the position of the part of interest relative to familiar bony landmarks and make appropriate adjustments in patient positioning and centering.

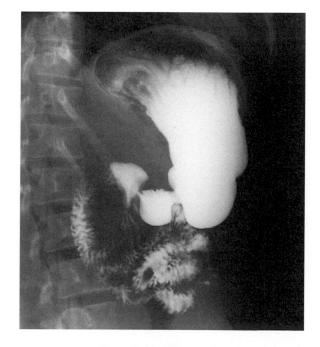

Figure 15–33. RAO stomach.

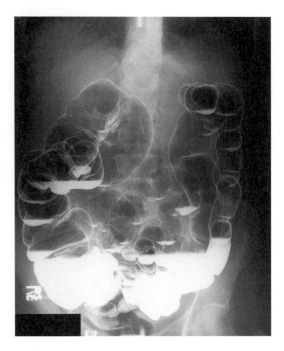

Figure 15–34. AP double-contrast large intestine, upright.

Small Bowel Series. Usually combined with an upper GI series, the small bowel series includes PA or AP projections of the abdomen to monitor the flow of barium through the small intestines. Although the PA projection positions the small intestines closer to the film and compresses the abdomen, spreading out the intestines and reducing tissue thickness, the AP projection is often performed because of the patient's condition. The first film is usually obtained approximately 15 minutes after the ingestion of contrast media; subsequent films are taken in 30-minute intervals for up to 2 hours or until the contrast media reaches the ileocecal junction, as directed by the radiologist; occasionally, additional films are needed beyond 2 hours. Lead markers indicating the amount of time that has elapsed since ingestion of the contrast should be included on each projection. Each film should be shown to the radiologist who will instruct the radiographer on when to obtain the next radiograph. When the barium passes through the ileocecal valve, the patient may need to be prepared for recumbent fluoroscopic examination and spots by the radiologist. Ice water, water-soluble gastrointestinal contrast media, or saline solution, ingested separately or mixed with the barium, can be used to stimulate peristalsis and complete the examination in less time.

Barium Enema. After the fluoroscopic examination has been completed, overhead films are obtained per department routine or radiologist instructions. Projections for a single-contrast barium enema may include AP, PA, RPO, LPO, left lateral, and axial rectosigmoid. Double (air)-contrast studies may also include decubitus and upright projections to better demonstrate the mucosal lining *(Figure 15–34)*. To include the entire large intestine, two films positioned crosswise may be needed; the first film should include the symphysis, with the second film overlapping the first and including the left colic flexure. When decubitus films are performed, radiolucent supports should be positioned under small patients to center the patient on the film.

After the patient has eliminated the barium, a postevacuation AP or PA radiograph is obtained; many routines also include a left lateral projection *(Figure 15–35)*. If the patient has not adequately eliminated the barium, a return trip to the rest room may be necessary with a repeat postevacuation film. Postevacuation films should be clearly marked with an appropriate lead marker.

ALTERNATE PROJECTIONS/PROCEDURES

As an alternative to the standard small bowel series, contrast media can be directly injected into the small bowel via a long tube; this examination is termed an **enteroclysis procedure** *(Figure 15–36)*. Although the procedure generally causes increased patient discomfort, takes longer, and carries an increased risk of bowel perforation when compared with the traditional small bowel series, it is ideal for patients with a clinical history of small bowel obstruction, Crohn's disease, or malabsorption disease. This examination is used to evaluate shape and form—not function—of the small bowel.

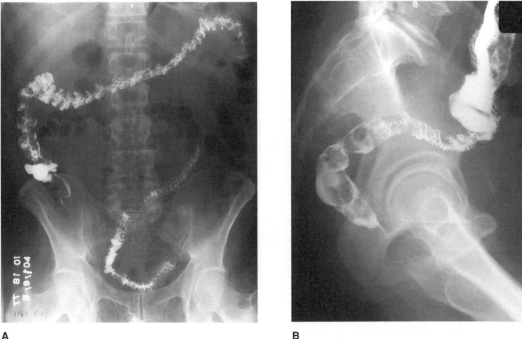

A   B

Figure 15–35. PA **(A)** and lateral **(B)** postevacuation barium enema projections.

Patient preparation is similar to that followed for the standard small bowel study; however, enemas are not recommended as some fluid may be retained in the small bowel. Under fluoroscopy, the patient is intubated with a special enteroclysis catheter; the end of the catheter is advanced to the area of the duodenojejunal junction. High-density barium is then injected into the catheter. To produce a double-contrast effect, methylcellulose can be injected after the barium. In addition to the spot films, conventional radiographs, such as AP, PA, oblique, and upright projections, may be requested. Patients should follow the postexamination instructions previously described.

Sialography is the radiographic examination of the salivary ducts following the injection of contrast media *(Figure 15–37)*. This examination may be performed to diagnose calculi, strictures in the ducts, sialectasia (dilation), fistulae, or mixed parotid tumors; it may also be performed preoperatively when pathology related to the salivary glands is known. Severe inflammation of the salivary ducts and a history of hypersensitivity to iodinated contrast medium would be contraindications to performing this examination.

Because the salivary ducts are small, they can be difficult to localize. To dilate the duct of interest and aid in its localization, the patient may be asked to suck on a piece of lemon. Once the duct is localized, the radiologist inserts a blunted butterfly needle or sialography catheter into it. The contrast medium, either an oil-based or water-soluble iodinated material, is injected manually or allowed to drip in at a continuous rate (hydrostatic technique). The patient feels pressure when the duct fills with contrast medium. Preliminary and postcontrast films of the mandible, including an AP or PA, lateral, and axiolateral oblique projections, are usually obtained. A tangential AP projection in which the patient's head is rotated toward the side of interest and the cheek is puffed out may be included in the series. At the completion of the procedure, the patient is once again asked to suck on a piece of lemon, causing the contrast media to be excreted along with the saliva.

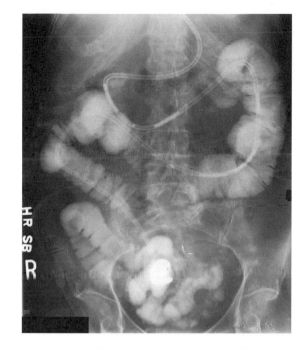

Figure 15–36. Enteroclysis examination of the small bowel.

PEDIATRIC PATIENTS

Radiographic examination of the pediatric patient's gastrointestinal tract is performed to identify a congenital abnormality or other pathology. These procedures are generally less complicated in the child when compared with the adult. Because there is little variation in location of the stomach and intestines, patient positioning is much easier. In addition, motility is usually faster and patient preparation in infants and young children is usually minimal *(Table 15–9)*.

Although the procedures are in some ways more simple, radiation protection is a greater consideration, however. Prior to fluoroscopy for an upper GI examination, a lead shield should be placed on the table under the patient's buttocks to shield the patient from the fluoro tube located under the table; lead shielding under the patient's head and neck will help protect anyone holding the patient. In addition, videotape and digital fluoroscopy can reduce the need for repeated fluoroscopy and minimize the number of overhead films requested.

The accessory equipment used for children varies depending on the patient's age. A feeding bottle and nipple are used for an infant, whereas a cup and straw should be used for an older child; a feeding catheter or syringe may also be used. Flexible enema tips are available for barium enemas. Rectal retention tips with inflatable cuffs are contraindicated for pediatric patients, as they may perforate the rectum or artificially distend the rectum in cases of Hirschsprung's disease.

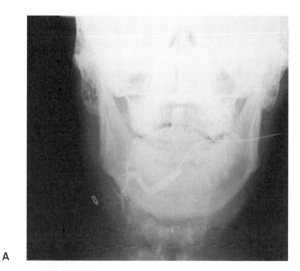

A

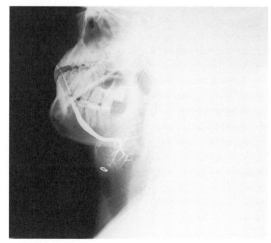

B

Figure 15–37. AP **(A)** and axiolateral oblique **(B)** projections for the submaxillary ducts.

Table 15–9. Summary of Pediatric Patient Preparation

Esophagram and upper GI	
0–2 years	NPO 3–4 hours
>2 years	NPO 6 hours
Barium enema	
0–2 years	No preparation
2–10 years	Low-residue diet evening meal; a mild laxative with water at bedtime[a]
>10 years	Same as for 2- to 10-year-olds; double the dose of laxative

Patients with Hirschsprung's disease should not undergo preparation for a barium enema. In addition, the referring physician should be consulted prior to preparation of patients with acute surgical conditions and/or inflammatory bowel diseases.
[a]A Pedifleet enema may be prescribed for the morning.

▶ *Special Breathing Techniques:*

- *Valsalva maneurer—while holding the breath on deep inspiration, the patient bears down as if trying to move the bowels*

- *Modified valsalva maneurer—with the mouth closed, the patient pinches the nose closed and tries to blow the nose*

- *Mueller maneurer—after exhaling, the patient tries to inhale against the closed glottis*

BREATHING INSTRUCTIONS

To reduce stress on the abdomen that could lead to involuntary motion, all radiographs of the alimentary canal are obtained during suspended expiration. Although typical breathing instructions are usually given, instructions for an esophagram are to instruct the patient to swallow a bolus of barium just prior to the exposure; the act of deglutition suspends respiration briefly on expiration. Instructing the patient to stop breathing, therefore, is not necessary and allows the exposure to be made before the esophagus empties.

Periodically, special breathing techniques are used to increase the intrathoracic and intraabdominal pressures. For the **Valsalva maneuver,** the patient is instructed to take in a deep breath, hold the breath in, and bear down as if trying to move the bowels; air is forced against the closed glottis. A **modified Valsalva maneuver** is accomplished by the patient pinching the nose closed, closing the mouth, and trying to blow the nose. To produce the reverse effect, the patient is instructed to exhale, then try to inhale against the closed glottis; this technique is called the **Mueller maneuver.**

EXPOSURE FACTORS

To adequately penetrate the barium for single-contrast studies of the stomach, small bowel, and large intestine, 100 to 120 kVp is recommended; higher-kVp techniques also permit a reduction in mAs with a shorter exposure time. Because the esophagus is relatively small and may not be completely filled with barium, 90 kVp penetrates the barium without overexposure. Radiographs for double- or water-soluble contrast studies should be obtained using 85 to 90 kVp to prevent overexposure of the thin coating of barium along the mucosal lining. The mAs required depends on patient size, type of x-ray generator, film/screen speed, type of grid, and amount of barium present. To minimize image blur as a result of peristaltic activity or spasm, relatively short exposure times should be used. Technical factors for children should be modified using the guidelines outlined in Chapter 3.

Although automatic exposure control is frequently used for overhead projections of the alimentary canal, the radiographer should understand that the wide variation in location of the organs of the digestion system may cause underexposed films. The colon, especially, can have a very unusual shape and position. If the barium-filled structures are not over the detectors, the resulting film may be underexposed. On the other hand, if a barium-filled structure is directly over the detector or widespread in the abdomen, such as in the small bowel, the radiograph may be overexposed.

In addition to setting exposure factors for overhead films, the radiographer must also set the kVp for any spot films taken during fluoroscopy. Generally, the kVp for fluoroscopy is set at the same kVp used for the overhead films; 100 to 120 kVp, therefore, is used for the single-contrast upper GI, small bowel, and barium enema examinations; 90 kVp can be used for the esophagram and double contrast studies. Please note that the kVp will need to be changed when performing both the esophagram and upper GI.

EQUIPMENT CONSIDERATIONS

A fluoroscopic unit is required for radiographic examination of the alimentary canal; a table capable of the 90° upright and the Trendelenburg positions is necessary for studies of the esophagus and stomach. A portable grid, or other device, is necessary for decubitus films. In addition, lead aprons and gloves and a compression paddle should be available during fluoroscopy. Sponges or other supports should also be available, if needed. Other ancillary equipment specific to each examination is listed in *Table 15–7.*

RADIOGRAPHIC POSITIONING OF THE DIGESTIVE SYSTEM

- ► AP ESOPHAGUS

- ► RAO ESOPHAGUS

- ► LATERAL ESOPHAGUS

- ► PA STOMACH (UPPER GI)

- ► AP STOMACH (UPPER GI)

- ► RAO STOMACH (UPPER GI)

- ► LATERAL STOMACH (UPPER GI)

- ► LPO STOMACH (UPPER GI)

- ► PA/AP SMALL BOWEL

- ► AP/PA COLON (PRELIMINARY, CONTRAST-FILLED & POSTEVACUATION)

- ► AP OBLIQUE COLON (RPO & LPO)

- ► AP AXIAL RECTOSIGMOID REGION

- ► LATERAL RECTUM (CONTRAST-FILLED & POSTEVACUATION)

- ► LATERAL DECUBITUS COLON (DOUBLE-CONTRAST STUDIES)

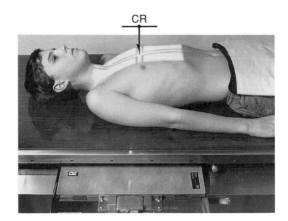

Figure 15–38. AP esophagus.

▶ AP ESOPHAGUS

Technical Considerations

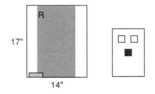

- Film size: 14 × 17 in. (35 × 43 cm) lengthwise.
- Grid required.
- 90 kVp.
- Collimate to an 8 in. field size crosswise and to film lengthwise.

Shielding

- Gonadal shielding should be used on all patients, especially children and adults of reproductive age.

Patient Positioning

- Assist the patient to the supine position on the radiographic table; arms should be comfortably positioned at the sides and knees flexed and supported by sponges or pillows. **Note:** This projection may also be obtained with the patient upright; however, the recumbent position allows for more complete filling of the esophagus; a comparable view may also be obtained with the patient prone.

Part Positioning

- Center the midsagittal plane to the midline of the table.
- Adjust the long axis of the patient parallel with the long axis of the table; the pelvis and shoulders should not be rotated.
- Set the exposure factors prior to administering contrast media.
- Turn the patient's head slightly, if necessary, to facilitate drinking the barium suspension.
- Position the cassette so the upper edge is 2 to 3 in. above the top of the shoulders *(Figure 15–38)*.

Central Ray

- Direct the central ray perpendicular to the midpoint of the cassette; the central ray should enter at the level of T5–6.

Breathing Instructions

- Instruct the patient to take 1 to 3 spoonfuls or several drinks of thick barium through a straw; the final spoonful or drink should be held in the mouth until instructed to swallow. **Note:** The exposure may also be made while the patient is continuously swallowing barium while drinking through a straw.
- Instruct the patient to take in a breath, blow it out, then swallow before taking in another breath; make the exposure immediately after the patient swallows (respiration is naturally suspended for approximately 2 seconds after swallowing). **Note:** Breathing instructions are unnecessary when the patient is continuously swallowing barium.

Image Evaluation

- The lower part of the neck, thoracic esophagus, and proximal stomach should be included in the collimation field.
- Asymmetry of the ribs and sternoclavicular joints indicates rotation.
- Barium should be evident in the full length of the esophagus.
- Exposure factors should be such that the barium is penetrated without being overexposed *(Figure 15–39)*.

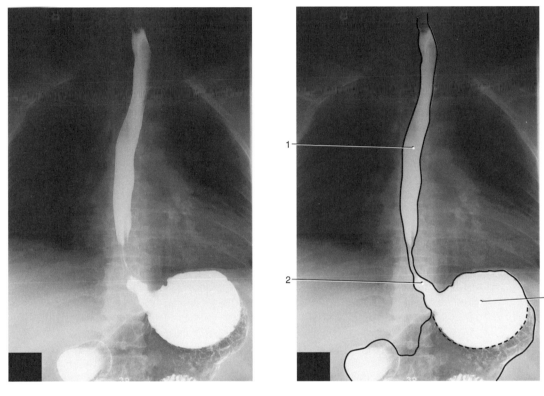

Figure 15–39. AP esophagus.

1. Esophagus	2. Cardiac antrum	3. Stomach, fundus

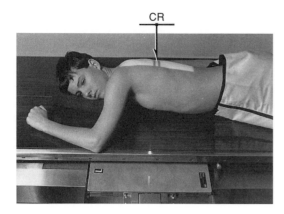

Figure 15–40. RAO esophagus.

▶ RAO ESOPHAGUS

Technical Considerations

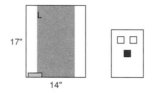

- Film size: 14 × 17 in. (35 × 43 cm) lengthwise.
- Grid required.
- 90 kVp.
- Collimate to an 8 in. field size crosswise and to film lengthwise.

Shielding

- Gonadal shielding should be used on all patients, especially children and adults of reproductive age.

Patient Positioning

- Assist the patient to the prone position on the radiographic table. **Note:** This projection may also be obtained with the patient upright; however, the recumbent position allows for more complete filling of the esophagus.

Part Positioning

- Rotate the patient to a 35° to 45° RAO position; adjust the patient's left arm and leg for support; asthenic patients must be rotated more than hypersthenic patients to project the esophagus anterior to the spine.
- Center the thorax so the plane passing approximately 2 in. to the left of the thoracic spinous processes is centered to the midline of the table.
- Adjust the long axis of the patient parallel with the long axis of the table.
- Position the cassette so the upper edge is 2 to 3 in. above the top of the shoulders *(Figure 15–40)*.

Central Ray

- Direct the central ray perpendicular to the midpoint of the cassette; the central ray should enter at the level of T5–6.

Breathing Instructions

- Instruct the patient to take 1 to 3 spoonfuls or several drinks of thick barium through a straw; the final spoonful or drink should be held in the mouth until instructed to swallow. **Note:** The exposure may also be made while the patient is continuously swallowing barium while drinking through a straw.
- Instruct the patient to take in a breath, blow it out, then swallow before taking in another breath; make the exposure immediately after the patient swallows (respiration is naturally suspended for approximately 2 seconds after swallowing). **Note:** Breathing instructions are unnecessary when the patient is continuously swallowing barium.

Image Evaluation

- The lower part of the neck, thoracic esophagus, and proximal stomach should be included in the collimation field.
- The esophagus should not be superimposed over the spine.
- Barium should be evident in the full length of the esophagus.
- Exposure factors should be such that the barium is penetrated without being overexposed *(Figure 15–41)*.

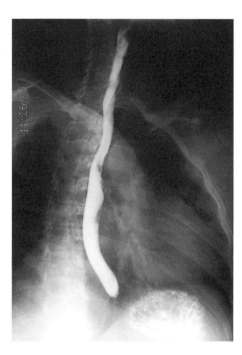

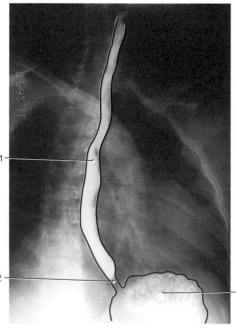

Figure 15–41. RAO esophagus.

1. Esophagus   2. Cardiac antrum   3. Stomach, fundus

▶ LATERAL ESOPHAGUS

Technical Considerations

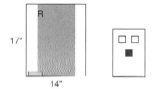

- Film size: 14 × 17 in. (35 × 43 cm) lengthwise.
- Grid required.
- 90 kVp.
- Collimate to an 8 in. field size crosswise and to film lengthwise.

Shielding

- Gonadal shielding should be used on all patients, especially children and adults of reproductive age.

Patient Positioning

- Assist the patient to the supine position on the radiographic table. **Note:** This projection may also be obtained with the patient upright; however, the recumbent position allows for more complete filling of the esophagus.

Part Positioning

- Rotate the patient to the right or left lateral position; the arms should be at right angles with the body, one directly over the other.
- Adjust the patient to a true lateral position; flex the knees and hips to a comfortable position.
- Center the midcoronal plane to the midline of the table.
- Adjust the long axis of the patient parallel with the long axis of the table.
- Position the cassette so the upper edge is 2 to 3 in. above the top of the shoulders *(Figure 15–42)*.

Central Ray

- Direct the central ray perpendicular to the midpoint of the cassette; the central ray should enter at the level of T5–6.

Breathing Instructions

- Instruct the patient to take 1 to 3 spoonfuls or several drinks of thick barium through a straw; the final spoonful or drink should be held in the mouth until instructed to swallow. **Note:** The exposure may also be made while the patient is continuously swallowing barium while drinking through a straw.
- Instruct the patient to take in a breath, blow it out, then swallow before taking in another breath; make the exposure immediately after the patient swallows (respiration is naturally suspended for approximately 2 seconds after swallowing). **Note:** Breathing instructions are unnecessary when the patient continuously swallows barium.

Image Evaluation

- The lower part of the neck, thoracic esophagus, and proximal stomach should be included in the collimation field.
- The esophagus should not be superimposed over the spine; posterior ribs should be superimposed.
- Barium should be evident in the full length of the esophagus.
- Exposure factors should be such that the barium is penetrated without being overexposed *(Figure 15–43)*.

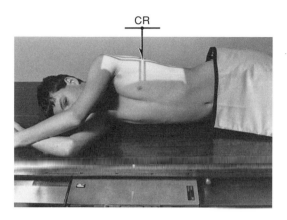

Figure 15–42. Lateral esophagus.

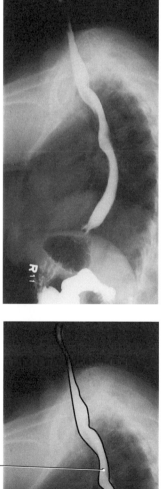

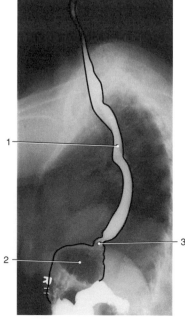

Figure 15–43. Lateral esophagus.

1. Esophagus   2. Stomach, fundus   3. Cardiac antrum

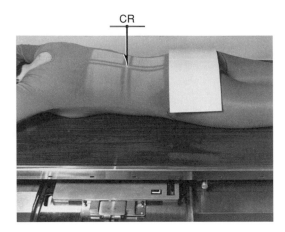

Figure 15–44. PA stomach, centered for 11 × 14-in. cassette.

► PA STOMACH (UPPER GI)

Technical Considerations

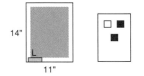

- Film size: 11 × 14 in. (28 × 35 cm) lengthwise, or 14 × 17 in. (35 × 43 cm) lengthwise, or 10 × 12 in. (24 × 30 cm) lengthwise. **Note:** Because the stomach lies more horizontally in hypersthenic patients, the cassette may be oriented transversely when appropriate.
- Grid required.
- 100–120 kVp (barium); 85–90 kVp (double or water-soluble contrast).
- Collimate to rib margins crosswise and to film lengthwise (14 × 17 in. film) or to allow ¹/₂ in. margins on smaller film sizes.

Shielding

- Gonadal shielding should be used on all patients, especially children and adults of reproductive age whenever smaller films are used.

Patient Positioning

- Assist the patient to the prone position on the radiographic table. Position the patient's arms comfortably on the table near the head. **Note:** This projection may also be performed with the patient erect; centering should be approximately 1 to 4 in. lower, with the greater adjustment used for asthenic patients.

Part Positioning

- Adjust the patient's body so there is no rotation.
- Center the midsagittal plane to the midline of the table (14 × 17-in. cassette) or 1 to 2 in. to the right of the table's midline for smaller cassettes (sagittal plane 1 to 2 in. left of the spine will be centered to the table). **Note:** Asthenic patients should be centered so their midsagittal plane corresponds with the midline of the table regardless of film size.
- Adjust the long axis of the patient to lie parallel with the long axis of the table (Figure 15–44).

Central Ray

- Direct the central ray perpendicular to the level of the duodenal bulb; the location of the duodenal bulb will vary depending on body habitus
  Sthenic. The central ray should enter at the level of L2, about 1 to 2 in. above the inferior margin of the ribs.
  Hypersthenic. The central ray should enter at the level of L1, about 3 to 4 in. above the inferior margin of the ribs. **Note:** To prevent superimposition of the pylorus and duodenal bulb in hypersthenic patients, the central ray can be directed 35° to 45° cephalad.
  Asthenic. The central ray should enter at the level of L3 (level of the inferior margin of the ribs).
- Center the cassette to the central ray.

Breathing Instructions

- Instruct the patient to take in a breath, blow it out, and hold it out during the exposure.

Image Evaluation

- The entire stomach and duodenum should be included within the collimated area; the diaphragm and small bowel should also be included when using larger films.
- The transverse processes of the vertebrae should be symmetrical.
- The pylorus and duodenal bulb should be centered lengthwise on the film.
- The barium should be adequately penetrated without overexposure *(Figure 15–45).*

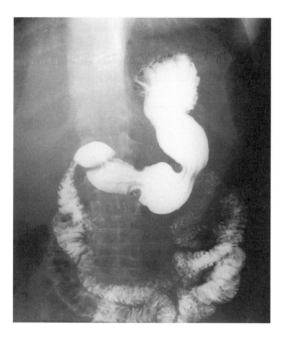 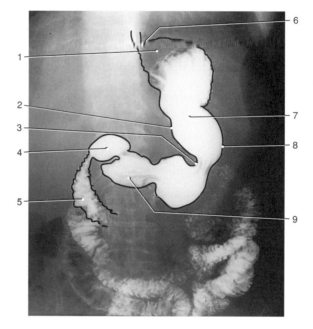

Figure 15–45. PA stomach.

1. Fundus	4. Duodenal bulb	7. Body
2. Lesser curvature	5. Duodenum	8. Greater curvature
3. Angular notch	6. Cardiac notch	9. Pyloric antrum

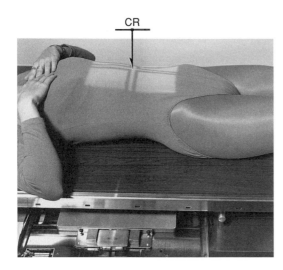

Figure 15–46. AP stomach, 10 × 12-in. cassette.

► AP STOMACH (UPPER GI)

Technical Considerations

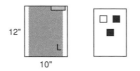

- Film size: 14 × 17 in. (35 × 43 cm) lengthwise or 11 × 14 in. (28 × 35 cm) lengthwise or 10 × 12 in. (24 × 30 cm) lengthwise. **Note:** Because the stomach lies more horizontally in hypersthenic patients, the cassette may be oriented transversely, when appropriate.
- Grid required.
- 100–120 kVp (barium); 85–90 kVp (double or water-soluble contrast).
- Collimate to rib margins crosswise and to film lengthwise (14 × 17-in. film) or to allow 0.5-in. margins on smaller film sizes.

Shielding

- Gonadal shielding should be used on all patients, especially children and adults of reproductive age whenever smaller films are used.

Patient Positioning

- Assist the patient to the supine position on the radiographic table; position the patient's arms comfortably on the table at the sides or with hands on upper chest. **Note:** This projection may also be performed with the patient erect; centering should be approximately 1 to 4 in. lower, with the greater adjustment used for asthenic patients.

Part Positioning

- Adjust the patient's body so that the ASISs are equidistant from the table.
- Center the midsagittal plane to the midline of the table (14 × 17-in. cassette) or 1 to 2 in. to the left of the table's midline for smaller cassettes (sagittal plane 1–2 in. right of the spine will be centered to the table). **Note:** Asthenic patients should be centered so their midsagittal plane corresponds with the midline of the table regardless of film size.
- Adjust the long axis of the patient to lie parallel with the long axis of the table *(Figure 15–46)*.

Central Ray

- Direct the central ray perpendicular to the level of the duodenal bulb; the location of the duodenal bulb will vary depending on body habitus:
    Sthenic. The central ray should enter at the level of L1, about halfway between the xiphoid process and the inferior margin of the ribs.
    Hypersthenic. The central ray should enter at the level of T12, about 3 to 4 in. above the inferior margin of the ribs.
    Asthenic. The central ray should enter at the level of L2, about 1 in. above the inferior margin of the ribs.
- Center the cassette to the central ray.

Breathing Instructions

- Instruct the patient to take in a breath, blow it out, and hold it out during the exposure.

Image Evaluation

- The entire stomach and duodenum should be included within the collimated area; the diaphragm and small bowel should also be included when using larger films.
- The transverse processes of the vertebrae should be symmetrical.
- The pylorus and duodenal bulb should be centered lengthwise on the film.
- The barium should be adequately penetrated without overexposure (Figure 15–47).

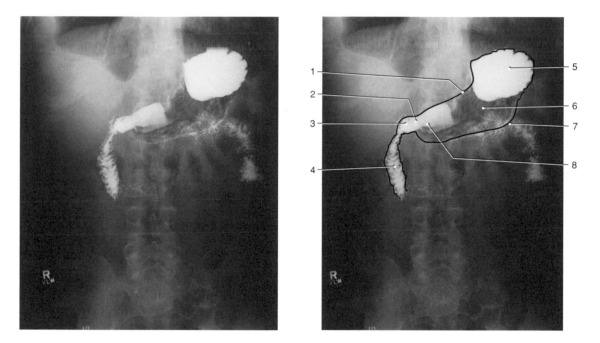

Figure 15–47. AP stomach and duodenum, 14 × 17-in. cassette.

1. Lesser curvature	4. Duodenum	7. Greater curvature
2. Pyloric orifice	5. Fundus	8. Pyloric antrum
3. Duodenal bulb	6. Body	

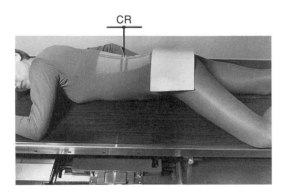

Figure 15–48. RAO stomach and duodenum.

▶ RAO STOMACH (UPPER GI)

Technical Considerations

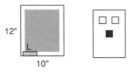

- Film size: 10 × 12 in. (24 × 30 cm) lengthwise or 11 × 14 in. (28 × 35 cm) lengthwise.
- Grid required.
- 100–120 kVp (barium); 85–90 kVp (double or water–soluble contrast).
- Collimate to allow 0.5-in. margins.

Shielding

- Gonadal shielding should be used on all patients, especially children and adults of reproductive age.

Patient Positioning

- Assist the patient to the prone position on the radiographic table; position the patient's right arm comfortably at the side and the left arm on the table near the head. **Note:** This projection may also be performed with the patient erect; centering should be approximately 1 to 4 in. lower, with the greater adjustment used for asthenic patients.

Part Positioning

- Elevate the patient's left shoulder and hip so the coronal plane forms a 40° to 70° angle with the table-top; generally, hypersthenic patients require more rotation than sthenic and asthenic patients to best demonstrate the pyloric canal and duodenum.
- Center the longitudinal plane passing midway between the vertebral column and elevated lateral margin of the thorax to the midline of the table *(Figure 15–48)*.
- Adjust the long axis of the patient to lie parallel with the long axis of the table.

Central Ray

- Direct the central ray perpendicular to the level of the duodenal bulb; the location of the duodenal bulb will vary depending on body habitus:

  Sthenic. The central ray should enter at the level of L2, about 1 to 2 in. above the inferior rib margin.

  Hypersthenic. The central ray should enter at the level of L1, about 3 to 4 in. above the inferior rib margin.

  Asthenic. The central ray should enter at the level of L3 (the level of the inferior rib margin).
- Center the cassette to the central ray.

Breathing Instructions

- Instruct the patient to take in a breath, blow it out, and hold it out during the exposure.

Image Evaluation

- The entire stomach and duodenum should be included within the collimated area; part of the diaphragm should also be demonstrated.
- The duodenal bulb and C-loop should be free of superimposition by the pylorus and seen in profile.
- The pylorus and duodenal bulb should be centered lengthwise on the film.
- The barium should be adequately penetrated without overexposure *(Figure 15–49)*.

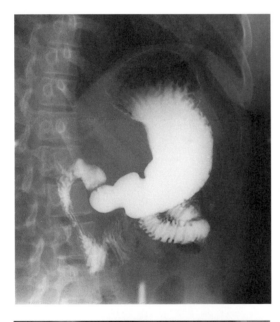

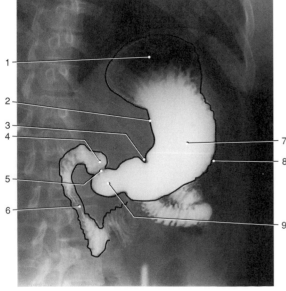

Figure 15–49. RAO stomach and duodenum.

1. Fundus	4. Duodenal bulb	7. Body
2. Lesser curvature	5. Pyloric orifice	8. Greater curvature
3. Angular notch	6. Duodenum	9. Pyloric antrum

► LATERAL STOMACH (UPPER GI)

Technical Considerations

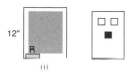

- Film size: 10 × 12 in. (24 × 30 cm) lengthwise or 11 × 14 in. (28 × 35 cm) lengthwise.
- Grid required.
- 100–120 kVp (barium); 85–90 kVp (double or water-soluble contrast).
- Collimate to allow 0.5-in. margins

Shielding

- Gonadal shielding should be used on all patients, especially children and adults of reproductive age.

Patient Positioning

- Assist the patient to the supine position on the radiographic table.

Part Positioning

- Rotate the patient to the right lateral position; the arms should be at right angles with the body, one directly over the other.
- Adjust the patient to a true lateral position flexing the knees and hips to a comfortable position.
- Center the plane midway between the midcoronal plane and anterior surface of the abdomen to the midline of the table.
- Adjust the long axis of the patient parallel with the long axis of the table *(Figure 15–50)*.

Central Ray

- Direct the central ray perpendicular to the level of the duodenal bulb; the location of the duodenal bulb will vary depending on body habitus:

   Sthenic. The central ray should enter at the level of L1, about halfway between the xiphoid process and the inferior margin of the ribs.

   Hypersthenic. The central ray should enter at the level of T12, about 3 to 4 in. above the inferior margin.

   Asthenic. The central ray should enter at the level of L2 about 1 in. above the inferior margin of the ribs.
- Center the cassette to the central ray.

Breathing Instructions

- Instruct the patient to take in a breath, blow it out, and hold it out during the exposure.

Image Evaluation

- The entire stomach and duodenal bulb should be included in the collimation field.
- The spine should be in a true lateral position; the vertebral bodies should appear "block-like."
- The stomach should be in the middle of the collimation field.
- On hypersthenic patients, the pylorus and duodenum should be demonstrated.
- Exposure factors should be such that the barium is penetrated without being overexposed *(Figure 15–51)*.

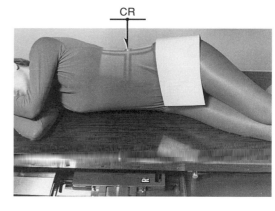

Figure 15–50. Lateral stomach and duodenum.

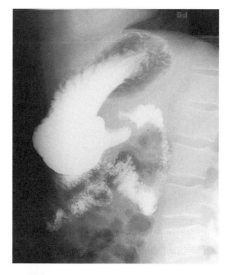

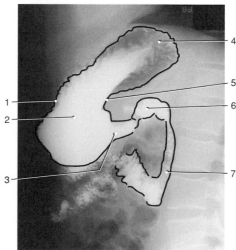

1. Greater curvature
2. Body
3. Pyloric antrum
4. Fundus
5. Lesser curvature
6. Duodenal bulb
7. Duodenum

Figure 15–51. Lateral stomach and duodenum.

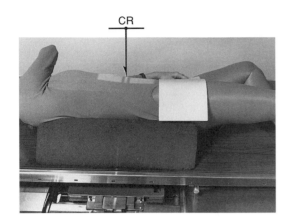

Figure 15–52. LPO stomach and duodenum.

► LPO STOMACH (UPPER GI)

Technical Considerations

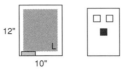

- Film size: 10 × 12 in. (24 × 30 cm) lengthwise or 11 × 14 in. (28 × 35 cm) lengthwise.
- Grid required.
- 100–120 kVp (barium); 85–90 kVp (double or water-soluble contrast).
- Collimate to allow 0.5-in. margins.

Shielding

- Gonadal shielding should be used on all patients, especially children and adults of reproductive age.

Patient Positioning

- Assist the patient to the supine position on the radiographic table. **Note:** This projection may also be performed with the patient erect; centering should be approximately 3 to 6 in. lower, with the greater adjustment used for asthenic patients.
- Adjust the long axis of the patient to lie parallel with the long axis of the table.

Part Positioning

- Elevate the patient's right shoulder and hip so the coronal plane forms a 40° to 70° angle with the tabletop; generally, hypersthenic patients require more rotation than sthenic and asthenic patients to best demonstrate the pyloric canal and duodenum.
- Position the patient's right arm either across the upper chest or at the side; a radiolucent support can be placed behind the patient for immobilization and patient comfort.
- Center the longitudinal plane passing midway between the vertebral column and left lateral margin of the thorax to the midline of the table *(Figure 15–52).*

Central Ray

- Direct the central ray perpendicular to the level of the duodenal bulb; the location of the duodenal bulb will vary depending on body habitus:
  Sthenic. The central ray should enter at the level of L1, halfway between the xyphoid process and the lower, lateral margin of the ribs.
  Hypersthenic. The central ray should enter at the level of T12, about 3 to 4 in. above the inferior margin of the ribs.
  Asthenic. The central ray should enter at the level of L2, about 1 in. above the inferior margin of the ribs.
- Center the cassette to the central ray. **Note:** The stomach is higher in this position than in the PA or RAO positions.

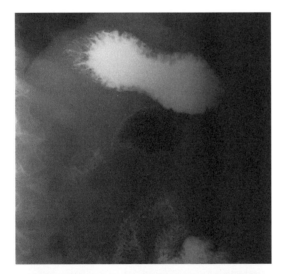

Breathing Instructions

- Instruct the patient to take in a breath, blow it out, and hold it out during the exposure.

Image Evaluation

- The entire stomach and duodenum should be included within the collimated area; part of the diaphragm should also be demonstrated.
- The duodenal bulb and C-loop should be free of superimposition by the pylorus and seen in profile.
- The pylorus and duodenal bulb should be centered lengthwise on the film.
- The barium should be adequately penetrated without overexposure *(Figure 15–53).*

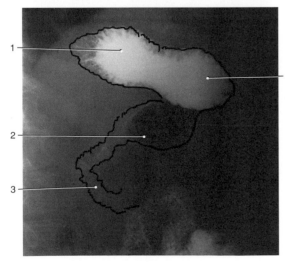

Figure 15–53. LPO stomach and duodenum.

1. Fundus	3. Duodenum	4. Body
2. Pyloric antrum		

► PA/AP SMALL BOWEL

Technical Considerations

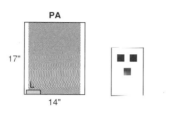

- Film size: 14 × 17 in. (35 × 43 cm) lengthwise.
- Grid required.
- 100–120 kVp (barium); 85–90 kVp (water-soluble contrast).
- Collimate to rib margins crosswise and to film lengthwise; a time marker indicating postingestion time should be placed within the field.

Shielding

- Gonadal shielding should be used on male patients, especially children and adults of reproductive age, as long as it does not compromise the examination.

Patient Positioning

- Assist the patient to the prone position on the radiographic table; position the patient's arms comfortably on the table near the head. **Note:** This projection may also be obtained with the patient supine.

Part Positioning

- Adjust the patient's body so there is no rotation.
- Center the midsagittal plane to the midline of the table *(Figure 15–54)*.
- With the patient lying as flat as possible, adjust the long axis of the patient to lie parallel with the long axis of the table.

Central Ray

- Direct the central ray perpendicular to the level of the duodenal bulb (L-2) for the first film (15-minute; the diaphragm should be included) *or* the level of the iliac crests for all subsequent films (30-minute and later).
- Center the cassette to the central ray.

Breathing Instructions

- Instruct the patient to take in a breath, blow it out, and hold it out during the exposure.

Image Evaluation

- The entire diaphragm and upper half of the pelvis should be included within the collimated area on the first film; the diaphragm may not be included on subsequent films.
- The transverse processes of the vertebrae should be symmetrical.
- The spine should be centered crosswise on the film.
- The barium should be adequately penetrated without overexposure.
- A time marker indicating postingestion time should be included within the collimation field but away from the intestines *(Figure 15–55)*.

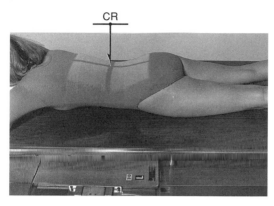

Figure 15–54. PA small bowel, initial film centered above the level of the iliac crests.

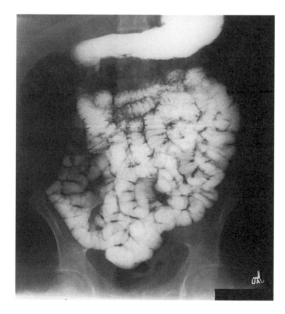

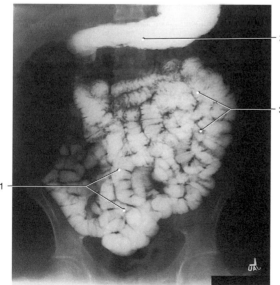

Figure 15–55. PA small bowel, 1-hour film; centering is slightly higher than the iliac crests due to patient size.

1. Ileum　　　　　2. Stomach　　　　　3. Jejunum

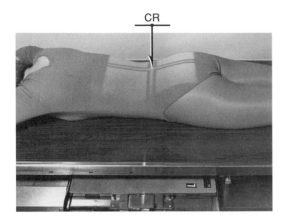

Figure 15–56. PA large intestine.

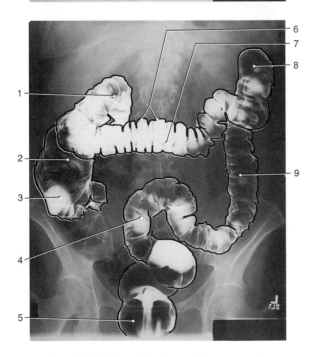

Figure 15–57. PA large intestine, double-contrast study.

▶ AP/PA COLON (PRELIMINARY, CONTRAST-FILLED & POSTEVACUATION)

Technical Considerations

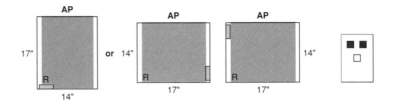

- Film size: 14 × 17 in. (35 × 43 cm) lengthwise or crosswise (2).
- Grid required.
- 100–120 kVp (barium); 85–90 kVp (double or water-soluble contrast; postevacuation).
- Collimate to rib margins crosswise and film lengthwise.

Shielding

- Gonadal shielding should be used on male patients, especially children and adults of reproductive age, as long as it does not compromise the examination.

Patient Positioning

- Assist the patient to the supine position on the radiographic table; position the patient's arms comfortably on the table near the head. **Note:** This projection may also be obtained with the patient prone *(Figures 15–56, 15–57).*
- Center the midsagittal plane to the midline of the table.
- Adjust the long axis of the patient to lie parallel with the long axis of the table.

1. Right colic (hepatic) flexure
2. Ascending colon
3. Cecum
4. Sigmoid (pelvic) colon
5. Rectum
6. Haustra
7. Transverse colon
8. Left colic (splenic) flexure
9. Descending colon

Part Positioning

• Adjust the patient's body so that the ASISs are equidistant from the table; the shoulders and pelvis should not be rotated *(Figure 15–58)*.

Central Ray

• Direct the central ray perpendicular to the level of the iliac crests; align the cassette to the central ray. **Note:** Large patients may require the use of two 14 × 17-in. cassettes positioned crosswise, the first to include the symphysis pubis and the second positioned with at least a 2- to 3-in. overlap of the first.

Breathing Instructions

• Instruct the patient to take in a breath, blow it out, and hold it out during the exposure.

Image Evaluation

• The entire large intestine should be included within the collimated area.
• The iliac crests should be symmetrical.
• The spine should be centered crosswise on the film.
• The barium should be adequately penetrated without overexposure.
• On a double-contrast study, barium will fill the transverse colon when the patient is prone and the ascending and descending colon when the patient is supine.
• An appropriate marker should be visible on the postevacuation film *(Figure 15–59)*.

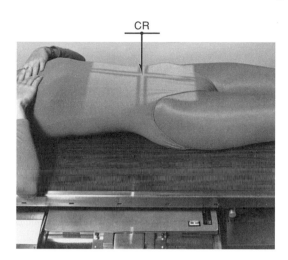

Figure 15–58. AP large intestine.

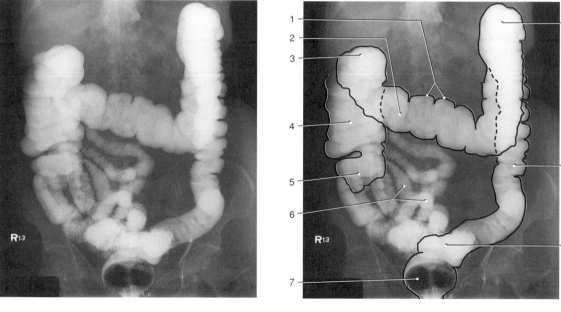

Figure 15–59. Large intestine, single-contrast study.

1. Haustra	5. Cecum	8. Left colic (splenic) flexure
2. Transverse colon	6. Ileum	9. Descending colon
3. Right colic (hepatic) flexure	7. Rectum	10. Sigmoid (pelvic) colon
4. Ascending colon		

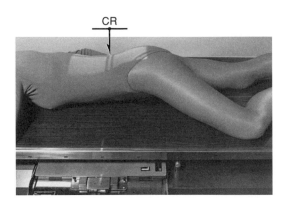

Figure 15–60. RAO large intestine; comparable to the LPO projection.

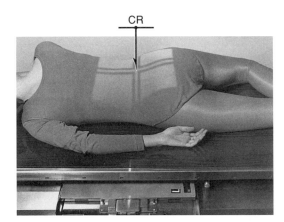

Figure 15–61. LAO large intestine; comparable to the RPO projection.

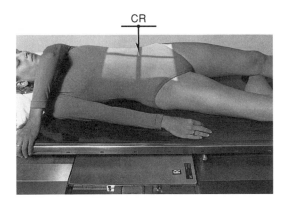

Figure 15–62. RPO large intestine.

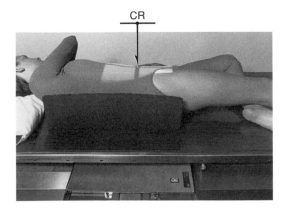

Figure 15–63. LPO large intestine.

► AP OBLIQUE COLON (RPO & LPO)

Technical Considerations

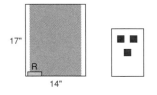

- Film size: 14 × 17 in. (35 × 43 cm) lengthwise.
- Grid required.
- 100–120 kVp (barium); 85–90 kVp (double or water-soluble contrast; postevacuation).
- Collimate to rib margins crosswise and to film lengthwise.

Shielding

- Gonadal shielding should be used on male patients, especially children and adults of reproductive age, as long as it does not compromise the examination.

Patient Positioning

- Assist the patient to the supine position on the radiographic table; position the patient's arms comfortably on the table near the sides. **Note:** These projections may also be obtained with the patient upright. The RAO/LAO projections may also be performed and provide comparable views *(Figures 15–60, 15–61)*.
- For the RPO, position the patient so the midsagittal plane is approximately 2 to 3 in. left of the midline of the table. **Note:** Both obliques will be obtained.
- Adjust the long axis of the patient to lie parallel with the long axis of the table.

Part Positioning

- Rotate the patient's hips and shoulders 35° to 45° toward the right side (RPO); the left arm should be brought across the upper chest and the left leg can be used for support.
- Adjust the centering so that the plane passing 2 to 3 in. medial to the elevated ASIS is centered to the midline of the table (the larger the patient, the more medial the centering).
- The LPO should be obtained by reversing all movements *(Figures 15–62, 15–63)*.

Central Ray

- Direct the central ray perpendicular to the level of the iliac crests.
- Center the cassette to the central ray. **Note:** Centering may have to be slightly higher on the RPO to include the splenic flexure regardless of body habitus; large patients may require the use of two 14 × 17-in. cassettes positioned crosswise, the first to include the symphysis pubis and the second positioned with at least 2- to 3-in. overlap of the first.

Breathing Instructions

- Instruct the patient to take in a breath, blow it out, and hold it out during the exposure.

Image Evaluation

- The entire large intestine should be included within the collimated area.
- The flexure on the elevated side should be demonstrated (RPO: splenic flexure, LPO: hepatic flexure).
- The large intestine should be centered crosswise on the film.
- The barium should be adequately penetrated without overexposure *(Figures 15–64, 15–65).*

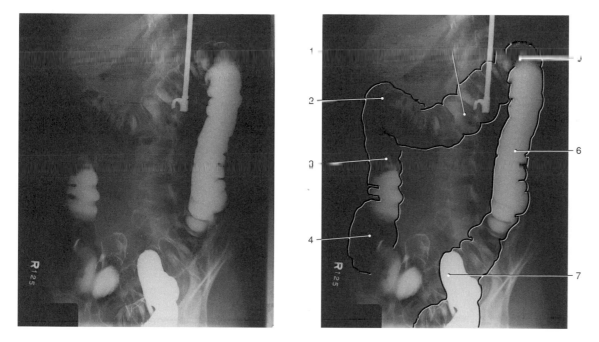

Figure 15–64. RPO large intestine.

1. Transverse colon
2. Right colic (hepatic) flexure
3. Ascending colon
4. Cecum
5. Left colic (splenic) flexure
6. Descending colon
7. Sigmoid colon

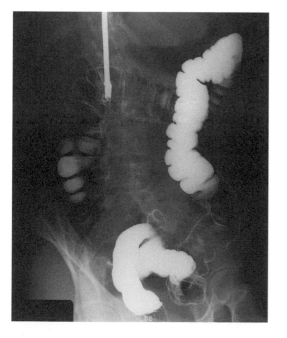
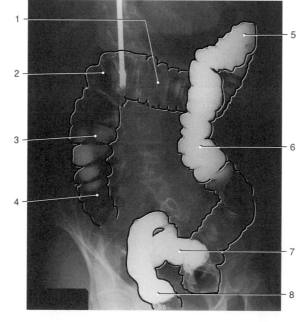

Figure 15–65. LPO large intestine.

1. Transverse colon
2. Right colic (hepatic) flexure
3. Ascending colon
4. Cecum
5. Left colic (splenic) flexure
6. Descending colon
7. Sigmoid colon
8. Rectum

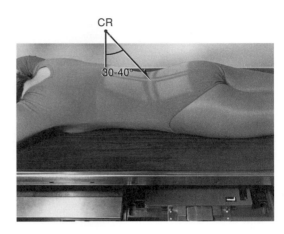

Figure 15–66. PA axial rectum and sigmoid colon.

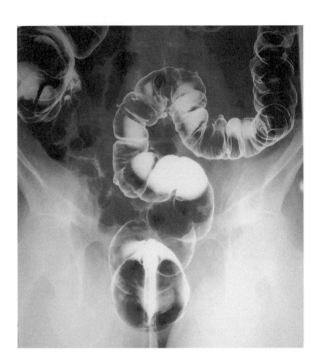

Figure 15–67. PA axial rectum and sigmoid colon.

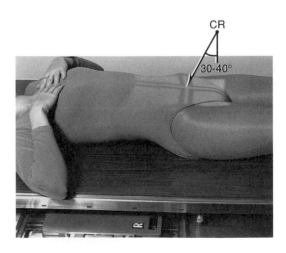

Figure 15–68. AP axial rectum and sigmoid colon.

▶ AP AXIAL RECTOSIGMOID REGION

Technical Considerations

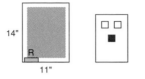

- Film size: 11 × 14 in. (30 × 35 cm) lengthwise or 14 × 17 in. (35 × 43 cm) lengthwise.
- Grid required.
- 100–120 kVp (barium); 85–90 kVp (double or water-soluble contrast; postevacuation).
- Collimate to allow 0.5-in. margins (small film) or to rib margins crosswise and film lengthwise (large film).

Shielding

- Gonadal shielding should be used on male patients, especially children and adults of reproductive age, as long as it does not compromise the examination.

Patient Positioning

- Assist the patient to the supine position on the radiographic table; position the patient's arms comfortably on the table near the sides or with hands on upper chest. **Note:** This projection may also be obtained with the patient prone *(Figures 15–66, 15–67)*. To better demonstrate a tortuous rectosigmoid area, the patient can be rotated 30° to 40° toward the left side (LPO).

Part Positioning

- Adjust the patient's body so the ASISs are equidistant from the table; the shoulders and pelvis should not be rotated *(Figure 15–68)*.
- Center the midsagittal plane to the midline of the table.
- Adjust the long axis of the patient to lie parallel with the long axis of the table.

Central Ray

- Direct the central ray 30° to 40° cephalad to a point approximately 2 in. inferior to the level of the ASISs (11 × 14 in.) or to the level of the ASISs (14 × 17 in.).
- Center the cassette to the central ray. **Note:** The central ray should be directed 30° to 40° caudad when the patient is prone.

Breathing Instructions

- Instruct the patient to take in a breath, blow it out, and hold it out during the exposure.

Image Evaluation

- The rectosigmoid region should be included within the collimated area.
- The iliac crests should be symmetrical.
- The spine should be centered crosswise on the film.
- The barium should be adequately penetrated without overexposure *(Figure 15–69)*.

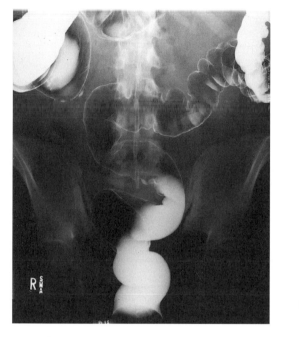 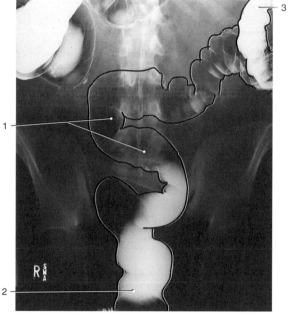

Figure 15–69. AP axial rectum and sigmoid colon.

1. Sigmoid colon   2. Rectum   3. Descending colon

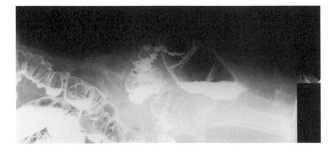

Figure 15–70. Cross-table lateral rectum, double-contrast study.

► LATERAL RECTUM (CONTRAST-FILLED & POSTEVACUATION)

Technical Considerations

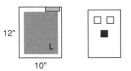

- Film size: 10 × 12 in. (24 × 30 cm) lengthwise.
- Grid required.
- 100–120 kVp (barium); 85–90 kVp (double or water-soluble contrast; postevacuation).
- Collimate to allow 0.5-in. margins.

Shielding

- Gonadal shielding should be used on male patients, especially children and adults of reproductive age, as long as it does not compromise the examination.

Patient Positioning

- Assist the patient to the left lateral position on the table. **Note:** This projection can also be obtained using a vertical grid device and a horizontal beam with the patient prone, especially when performing a double-contrast study *(Figure 15–70).*

Part Positioning

- Adjust the thorax and pelvis to a true lateral position; the right leg should be directly over the left leg.
- Center the plane 2 in. posterior to the midcoronal plane to the midline of the table.
- Flex the knees and hips to a comfortable position; position the arms at a 90° angle with the body *(Figure 15–71).*

Central Ray

- Direct the central ray perpendicular to the level of the ASIS.
- Center the cassette to the central ray.

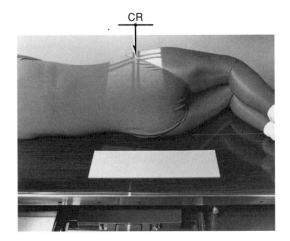

Figure 15–71. Lateral rectum.

Breathing Instructions

• Instruct the patient to take in a breath, blow it out, and hold it out during the exposure.

Image Evaluation

• The entire rectosigmoid region should be included within the collimated area.
• The femoral heads should be superimposed.
• The barium should be adequately penetrated without overexposure *(Figure 15–72)*.

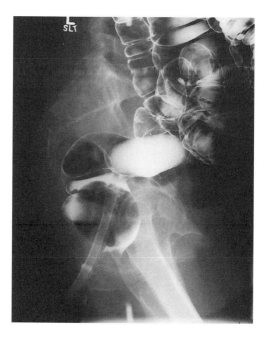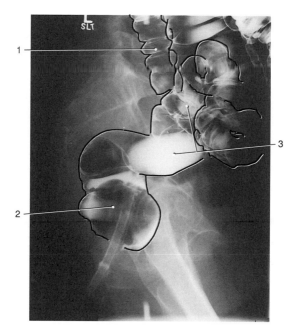

Figure 15–72. Lateral rectum.

1. Descending colon   2. Rectum   3. Sigmoid colon

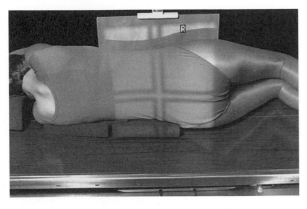

Figure 15–73. Left lateral decubitus large intestine, double-contrast study.

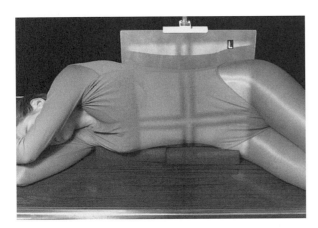

Figure 15–74. Right lateral decubitus large intestine, double-contrast study.

► LATERAL DECUBITUS COLON (DOUBLE-CONTRAST STUDIES)

Technical Considerations

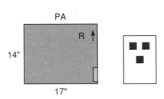

- Film size: 14 × 17 in. (35 × 43 cm) lengthwise with the patient.
- Grid required.
- 85–90 kVp.
- Collimate to the abdominal walls crosswise and to film lengthwise.

Shielding

- Although shielding can be difficult for decubitus projections, a shadow shield or lead drape can be used to shield male patients.

Patient Positioning

- Assist the patient to the left lateral decubitus position on the table or stretcher; the right leg should be directly over the left leg and the right arm should be directly over the left; AP or PA projections can be performed.
- Extend the arms upward so the elbows are near the face.

Part Positioning

- Adjust the thorax and pelvis to a true lateral position; check for rotation by standing at the head or foot of the patient and making sure the shoulders and hips are superimposed.
- A vertically positioned grid cassette should be positioned so it is centered to the level of the iliac crests.
- The patient should be elevated on radiolucent supports, as necessary, to align the midsagittal plane of the patient to the midline of the film (Figure 15–73).
- The right lateral decubitus projection should be obtained by reversing the patient position (Figure 15–74).

Central Ray

- Direct the central ray horizontally to the midline of the grid.

Breathing Instructions

- Instruct the patient to take in a breath, blow it out, and hold it out while the exposure is being made.

Image Evaluation

- The entire large intestine should be included within the collimation field.
- Asymmetry of the iliac crests indicates rotation of the pelvis; if the shoulders are not lateral, the ribs will be asymmetrical.
- Unless pathology is present, the spine should be fairly straight and centered to the film *(Figures 15–75, 15–76)*.

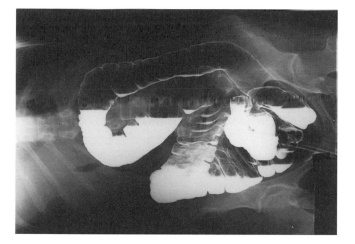 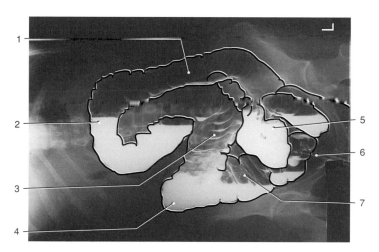

Figure 15–75. Right lateral decubitus large intestine, double-contrast study.

1. Descending colon
2. Left colic (hepatic) flexure
3. Transverse colon
4. Right colic (splenic) flexure
5. Sigmoid colon
6. Rectum
7. Ascending colon

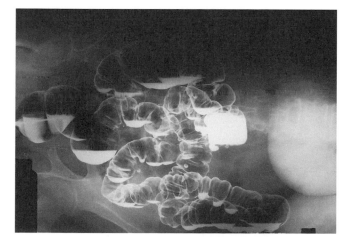 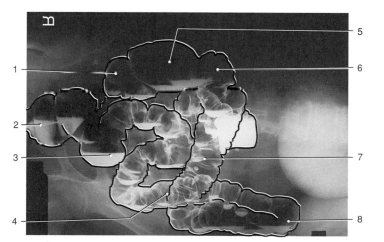

Figure 15–76. Left lateral decubitus large intestine, double-contrast study.

1. Cecum
2. Rectum
3. Sigmoid colon
4. Descending colon
5. Ascending colon
6. Right colic (hepatic) flexure
7. Transverse colon
8. Left colic (splentic) flexure

$\mathcal{S}$UMMARY

► Contrast media are administered either orally, rectally, or through a special tube for the various radiographic examinations of the digestive system.

► All radiographic examinations of the alimentary canal use fluoroscopy at some point during the procedure.

► For radiography of the digestive system, the patient must complete an appropriate pre-examination preparation to ensure that the structures of interest are free of food and/or stool.

► The acquisition and documentation of a pertinent patient history are important for diagnosis and patient safety and should include information about previous surgery or related procedures such as sigmoidoscopy and colonoscopy.

► Because gastrointestinal studies may be lengthy and somewhat uncomfortable for the patient, the radiographer must clearly explain the entire procedure to the patient, including what can be expected and the length of the examination.

► Although ostomy patients usually have radiographic examinations in which contrast is administered through the stoma, some may also have barium given rectally.

► Postexamination instructions are important to prevent fecal impaction, which could lead to bowel obstruction.

► In addition to gathering the necessary supplies for the specific examination, the fluoroscopic unit must be prepared.

► A scout film is obtained prior to fluoroscopy to evaluate patient preparation and the presence of obvious pathology.

► Radiographic examinations of the esophagus and stomach usually include AP/PA, RAO, and lateral projections.

► Projections for a small bowel series are obtained at timed intervals following the ingestion of contrast media.

► Although single-contrast radiographic examination of the large intestine may include AP/PA, oblique, axial, and lateral projections, double-contrast examinations generally include lateral decubitus projections.

► Accessory equipment used for pediatric gastrointestinal procedures should be age appropriate.

► Minimizing radiation exposure is a primary consideration when performing gastrointestinal radiography on children.

► To reduce the risk of involuntary motion, gastrointestinal radiographs are obtained during suspended expiration.

► To penetrate the barium, 100 to 120 kVp is recommended for single-contrast studies of the stomach, small bowel, and colon; 85 to 90 kVp should be used for double-contrast examinations in which a thin layer of barium coats the mucosal lining.

► A grid device is required for all radiography of the gastrointestinal system.

QUESTIONS FOR CRITICAL THINKING & APPLICATION

1. If a patient was diagnosed with a malabsorption problem, what part of the alimentary canal is most likely to be at fault? What kind of symptoms will the patient exhibit?

2. How does a hiatal hernia occur? What structures are affected? Describe its appearance radiographically.

3. Outline the anatomic differences between the small and large intestines. How to each anatomic demonstrated radiographically?

4. Define *appendicitis*. If a patient was being evaluated for possible appendicitis, where would he or she most likely experience pain? What is the relationship between a ruptured appendix and peritonitis?

5. After the administration of barium sulfate, where would the contrast medium most likely be demonstrated on AP and PA projections of the stomach? In a double-contrast barium enema (barium sulfate and air), where would the barium sulfate settle on AP and PA projections?

6. A very ill patient scheduled for an upper GI series has been brought to the department on a stretcher. Describe how the room should be prepared.

7. Patient preparation for a barium enema is extensive. Explain how poor preparation can affect the outcome of the examination.

8. Although patient communication is an integral component of any radiographic examination, it is especially important for gastrointestinal radiography. Demonstrate how you would explain a barium enema examination to an elderly patient who had never been to the hospital prior to this examination. How would you explain this to a deaf patient or one who does not speak your language?

9. State two reasons why the prone position might be preferred over the supine position for radiography of the small bowel.

10. A patient with a colostomy in the descending colon has been scheduled for a colon examination. Barium must be administered through the stoma. Describe how you would approach the patient and discuss complications relative to routine positioning that may be encountered.

FILM CRITIQUE

Name this projection.

Describe how this patient was positioned *(Figure 15–77)*.

What anatomy should be demonstrated on this projection?

Was the patient positioning accurate?

Was patient centering accurate?

Were technical factors appropriate?

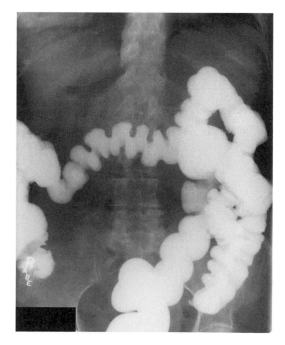

Figure 15–77

16

BILIARY SYSTEM

► OBJECTIVES

Following the completion of this chapter the student will be able to:

- Given diagrams or radiographs, name and describe the anatomy of the biliary system, to include the liver, gallbladder, and ducts.

- Discuss the orientation of the gallbladder according to body habitus, physical position, and respiration.

- Identify the functions of each of the structures in the biliary system.

- Describe the relationship of the pancreas with the biliary system.

- Discuss the use of contrast media in radiographic examinations of the biliary system, to include type and route of administration.

- State the criteria used to determine positioning accuracy on radiographs of the biliary system and evaluate radiographs of the biliary system in terms of positioning, centering, image quality, radiographic anatomy, and pathology.

- Define terminology associated with the biliary system, to include anatomy, procedures, and pathology.

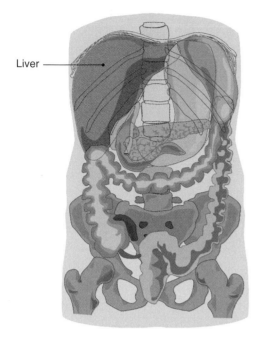

Figure 16–1. Location of liver in right upper quadrant of the abdomen.

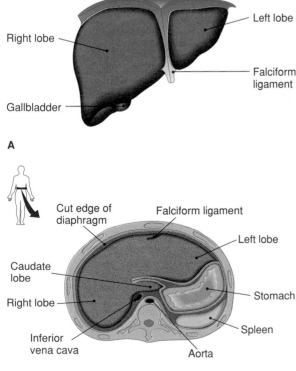

A

B

Figure 16–2. Liver: **(A)** anterior view, **(B)** sectional view.

▶ ANATOMY OF THE BILIARY SYSTEM

The biliary system refers to those structures concerned with the production, storage, and movement of bile. Such structures include the liver, gallbladder, and various biliary ducts *(Table 16–1).*

LIVER

The liver is a large, wedge-shaped organ located in the upper abdomen just inferior to the diaphragm. Although the majority of it lies in the right upper quadrant above the right kidney, the liver does cross the midline of the body to extend into the left upper quadrant *(Figure 16–1).* With the exception of its posterior surface, most of the organ is covered by visceral peritoneum. The liver is the body's largest solid organ, weighing approximately 3 pounds (1.4 kg) and contributing to 2.5% of the body's total weight. *Table 16–2* summarizes the average dimensions of the liver.

The liver is divided into two major **right and left lobes** and two minor **caudate and quadrate lobes.** The large right lobe is separated from the smaller left lobe by the **falciform** (FAL-si-form) **ligament.** This mesentery cord extends from the inferior aspect of the diaphragm through a fissure between the major lobes to help suspend the liver in the upper abdomen *(Figure 16–2).* The minor lobes are much smaller than either the right or left lobe. In fact, it is thought that the minor lobes are actually divisions of the right lobe. The caudate lobe is located on the posterior side of the liver behind the right lobe. The quadrate lobe lies on the inferior surface of the liver. These lobes are identified in *Figure 16–3.*

The functional component of the liver, the **parenchyma** (pah-RENG-ki-mah), is composed of numerous tiny lobules. That is, each lobe of the liver is subdivided into microscopic functional units called **liver lobules.** These hexagon-shaped units are comprised of **hepatocytes,** or liver cells (*hepato* = "liver"), which absorb nutrients and remove toxic materials from the blood circulating through the liver, in addition to producing bile. The hepatocytes are specialized cells that have the ability to partially regenerate if injured. Tiny bile capillaries called **canaliculi** (kan-ah-LIK-ū-lī) form a network of ducts around the hepatocytes. The tiny ducts continually unite to form larger ducts in each lobe, which eventually form the right and left hepatic ducts that drain the bile from the liver *(Figure 16–4).*

The hepatocytes in the liver manufacture approximately 1 qt (1 L) of bile per day. This fluid plays an important role in the emulsification, absorption, and digestion of ingested fats. **Bile** is a liquid substance composed mainly of bile salts, bile pigments, cholesterol, and water. The bile pigments are responsible for its characteristic yellowish color. The bile salts facilitate the absorption of fats. Approximately 80% of the bile salts are absorbed in the small intestine, transported to the liver, and recycled as a component of bile once again. Cholesterol, a steroid alcohol synthesized by the liver, is a precursor of bile acids and steroid hormones. It is often a main component of gallstones.

Table 16–1. Production and Movement of Bile Within the Biliary System

Liver	Manufacture of bile by hepatocytes in liver
↓	
Right and left hepatic ducts	Hollow tubes that drain the bile from the main lobes of the liver
↓	
Common hepatic duct[a]	Larger duct formed by union of right and left hepatic ducts
↓	
Cystic duct	Duct that conveys bile into the gallbladder
↓	
Gallbladder	Expandable sac that functions to store and concentrate bile
↓	
Cystic duct	Same duct as before; also functions to convey bile out of the gallbladder
↓	
Common bile duct	Duct formed by junction of common hepatic duct with cystic duct; transports bile to the duodenum
↓	
Hepatopancreatic ampulla	Short, dilated area at distal portion of common bile duct where it merges with pancreatic duct
↓	
Hepatopancreatic sphincter	Round muscle at opening of hepatopancreatic ampulla into descending portion of duodenum
↓	
(Duodenum of small intestine)	

[a]At this point, bile may go directly into common bile duct, bypassing the cystic duct and gallbladder.

Table 16–2. Average Dimensions of the Liver

Width (transverse)	21.6 cm	8.5 in.
Height (vertical)	16.5 cm	6.5 in.
Depth (anteroposterior)	11.4 cm	4.5 in.

The liver is a highly vascular structure. Blood is supplied to it via the hepatic artery and the portal vein. Both of these vessels enter the liver at the **porta hepatis,** which literally translates as "gate to the liver." This transverse fissure is located on the posteroinferior surface of the liver at the junction of the right, caudate, and quadrate lobes. It is sometimes referred to as the **hilus** of the liver and is demonstrated in *Figure 16–3.*

In addition to the production of bile, the liver performs approximately 200 functions, including metabolic and regulatory roles. It receives roughly 25% of the total cardiac output via the hepatic artery. Old, worn out, and/or damaged red blood cells are removed from circulation, along with pathogens and toxins. As the portal vein brings blood to the liver from the digestive tract, pancreas, and spleen, nutrients are removed from the bloodstream and vitamins A, D, K, and E are absorbed and stored in the liver. Because the functions of the liver are essential to life, any disease that damages the liver and/or diminishes liver function represents a significant risk to a person's well-being.

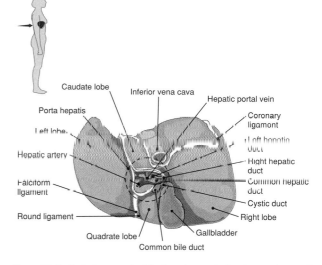

Figure 16–3. Posterior aspect of the liver demonstrating the quadrate and caudate lobes, as well as the porta hepatis.

GALLBLADDER

The gallbladder is a small, hollow sac located in the right upper quadrant of the abdomen. On a lateral view, the gallbladder is seen lying just anterior to the midcoronal plane of the body *(Figure 16–5)*. It lies in a shallow depression on the posteroinferior surface of the liver. The bottom of the gallbladder is usually suspended lower than the inferior margin of the liver and lies approximately at the level of the ninth costal cartilage *(Figure 16–6)*. The exact position of the gallbladder, however, is variable, depending largely on a person's body habitus (asthenic or hypersthenic), physical position (upright or recumbent), and respiration (inspiration or expiration). The gallbladder in a hypersthenic individual is usually located higher, transversely, and more laterally. The gallbladder in an asthenic individual hangs low and close to the spine *(Figure 16–7)*.

The three main parts of the gallbladder are the fundus, body, and neck. The **fundus** is the rounded distal portion. The **body** is simply the middle portion of the organ. The **neck** is the superior constricted area

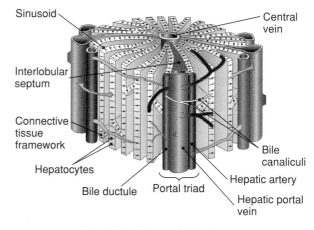

Figure 16–4. Diagram of a liver lobule.

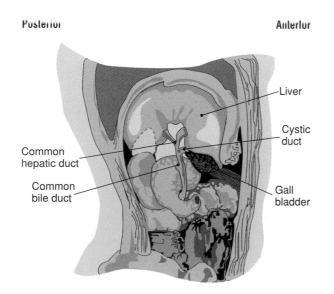

Figure 16–5. Location of the liver, gallbladder, and bile ducts, as demonstrated on a sagittal view of the abdomen.

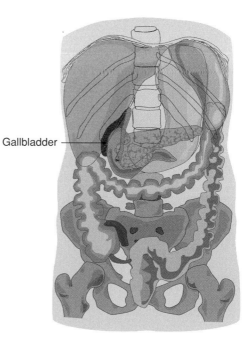

Figure 16–6. Location of gallbladder in the right upper quadrant of the abdomen.

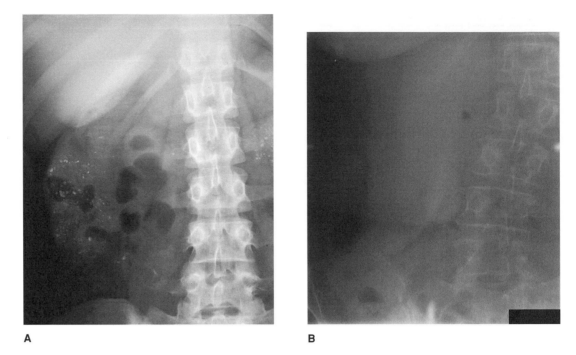

A

B

Figure 16–7. Relative position of the gallbladder is affected by body habitus. Notice that the gallbladder is located higher and more laterally on a hypersthenic patient **(A)** and lower and more medially on a hyposthenic/asthenic patient **(B)**.

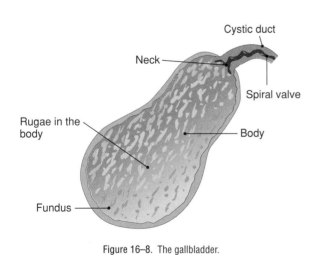

Cystic duct

Neck

Spiral valve

Rugae in the body

Body

Fundus

Figure 16–8. The gallbladder.

that is continuous with the cystic duct *(Figure 16–8)*. The gallbladder has muscular walls that enable it to contract and expand as needed. At its fullest, the gallbladder measures approximately 1 in. (2.5 cm) wide and 3 to 4 in. (7 to 10 cm) long and assumes the shape of a pear. It can hold roughly 40 mL of bile. The inner mucosal lining falls into folds called **rugae** when the gallbladder is empty. These are similar in appearance to the folds in the lining of the stomach. The outer surface of the gallbladder is covered by visceral peritoneum.

The gallbladder functions to store and concentrate bile. If bile is not immediately needed to aid in digestion, it is stored in the gallbladder where water and ions are absorbed by capillaries in the mucosa, leaving an increased concentration of bile salts. As the composition of bile changes, it can actually become ten times more concentrated than its original state. **Choleliths** (KŌ-lē-liths), or gallstones, may form in the event that too much water is absorbed or if the cholesterol in the bile becomes too concentrated *(Figure 16–9)*. When the bile is needed for digestion, the walls of the gallbladder contract, expelling the bile out of the gallbladder through the cystic duct.

BILIARY DUCTS

Bile is transported through a system of biliary ducts located on the midcoronal plane of the body, as demonstrated in *Figure 16–5*. As stated previously, the small ducts in the liver lobules combine to form larger ductules and ducts. The **right and left hepatic ducts** drain the bile from the major lobes of the liver. As they leave the liver at the porta hepatis, they unite to form the **common hepatic duct,** which is approximately 1.5 in. (3–4 cm) long. The **cystic duct** extending from the gallbladder is also 1.5 in. (3–4 cm) long. It merges with the common hepatic duct to form the **common bile duct,** which is about 3 in. (7.5 cm) long. The common bile duct travels inferiorly toward the duodenum. At its distal end, it usually converges with the **pancreatic duct** from the pancreas to become a slightly expanded area known as the **hepatopancreatic ampulla** (ampulla of Vater). At this point, the duct enters the descending portion of the duodenum through the **hepatopancreatic sphincter** (sphincter of Oddi). This sphincter is a ringlike muscle that has the ability to open and close on stimulation. **Duodenal papillae** are present at the site of the sphincter. These are nipplelike projections of the duct into the lumen of the duodenum *(Figure 16–10)*. Because the papillae cause this area to be slightly constricted, choleliths may obstruct the opening and impede the flow of bile, resulting in pressure and intense pain.

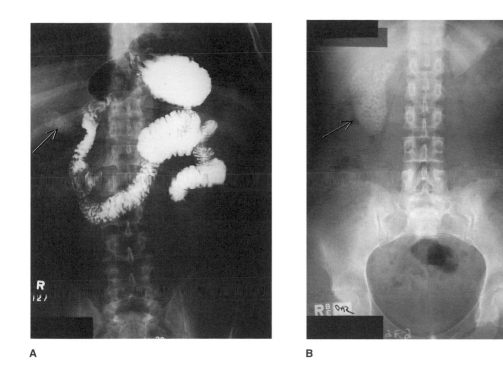

A **B**

Figure 16–9. **(A)** Calcifications are seen in the gallbladder without the aid of a cholecystopaque on a small bowel film. **(B)** Gallstones are also demonstrated on the cholecystogram.

PHYSIOLOGY

Although bile is manufactured continuously by the liver, it is not usually permitted to flow freely down the bile ducts and into the duodenum. The hepatopancreatic sphincter is securely closed except when an individual is eating. This causes the bile to back up the common bile duct, through the cystic duct, and into the gallbladder, where it is stored and concentrated until it is needed. When chyme moves into the duodenum from the stomach after the individual ingests food, the cells of the intestinal mucosa are stimulated to secrete **cholecystokinin (CCK)** (kō-le-sis-tō-KĪ-nin) into the bloodstream. In addition to producing a feeling of fullness, this hormone prompts the gallbladder to contract and expel bile. It also stimulates the pancreas to secrete pancreatic juice and causes the hepatopancreatic sphincter to relax, permitting the flow of both bile and pancreatic juice into the duodenum where they mix with the food substances. The enzymes in the pancreatic juice break down proteins, carbohydrates, and fats in food. Bile is responsible primarily for the **emulsification** (ē-mul-si-fi-KĀ-shun) of fats; that is, it breaks the large lipid globules apart into smaller particles that can be more readily digested and absorbed. It also facilitates the absorption of cholesterol *(Figure 16–11)*.

The amount of cholecystokinin released into the bloodstream increases when the chyme in the duodenum contains an increased amount of fat. Consequently, more bile is expelled from the gallbladder and transported to the small intestine. This has a widespread effect as the increased amount of bile results in more bile salts being reabsorbed into the bloodstream, which in turn causes an elevation in bile production by the liver.

PANCREAS

The pancreas (PAN-krē-as) is not part of the biliary system. It is included in this chapter because, like the liver and gallbladder, it is an accessory organ of digestion. It actually is a dual gland, having two different types of tissue and exhibiting both exocrine and endocrine properties. It is approximately 5 to 6 in. (12 to 15 cm) in length and 1 in. (2.5 cm) thick, and weighs 3 oz (80 g). It is an elongated structure that spans the right and left upper quadrants of the abdomen. Located behind the stomach, it is a retroperitoneal gland consisting of three main parts: a head, body, and tail *(Figure 16–12)*. The large head is situated in the C-loop of the duodenum, whereas the body and tail taper toward the spleen. Because of its proximity to the

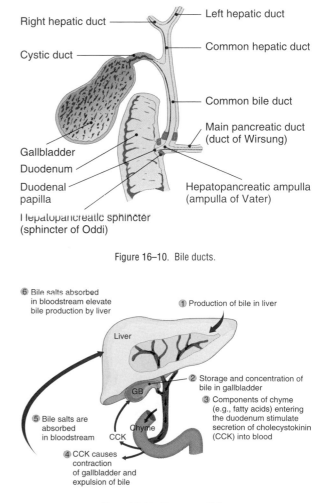

Figure 16–10. Bile ducts.

Figure 16–11. Transport of bile.

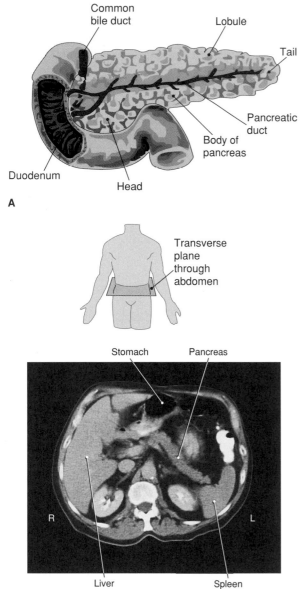

A

B

Figure 16–12. The pancreas **(A)** can be demonstrated on an axial CT image of the abdomen **(B)**.

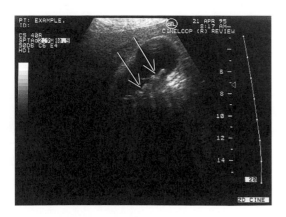

Figure 16–13. Sonogram of the gallbladder. Note the presence of stones.

stomach, duodenum, and bile ducts, any enlargement of the pancreas resulting from pathology exerts pressure on those structures, possibly distorting their natural shape.

Structurally, approximately 99% of the pancreas is exocrine in nature, being composed of clusters of cells known as **acini** (AS-i-nī) (singular, acinus) which are connected to small ducts. These cells secrete up to 1.6 qt (1500 mL) of pancreatic juice per day. The pancreatic juice, which is a mixture of fluid digestive enzymes, is transported to the duodenum via the **main pancreatic duct** (duct of Wirsung), which usually merges with the common bile duct at the hepatopancreatic ampulla. Occasionally, an accessory duct is present in the head of the pancreas and enters the duodenum approximately 1 in. (2.5 cm) superior to the hepatopancreatic sphincter. Once in the duodenum, the enzymes in the pancreatic juice mix with the food to aid in the digestive process.

The remaining 1% of pancreatic tissue comprises endocrine cells called **pancreatic islets** or the **islands of Langerhans.** Because these cells are ductless, their secretions are absorbed directly into the bloodstream. Glucagon and insulin, hormones secreted by these cells, play an significant role in the metabolism of carbohydrates.

► PROCEDURAL CONSIDERATIONS

Radiographic examination of the biliary system includes studies of both the gallbladder and the biliary ducts. For years, the oral cholecystogram (OCG) was the examination of choice for identifying calculi or other gallbladder-related problems. Today, ultrasonography frequently replaces the oral cholecystogram in most hospitals.

There are several methods for evaluating the biliary ducts, depending on the situation. The more common procedures are described. Because intravenous cholangiography has been replaced by sonography *(Figure 16–13),* it is not discussed in this text. Radiographic examinations of the biliary system are named for the route of contrast administration and the structures examined.

ORAL CHOLECYSTOGRAPHY

Cholecystography (ko-le-sis-TOG-rah-fe) is the term used to describe radiography of the gallbladder. This examination is typically performed to detect cholelithiasis (stones), cholecystitis, masses, biliary stenosis, or abnormal growth relative to the gallbladder, but is contraindicated for patients with pyloric obstruction, malabsorption syndrome, severe jaundice, liver dysfunction, or hypersensitivity to iodinated contrast media. Because vomiting and/or diarrhea may result in little or no absorption of the contrast medium, these symptoms may be reason to cancel or postpone the procedure.

The radiographic procedure usually consists of two or three overhead films and upright fluoroscopic spots; a decubitus projection is sometimes substituted for the upright spots. To evaluate the contracting ability of the gallbladder, a fatty meal, either egg nog or a commercially prepared substitute, may be administered orally to the patient. Approximately 15 to 20 minutes later, a post-fatty meal film is obtained with the patient in the right posterior oblique position to facilitate drainage of the gallbladder.

Patient Preparation

Patient preparation for an OCG must begin prior to the day of the actual examination. The patient is usually instructed to eat fatty foods for 1 to 2 days prior to the study. On the eve of the examination, however, the patient should eat a fat-free meal and ingest a single dose of oral cholecystopaque, usually 4 to 6 tablets, 2 to 3 hours afterward; some department protocols routinely require that a double dose of contrast be given, 6 pills on each of two consecutive nights (12 pills total). After ingestion of the cholecystopaque tablets, the patient should refrain from eating; drinking small amounts of water is usually permitted as long as this does not conflict with another examination being performed on the same day (such as an upper GI study). In some departments, a cleansing enema may also be part of the routine preparation. Because laxatives could cause the cholecystopaque tablets to be eliminated before the contrast can be absorbed, laxatives should be avoided for 24 hours prior to ingestion of contrast medium.

On the day of the examination, the patient should be instructed to remove all clothing and put on a patient gown. A pertinent patient history should be obtained to determine whether the prescribed diet was followed, if the cholecystopaque tablets were ingested, and whether vomiting or diarrhea occurred; information about any previous relevant surgery should also be obtained *(Figure 16–14).* Although it is rare, there have been instances in which patients have prepared for an oral cholecystogram years after having

---

History Sheet: Oral Cholecystography

Patient Name: _____ Age: _____

Date: _____ X-ray No.: _____ Pregnant? _____

Symptoms (check all that apply):

_____ Nausea   _____ Abdominal pain

_____ Vomiting   _____ Dyspepsia

Abdominal Surgical History: _____

Exam Preparation: _____

Type and Amount of Contrast Ingested: _____

Description of Diet During Previous 24 Hours: _____

_____

Any Laxatives During Previous 24 Hours? _____

Any Vomiting? _____ Diarrhea? _____

Severity and Duration: _____

If Yes, Please describe _____

Bilirubin Count (if known): _____

Additional Comments: _____

_____

_____

_____

Technologist: _____ Radiologist: _____

Figure 16–14. History sheet for oral cholecystography.

had a cholecystectomy! Vomiting that occurs within 2 hours of ingestion of the contrast and/or diarrhea may result in a poorly visualized gallbladder.

Room Preparation

Preliminary overhead scout and spot films are obtained with the table in the horizontal or upright position. After the overhead OCG films have been reviewed by the radiologist, upright fluoroscopic spot films are usually obtained. The radiographic table must be in the 90° upright position for this purpose; the lead protective curtain on the fluoro tower should be positioned to provide maximum protection for the fluoroscopist. A fatty meal should be available to assess function, if requested by the radiologist. Because patients with gallbladder disease are often nauseous, an emesis basin should be available.

Positioning Considerations

Although initial OCG radiographs are usually obtained with the patient recumbent, they may also be obtained with the patient upright. The first film is usually considered the "scout," because the gallbladder varies in location and does not always visualize. For this reason, the scout is often obtained using a 14 × 17-in. cassette. If the gallbladder is visualized on the scout film, localization films are obtained with the patient in the prone and LAO positions. To place the gallbladder closer to the film, the PA projection is performed; the LAO projection is used to move the gallbladder away from the spine and any bowel gas that may obscure it. Because the gallbladder lies very close to the spine in asthenic patients, these patients must be rotated more than hypersthenic patients, whose gallbladders lie more laterally. Right lateral decubitus or upright projections are usually obtained for stratification of stones *(Figure 16–15)*.

► Related Terminology

acholia (ah-KŌ-lē-ah)—failure to secrete bile

biliary (BIL-ē-ā-rē)—pertaining to bile

biliary calculus (BIL-ē-ā-rē KAL-ku-lus)—gallstone; same as a cholelith

biliary stenosis (BIL-ē-ā-rē ste-NŌ-sis)—narrowing or constriction of any of the biliary ducts that blocks the flow of bile

bilirubin (bil-ē-ROO-bin)—orange- or yellow-colored bile pigment produced from the hemoglobin of red blood cells; an increased level in the blood may indicate liver and gallbladder disease

cirrhosis (si-RŌ-sis)—degenerative disease of the liver in which the liver cells are progressively destroyed

cholangitis (kō-lan-JĪ-tis)—inflammation of the bile ducts

chole- (KŌ-lē)—prefix denoting bile

cholecystectomy (kō-lē-sis-TEK-tō-mē)—surgical removal of the gallbladder

cholecystitis (kō-lē-sis-TĪ-tis)—inflammation of the gallbladder

cholecystopaque (kō-iē-SIS-tō-pak)—iodinated contrast medium used in radiographic procedures of the biliary tract

choledochus (kō-LĒD-ō-kus)—another name for the common bile duct

cholelithiasis (kō-lē-li-THĪ-ah-sis)—condition of having gallstones

cholelithotomy (kō-lē-li-THOT-ō-mē)—incision into the biliary tract, including the gallbladder, for the removal of gallstones

cholelithotripsy (kō-lē-LITH-ō-trip-sē)—procedure in which sound waves are used to crush gallstones

cholesteremia (kō-les-ter-Ē-mē-ah)—abnormal condition in which there is an increased amount of cholesterol in the bloodstream

hepatitis (hep-ah-TĪ-tis)—inflammation of the liver

hepatomalacia (hep-a-tō-mah-LĀ-shē-ah)—abnormal softening of the liver

hepatomegaly (hep-ah-tō-MEG-a-lē)—abnormal condition in which the liver is enlarged

jaundice (JAWN-dis)—abnormal condition in which the tissues, including skin and sclera of the eyes, are yellowish from a high concentration of bilirubin in the bloodstream and bile pigment deposits in the bloodstream

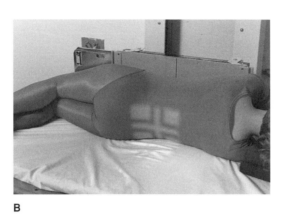

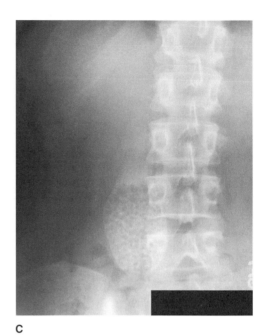

A   B   C

Figure 16–15. Upright **(A)** and right lateral decubitus **(B)** positioning may be used to demonstrate stratification of stones in the gallbladder, PA upright gallbladder (cholecystogram) **(C)**.

CHOLANGIOGRAPHY

Cholangiography (ko-lan-jē-OG-rah-fē), radiographic examination of the biliary ducts, generally involves direct injection of contrast media into the bile ducts to evaluate the patency or condition of the ducts and/or the presence of stones. The procedure can be performed in surgery, through a biliary drainage tube following surgery, through a long, slender needle passed directly into the biliary ducts, or by using a fiberoptic endoscope passed into the mouth and through the hepatopancreatic ampulla. The intravenous cholangiogram, accomplished via intravenous injection of iodinated contrast, is rarely, if ever, performed today, having been replaced by ultrasound, percutaneous transhepatic cholangiography, and endoscopic retrograde cholangiopancreatography.

The **operative cholangiogram** is a surgical procedure often performed to assess patency of the ducts following the removal of biliary stones and/or the gallbladder *(Figure 16–16)*. The traditional procedure generally includes one or more AP or RPO projections following the direct injection of contrast media into the common bile duct. The surgeon administers the contrast media and instructs the technologist when to make the exposure. Because the patient is usually draped for surgery prior to the radiographer's entry into the surgery suite, the radiographer should consult with the anesthetist or other member of the surgical team to determine patient size for accurate technical factor selection. C-arm fluoroscopy may also be used, replacing the traditional overhead films. In either case, knowledge of sterile procedure and sterile areas in the surgical suite is vitally important to preventing contamination of the sterile field.

T-tube cholangiography, also called **postoperative** or **delayed cholangiography,** is performed on a patient postoperatively to demonstrate the patency of the ducts, presence of calculi or other pathology, and status of the hepatopancreatic ampulla *(Figure 16–17)*. During surgery, a small T-shaped tube is positioned so the cross of the "T" is in the common bile duct and the bottom of the "T" extends through the wall of the patient's abdomen for drainage. One day prior to the examination, the tube should be clamped off to allow the ducts to fill with bile, eliminating any air bubbles, which may look like cholesterol stones radiographically. On the day of the procedure, the patient may receive a cleansing enema about 1 hour before the examination; the meal preceding the examination should be withheld.

Following universal precautions, the radiologist injects, in fractional doses, a relatively low-density, water-soluble contrast medium through the tubing; progress is monitored fluoroscopically. Fluoroscopic spot and conventional films are obtained per radiologist request. Any residual stones may be removed by the radiologist with the use of a basket catheter.

Right hepatic duct   Common hepatic duct
Left hepatic duct   Cystic duct

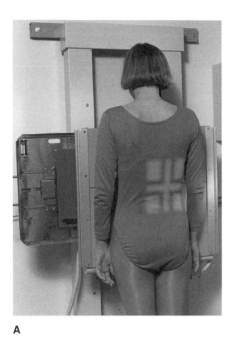

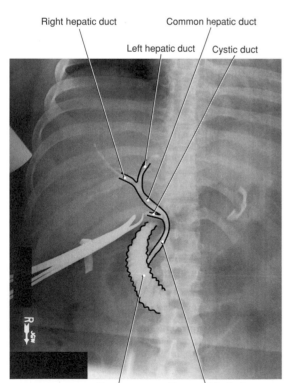

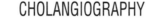

Duodenum   Common bile duct

Figure 16–16. Operative cholangiogram demonstrating patency of the biliary ducts.

Percutaneous transhepatic cholangiography (PTC) may be performed when the patient is jaundiced and dilation of the biliary ducts is evident on CT or ultrasound images *(Figure 16–18)*. It is the most invasive of the nonsurgical procedures, as it involves insertion of a long, thin-walled needle (a Chiba or "skinny" needle is recommended) through the liver, directly into the bile duct. To prevent possible infection, the examination is performed using sterile procedure; the patient's right side is surgically scrubbed and draped. Using fluoroscopy to monitor the procedure, the radiologist inserts the needle and slowly injects the contrast media. If necessary, the radiologist may extract any visible stones using a special basket catheter. Fluoroscopic spot films are obtained as needed.

Endoscopic retrograde cholangiopancreatography (ERCP) is an alternate procedure used to diagnose biliary and pancreatic pathologic conditions *(Figure 16–19)*. Under fluoroscopic guidance, a therapeutic endoscope is passed through the mouth to the hepatopancreatic ampulla (usually by a gastroenterologist). A topical anesthetic sprayed onto the patient's throat eases passage of the endoscope. After the endoscope reaches the ampulla, a small cannula is passed through the endoscope, directly into the ampulla. Contrast is then administered retrograde into the common bile duct; a diluted contrast is generally recommended when small stones are suspected. Stones, if present, can then be extracted and tumors can be biopsied during this procedure; spot films may be taken. Sonography of the upper abdomen is often performed prior to the examination to rule out the possibility of pseudocysts, as injection of contrast media into a pseudocyst may cause it to rupture. Because the topical anesthetic causes temporary pharyngeal paralysis, patients are usually prohibited from ingesting food or drink for at least 1 hour after the examination. To minimize irritation to the stomach and small bowel, food may also be withheld for up to 10 hours.

Patient Preparation

Patients preparing for T-tube cholangiography, PTC, or ERCP should remove all clothing and put on a patient gown; the radiographer is not responsible for preparing a patient for operative cholangiography. A history form similar to that in *Figure 16–14* can be used. Because iodinated contrast media is used, hypersensitivity should be determined prior to starting the examination; hypersensitivity, however, is not necessarily a contraindication to ERCP. Because PTC is considered a sterile procedure, the area in which the needle enters must be surgically scrubbed; sterile drapes should then be placed around the site prior to needle insertion.

Room Preparation

Although the various cholangiographic procedures are very different, some of the supplies are the same *(Table 16–3)*. Sterile trays with the necessary equipment are often prepackaged in house or purchased commercially. The availability of contrast media used for the operative cholangiogram is the responsibility of the surgical team. Because percutaneous transhepatic cholangiography is performed using a sterile field, the lead drape on the fluoro tower must be moved to prevent contamination. The gastroenterologist performs the ERCP; a nurse assistant is often responsible for providing a tray with the necessary equipment, as well as the endoscope used for the procedure.

Positioning Considerations

For an operative cholangiogram, AP and/or 15° to 20° RPO projections are obtained of the patient's right upper quadrant, per physician's request. Prior to entry into the surgery suite, care must be taken to ensure that the mobile unit is clean and operating correctly. Inside the surgical suite, the radiographic tube should be positioned to avoid angling into the grid, producing unwanted grid lines and an underexposed film. A C-arm fluoroscopic unit may also be used to perform this examination, according to department protocol and surgeon preference.

Prior to starting T-tube cholangiography, a scout film is generally taken of the right upper quadrant. This first film may be obtained with the patient supine or in the RPO position, per department routine or radiologist request. Prior to injection of contrast, the patient should be placed in the RPO position with a radiolucent support used for immobilization. Films are obtained at the direction of the radiologist.

While performing percutaneous transhepatic cholangiography, a scout film may not be necessary. The patient may be positioned supine or in the RPO position; fluoroscopic spot films are obtained under the direction of the radiologist.

Endoscopic retrograde cholangiopancreatography is performed by a gastroenterologist. The radiographer's primary responsibilities usually include providing radiation protection apparel for personnel in the room, operating the fluoroscopic unit, obtaining spot films per instruction, and assisting as necessary.

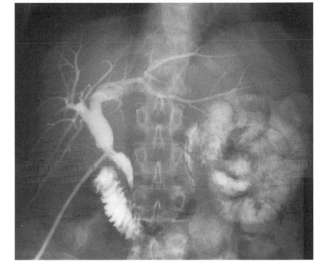

Figure 16–17. T-tube cholangiogram. Notice the cross of the T in the common bile duct.

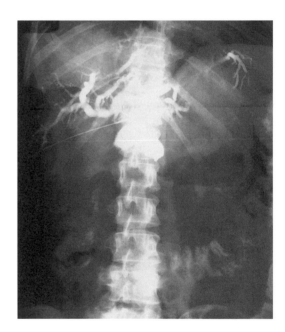

Figure 16–18. Percutaneous transhepatic cholangiogram.

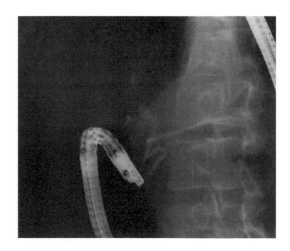

Figure 16–19. Radiographic spot film of an endoscopic retrograde cholangiopancreatogram (ERCP).

493

► *Gallstones*

Gallstones are also known as choleliths or biliary calculi. Eighty percent of these stones are formed from a combination of calcium, cholesterol, and bile pigments; however, stones can have different compositions and may be pure cholesterol or bile pigment in nature.

The population at higher risk for forming gallstones are women over the age of 40, especially if they are overweight, pregnant, or taking oral contraceptives. Native Americans are also in the high-risk group.

Gallstones are usually diagnosed during ultrasound examination or oral cholecystography (OCG). Only 20% of gallstones have sufficient calcium present to be visualized without the aid of contrast medium in the gallbladder.

The traditional method of treatment has been surgical removal (cholecystectomy); however, current treatment techniques include dissolving the stones with drug therapy, vaporizing them with lasers, pulverizing them with lithotripsy (shock-wave therapy), and removing them orally during endoscopic retrograde cholangiopancreatography.

Table 16–3. Supplies for Radiographic Examinations of the Biliary System

Oral cholecystography	Fatty meal
	Emesis basin
T-tube cholangiography	Sterile basin
	Sterile water
	Contrast medium
	Syringe with needle
	Disposable gloves
	Hemostat
	Emesis basin
Percutaneous transhepatic cholangiography	Disposable sterile gloves (at least two pair)
	Sterile basin
	Sterile water
	Contrast medium
	Syringe with needle
	Chiba or "skinny" needle
	Surgical scrub/solution for skin prep
	Sterile towels for draping
	Hemostat
	Emesis basin
Endoscopic retrograde cholangiopancreatography	Fiberoptic endoscope
	Oral anesthetic
	Contrast medium
	Disposable sterile gloves
	Sterile towels
	Emesis basin

OTHER PROCEDURAL CONSIDERATIONS

Breathing Instructions

Projections of the biliary system should be obtained during suspended expiration, as the patient is more relaxed. Inspiration is not recommended as it places the patient under greater strain and moves the gallbladder 1 to 3 in. inferiorly, which may affect part centering. The exposure should be made approximately 2 seconds after the patient stops breathing to minimize peristaltic motion.

Exposure Factors

Because the contrast media used for examination of the biliary system is not very dense, a moderate kilovoltage of 65 to 75 kVp should be used to enhance subject contrast. For fluoroscopic spots, the kilovoltage should be set no higher than 80 on the control panel; higher kVp results in poor radiographic contrast. The mAs required for overhead films depends on patient size, type of x-ray generator, film/screen speed, type of grid, and pathologic conditions that may be present.

Equipment Considerations

A radiographic table with a grid is required for all examinations of the biliary system that are performed in the radiology department. For operative cholangiography performed on a table without a grid, a portable grid is needed. A fluoroscopic unit is required for T-tube cholangiography, PTC, ERCP, and upright OCG spot films. A radiolucent support should be available for the RPO position. Other ancillary equipment is listed in *Table 16–3.*

RADIOGRAPHIC POSITIONING OF THE BILIARY SYSTEM

- ► PA GALLBLADDER (ORAL CHOLECYSTOGRAM)

- ► LAO GALLBLADDER (ORAL CHOLECYSTOGRAM)

- ► RIGHT LATERAL DECUBITUS GALLBLADDER (ORAL CHOLECYSTOGRAM)

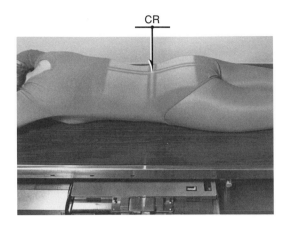

Figure 16–20. PA gallbladder, abdominal scout using 14 × 17-in. cassette.

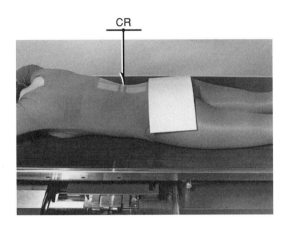

Figure 16–21. PA gallbladder, localized view using 10 × 12-in. cassette.

► PA GALLBLADDER (ORAL CHOLECYSTOGRAM)

Technical Considerations

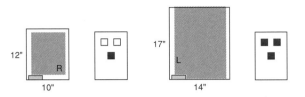

- Film size: 14 × 17 in. lengthwise (scout); 10 × 12 in. lengthwise (localized).
- Grid required.
- 65–75 kVp.
- Collimate to the abdominal walls laterally and to film size lengthwise (scout) or enough to allow 0.5-in. margins (localized).

Shielding

- Male patients should be shielded for the scout film according to department policy; all patients, especially those capable of reproduction, should be shielded for localized films.

Patient Positioning

- Assist the patient to the prone position on the table with a small pillow to support the head. **Note:** This projection can also be obtained with the patient standing facing an upright grid device.

Part Positioning

Abdominal Scout (14 × 17-in. Cassette)
- Center the midsagittal plane to the midline of the table and parallel with the long axis of the table *(Figure 16–20)*.

Localized View (10 × 12-in. Cassette)
- Center the sagittal plane midway between the spine and lateral margin of the right ribs to the midline of the table and parallel to the long axis of the table *(Figure 16–21)*.

Central Ray

Abdominal Scout (14 × 17-in. Cassette)
- Direct the central ray perpendicular to the level of the iliac crests; center the cassette to the central ray; tall patients may require centering as much as 2 to 3 in. above the iliac crests.

Localized View (10 × 12-in. Cassette)
- Direct the central ray perpendicular to the level of L2, approximately 0.5 to 1 in. above the inferior margin of the ribs (sthenic patients); center the cassette to the central ray. **Note:** Centering for hypersthenic patients should be approximately 2 in. higher and more lateral than stated; centering for asthenic or erect patients should be 1 to 2 in. lower.

Breathing Instructions

- Instruct the patient to take in a breath, blow it out, and hold it out during the exposure.

Image Evaluation

Abdominal Scout (14 × 17-in. Cassette)
- The symphysis pubis and lateral margins of the lower ribs should be seen within the collimated area; the symphysis pubis may not be seen, however, on very tall patients on which the centering has been moved upward.
- Unless pathology is present, the vertebral column should be straight and centered to the film.
- Asymmetry of the iliac crests and ischial spines indicates rotation of the pelvis.

- High contrast should be seen within the vertebrae and iliac crest; the gallbladder, if demonstrated, should also have high contrast *(Figure 16–22)*.

Localized View (10 × 12-in. Cassette)

- The gallbladder should be centered within the collimated area; the area of the biliary ducts should also be included.
- Unless pathology is present, the spine should be straight and demonstrated near the medial border of the radiograph; spinous processes should be seen at the midline of the vertebral column.
- High contrast should be seen within the vertebrae; the gallbladder, if demonstrated, should also have high contrast *(Figure 16–23)*.

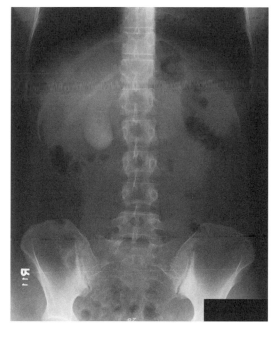 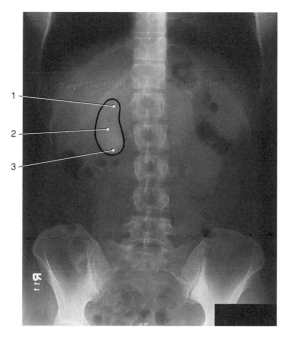

Figure 16–22. PA gallbladder, abdominal scout.

| 1. Neck | 2. Body | 3. Fundus |

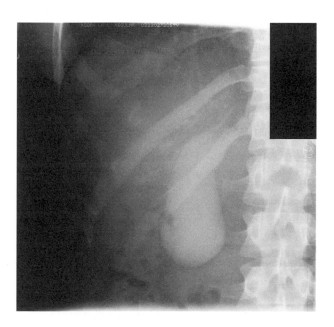

Figure 16–23. PA gallbladder, localized upright position.

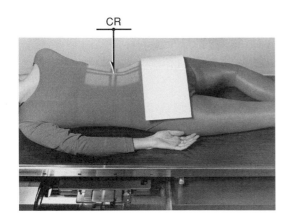

Figure 16–24. LAO gallbladder, recumbent.

► LAO GALLBLADDER (ORAL CHOLECYSTOGRAM)

Technical Considerations

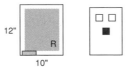

- Film size: 10 × 12 in. or 8 × 10 in. lengthwise.
- Grid required.
- 65–75 kVp.
- Collimate to allow 0.5-in. margins on all sides.

Note: The reverse oblique, the RPO, is usually preferred for T-tube and percutaneous transhepatic cholangiography; it is also used for patients unable to assume the LAO position.

Shielding

- Gonadal shielding should be used on all patients, especially patients capable of reproduction.

Patient Positioning

- Assist the patient to the prone position on the table with a small pillow to support the head; the left arm should be at the side with the right arm near the head. **Note:** This projection can also be obtained with the patient standing facing an upright grid device.

Part Positioning

- Rotate the patient to a 15° to 40° LAO position; the patient's right arm and leg can be used for support. **Note:** Very thin patients must be rotated more than hypersthenic patients to move the gallbladder away from the spine.
- Center the sagittal plane midway between the spine and lateral margin of the right ribs to the midline of the table.
- Adjust the long axis of the patient to lie parallel with the table *(Figure 16–24)*.

Central Ray

- Direct the central ray perpendicular to the level of the last rib; center the cassette to the central ray. **Note:** Centering for hypersthenic patients should be approximately 2 in. higher and more lateral than stated; centering for asthenic patients should be 1 to 2 in. lower.

Breathing Instructions

- Instruct the patient to take in a breath, blow it out, and hold it out during the exposure.

Image Evaluation

- The gallbladder should be centered within the collimated area; the area of the biliary ducts should also be included.
- Unless pathology is present, the spine should be straight and demonstrated near the medial border of the radiograph.
- The gallbladder should be demonstrated away from the vertebral column.
- High contrast should be seen within the vertebrae and iliac crest; the gallbladder, if demonstrated, should also have high contrast *(Figure 16–25)*.

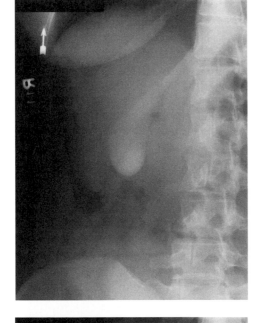

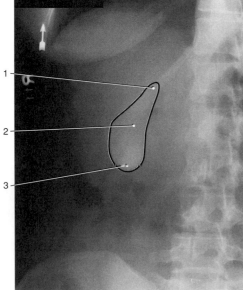

Figure 16–25. LAO gallbladder, upright.

1. Neck   2. Body   3. Fundus

► RIGHT LATERAL DECUBITUS GALLBLADDER (ORAL CHOLECYSTOGRAM)

Technical Considerations

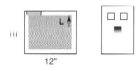

- Film size: 10 × 12 in. crosswise.
- Grid required.
- 65–75 kVp.
- Collimate to allow 0.5 in. margins on all sides.

Shielding

- Gonadal shielding should be used on all patients, especially those capable of reproduction.

Patient Positioning

- Turn the radiographic table to the 90° upright position; a wall unit may also be used.
- Assist the patient to the right lateral position on a stretcher; the right arm can be used to support the head. **Note:** This projection can also be obtained using a grid cassette with the patient lying in the right lateral position on the table.

Part Positioning

- Position the stretcher against the upright table or grid device so the patient is facing away from the film; the patient's abdomen should be as close to the grid device as possible. **Note:** It may be easier to position hypersthenic patients for an AP projection.
- Move the stretcher so the level of the last rib corresponds with the midline of the grid device. **Lock the stretcher wheels!**
- Adjust the pelvis and thorax to a true lateral position *(Figure 16–26)*.

Central Ray

- Direct the central ray horizontally to the grid device through the plane passing halfway between the lateral margin of the right ribs and the spine; center the cassette to the central ray. **Note:** When using a portable grid, it may be necessary to elevate the patient on a radiolucent support to ensure the entire gallbladder is included on the radiograph.

Breathing Instructions

- Instruct the patient to take in a breath, blow it out, and hold it out during the exposure.

Image Evaluation

- The gallbladder and spine should be seen within the collimated area.
- Unless pathology is present, the spine should be straight.
- The gallbladder should be demonstrated away from the vertebral column.
- High contrast should be seen within the vertebrae; the gallbladder, if demonstrated, should also have high contrast *(Figure 16–27)*.

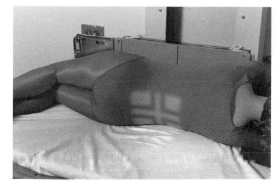

Figure 16–26. Right lateral decubitus gallbladder.

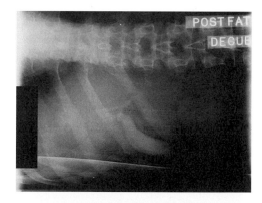

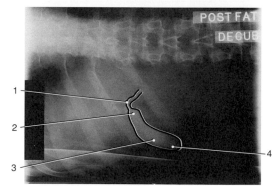

1. Cystic duct   3. Body of gallbladder   4. Fundus of gallbladder
2. Neck of gallbladder

Figure 16–27 . Decubitus gallbladder, post-fatty meal. *(Courtesy Dorothy A. Saia, BS, RT(R)).*

$\mathcal{S}$UMMARY

▶ Oral cholecystography may be performed to identify calculi and other pathology of the gallbladder; ultrasonography is frequently substituted for the routine oral cholecystogram.

▶ Patient preparation for an oral cholecystogram begins 1 to 2 days prior to the radiographic examination and includes a fatty diet followed by a fat-free meal and ingestion of oral contrast medium the evening before the examination.

▶ Cholangiography, radiographic examination of the biliary ducts, can be performed in surgery (operative), via a biliary drainage tube following surgery (T-tube or delayed), or through a long, slender needle passed directly into the biliary ducts (percutaneous transhepatic).

▶ To ensure visualization of small stones, the contrast medium used for cholangiography is often low density.

▶ The biliary ducts can also be examined using a fiberoptic endoscope that passes from the mouth to the hepatopancreatic ampulla (endoscopic retrograde cholangiopancreatography).

▶ For the oral cholecystogram, a "scout" film is usually obtained using a 14 × 17-in. cassette to locate the gallbladder and assess visualization.

▶ All radiographs of the biliary system should be obtained during suspended expiration.

▶ To enhance subject contrast, 65 to 75 kVp is recommended for all radiography of the biliary system; fluoroscopic spots should be obtained using no more than 80 kVp.

$\mathcal{Q}$UESTIONS FOR CRITICAL THINKING & APPLICATION

1. If a patient has a cholecystectomy, is bile still manufactured by the liver? If so, what happens to it as it can no longer be stored in the gallbladder? Why must a patient modify his or her fat intake after a cholecystectomy?

2. Scientists are trying to synthetically reproduce the hormone cholecystokinin. Why would this chemical be marketed as a weight-loss product?

3. A patient with a history of a "gallbladder attack" has an oral cholecystogram performed that reveals the presence of gallstones. Generally, where in the abdomen would the patient have experienced pain during the attack? What would cause pain in such an "attack"?

4. How does a contrast medium taken orally for a cholecystogram find its way to the gallbladder causing it to visualize?

5. Newborn infants often appear jaundiced and in fact may have a condition known as neonatal (physiologic) jaundice. What causes this condition? How is it treated?

6. Hypersensitivity to iodine is not necessarily a contraindication to endoscopic retrograde cholangiopancreatography. Explain why.

7. Why might knowledge of the patient's bilirubin count be important information when performing an oral cholecystogram?

8. When asked about vomiting or diarrhea, the patient scheduled for an oral cholecystogram tells you he vomited several hours after taking the pills and had mild diarrhea in the morning. Describe how you would proceed.

9. When obtaining the patient history, you discover that your patient did not accurately follow all of the preexamination instructions and ate a light breakfast that included toast with butter prior to her oral cholecystogram. What implications could this have on the success of the procedure?

10. A hypersthenic patient has been scheduled for an oral cholecystogram. Where would you expect the gallbladder to be located? What are the considerations for performing the LAO projection?

FILM CRITIQUE

Given this scout film taken prior to localized spot films of the gallbladder *(Figure 16–28),* state the amount of patient rotation you would use for the LAO projection and describe, using bony landmarks, how would you localize the gallbladder for this projection?

Was patient positioning and alignment for this AP projection accurate?

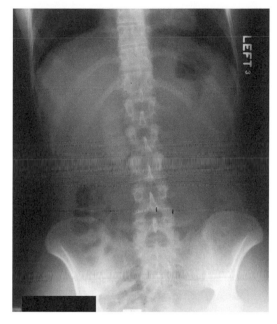

Figure 16–28.

MAMMOGRAPHY

ANGELA M. PICKWICK, MS, RT(R)(M)

▶ OBJECTIVES

Following the completion of this chapter the student will be able to:

- Given diagrams or radiographs, name and describe the anatomy of the breast.

- Define terminology associated with breast imaging, to include anatomy, procedures, and pathology of both the male and female breast.

- Describe the basic and recommended routine projections of the breast.

- Discuss the alternate projections of the breast for imaging "hard to demonstrate" lesions.

- Describe procedural modifications for patients who have an unusual body habitus, physical limitations, or breast augmentation.

- State the criteria used to determine positioning accuracy on radiographs of the breast and evaluate radiographs of the breast in terms of positioning, centering, image quality, radiographic anatomy, and pathology.

- Describe the process of needle localization for biopsy procedures.

- Describe the procedure for imaging breast biopsy specimens.

- Explain the importance of critical quality assurance and control related to breast imaging.

With one in every eight women developing breast cancer today, breast imaging has become very highly visible in the public domain. A woman's best defense against this disease is a monthly breast self-examination, a clinical examination of the breasts by her physician, and the mammogram. With improved dedicated radiographic units, film/screen combinations, and knowledge in the area of breast imaging, many lives can be saved through the early detection of this life-threatening disease. Governmental agencies and professional organizations within the field of radiology have joined forces to try to ensure that breast imaging services across the United States provide high-quality images for optimum interpretation by the radiologist. Along with early detection and treatment, it is hoped this effort will decrease the number of women who die from breast cancer each year.

With much detailed information and guidelines provided to experienced radiographers for optimum imaging, this chapter provides only content at an entry level for the student radiographer. Should the reader desire to become specialized in this area of radiography, there may be several requirements. Further clinical experience, study, and perhaps ARRT certification in this area may be required. It is critically important for the student radiographer to understand the unique considerations for this radiographic specialty. Therefore, the psychological aspects of working with both female and male patients will be addressed, as well as the technical aspects of operating dedicated units with very specific components and strict processing quality control guidelines. Although the focus of this chapter is positioning, it is important to include the distinct technical differences in producing quality mammograms in contrast to the technical aspects of other radiographic examinations. The very critical technique and art of mammographic positioning and variations of the mammographic procedure are presented along with the complementary imaging modalities. The future of breast imaging is also discussed.

Throughout this chapter, the terms *breast imaging* and *mammography* are used interchangeably, as are the terms *projection* and *view*. This may be confusing for some students; however, in viewing the mammogram, the films are hung on the viewbox in the same orientation as they were taken. For example, a right lateral projection of the breast is displayed on the viewbox in the same orientation as if we were looking at the patient's right breast positioned in the unit under compression. This is different from regular radiography, where films are hung on the viewboxes as if the viewer was facing and observing the patient (ie, a PA projection of the chest is hung so the viewer sees an AP view of the chest, with the heart on the patient's left and viewer's right). By experiencing how the films are taken and observing this viewing process, the student radiographer is assisted in understanding this concept fully.

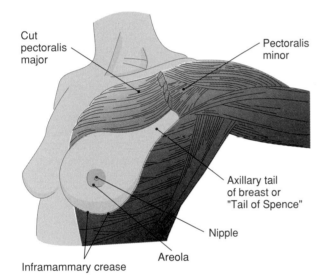

Cut pectoralis major
Pectoralis minor
Axillary tail of breast or "Tail of Spence"
Nipple
Areola
Inframammary crease

Figure 17–1. Anatomy of the breast and its relationship to the chest muscle.

▶ ANATOMY OF THE BREAST

It is important to know the basic anatomy of the breast to obtain the most diagnostic mammogram possible. Recognizing the critical landmarks and using them to optimize positioning the breast in each of the projections will greatly benefit the patient by adequately demonstrating various pathologic conditions.

The breast, or mammary (lactation) gland, is found in both the male and the female of the human species. In the female, it serves as an accessory reproductive organ for milk secretion for the nourishment of offspring. Being a conical structure, the breast attaches posteriorly to the anterior chest wall at the pectoralis major muscle *(Figure 17–1)*. The breasts extend approximately between the second and seventh ribs, and in the lateral dimension between the sternum and axillary region. The **nipple,** located at the most anterior or distal region, is surrounded by the **areola** (ah-RE-o-lah), an area where the skin is more darkly pigmented. The areola is composed of sebaceous glands and, on the circumference, by several hair follicles. Being thicker toward the base of the breast, the skin becomes thinner as it reaches the apex, or nipple region. The skin contains sebaceous and sweat glands, as well as hair follicles. Skin pores can often be seen on the mammogram. A very important landmark, the **inframammary crease,** is the convergence of the inferior aspect of the breast and the anterior chest wall.

Internally, nerves, blood vessels, and lymphatic vessels supply the breast tissue. The lymphatics drain the breast posteriorly from the nipple to nodes in the axillary regions and to several internal mammary nodes *(Figure 17–2)*. The importance of the lymphatics relates to how easily breast cancer cells can spread to other areas of the body. The axillary nodes are in contact with the extension of breast tissue called the **axillary tail** or **tail of Spence.** Unfortunately, this contact makes the lymphatic system an excellent transport mechanism for these deadly cells, as the axillary tail is located in the upper, outer quadrant of the breast from which a large number of cancers arise. Blood vessels that supply the breast, especially veins, can also be seen on the mammographic films. In later years, small calcifications may appear in the vessels, but usually do not indicate anything of a serious nature.

About 15 to 20 glandular lobes compose the breast and are separated by dense connective tissue and fat, or adipose tissue. Apart from supporting the glandular lobes, these **suspensory ligaments,** also known as **Cooper's ligaments,** support the entire breast weight by attachments that extend from the pectoralis

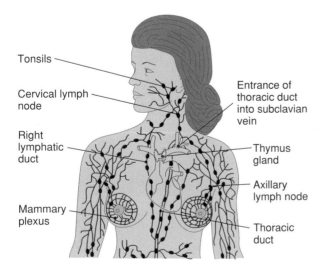

Tonsils
Cervical lymph node
Right lymphatic duct
Mammary plexus
Entrance of thoracic duct into subclavian vein
Thymus gland
Axillary lymph node
Thoracic duct

Figure 17–2. Lymphatic vessels in the chest region.

major muscle fascia to the skin anteriorly *(Figure 17–3)*. In the later years, these ligaments become weakened and the breasts "droop" from the normal position they once had in younger years. It is a challenge to the radiographer to perform diagnostic mammography, as size and shape of the thorax and breasts vary greatly from patient to patient.

Composition and density of the breast can be affected by many factors, including age and body fat composition. As puberty approaches and prior to the first pregnancy, the female breast becomes very dense from the abundance of fibroglandular tissue which develops from the effects of the ovarian hormones. This **fibroglandular type** of breast can also be seen in **nulliparous** (nu-LIP-ah-rus) females, those who have never had children. In this type of patient, the lobes of glandular tissue enlarge, the ducts become larger, and some body fat is deposited. This type of dense fibroglandular tissue requires more radiographic expo-sure. In practice, if the the first part of her reproductive and adult progum to the breast loses much of its fibroglandular characteristics and becomes more fatty replaced, resulting in a **fibroglandular fatty breast.** This average type of breast tissue is slightly easier to penetrate on the mammogram, so less exposure is required to achieve a diagnostic film than on the fibroglandular breast. The last category is the **postmenopausal breast.** Here the breast is primarily fatty replaced as there has been measurable atrophy of the glandular tissue, and is therefore very easily penetrated. Care must be taken not to overpenetrate the breast in this category *(Figure 17–4)*.

Breasts of nulliparous women tend to be very dense, but in women with multiple pregnancies, the breast loses its glandular tissue, especially in those who have breast-fed their children. The fatty replacement of the breast begins from the posterior aspect of the breast to the anterior, extending into the lateral region. Aside from age, parity and medications (especially hormones) affect breast density. Women who have experienced menopause and have declining hormonal levels have even less glandular tissue. In contrast to this, the postmenopausal patient who is undergoing hormone replacement therapy has a breast that is somewhat denser and radiographically appears like that of a younger woman. It is critically important to record these factors on the patient's history sheet to provide appropriate exposure factors and proper centering to yield diagnostic films that can be accurately interpreted.

The actual anatomy of the breast, specifically the inframammary crease, nipple, and pectoralis muscle, becomes quite useful and critical for positioning the breast accurately in each of the projections. **Breast mobility** is a concept that must be understood to correctly position the breast and enhance compression. It also contributes to the maximum visualization of the breast on the mediolateral oblique projection. The breast has some mobility at the lateral and inferior margins, unlike the medial and superior margins. Elevation of the breast, from the inframammary crease upward toward the superior aspect, allows for more effective compression on the craniocaudad projection. Likewise, the lateral mobility allows the radiographer to position the cassette parallel to the pectoralis muscle and enhance the compression in the mediolateral oblique projection. Therefore, placing the mobile part of the breast on the immobile part of the unit and the immobile part of the breast against the movable compression device helps to place as much breast tissue as possible on the film. This action prevents superior breast tissue from being sacrificed when the compression device moves inferiorly against the chest wall on the craniocaudad projection. It applies again to the medial aspect of the breast when the device moves laterally across the sternal area on the mediolateral oblique projection. These aspects are addressed later in the chapter.

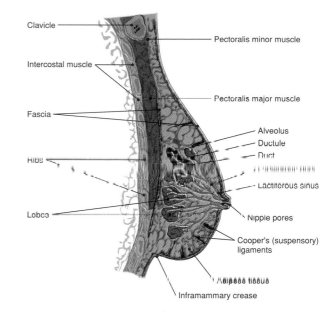

Figure 17–3. Sectional image of the breast demonstrates the suspensory ligaments.

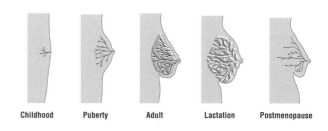

Figure 17–4. Different types of breast tissue.

BREAST PATHOLOGY

Mammography is excellent for imaging many abnormalities of the breast. Changes in symmetry of breast tissue density, architectural or ductal patterns, contour, or skin thickening can be demonstrated. Masses, calcifications, and dilation of veins or ducts can also be visualized. The most frequently seen process in menstruating women is that of fibrocystic changes in the breast, which make the breast radiographically dense as a result of multiple cysts within the breast tissue. Although some of these pathologies are benign, others are malignant and often fatal. Despite correlating the images with the clinical history, biopsy with clinical laboratory evaluation is the only method of verifying a diagnosis so appropriate treatment can be rendered. The radiographer provides optimum service for the patient if he or she begins to recognize demonstrable pathology and then relates symptoms and history to use appropriate positioning and technical factors.

▶ PROCEDURAL CONSIDERATIONS

Breast imaging is a very challenging area of radiography. Because the attitudes relating to breast examination and handling of the breasts may be more complex and sensitive, the radiographer should be mindful that some psychological considerations are of great importance in working with a patient to achieve a high-

▶ Related Terminology

biopsy (BĪ-op-se)—pathologic examination of body tissue that has been removed from the body

carcinoma (kar-se-NŌ-mah)—malignant neoplasm or growth that appears radiographically dense, is frequently of irregular shape, and comprises epithelial cells that tend to metastasize easily to surrounding tissue

fibroadenoma (fī-brō-adn-O-mah)—frequently seen in women under the age of 30, a radiographically dense, encapsulated, round, and movable benign tumor that develops from epithelial and fibroblastic tissue brought on by higher than normal estrogen levels

fibrocystic changes (disease)—development of benign cystic spaces within the ducts from monthly hormone fluctuations that cause cysts to form throughout the breast tissues that might mask or hide other malignant tumors

fine-needle aspiration (FNA)—biopsy technique using a fine needle to remove cells from a localized breast lesion for pathologic evaluation

gynecomastia (jin-e-kō-MAS-te-ah)—most common disorder that results in excessive development of the male breast from physiologic, hormonal, or pharmacologic causes

hormone replacement therapy (HRT)—prescribing of hormones for postmenopausal women to maintain their hormone levels to decrease symptoms and complications that could arise from declining estrogen levels

intraductal papilloma (pap-i-LŌ-mah)—benign, lobulated neoplasm, composed of benign epithelial tissue and located in the walls of ducts of the breast with a "berrylike" shape

lactation—milk secretion from the breast

lumpectomy—removal of a tumor without excision of surrounding tissue and lymph nodes

Mammography Quality Standards Act (MQSA)—legislation passed in Congress in October 1994 to improve and standardize optimum quality of mammography

mastectomy (mas-TEK-tah-mē)—removal of the breast

mastitis (mas-TĪ-tis)—inflammation of breast tissue

mastorrhagia (mas-to-RA-je-ah)—copious discharge of blood from the breast

microcalcifications—minute calcium deposits in the breast that could possibly indicate the presence of malignancy, although they can be benign

multiparity—condition of having had more than one pregnancy that resulted in offspring alive or stillborn

nulliparity—condition of not having ever been pregnant

parity—condition of being pregnant and delivering a child

symmetry—similarity in size, shape, and composition of anatomy so that one side of the body, or the breasts in this case, is a "mirror image" of the other side

Table 17–1. Guidelines for Performing Mammography on Symptom-free Women[a]

- American Cancer Society—yearly mammograms beginning at age 40
- American College of Radiology—yearly or alternate-year mammograms beginning at age 40

[a]These guidelines are current as of May, 1997, but are under review by ACS and ACR.

quality study. It is necessary to treat the patient with sensitivity and respect, as the radiographer does not know what prior experiences may interfere with obtaining an adequate study.

Another area of concern for most patients is the effect of radiation on the breast and associated cancer risks. Many patients ask the radiographer, "Is the radiation harmful to me? Can I get cancer from this mammogram?" The study of radiation biology, in groups of people such as the survivors of the atomic bombs in Japan and patients from the 1940s and 1950s treated with high doses of ionizing radiation for various disease processes, has provided knowledge that radiation can provoke breast cancer. Mammography patients, however, were not among these groups. With the low levels of radiation used in medical imaging and the improved equipment and film/screen systems, the benefits of mammography outweigh the risks. Some data indicate that breast exposure later in life is safer than in the younger years. The reason for this might be that the postmenopausal breast has more fatty replacement tissue and declining fibroglandular tissue; it is the glandular tissue that is so sensitive to radiation. The research surrounding this issue progresses today. Even though the American College of Radiology (ACR) recommends that the average dose not exceed 0.3 rad per projection, most sites average 0.1 rad per projection. Considering there are four standard projections in a mammogram, 0.4 to 1.2 rad seems to be the average glandular dose to the patient.

Mammograms are performed on patients with symptoms (*diagnostic*) and without symptoms (*screening*). The American Cancer Society and the American College of Radiology have established guidelines for mammography on women without symptoms. These guidelines are illustrated in *Table 17–1*.

These guidelines are not universally accepted. Deviation from the guidelines depends on the patient's medical history. It is the responsibility of the patient and her physician to make the final decision on how routinely this examination is performed. Although these guidelines are based on assumptions that benefit outweighs risk, the debate continues. Some researchers suggest that mammography under age 50 is not worthwhile, whereas others feel that younger patients with more aggressive diseases can be detected and helped earlier. In any case, it is the responsibility of the radiographer performing mammography to employ all the methods available to minimize excess dose to the patient. Being knowledgeable in the areas of patient care, equipment, exposure, positioning, and film processing will ensure optimum patient care with respect to providing diagnostic images at the lowest possible dose.

PATIENT PREPARATION

When beginning the mammographic procedure, it is important to be professional and reassuring as the patient's anxiety level may be high. Radiographers should introduce themselves to the patient to begin establishing a trusting relationship for accomplishing the procedure. Using the sense of touch when accompanying the patient to the dressing room, as well as before you begin the procedure itself, may relieve a little of the anxiety before actually positioning the breast on the radiographic unit. Voice modulation and clear instructions let patients know that they are your primary focus and begin to build a sense of trust. The radiographer needs to be proficient in responding to basic first aid, as occasionally a patient's anxiety may cause him or her to feel faint or even hyperventilate. Displaying confidence when working with the patient helps the patient feel more comfortable about having the examination performed.

Male patients cannot be overlooked. Although the majority of mammograms are performed on females, males are not exempt from developing breast diseases. Development of pathologies such as gynecomastia, cysts, hematomas, abscesses, enlarged lymph nodes, fibroadenomas, intraductal papillomas, and even cancer may lead to a mammographic examination. Just as the radiographer needs to be sensitive to the female patient, the male patient may be equally apprehensive. The first cause of anxiety results from a man coming to a "women's center" for a "woman's" procedure. If possible, the male patient should complete his preprocedural referral and insurance information away from the waiting room of female patients. Likewise, it may be feasible to have the male patient enter the radiographic room from a location where he is least likely to meet a female patient in her gown. Embarrassment is not limited to the female sex. Most men are just as modest as women and are very shy about having the examination performed. Males should also have the procedure, including the importance of breast compression, explained to them.

Prior to arrival at the radiology facility, the patient should have been instructed to refrain from using deodorant, perfumes, lotions, or powders of any kind on the breast, chest, or underarm areas. Components of these products may cause unwanted artifacts on the resultant breast images that may be mistaken for unfortunate pathologic conditions. After being identified and proceeding to a changing area, the patient

MAMMOGRAPHY PATIENT INFORMATION SHEET

Patient Name:_____ Date: _____

Birth Date:_____ Radiology Number: _____

Referring Physician: _____

Mammogram History:

Previous mammogram _____ yes _____ no

If yes, date: ___/___/___ , Location: _____

Last clinical breast exam: ___/___/___

Practice breast self-exam _____ monthly _____ occasionally _____ not at all

Current Symptoms: _____ None			
	R	L	How Long?
Pain	_____	_____	_____
Dimpling	_____	_____	_____
Nipple Retraction	_____	_____	_____
Nipple Discharge	_____	_____	_____

Menstrual History:	Date
Menarche_____	_____
Menopause _____	_____
Date of Last Period:	_____
Nursed within 6 mos. (Y/N)	_____
Uterus Removed (Y/N)	_____
Ovaries Removed (Y/N)	_____

Previous Breast Problems: _____ None			
	R	L	How Long?
Cancer	_____	_____	_____
Lumpectomy	_____	_____	_____
Mastectomy	_____	_____	_____
Radiation	_____	_____	_____
Chemotherapy	_____	_____	_____
Aspiration	_____	_____	_____
Biopsy	_____	_____	_____
Reduction	_____	_____	_____
Implants	_____	_____	_____

Family History of Breast Cancer: _____ None	
	Age
Mother	_____
Sister	_____
Aunt	_____
Daughter	_____
Grandmother	_____

Personal History of Cancer: yes _____ no _____

If yes, site: _____ date: _____

Medication: _____ None	
	How Long?
Female Hormones	_____
Birth Control	_____
Fertility Drugs	_____
Other	_____

Childbirth History: _____ None	
Number of Pregnancies	_____
Age at First Delivery	_____
Number of Full Term Deliveries	_____

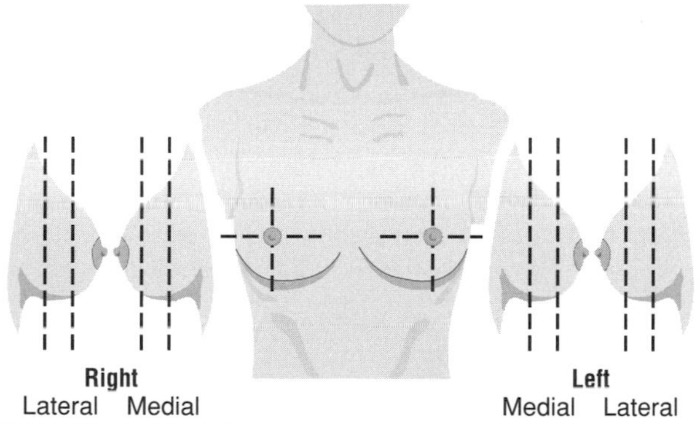

Right — Lateral Medial

Left — Medial Lateral

If Diagnostic, Reason for Exam:

Technologist's Remarks:

Technologist's Signature: _____

Figure 17–5. Sample history sheet for mammography. *(Courtesy of St. Luke Hospital, Ft. Thomas, Kentucky.)*

should be questioned about whether he or she followed these instructions. If not, the patient should be directed to a rest room, given appropriate soap, water, and towels, and instructed to wash the unwanted materials from the examination areas. The patient should then be instructed to remove all articles of clothing and jewelry from the chest region. Even though the unclothed breast is imaged during the radiographic examination, a gown should be provided for the patient's modesty. This gown should open in the front for ease of positioning when the patient's examination begins.

A thorough patient history should be obtained and recorded prior to imaging the breasts (*Figure 17–5*). Even though there is no standardized history sheet across the field of radiology, the following aspects of the patient's history are important in assisting the radiographer in evaluating the density of the breast and the appropriate technical factors to produce a high-quality radiograph. Other than the patient's

Table 17–2. Clinical Signs of Breast Cancer

The following clinical signs may indicate a malignancy,
especially when more than one is present.

- Lump
- Thickening of breast tissue
- Swelling
- Dimpling or puckering
- Distortion of shape or size
- Retraction or scaliness of nipple
- Pain or tenderness
- Nipple discharge
- Redness or persistent skin irritation

demographic information, birth date, and name of the referring physician, the following aspects are answered by the patient or asked by the radiographer:

- Description of the symptoms and location of the area of concern, including duration
- Family history of breast cancer or any other kind of cancer
- Personal history of breast cancer or any other kind of cancer
- Location and time of previous breast surgeries, biopsies, or cyst aspirations, and pathologic results
- Parity/history of breast-feeding
- Date of last menstrual period and regularity of menses
- Medications taken daily, especially hormone replacement therapy
- Date of previous clinical breast examination and Pap smear by a physician
- Last mammographic study and location of films

Considerations that might be added to the radiographer's section of the procedural/history sheet include:

- Presence of tattoos, scars, nevi, skin tags, or other skin abnormalities
- Documentation of scars or location of symptoms on a diagrammatic representation of the patient's chest and breast regions
- Other pertinent information for the radiologist as determined by the radiographer

A signature line should be included at the bottom of the history sheet. *Figure 17–5* provides an example of a history form that may be used. Once the patient has completed the history sheet and has been informed of the critical importance of breast compression as part of the procedure, she or he should sign the form to indicate the understanding of the procedure. Should the patient not be able to tolerate adequate compression, then this information should also be documented on the radiographer's section of the history sheet. In some settings, the radiographer is also certified to perform a clinical breast examination on the patient. Documentation of this should also be given to the radiologist interpreting the mammogram, along with the history sheet, to assist in an accurate interpretation. *Table 17–2* identifies clinical signs that may contribute to accurate diagnosis.

The location of symptoms or abnormalities should be documented on the history sheet with the use of a localization method. Either the clock method or the quadrant method of localization may be used, although the clock method *(Figure 17–6)* is somewhat confusing as the "3 o'clock" location on the medial aspect of the right breast is not at the same location on the left breast. It may be preferable, therefore, to use the quadrant method *(Figure 17–7)* to keep the description of symptoms uniform. Each breast has the same quadrants relative to uniform relationship to anatomic regions.

It is very important for the patient to have any previous mammogram available for comparison with each study that succeeds it. If the patient has not returned to the imaging site of the initial study, then she or he should make every effort to bring the radiographs or have them sent from the previous facility to the new site for comparison. This practice is quite common with the changes in reimbursement policies and patients frequently changing their insurance or HMOs. It is extremely important for the interpreting radiologist to have the previous mammogram to look for changes that have occurred since the last examination. Some breast architecture is normal for one patient but perhaps not for another; therefore, changes might be easily misinterpreted without being able to use previous examinations for comparison. If no preceding films are available and a suspicious area is present, additional views or a follow-up study may be required within the next 3 to 6 months following the mammogram.

When the patient enters the examination room, the radiographer should explain the entire procedure, including the operation of the equipment, to the patient. It is possible that the patient has heard others' experiences with the examination and may be apprehensive. Most patients do not fully understand the concept and importance of maximum breast compression and how the radiographic unit is used to accomplish it. Communication with the patient is of key importance as correct positioning of the breast in any projection may be the difference between an accurate and an inaccurate interpretation.

On completion of the entire procedure, the patient should be informed as to when and from whom the results of the mammogram can be acquired. She should be told the time frame in which her referring physician will receive the report and asked what understanding she has about getting the results. The patient should call her physician's office for the results if no clear instructions were given prior to the procedure.

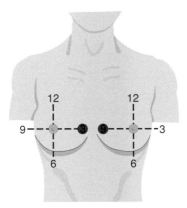

Figure 17–6. Clock method of localization.

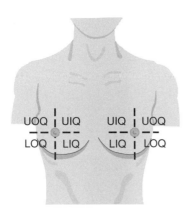

Figure 17–7. Quadrant method of localization.

ROOM PREPARATION

It is very important to prepare the radiographic room prior to the patient's entrance to avoid increasing the patient's anxiety. The dedicated mammographic unit *(Figure 17–8)* should be turned on with the tube appropriately warmed up. The face of the cassette holder, compression device, and other surfaces that come into contact with the patient should be cleaned with a disinfectant solution before the next patient's examination begins. A cassette should be inserted into the cassette holder and lead markers correctly placed to indicate the right or left breast and the view being produced. An appropriate number of cassettes should be available to perform the study without interruption.

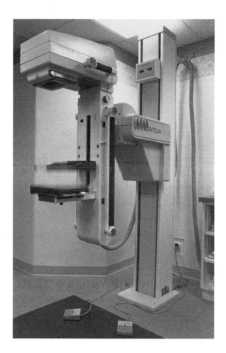

Figure 17–8. Mammographic unit.

POSITIONING CONSIDERATIONS

Radiographic examination of the breast is used to demonstrate the architecture of the breast and possible pathology. The recommended or routine projections of the breast serve to provide views of the entire breast in two dimensions to localize a mass or lesion. Correct positioning of the breast is required for accurate diagnosis. Routinely, the **craniocaudad (CC)** and **mediolateral oblique (MLO)** projections are obtained separately on each breast (four projections for the patient with two breasts). To obtain the craniocaudad projection, the film tray is elevated to the level of the inframammary crease. If the film tray is too high, inferior and posterior tissue will not be seen, and if the tray is too low, the breast will droop and superior and posterior tissue will be missed. Once the film tray is at the correct height, the breast being examined is then gently lifted and pulled forward onto the film holder. The patient should be rotated slightly to ensure that the medial and posterior breast tissue is demonstrated. If the medial side is not imaged on the craniocaudad projection, it may not be included in the examination. Pectoralis major muscle will be seen on at least 20% of the patients.

The mediolateral oblique projection is obtained with the C-arm turned 30° to 70°, depending on the patient size; very thin patients generally require a greater angle than overweight patients. The angle of the C-arm should match the angle of the patient's pectoralis major muscle to include all the glandular tissue *(Figure 17–9)*. On most patients, the pectoralis major muscle should be seen down to the level of the nipple.

Because the nipple may be mistaken for a lesion that is not present, the nipple should be in profile whenever possible. Breast tissue should not be sacrificed, however, to get the nipple in profile. If it is impossible to get the nipple in profile, this should be documented on the history sheet. A second projection of the anterior aspect of the breast with the nipple in profile may be requested, if needed.

The radiographer must strive to include maximum breast tissue on the radiograph, while applying adequate breast compression to produce a high-contrast, high-resolution image. A hard plexiglass plate is used to compress the breast. Breast compression can easily be accomplished by using a foot pedal, which allows the radiographer to use both hands to position the patient's breast tissue optimally. The machine will apply anywhere from 25 to 35 pounds of pressure to the breast. Compression may also be applied manually. Because it requires the use of one hand, however, the radiographer only has the other hand with which to do the positioning of the breast. Compression should only be applied sufficiently to cause the breast to feel taut to the fingertips at contact. Some patients will feel some discomfort, but none should feel real pain. The patient should be encouraged to relax her or his muscles so that maximum breast tissue can be demonstrated. This concept is especially true for the mediolateral oblique position, which is the most helpful because it shows all aspects of the breast from the inframammary crease to the tail of the breast.

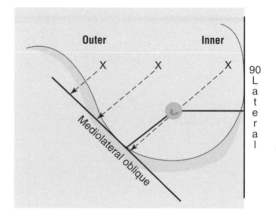

Figure 17–9. Mediolateral oblique versus 90° lateral positioning.

Adequate Breast Compression
- Flattens and separates breast structures, minimizing superimposition
- Decreases OID by decreasing tissue thickness, thereby improving visibility of detail
- Reduces radiation exposure caused by decreased tissue thickness
- Immobilizes the patient
- Produces a more uniform density

When performing mammography on either a small-breasted woman or a male patient where breast tissue may be minimal, it may be difficult to bring the breast tissue forward without the compression device striking the radiographer's hand before the device reaches the breast. Even though commercially available instruments can be purchased, a simple flexible rubber spatula can be used to bring the breast tissue onto the cassette holder when the radiographer's fingers will no longer fit between the compression device and the cassette holder.

As a final comment regarding compression, the patient should never be left in the unit with compression longer than the time it takes to step behind the leaded glass barrier and make the exposure. Many units allow the radiographer to release the compression from the control panel at the conclusion of the exposure without having to do it manually on the unit. This immediately takes the pressure off the breast so

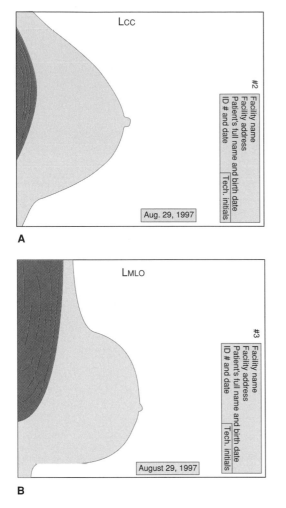

A

B

Figure 17–10. Note the use of the lead markers to indicate the breast being examined and the projection. **(A)** Craniocaudad. **(B)** Mediolateral oblique.

Table 17–3. Appropriate Abbreviations for Mammographic Projections

Routine projections	
Craniocaudad	CC
Mediolateral oblique	MLO
Alternate projections	
Caudocranial	FB (meaning "from below")
Lateromedial oblique	LMO
Projections for "hard to demonstrate" lesions	
Exaggerated craniocaudad	XCCL
Cleavage	CV
Axillary tail	AT
Roll medial	RM
Roll lateral	RL
Tangential	TAN
90° mediolateral	ML
90° lateromedial	LM
Spot compression	Usually identified by small paddle
Magnification	M
Implant displaced	ID

Adapted from the American College of Radiology Labeling Codes.

the patient can relax. Sometimes it may be necessary to release it by hand on the unit. This is acceptable, but not the quickest assistance to the patient, who may be both uncomfortable and anxious.

Labeling of the breast image is extremely important. The American College of Radiology has provided guidelines for uniformity of labeling so that the radiographs are not lost or misinterpreted, as mammograms may travel between facilities. *Table 17–3* lists the various abbreviations indicating the view being presented. It is assumed that the student already understands the concept of placement of a right or left marker on the cassette for the purpose of identifying the appropriate side of the body being examined.

The labeling should be permanent and provide the facility name, patient name (both first and last names), patient's distinctive identification number or date of birth, and date of the examination. Lead markers must be used to indicate the projection (ie, CC or MLO) and the lateral (ie, right or left). These markers should be placed on the cassette or cassette holder adjacent to the breast and closest to the axillary aspect. The initials of the radiographer performing the examination should be placed either on the cassette and exposed on the film or on the area of the patient's identification. Even though flash cards are not yet required for the patient/facility data, they are strongly recommended because they are permanently imprinted on the radiograph. Each cassette should be identified with small numbers so that artifacts may be traced and regular cleaning can be documented. Separate date stickers are recommended by the American College of Radiology for facilitating reading of the date with overhead, not transmitted, light. Documenting technical factors is recommended also so that comparison films can be done with accuracy in the future *(Figure 17–10)*.

Gonadal shielding should be used on all patients, especially those of reproductive age, even though the central ray is often being directed 90° from the patient's torso in some projections. The lead apron should be placed around the waist so the abdomen's anterior aspect is shielded. Should the dedicated unit be used to position in an alternate way to accommodate body habitus or physical limitations, the central ray may point directly to the abdominal region. The patient's head is turned away from the side being examined as a result of proper positioning; this also assists in radiation protection as the eyes are turned away from the beam.

ALTERNATE PROJECTIONS/PROCEDURES

Supplementary or advanced projections are taken when patients cannot assume the positions for the routine projections or when a lesion is not able to be included on the routine images. The **caudocranial** projection can be obtained when a patient cannot assume the position for the standard craniocaudad projection. The position of the mammographic unit can be modified to a certain degree to accommodate the patient's body build or lack of mobility. For example, for an older patient whose spine has become very kyphotic or one who has a pacemaker, it may be difficult to get the breast on the cassette holder with adequate compression. A possible solution is to turn the C-arm 180° so the x-ray tube is below and the cassette holder is at the cranial aspect. The breast then is positioned so the cassette holder is placed at the most superior aspect of the breast, snugly against the chest wall, while the compression device elevates the infra-

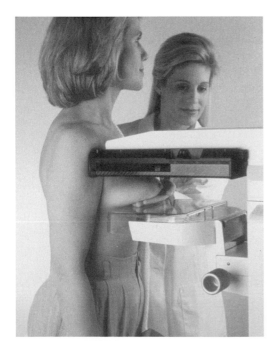

Figure 17–11. Caudocranial (FB) position. *(Courtesy of LORAD, a subsidiary of Trex Medical Corporation.)*

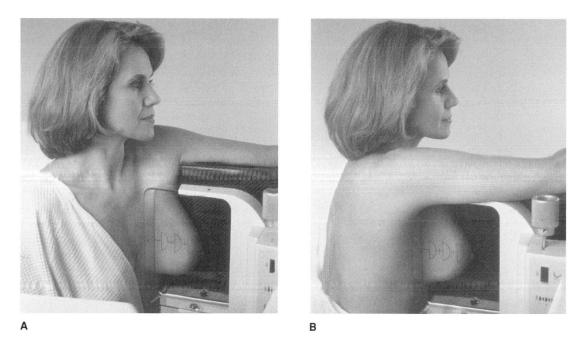

A   B

Figure 17–12. Mediolateral **(A)** and lateromedial **(B)** positions.*(Photos courtesy of LORAD, a subsidiary of Trex Medical Corporation.)*

mammary margin to complete the compression of the breast against the holder. To accomplish this, the patient must be able to straddle the tube head *(Figure 17–11)*. This accommodation is referred to as the **caudocranial** or **FB** ("from below") projection. This projection may also be used to image a small breast or a male breast or to localize a lesion in the inferior portion of the breast prior to surgery.

True 90° **mediolateral** or **lateromedial** projections are sometimes obtained to complement the mediolateral oblique projection to verify a finding that may be demonstrated on the routine craniocaudad and/or mediolateral oblique projections. To localize a lesion in the third dimension in the breast, a 90° mediolateral or lateromedial projection can demonstrate whether the lesion is in the medial or the lateral aspect of the breast *(Figure 17–12)*. For example, a lesion in the upper inner quadrant of the breast that appears below the nipple on the mediolateral oblique will appear above the nipple on the 90° mediolateral projection if the lesion is in the medial aspect of the breast. Conversely, if the lesion is located in the lower aspect of the breast on the mediolateral oblique projection and appears below the nipple on the 90° lateral projection, then the lesion is located in the lateral portion of the breast *(Figure 17–13)*. If the lesion is seen in about the same position in both the mediolateral oblique and 90° lateral projections, then it can be assumed that the lesion is in the central region of the breast.

A **tangential** projection provides a view of the area in question without superimposition of tissue over a lesion. It aids in determining if calcifications are within the breast or on the surface of the skin. Just as in general radiography, the "skimming" effect of the central ray across the area marked by the lead marker produces an image that will assist in separating a palpable mass from surrounding dense breast tissue. The radiographer must firmly hold the breast with the marker in profile as the compression is applied.

Breast tissue can be rolled medially or laterally so previously superimposed tissues in the craniocaudad projection do not appear in the same region. This can be accomplished by rolling the breast tissue between the hands and placing the breast on the cassette holder with compression for another craniocaudad projection. The radiographer should stand on the medial side of the affected breast and, with one hand on the cranial aspect breast, roll the superior tissue to the medial side while the other hand, positioned under the abreast, rolls the inferior tissue laterally. The compression is then applied to the breast so as to keep the tissue from being superimposed, as it was on the original craniocaudad projection. If one wants to see the superior tissue rolled to the lateral side, the radiographer's position is reversed and the roll is accomplished from the lateral side of the patient *(Figure 17–14)*.

An **exaggerated craniocaudad** projection is used when a lesion is suspected in the lateral aspect of the breast and cannot be adequately imaged on the conventional craniocaudad projection. In about 10% of all patients, the tail of Spence, or axillary tail, wraps around the pectoralis major muscle and cannot be adequately demonstrated on the standard craniocaudad projection. In this case, the patient's body must be rotated about 45° so the lateral aspect of the breast is placed on the cassette holder. The C-arm can be angled 5° toward the lateral side so as to avoid the compression of the humeral head of the shoulder *(Figure 17–15)*.

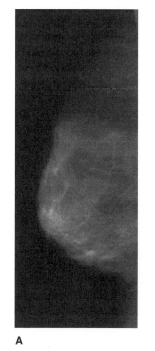
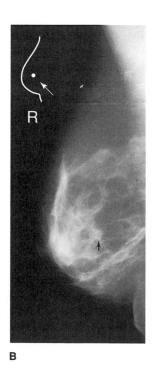

A   B

Figure 17–13. Mediolateral projection **(A)** performed to evaluate a suspicious area **(B)** seen on the mediolateral oblique view.

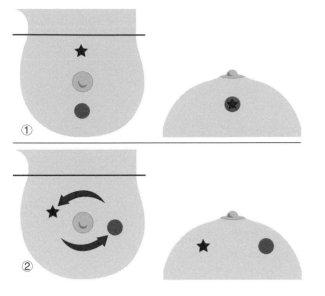

Figure 17–14. Rolled position.

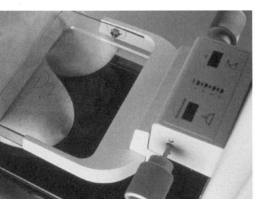

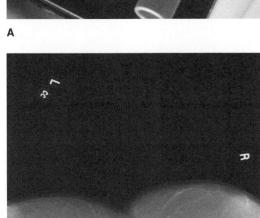

Figure 17–16. Patient positioned for cleavage position **(A)**; cleavage projection **(B)**. *(Photo courtesy of Trex Medical Bennett Division. Radiograph courtesy of Community Radiology Associates, Inc.)*

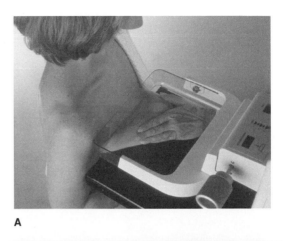

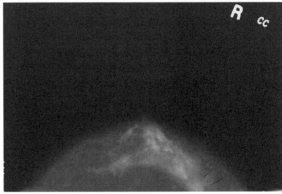

Figure 17–15. Patient positioned for exaggerated CC position **(A)**. *(Courtesy of LORAD, a subsidiary of Trex Medical Corporation.)* Craniocaudad projection **(B)** compared to the exaggerated CC position **(C)**. *(Radiographs courtesy of Community Radiology Associates, Inc.)*

To visualize the most medial breast tissue, a **cleavage** projection can be performed. Both breasts are placed on the cassette holder as for the craniocaudad projection. This positioning is most easily accomplished from behind the patient by lifting both inframammary margins and placing both breasts on the cassette holder. Instructing the patient to grasp the holder from beneath and pull the chest wall tightly against the edge of the compression device ensures that all the tissue is included. The patient's head should be turned to one side; assist the patient in assuming the best position possible. Depending on the size of the breast and the position of the photocells, a manual technique may be required *(Figure 17–16)*.

Spot compression is performed using a smaller compression device or paddle to allow the area of interest to be more compressed and, therefore, less superimposed. It is critical to localize the area of interest from the initial craniocaudad projection so that the area is in the center of the small compression paddle. It is also important to use compression enthusiastically to obtain the best possible image of the lesion without superimposition *(Figure 17–17)*.

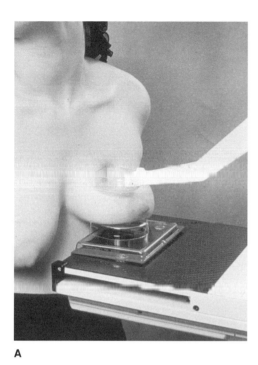

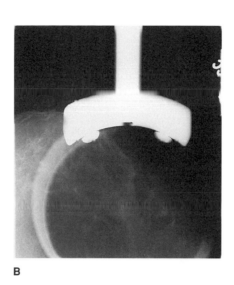

A   **B**

Figure 17–17. Patient positioned for spot image **(A)**; localized spot projection **(B)**. *(Photo courtesy of Trex Medical Bennett Division. Radiograph courtesy of Community Radiology Associates, Inc.)*

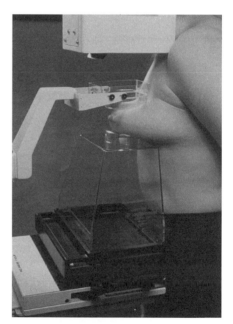

A

B

Figure 17–18. Patient correctly positioned for magnification view **(A)**. Magnified craniocaudad projection **(B)**. *(Photo courtesy of American Mammographics MammoSpot®, Chattanooga, TN. Radiograph courtesy of Community Radiology Associates, Inc.)*

To evaluate calcifications or architectural detail within the breast, **magnification** is very helpful. The small focal spot must be used to resolve the minute detail that small calcifications provide. A grid is not used because the increased OID provides an "air gap" that absorbs the scatter. As a result of this increased OID, the exposure time is longer than that for the standard projections, so it is vitally important that the patient hold her breath through the entire exposure to avoid motion artifact. It is customary to use the small compression paddle, and image only the area of interest, not the entire breast *(Figure 17–18)*.

By modifying methods and using mammographic accessory devices, radiographers can provide patients with more diagnostic services that may benefit them in treating their medical conditions. Procedures such as needle localization and biopsy complement the basic mammogram and can be performed easily by using either existing equipment or specialized units. These procedures should not be intimidating. If the basics of routine mammography are understood and performed with confidence, then departure from the routine should not be an obstacle to competent execution of the specialty examinations.

Mammography of the Augmented Breast

Demonstrating the normal breast tissue in the patient with augmented breasts can present the radiographer with a challenge. If the mechanics of displacing the prosthesis against the chest wall are understood by the radiographer, then the task is made a little easier. If the patient has little body fat, especially around the prostheses, it may not be feasible to perform the standard mammogram. Depending on her symptoms in this case, the patient may be a candidate for a breast MRI. On the other hand, if the patient has adequate body fat, displacement views can be obtained with little difficulty. A total of eight films are required, two sets each of the bilateral craniocaudad and mediolateral oblique projections. One set is done with manual technique, slight compression, and the implants in place to demonstrate the posterior aspect of the natural breast tissue *(Figure 17–19)*. The second set is done with automatic exposure control, regular compression, and the implants displaced, demonstrating the anterior portion of the natural breast tissue *(Figure 17–20)*. This technique, developed Dr. G. William Eklund, has enhanced the diagnosis of lesions in the patient with augmentation when mammography is not a viable option to evaluate the natural breast tissue.

Galactography

Galactography is demonstration of the collecting ducts surrounding the nipple region by injection of contrast medium through the orifice of the collecting ducts. This procedure can also be referred to as ductography, as it is intraductal pathology that is demonstrated. The patient usually presents with nipple discharge

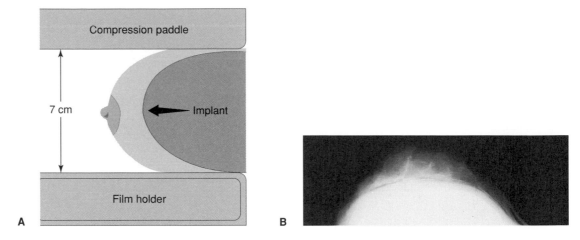

Figure 17–19. Compression used with the augmented breast **(A)**; craniocaudad projection with prosthesis **(B)**. *(Radiograph courtesy of Community Radiology Associates, Inc.)*

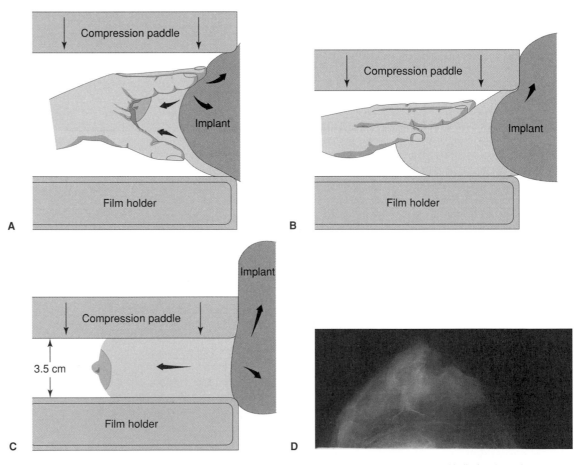

Figure 17–20. Displaced prosthesis with compression of only the breast **(A,B,C)**; craniocaudad projection with displaced prosthesis **(D)**. *(Radiograph courtesy of Community Radiology Associates, Inc.)*

and has symptoms related to an inflammatory process; abnormal discharge from the nipple may be an indication of breast cancer. Evaluation of the distal lactiferous ducts is relatively simple. Good use of sterile technique and Universal Precautions should be used during all phases of the procedure.

A tray containing several small sterile syringes (1.0–5.0 mL), several 27- to 30-gauge blunt-end cannulas (such as those used for sialography), water-soluble contrast medium, topical cleansing agent, gauze pads, and sterile gloves should be assembled ahead of time. The procedure should be carefully explained to the patient; routine mammography films should be available for comparison. With the patient either supine or seated erect, the nipple is cleansed with an antiseptic solution. The blunt needle is introduced by the radiologist into the dilated orifice of the nipple and a small amount of the contrast medium is injected. The amount injected varies from patient to patient, but is usually 1 to 3 mL. To determine if the ducts have filled adequately, the patient is asked to tell the radiologist when the breast feels tight or full. When the patient indicates fullness, the injection is terminated so as to not rupture the ducts and cause extravasation outside the ducts into the surrounding tissue. Should this happen, the patient will feel much discomfort. Immediately after the injection, the cannula is carefully taped to the side of the breast and craniocaudad and mediolateral projections are performed without compression or change in exposure factors; compression may cause the contrast medium to be expressed from the breast. After the mammograms have been obtained the cannula is removed and the patient is told what to expect with respect to discharge of the contrast medium from the breast. A gauze pad may be given to the patient for inside the brassiere to prevent staining by secretions and contrast medium.

Magnification projections may be requested for improved visualization on one or both of these projections. This procedure demonstrates not only locations of lesions, but also the number of lesions present, thereby possibly eliminating any diagnostic surgical procedure for the patient. If the study is positive and the lesion must be removed, the resultant films could be used for preoperative planning *(Figure 17–21)*.

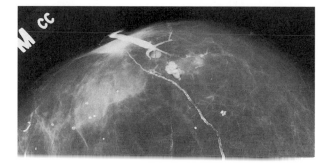

Figure 17–21. Galactogram; note the raspberry-shaped benign papilloma. *(Radiograph courtesy of Community Radiology Associates, Inc.)*

Needle Localization for Biopsy

The dedicated unit or a specialized stereotactic table may be used in a biopsy procedure either to confirm a malignancy or to localize a lesion requiring surgical excision. This can be accomplished with a gunlike device for a core biopsy or simply a fine needle for aspiration of cells *(Figure 17–22)*. Specialized table units for this purpose either have their own generator or share a generator with the radiographic unit. Frequently the images produced are digital images with much improved resolution for localizing minute calcifications. Stereotactic capabilities allow for localizing a lesion in three dimensions with greater precision and accuracy.

Specimen Imaging

Imaging of the breast specimen after the lesion has been excised from the patient's breast is quite common. When the specimen arrives in the radiology department, it should be radiographed on the dedicated unit; Universal Precautions should be followed. The specimen itself should be placed on the cassette tunnel or holder and compression should be applied. The grid does not need to be used because the specimen is much smaller than the entire compressed breast. The kVp range should be less than that for routine mammography, approximately 22 to 24 kVp. This is only a guideline, as units vary from vendor to vendor and calibration varies between units. It is not uncommon to use threads and/or needles to mark the specific areas of a tissue mass or to indicate the presence of calcifications *(Figure 17–23)*. These indicators are placed earlier in a needle localization procedure prior to surgery. They assist the surgeon, pathologist, and radiologist in making an accurate determination as to whether the entire tissue in question has been excised during the surgical procedure. Magnification is commonly used in this application also. The factor of magnification is usually between 1.5 and 2.0 times. A magnification factor any higher than 2.0 will lead to unsharpness of the periphery of the lesion itself.

The radiologist and pathologist should compare the specimen with the routine mammogram to ensure that the surgeon has surgically removed the entire extent of the lesion. This should be done expediently as the patient is most likely still under anesthesia until the surgical procedure has concluded.

Ancillary and Complementary Modalities

There are other imaging techniques that assist in interpretation and complement the radiographic examination of the breast. **Ultrasound** can be used to differentiate between solid and cystic masses, evaluate palpable masses in young patients, evaluate masses that are not included on a breast image or that are not well demonstrated on a radiographically dense breast, and assist in rare aspiration/biopsy procedures if radiographs are not helpful.

Despite being an expensive technology, **MRI** has become especially useful in patients with breast augmentation when leakage or rupture is suspected. Mammography has limited application in these patients unless silicone has extravasated and is still close to the implant. Mammography also does not allow visualization of the inside of the silicone capsule for evaluation. It is equally important to evaluate the normal breast tissue that encompasses the prostheses. Aside from the augmentation application, MRI demonstrates breast tissue in those patients whose breasts are too dense to yield mammographic images of diagnostic quality. MRI provides hope that malignancy can be discovered in these patients; both unenhanced and enhanced images using a contrast medium should be obtained to highlight malignant lesions. Fat necrosis and/or scarring in postsurgical patients can be distinguished from new or recurrent malignant lesions using this imaging modality. Despite all of these indications for using MRI to image the breast, however, the high cost of these scans does not merit use of MRI as a screening method. So for the present time, film/screen mammography remains the primary screening tool for breast disease.

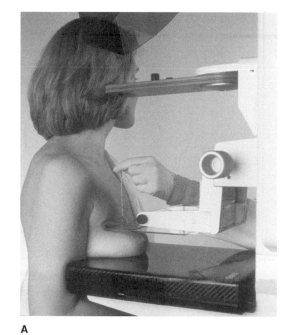

A

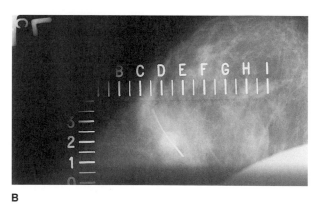

B

Figure 17–22. Needle localization using traditional mammography unit. *(Photo courtesy of LORAD, a subsidiary of Trex Medical Corporation.)*

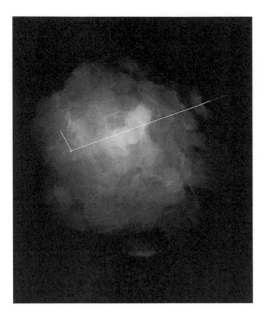

Figure 17–23. Breast specimen. *(Radiograph courtesy of Community Radiology Associates, Inc.)*

Digital Mammography

The future of breast imaging lies in utilization of computers to assist in constructing breast images. Currently used in some biopsy units, digital mammography is helpful in enhancing low-contrast structures within the breast, including microcalcifications. The computer can be programmed to assist the radiologist in interpreting the examination by detecting patterns in the breast tissue that are characteristic of malignancies.

Other Developing Breast Imaging Techniques

Apart from the methods discussed, several other alternative imaging techniques are being pursued. Research involving breast scintigraphy, CT laser mammography, and Doppler ultrasound has begun. Breast scintigraphy is performed following the injection of a radionuclide that enhances breast lesions that may be biopsied for malignancy, including axillary nodes that may contain malignant cells.

BREATHING INSTRUCTIONS

To minimize the possibility of motion artifacts on the radiographs, the patient should be instructed to suspend respiration for the exposure. The patient should not take in a deep breath, as this action may cause a motion artifact or result in movement of breast tissue out of the compression device.

EXPOSURE FACTORS

As each mammographic unit is calibrated differently and every patient's breast composition is unique, technical factors are not given for each projection discussed. It should be noted that the amount of tissue compression, expected density of the breast, which is estimated from the patient history, and assessment of tissue by feel when positioning greatly assist in exposure factor selection. One must be knowledgeable about appropriate use of exposure factors to minimize noise and demonstrate early lesions as soon as they are large enough to be visualized. This aspect is critical as exposure factors can either enhance or degrade the diagnostic quality of the mammogram. Because there is very little inherent subject contrast in the breast tissue, exposure factors must be appropriately selected. Appropriate kVp ranges from 25 to 30 and automatic exposure control are usually used to ensure films of similar density.

Automatic exposure control (AEC), or phototiming, is commonly used in film/screen mammography. The ionization chamber must be calibrated to coincide with the film/screen combination and film processing being used. When preparing equipment for the patient, it is necessary to make sure that the cassette holder is connected to the AEC receptacle. The "backup" timer on the control panel should be set so that the exposure is terminated when the maximum mAs is reached. With AEC, consistent exposures can be made to ensure image quality. Manual techniques can also be used; however, there is a greater chance for error in technique. A mammographer is limited to manual techniques when imaging augmented breasts.

The most critical aspect of using AEC is accurate positioning. Just as in regular radiography, if the center of the structure is not centered over the center of the photocells, the exposure is either under- or overexposed, thereby necessitating a repeat exposure. The appropriate photocell must be selected for the size of breast being imaged, placing the photocell under the densest portion of the breast *(Figure 17–24)*.

For accurate placement of photocells, the radiographer must know where to expect dense tissue in the breast. Even though common sense might indicate the photocell selected should be more posterior as the breast may seem anatomically thicker there, it is actually the approximate anterior third of the breast to which the photocell must be adjusted. The photocell position options, of which there are three, function also in the sense of matching the cells to breast size. For example, the cell closest to the chest wall would be used on a breast that is very small and extends a very short distance onto the cassette holder. In contrast, the cell furthest away from the chest wall would be selected for a large breast, which extends further forward and covers the majority of the cassette surface.

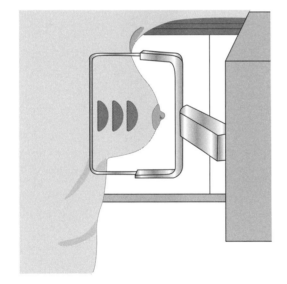

Figure 17–24. Position of the photocells on the mammographic unit is sometimes represented on the compression device.

EQUIPMENT CONSIDERATIONS

A dedicated mammography unit is used to obtain diagnostic radiographs from which high-quality images lead to an optimum and accurate diagnosis. The challenge of producing high-quality images results from the necessity of maximizing soft tissue structure resolution, while keeping the patient dose to a minimum because it is known that radiation can induce cancers. Several components assist the mammographer in positioning; the unit itself is equipped with an x-ray tube and filtration appropriate for demonstrating the fine tissue structures in the human breast. This, coupled with a film/screen, low-dose imaging system, allows the radiologist to view the resultant images with confidence. It is important to understand the makeup of the imaging system to obtain the best images possible.

Mammography Unit

The mammography unit is mobile and can be placed in any position in the examination room. It is equipped with various locks to accommodate the height and flexibility of the patient. The tube and cassette holder can be raised and lowered to the patient's height for craniocaudad/caudocranial views, with the central ray directed perpendicular to the image receptor. The x-ray tube and image receptor are situated on opposite ends of a C-arm that can be rotated around a horizontal axis for obtaining mediolateral or lateromedial views. Should the radiographer need to obtain a mammogram on a patient in a wheelchair, the entire tube–receptor component (C-arm) can be moved, on some units, in a longitudinal direction to the right or left, much the same as the general radiographic x-ray tube along the long axis of the radiographic table *(Figure 17–25)*.

Assembly of the tube and filtration leads to images of high diagnostic quality. Fractional focal spots from 0.1 to 0.4 mm are available to obtain radiographs of maximum quality in terms of image sharpness and definition. If magnification images are to be performed, then the 0.1-mm focal spot is required. Anode targets, whose angle can range from 10° to −9° degrees, can be made of tungsten, molybdenum, or rhodium. Stationary anodes can be found in older units; however, modern mammography units have rotating anodes. Many current units usually have two anode targets, tungsten and molybdenum, with the molybdenum target producing a lower-energy x-ray beam for much better soft tissue detail. The window, or tube exit port through which the beam exits the tube, is constructed of beryllium or borosilicate glass. These low-atomic-number materials minimize attenuation of the low-energy beam. Filtration is minimal in this system to maximize the application of the low-energy beam to produce soft tissue images. Added molybdenum filtration, equivalent to 0.5 mm of aluminum, is used in addition to the beryllium window to filter out the low-end spectrum and harden the beam. The added filtration is most effective when it is constructed of the same material as the anode target. The degree of resolution desirable in breast images is 11 to 13 line pairs per millimeter. This aspect is critical when the radiologist is trying to visualize small calcifications which may be approximately 500 μm in size.

The location of the tube on the unit is of great value to the radiographer in two respects. First, it allows for ease of positioning, as a large part of the tube housing is away from the patient's head. Second, use of the "heel effect" is maximized. The tube housing is tilted on the top of the frame, positioning the cathode over the chest wall (anode pointing toward the body) and directing the best part of the beam through the thicker breast tissue adjacent to the pectoralis region *(Figure 17–26)*. Despite having uniform compression of the breast tissue, this allows the effective focal spot to provide a useful beam to cover the entire 10 × 12-in. cassette area.

The x-ray generators used in mammographic units are comparable to those used in general radiographic units. They can be single- or three-phase units, as well as the high-frequency generator, which is rapidly becoming the standard. Several advantages to using a high-frequency generator are beyond the scope of this discussion, but two deserve mention: good reproducibility of exposure and phototimer. Quantity and quality of the beam are improved over the three-phase generator, which are important considerations in mammography. By use of time and mA together, a lower kVp can be used on the exposure, thereby improving resolution of the image and providing high-contrast images. This factor is important when the images must delineate soft tissue structures that do not vary much from each other in attenuation of the beam. Three-phase and high-frequency generators allow exposures to be made in the 20 to 30 kVp range. This range is adequate for demonstration of the minute structures of the breast and demonstrates differences between normal and abnormal breast tissues.

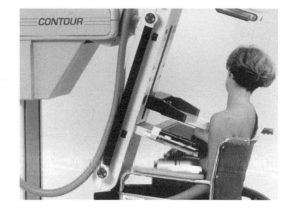

Figure 17–25. Accommodations can be made for patients unable to stand. *(Courtesy of Trex Medical Bennett Division.)*

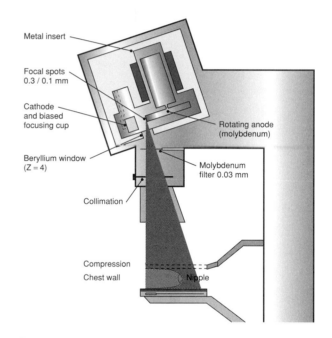

Figure 17–26. The tube housing is tilted so that the cathode is positioned over the chest wall, thus the anode-heel effect.

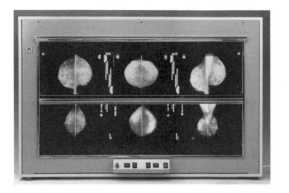

Figure 17–27. Mammographic examination correctly displayed on the illuminator. *(Photo courtesy of Broadwest Corporation.)*

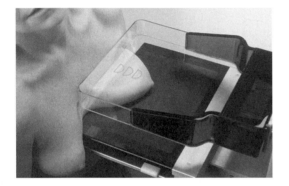

Figure 17–28. Compression device on a mammographic unit. *(Courtesy of LORAD, a subsidiary of Trex Medical Corporation.)*

Beam Limitation

To achieve the best detail possible, beam limitation is accomplished by using lead diaphragms at the exit of the tube or lead shutters in a collimation device. Diaphragms vary in size according to the cassette size or image receptor being used. The collimator can also be adjusted to limit the beam to the exact cassette size employed. In using either device, there should be no transparent borders or edges on the resultant breast image as the extraneous light from the viewbox will make it difficult for the radiographer and radiologist to view the breast image. This concept seems to be a paradox because it is known that beam limitation or collimation enhances subject contrast, but in this application, despite it being helpful in increasing contrast of the image, collimation is not limited strictly to the breast field but instead is "opened up" to the cassette size being used. This is not a problem as dose and image quality are not significantly affected by any scatter radiation from ionizations in the surrounding air. It is also highly recommended that the radiologist viewing the mammographic study mask the images so that no extraneous light from the viewboxes appears around the periphery of the 8 × 10-in. or 10 × 12-in. radiographs *(Figure 17–27)*.

Scatter radiation within a large or thick breast leads to deterioration of the image and results in decreased image contrast. To counteract this effect, grids are used to absorb scatter radiation in imaging of thicker breasts to enhance contrast, in tandem with low kVp. Although image quality is improved by the use of the 5:1 or 6:1 linear grids, patient dose is also increased, but is considered to be within acceptable limits. Grids can be stationary, as in a 3.5:1 grid, or reciprocating, as in the 5:1 grid. The latter provides better "cleanup" of scatter radiation. The grid itself consists of lead strips separated by carbon fiber interspaces. When the grid moves or oscillates, it blurs the grid line pattern. The grids are focused so that SIDs of 50 to 80 in. can be used without artifacts. The mammographer must be sure that the cable or connection for utilization of the grid is attached to the receptacle on the mammographic unit to provide power to oscillate the grid. Breasts that are compressed to 2 cm or less may be in little need of grid techniques.

Compression

Compression serves several important purposes. One is to flatten the breast, thereby separating the structures and avoiding superimposition. By decreasing the height of the breast tissue, the structures are brought closer to the image receptor, thus decreasing the OID and improving detail visibility. An added benefit of decreasing the thickness of the breast tissue is a reduction in the amount of radiation needed to penetrate the tissue, as the breast is thinner than it would be if no compression or improper compression were used. The last purpose is that of immobilization. With the breast compressed, the patient is assisted in holding still until the exposure has been made, eliminating the possibility of motion artifact.

Because compression plays a key role in optimum imaging, a stiff plexiglass device needs to be used appropriately to achieve homogeneous compression across the entire breast. The part of the device that makes contact with the chest wall should be at least 1 in. high and form a 90° angle with that part that makes contact with the breast tissue to apply compression *(Figure 17–28)*. The device or paddle size is selected to match the size of the cassette that is to be used. Placement of the compression paddle at a right angle to the chest wall assists in providing a uniform thickness of breast tissue, thereby providing a more optically homogeneous density across the breast image. Smaller specialized paddles can be used for cone-down spot compression of areas of interest.

The compression is applied either pneumatically or manually. Because 25 to 35 pounds of pressure is applied to the breast tissue for adequate compression, it may be uncomfortable for the patient. The level of discomfort may vary with the patient's menstrual cycle, hormone therapy, and intake of caffeine. It is critically important to instruct the patient in the benefits of compression and gain the patient's cooperation in the examination process. The patient can be asked to tell the radiographer when the pressure starts to become slightly uncomfortable. At that time, the radiographer can tap the breast tissue to check for tautness and adequate compression. The final decision to apply more compression, if necessary, rests with the radiographer, as the patient will sometimes be anxious and intolerant of compression.

Accessory Devices

Components can be used with the dedicated mammographic unit to assist in obtaining special views of the breast tissue in question. Attachments allow for the magnification, spot compression, and localization of lesions. Magnification views, which can increase the area of interest by 1.5 to 2 times the original tissue area, can be accomplished either with or without a compression device and require that a small focal spot of 0.2 mm or less be used. This view allows the radiographer and radiologist to see better resolution of the tissue, especially small microcalcifications that may represent malignancy. Coincidental findings may appear on the magnification view that would not have been demonstrated on the routine projections without magnification. With the "platform" attachment, an air gap is created, reducing scatter and therefore eliminating the need for a grid. It is critical that the patient fully cooperate with suspended respiration and remain motionless to avoid motion artifacts, as the exposure time will be increased. Magnification views are not routinely obtained because the dose to the patient is increased by a factor of 2 to 3. Spot compression is another diagnostic tool, a small, round plexiglass paddle is used to compress the area of interest, thereby decreasing superimposition of structures that cannot be easily seen free of superimposition in the routine views *(Figure 17–29)*. A slight increase in technique is required as close collimation to the compressed region is necessary to improve contrast and detail.

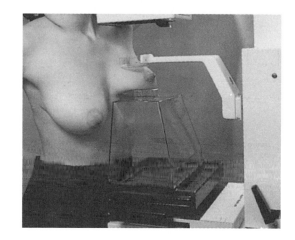

Figure 17–29. Spot paddle in place with patient positioned on a magnification platform. *(Photo courtesy of American Mammographics.)*

Image Receptors

Without appropriate film/screen combinations and satisfactory operation of processing equipment, the best mammographer can end up with less than adequate images. Historically speaking, the progression of image receptors has been steady since the advent of mammography in the late 1950s, when direct exposure film was used. Direct exposure film required long exposure times, which made motion artifacts common and gave patients doses to the breast that today would be unthinkable. Xeromammography was an improvement over the direct exposure film and reduced the dose significantly. Development of a single-screen cassette and single-emulsion film led us to today's imaging techniques. Through these developments, the dose to the patient has decreased significantly since breast imaging became more widespread in the 1950s.

Today, film/screen systems are especially designed for mammography. It is critical to employ such a system that provides the highest-quality image at the lowest patient dose. The sensitivity of the color spectrum of the film needs to match the color that the intensifying screen emits inside the cassette. The way these two components are used together is critical. Because the cassette has only one screen, it is essential for the mammographer to load the cassette so the film emulsion is adjacent to the intensifying screen in the cassette *(Figure 17–30)*. The cassette itself is made so that it attenuates very few of the x-ray photons and allows contact between the film and the intensifying screen. This ensures good detail of the structures within the breast. The integrity between the screen and film for good film/screen contact needs to be monitored on a semiannual basis with a fine wire-mesh screen to ensure that there is no loss of detail as a result of poor contact. As dirt inside the cassette can contribute to poor contact, intensification screens in this system need to be cleaned weekly. This requirement by the American College of Radiology demands cleaning of cassettes on a much more frequent basis than those cassettes used for general radiography. Eliminating any possibility of loss of detail by image blurring in the image receptor benefits the patient by producing a high quality image for the radiologist to interpret.

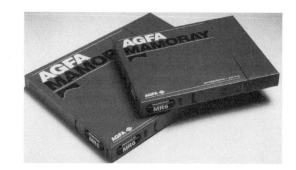

Figure 17–30. Special, single-emulsion film is used for mammography. *(Courtesy of Agfa Division, Bayer Corporation.)*

IMAGE PROCESSING

Quality assurance and processor quality control are absolutely essential in producing quality images. The best positioning skills are not useful if the images are not appropriately processed. Guidelines, as determined by the Mammography Quality Standards Act and the American College of Radiology, provide criteria that exceed criteria for processing of other radiographic studies done in a diagnostic radiology department. The optimum situation is to have a dedicated darkroom and processor for processing of mammographic images, although it is not mandatory.

Darkroom cleanliness is a must. Artifacts must be prevented so visible pathology on the mammogram is not obliterated. The counters and feedtray need to be cleaned each morning, prior to the first patient, to prevent artifacts on the radiographs. Processors must be cleaned regularly and maintained with fresh chemistry that matches the type of film used. Extended cycle processors, which require single-emulsion films to spend more time in the developer to enhance contrast, are preferred, although they are not currently the industry standard. Daily film sensitometry is required and documentation of results must be kept on file to demonstrate constant monitoring of processing parameters for detection of any change in film speed and contrast. Changes in chemistry temperature and/or in replenishment rates and dilution are just a few of the possible causes of inadequate processing of images. This process assists the radiographer in identifying problems before they happen, ensuring high-quality films. Should an incident occur during the workday, the problem must be resolved before any other films are taken. A good quality assurance program allows the highest-quality examination possible, thereby providing a more accurate interpretation.

RADIOGRAPHIC POSITIONING OF THE BREAST

- ► CRANIOCAUDAD (CC) BREAST

- ► MEDIOLATERAL OBLIQUE (MLO) BREAST

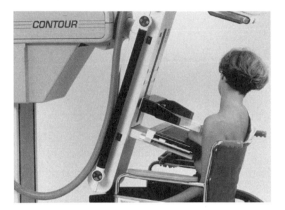

Figure 17–31. Routine craniocaudad positioning is modified for the seated patient. *(Photo courtesy of Trex Medical Bennett Division.)*

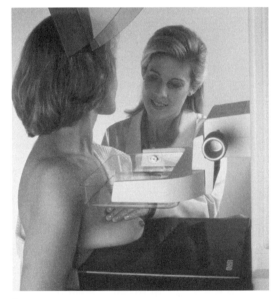

A

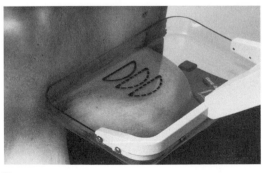

B

Figure 17–32. Craniocaudad position. (**A** *courtesy of LORAD, a subsidiary of Trex Medical Corporation*; **B** *courtesy of Agfa Division, Bayer Corporation.)*

► CRANIOCAUDAD (CC) BREAST

Technical Considerations

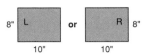

- Film size: 8 × 10 in. or 10 × 12 in., depending on breast size.
- Grid recommended for compressed breasts greater than 2 cm.
- 25–30 kVp.
- AEC usually recommended except for augmented breasts; cell position and selection depend on breast.
- Collimate to cassette size using collimator or diaphragm.

Shielding

Gonadal shielding should be used on all patients, especially those of reproductive age; turn the patient's head away from the side being examined.

Patient Positioning

- Assist the ambulatory patient to the standing erect position in front of the dedicated mammography unit; when necessary, the patient may be seated *(Figure 17–31)*.
- Instruct the ambulatory patient to assume a comfortable stance with feet apart and the body weight balanced.
- Adjust the unit to the level of the patient's inframammary crease when the breast is elevated; the patient should not have flexed knees or be standing on tiptoes. **Note:** This technique enhances compression from below so the compression device does not have to do all the compression from above, which could sacrifice inclusion of superior breast tissue.

Part Positioning

- Elevate the breast so the inframammary crease is at its maximum level, adjusting the level of the cassette holder so the top edge is at the level of the inframammary crease; the patient's inframammary crease should be firmly against the cassette's edge. **Note:** The radiographer should be standing on the breast's medial aspect when positioning for this projection.
- Using both hands, one below the breast and one above, pull the breast tissue away from the chest wall and place it on the surface of the cassette holder with the nipple centered crosswise on the cassette.
- Turn the patient's head away from the side being examined to allow the patient to lean in for inclusion of more superior breast tissue.
- Using one hand to smooth the lateral breast tissue to avoid skin folds and the other to rest on the patient's shoulder and adjust the skin over the clavicle and reduce the "pulling sensation" while lowering the compression device onto the breast until the breast tissue is taut to the touch; make sure no breast tissue slips off the cassette.
- Position the opposite breast over the corner of the cassette holder to ensure maximum medial breast tissue of the breast being imaged.
- Instruct the patient to raise the arm of the side not being examined and place it forward on the handlebar of the unit; the arm of the examined side should be at the side with the arm externally rotated *(Figure 17–32)*.

Central Ray

- Direct the central ray perpendicular to the breast and cassette.

Breathing Instructions

- Instruct the patient to suspend respirations during the exposure. **Note:** Deep inspiration may cause motion artifact and/or movement of breast tissue resulting in a positioning error.

Image Evaluation

- Proper labeling, as required by the American College of Radiology, should be evident.
- The nipple and medial and lateral breast tissue should be included within the collimated area; the pectoralis major muscle is seen approximately 20% of the time.
- The nipple should be centered crosswise on the film and should be in profile, if possible.
- Appropriate exposure should demonstrate high image contrast and good detail resolution.
- Dense tissue should be adequately penetrated.
- There should be no evidence of motion or other artifacts *(Figures 17–33)*.

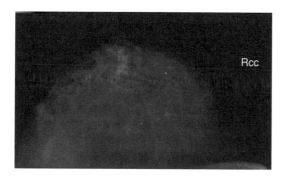

Figure 17–33. Craniocaudad projection. *(Courtesy of Community Radiology Associates, Inc.)*

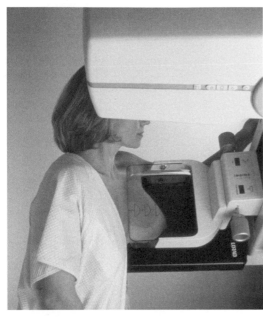

A

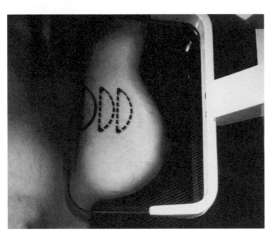

B

Figure 17–34. Mediolateral oblique position. (**A** *courtesy of LORAD, a subsidiary of Trex Medical Corporation*; **B** *courtesy of Agfa Division, Bayer Corporation.*)

► MEDIOLATERAL OBLIQUE (MLO) BREAST

Technical Considerations

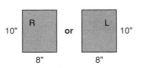

- Film size: 8 × 10 in. or 10 × 12 in., depending on breast size.
- Grid recommended for compressed breasts greater than 2 cm.
- 25–30 kVp.
- AEC usually recommended except for augmented breasts; cell position and selection depend on breast.
- Collimate to cassette size using collimator or diaphragm.

Shielding

- Gonadal shielding should be used on all patients, especially those of reproductive age; turn the patient's head away from the side being examined.

Patient Positioning

- Turn the C-arm 90° from the position used for the craniocaudad position.
- Assist the ambulatory patient to the standing erect position in front of the dedicated mammography unit; a patient who must sit should be seated to the side of the cassette holder.
- Instruct the ambulatory patient to assume a comfortable stance with feet apart and the body weight balanced; the shoulder muscles should be relaxed when positioning for this projection.
- After assessing the angle of the patient's pectoralis muscle with the flattened hand, elevate the breast toward the lateral side and adjust the angle of the tube and cassette to match the muscle angle (thin or small-breasted patients usually require approximately 60°–70°, whereas heavier patients with larger breasts usually need a 30°–60° angle).

Part Positioning

- Elevate and gently pull the breast upward and outward, placing the lateral side of the breast against the cassette holder; the radiographer should stand on the medial aspect of the breast.
- Position the axilla over the superior corner of the cassette holder; place the hand of the same arm on the handlebar with the elbow relaxed.
- Without letting go of the breast, lower the compression device onto the breast, making sure that no tissue slips out from the cassette until the skin is taut to touch; compression should adequately support the anterior breast tissue, preventing sagging and distortion of the ductal architecture.
- As the compression is applied, use one hand to smoothe the anterior breast tissue to avoid skin folds and position the other hand on the patient's sternum to adjust the skin over the sternum and clavicle and reduce the "pulling sensation" *(Figure 17–34).*

Central Ray

- Direct the central ray perpendicular to the breast and cassette.

Breathing Instructions

- Instruct the patient to suspend respirations during the exposure. **Note:** Deep inspiration may cause motion artifact and/or movement of breast tissue resulting in a positioning error.

Image Evaluation

- Proper labeling, as required by the American College of Radiology, should be evident.
- The nipple, pectoralis major muscle, and inframammary crease should be included within the collimated area.
- There should be no drooping of the anterior aspect of the breast (referred to as "camel's nose").
- The pectoralis major muscle should be seen down to the level of the nipple on most patients.
- Measurement of the distance from the posterior breast to the nipple line should be approximately the same as that measured in the craniocaudad position.
- Appropriate exposure factors should demonstrate high image contrast and good detail resolution.
- Dense tissue should be adequately penetrated.
- There should be no evidence of motion or other artifacts *(Figure 17–35)*

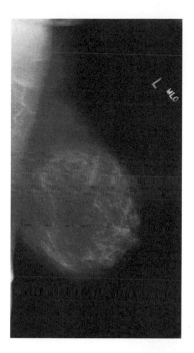

Figure 17–35. Mediolateral oblique projection. *(Courtesy of Community Radiology Associates, Inc.)*

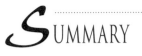

SUMMARY

▶ Radiographic examination of the breast must be performed with the utmost attention to detail considering the sensitivity of dealing with this body part and the way in which optimum imaging must be accomplished.

▶ The patient should be physically and mentally prepared for the examination, being treated with respect and care.

▶ The radiographer must be competent in proper positioning and communication skills.

▶ The routine mammography series includes the craniocaudad and mediolateral oblique projections of both breasts.

▶ Optional projections, such as the 90° mediolateral, the exaggerated craniocaudad, and the tangential projections, may be performed to further evaluate a suspicious area.

▶ Each mammogram should be evaluated using standard criteria; variations from the routine procedure should be performed with the same competency as a routine mammogram.

▶ Alternate procedures are required to evaluate augmented breasts, the collecting ducts, and locations of masses.

▶ The kVp range for mammography is usually 25 to 30; automatic exposure control is recommended to ensure consistency and minimize repeat radiographs.

▶ A dedicated mammography unit must be used when performing mammograms.

▶ Quality assurance, which includes processor monitoring, must be performed on a regular basis to ensure optimum diagnostic images.

▶ The patient should leave the facility with some understanding of how the results will be communicated to her or him.

QUESTIONS FOR CRITICAL THINKING & APPLICATION

1. Why does the shape of the breast influence the positioning of the breast?
2. Why does age of the patient and parity history influence the technical factors used to make the exposure?
3. How can you achieve a diagnostic craniocaudad projection on a kyphotic patient?
4. If a lesion is seen in the lateral aspect of the breast in the craniocaudad projection, where will it be seen in the mediolateral oblique projection? Where would it be on the 90° mediolateral?
5. Explain why automatic exposure devices are not recommended when performing mammography on patients with breast prostheses.

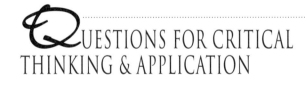

FILM CRITIQUE

Criteria for evaluating mammograms are very important.

Evaluate this mediolateral oblique for accurate positioning (*Figure 17–36*).

What criteria did you use?

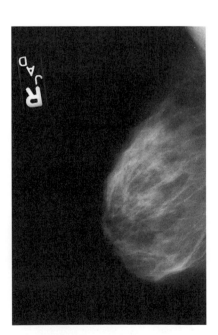

Figure 17–36.

18

CARDIOVASCULAR SYSTEM

MARYANN NESTHEIDE, BS, RT(R)(CV)

► OBJECTIVES

Following the completion of this chapter the student will be able to:

- Identify the major components of the cardiovascular system, to include their location and function.

- Discuss the relationship between the cardiovascular and lymphatic systems.

- Discriminate between veins and arteries with respect to size, location, and blood flow.

- Discuss radiographic examination of the cardiovascular system, including pre- and postprocedural patient care for angiographic procedures, and the Seldinger technique.

- Discuss what is meant by an "interventional" procedure.

- List and describe the equipment commonly used for angiographic procedures.

- Define terminology associated with the cardiovascular system and special radiographic procedures, to include anatomy and pathology.

The cardiovascular system: Heart

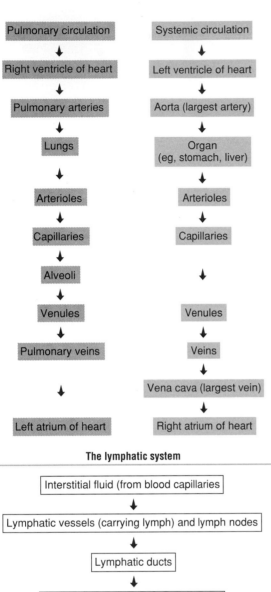

Figure 18–1. The circulatory system.

► ANATOMY OF THE CARDIOVASCULAR SYSTEM

The circulatory system is a complex transportation system that provides valuable oxygen and nutrients to every cell throughout the human body. The circulatory system consists of two distinct systems, cardiovascular and lymphatic, which transport fluid in a continuous directional flow *(Figure 18–1)*.

The cardiovascular system is subdivided into the systemic circulation and the pulmonary circulation *(Figure 18–2)*. The **systemic circulation** begins with the left ventricle of the heart and includes circulation to the entire body except the lungs. As the left ventricle pumps, the oxygenated blood travels out into the aorta and major arterial systems of the body. Arteries carry the oxygenated blood from the heart. The arterial walls consist of three layers which are, from the inside out, **tunica intima, tunica media,** and **tunica externa** or **adventitia** *(Figure 18–3)*. These layers form a strong, muscular structure that transports oxygenated blood through the high-pressure arterial system. As the blood travels, the arteries continue to divide and decrease in size into minute vessels called **arterioles.** The arterioles divide further into **capillaries** *(Figure 18–4)*. Arteries bring oxygenated blood and nutrients to the capillary beds where the exchange of oxygen and nutrients occurs. The by-products of cellular metabolism are discarded in the tissue fluid. The capillaries consist of thin walls through which oxygen and nutrients can be absorbed slowly, and waste products filtered out. The small capillaries join together to form **venules,** the beginning branches of the veins. They continue to unite to form larger **veins,** which are the pathway for deoxygenated blood flowing back to the right atrium of the heart. On average, a complete circuit of blood circulating through the body takes only 23 seconds (about 27 heartbeats) *(Figure 18–5)*.

The **pulmonary circulation,** which delivers blood only to the lungs, begins in the right ventricle of the heart. Blood is pumped from the right ventricle through the right and left pulmonary arteries into the lungs. It is here in the lungs that carbon dioxide is exchanged for oxygen. Blood is then transported through the pulmonary veins into the left atrium of the heart, which squeezes its blood into the left ventricle to begin the systemic circulation as previously described. It should be noted that the pulmonary arteries are the only arteries in the body that carry deoxygenated blood. Correspondingly, the pulmonary veins are the only veins that carry oxygenated blood *(Figure 18–6)*.

As the pressure in the venous system is substantially lower than that in the arterial system, the movement of the blood in the venous system is facilitated by the contraction of skeletal muscles in the walls of the veins. The contractions provide enough force to aid the flow of blood back to the heart. There are valves located inside larger veins that prevent backward flow of blood *(Figure 18–7)*. Although veins comprise the same three layers as arteries, their walls do not need to be as thick because venous pressure is low.

Cardiovascular anatomy in specific regions of the body is discussed throughout the Procedural Considerations section of this chapter as particular procedures are addressed.

The **lymphatic** (lim-FAT-ik) **system** is often thought to be a component of the cardiovascular system; however, it is a distinct system consisting of lymphatic vessels, lymph nodes, and organs (ie, tonsils, thymus gland, and spleen) that parallels the cardiovascular system *(Figure 18–8)*. It functions to filter cellular waste products from the blood, return interstitial fluid to the bloodstream, and help the body ward off infections. In the tissue space, clear interstitial (intercellular) fluid leaks out of the blood capillaries and passes through the permeable membrane of the **lymphatic vessels,** at which point it is then called **lymph.**

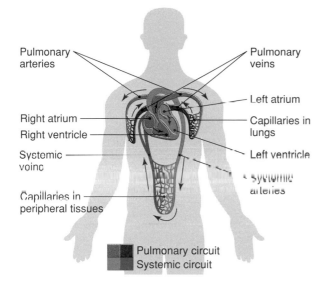

Pulmonary arteries

Pulmonary veins

Right atrium

Left atrium

Right ventricle

Capillaries in lungs

Systemic veins

Left ventricle

Systemic arteries

Capillaries in peripheral tissues

Pulmonary circuit
Systemic circuit

Figure 18–2. Overview of the circulatory system.

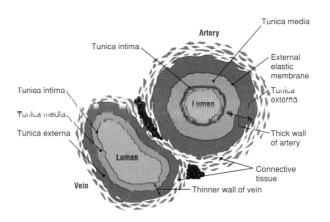

Tunica media

Artery

Tunica intima

Tunica intima

External elastic membrane

Tunica media

Lumen

Tunica externa

Tunica externa

Lumen

Thick wall of artery

Vein

Connective tissue

Thinner wall of vein

Figure 18–3. "Pipelines" of the cardiovascular system: comparison of artery and vein.

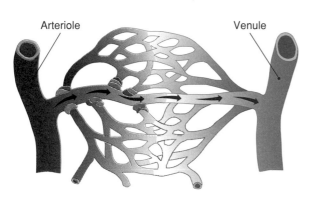

Arteriole

Venule

Figure 18–4. Capillary bed.

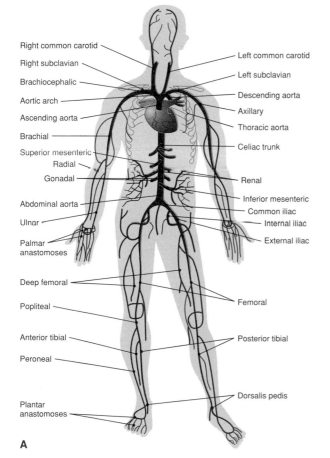

Right common carotid

Left common carotid

Right subclavian

Left subclavian

Brachiocephalic

Descending aorta

Aortic arch

Axillary

Ascending aorta

Thoracic aorta

Brachial

Celiac trunk

Superior mesenteric

Radial

Gonadal

Renal

Inferior mesenteric

Abdominal aorta

Common iliac

Ulnar

Internal iliac

Palmar anastomoses

External iliac

Deep femoral

Popliteal

Femoral

Anterior tibial

Posterior tibial

Peroneal

Plantar anastomoses

Dorsalis pedis

A

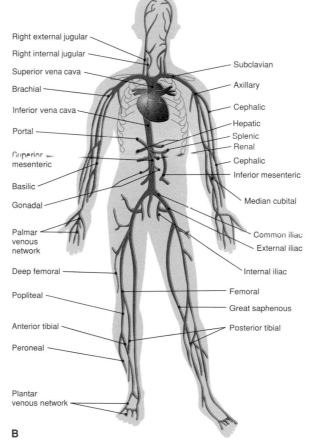

Right external jugular

Right internal jugular

Subclavian

Superior vena cava

Brachial

Axillary

Inferior vena cava

Cephalic

Portal

Hepatic

Splenic

Superior mesenteric

Renal

Cephalic

Basilic

Inferior mesenteric

Gonadal

Median cubital

Palmar venous network

Common iliac

External iliac

Internal iliac

Deep femoral

Popliteal

Femoral

Great saphenous

Anterior tibial

Posterior tibial

Peroneal

Plantar venous network

B

Figure 18–5. Cardiovascular system: **(A)** arterial anatomy, **(B)** venous anatomy.

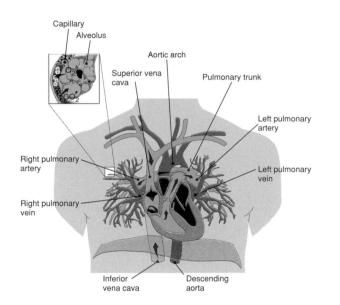

Figure 18–6. Pulmonary circulation.

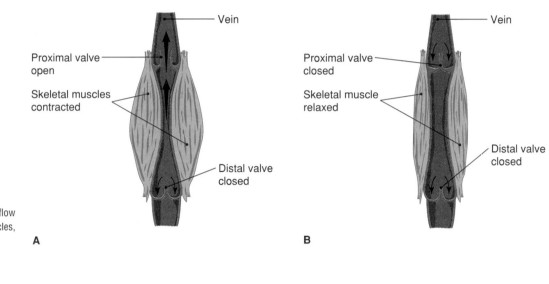

Figure 18–7. The contraction of skeletal muscles aids in the flow of blood through the veins. **(A)** Contracted skeletal muscles, **(B)** relaxed skeletal muscles.

A

B

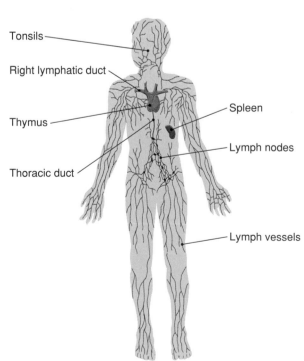

Figure 18–8. Lymphatic system.

The lymphatic vessels have one-way valves so that fluid flows in the direction of the heart much the same as blood in the veins flows. This lymph fluid is transported in the lymphatic vessels to the **lymph nodes,** which are clustered throughout the body. It is in the lymph nodes that bacteria are filtered out and pathogens are destroyed to help purify the blood. The lymphatic vessels are also responsible for transporting the lymph fluid back to the venous system, as they drain into either the right lymphatic duct or the thoracic duct, both of which in turn drain into the subclavian veins.

► PROCEDURAL CONSIDERATIONS

Angiography is the study of the vessels of the body. With the injection of contrast material into a blood vessel, a diagnosis can be made to help improve a patient's condition. The special procedures laboratory of today not only performs angiograms of the vessels within different systems of the body; it is also involved in many therapeutic procedures that can often substitute for surgery.

DIAGNOSTIC PROCEDURES

Angiographic examinations are frequently performed for diagnostic purposes. Indications may be specific to the particular area under examination, such as demonstration of a vascular tumor in a renal arteriogram. Angiographic procedures demonstrate aneurysms, arteriovenous malformations, and stenoses. In the case of trauma, injury to the vascular system may be evaluated.

The general procedure followed for angiography involves accessing the vessel of interest by using the Seldinger technique and feeding a catheter over a guidewire to the site. Water-soluble iodinated contrast medium is then injected, and the opacified vessels are filmed rapidly through the use of cinefluoroscopy or rapid film changers.

THERAPEUTIC PROCEDURES

In addition to many diagnostic examinations, therapeutic procedures are also undertaken in the special procedures laboratory.

The use of **thrombolytic** (throm-bō-LIT-ik) **agents** has increased over the years with the advance of medical techniques and therapy. Thrombolytic agents such as streptokinase and urokinase are medications used to dissolve an arterial blood clot that has occluded a blood vessel. Blood clots can form in any blood vessel of the body. When a blood vessel is occluded, the tissue normally supplied by that blood vessel begins to die. In the cardiac catheterization laboratory, thrombolytic agents may be infused into a coronary artery to stop a heart attack. In the special procedures laboratory, thrombolytic agents can be infused down the femoral artery to salvage the lower limb. In cases of acute thrombosis, streptokinase or urokinase is infused over a long period to dissolve the blood clot and restore blood flow, saving the distal tissue; however, there are many contraindications prohibiting the administration of thrombolytic agents, such as active bleeding, recent cerebrovascular accident, and any recent surgery. The use of thrombolytic agents places the patient at high risk for bleeding complications, but that must be weighed against the chance of heart attack or loss of a limb.

Just as individuals develop clots in the arterial system, clots can develop in the venous system. Typically, pulmonary emboli and deep vein thromboses have been treated with intravenous heparin and longterm coumadin therapy; however, there are many patients in whom this anticoagulation therapy is contraindicated. The problem of their treatment has been successfully addressed by using **vena cava filters.** Vena cava filters were once inserted in the operating room, which meant an involved surgical procedure and longer hospital stay. Now these filters are placed during a procedure in the special procedures laboratory. The vena cava filters can be introduced via the right and left femoral veins and internal jugular vein with the percutaneous method. An inferior vena cavagram is performed to document the position of renal veins and size of the inferior vena cava (IVC). As various types of filters are available, the type and size of filter is chosen based on need, ease of use, and effectiveness. Two examples of vena cava filters are illustrated in *Figure 18–9*. Once deployed in the IVC, this filter should trap clots before they can travel to the lungs or elsewhere in the body.

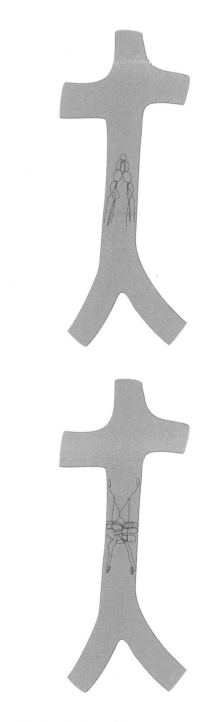

A

B

Figure 18–9. Greenfield **(A)** and bird's nest **(B)** are two examples of vena cava filters.

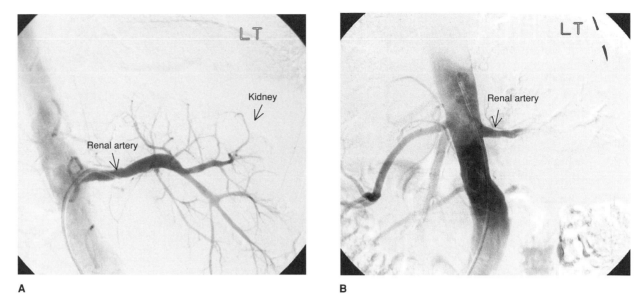

Figure 18–10. Renal arteriogram using embolization therapy. **(A)** Pre-embolization. **(B)** Postembolization. *(From Gronefeld D, Koscielicki T. Selected Pathological Conditions Affecting the Kidneys. Seminars in Radiologic Technology. 1996; 4/3; 120–135, with permission.)*

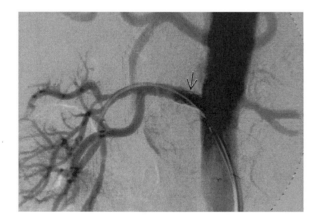

Figure 18–11. Renal arteriogram demonstrating a stent in the renal artery. *(From Gronefeld D, Koscielicki T. Selected Pathological Conditions Affecting the Kidneys. Seminars in Radiologic Technology. 1996; 4/3; 120–135, with permission.)*

The special procedures laboratory is also involved in **embolization therapy.** Embolization is used in the event of excess hemorrhage from trauma or when a vascular tumor needs to be surgically removed. In the case of gastrointestinal bleeding, the radiologist must identify the source of bleeding by performing an angiogram. Once the source is pinpointed, the radiologist can deliver the embolization agent. The most common agents used in embolization are the gelatin sponge (Gelfoam), metallic coils, detachable balloons, and alcohol. Once an agent is in place, blood adheres to it, forming a clot, which in turn should control or stop the bleeding. In the event of a vascular tumor on a kidney, renal infarction can be accomplished through embolization. The surgery to remove such a tumor can be very difficult and cause the patient to lose a great deal of blood. Prior to the surgery, a renal angiogram is performed to visualize the tumor's blood supply. The radiologist can use any of the above agents to occlude blood flow to the tumor, severely reducing or occluding the blood supply. The following day, the surgeon can remove the kidney and tumor successfully, with the patient sustaining very little blood loss *(Figure 18–10).*

Stents are used in both the special procedures laboratory and the cardiac catheterization laboratory to restore normal blood flow to an area. Stents consist of a stainless-steel tube mounted on an angioplasty balloon *(Figure 18–11).* The stent is carefully placed across the area of stenosis in an artery. Once the stent is in place, the balloon is inflated and the stent deployed. The balloon forces the stent into the wall of the vessel to push the stenosis or tumor out of the way of normal flow. Stents can be deployed in the aorta and the renal, subclavian, iliac, and femoral arteries. Biliary stents are used in the biliary tree when strictures or tumors obstruct biliary flow.

PATIENT CARE

Preparation

Before any invasive procedure is performed on a patient, certain preparations are required. First, the patient must consent to the procedure by signing an informed consent document. An explanation of the procedure, the reason it is needed, and possible complications should be given to the patient. A procedure cannot be performed if a mentally competent patient refuses to give his or her consent. Second, certain blood tests need to be completed to assess the patient's anticoagulation state, renal function, and potassium level. Any past allergic reactions to contrast media and/or any other allergies should be investigated.

The patient should have nothing by mouth (NPO) for 6 to 8 hours prior to the procedure. Intravenous access is started before the examination and preoperative medications are administered. Because many patients are anxious when having any invasive procedure performed, intravenous narcotics can be given by the radiologist or nurse on the physician's order. The patient can be premedicated with steroids or antihistamines to reduce the severity of a possible reaction to the contrast medium. As the patient will have had some intravenous drugs and is undergoing an invasive examination, physiologic monitoring is mandatory. Electrocardiogram (ECG), pulse oximetry, and automatic blood pressure measurements are recommended. There should also be emergency equipment (ie, crash cart) in the room or in close proximity in case of life-threatening situations.

Catheterization

To study the arterial or venous system, there needs to be access to the vessel. The most common site for arterial studies is the common femoral artery. The femoral artery can be palpated in the groin area. Using the **Seldinger technique,** arterial access can be accomplished *(Figure 18–12)*. In this approach, the radiologist, using an 18-gauge needle, punctures the skin of the groin area over the femoral pulse **(A),** removes the stylet of the needle, and slowly withdraws the needle until pulsating blood flows from the needle **(B).** A guidewire is then inserted into the needle and up into the common femoral artery **(C).** The needle is removed, leaving the wire in the artery **(D).** A plastic sheath inserted into the artery over the wire allows for the introduction of specialized catheters **(E, F).**

If there is a known or suspected occlusion of the femoral or iliac arteries, the radiologist can also gain access via the brachial or axillary arteries. These arteries are also accessed using the Seldinger technique. By use of the Sones technique, the brachial artery can be surgically exposed (cutdown) and a catheter inserted for the study. After the procedure, the artery must then be surgically repaired. Usually the left brachial or left axillary artery is chosen because the probability of stroke is less than with using the right side. Only the vertebral artery is crossed when passing the catheters down the subclavian artery into the abdominal aorta. The right carotid and right vertebral arteries are crossed with the introduction of catheters from the right side, placing both vessels at risk for emboli *(Figure 18–13)*.

No matter what approach is used, the area of interest must be prepared in a sterile manner. After the area is shaved, it is scrubbed with an approved solution to clean the skin of dirt, loose skin, oils, or transient microbes. The area is then draped with sterile towels and sheets. The purpose of the drape is to create a sterile field around the incision site. Sheets with a small opening and a self-adhesive circle are commonly used to drape the site and cover the patient from head to toe. The radiologist and the radiographer assisting in the procedure must wear sterile gloves, gown, mask, and eye protection to safeguard the patient from infection as well as to protect themselves from blood and bodily fluids.

Postprocedural Care

Postprocedurally, the arterial or venous sheath must be removed. Manual or mechanical pressure can be applied to the incision site to achieve hemostasis, which usually occurs in 10 to 15 minutes. If a hematoma is present, it should be noted in the patient's chart and circled with ink. The patient is sent to his or her room and watched closely by the attending nurse for up to 24 hours. Depending on the procedure and the patient's condition, the patient may go home the same day or be released the morning following the examination.

EQUIPMENT CONSIDERATIONS

For most angiographic procedures, the use of guidewires and catheters is necessary. **Guidewires** are required for the safe insertion, positioning, repositioning, and exchanging of catheters. They are typically made of a stainless-steel coil of wire that is supported internally by a fixed or movable core wire. The first 5- to 15-cm portion of the wire is flexible to ensure the safety of insertion. The typical length of a guidewire is 145 cm (57 in.) with its diameter ranging from 0.025 to 0.065 in. Exchange wires may run up to 300 cm in length. These wires are used to change catheters without losing the position of the wire in an area of interest *(Figure 18–14)*.

Catheters come in a wide range of shapes and sizes. Catheters are long, hollow, thin tubes having either a single end hole or multiple holes along the distal tip. They are used to deliver contrast media and other devices to a specific location inside the body. A catheter's outside diameter is measured by the French size (1F = 0.013 in. = 0.33 mm). Catheter sizes available in the special procedures laboratory may range from 3F to 8F. The shape of a catheter is preformed by the manufacturer to help in engaging different blood vessels. For example, a pigtail catheter has a curled distal tip with multiple side holes and is used in the aorta, whereas a cobra catheter has a gentle angle at the distal tip with just one end hole which helps when selecting renal or mesenteric arteries. The special procedures laboratory is filled with a variety of catheters that enable the radiologist to examine any blood vessel of the body *(Figure 18–15)*.

To make the blood vessels radiopaque, **contrast medium** must be injected. In the past, an iodine-based ionic contrast medium was used, but today with the advent of new agents, nonionic contrast medium may be used exclusively in many laboratories. The nonionic contrast medium has many advantages, as discussed in Chapter 13. Injection of ionic contrast medium for angiograms, especially of the extremities, can be quite painful. With nonionic contrast medium, the patient's discomfort level has been greatly reduced. Prior to the examination, the patient should be questioned about his or her allergy history. During the examination, a problem with clotting can occur with the use of contrast medium. The radiologist must be careful to constantly flush the contrast medium from the catheter to avoid blood clotting in its presence.

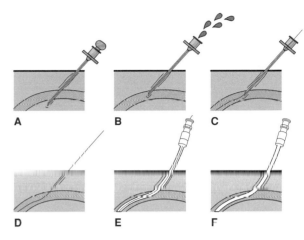

Figure 18–12. The Seldinger technique.

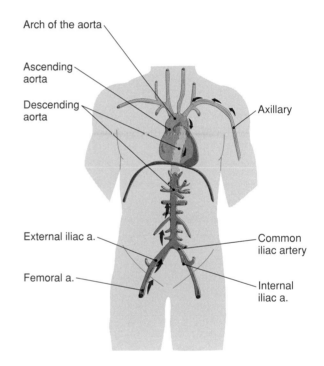

Figure 18–13. Placement of a catheter in the abdominal aorta is accomplished after accessing the femoral artery (large arrows) or the axillary artery (small red arrows).

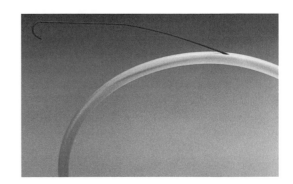

Figure 18–14. A guidewire is typically a stainless steel coil of wire.

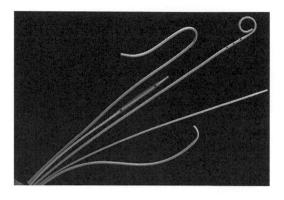

Figure 18–15. Note the assortment of tips on the catheters.

▶ Related Terminology

anastomosis (ah-nas-tō-MŌ-sis)—connection or communication between two vessels or organs that may occur naturally as in the circle of Willis, develop pathologically, or be surgically created

aneurysm (AN-ū-rizm)—weak area in a vessel's wall that causes it to balloon outward

angina (an-JĪ-nah or AN-ji-nah)—acute paroxysmal pain, usually in the chest, caused by myocardial ischemia

anomaly (ah-NOM-ah-lē)—deviation from the norm, such as malformation or absence of anatomic structures; the anomaly may be developmental, occurring in the embryo

arteriosclerosis (ar-tē-rē-ō-skle-RŌ-sis)—hardening of the arteries; abnormal condition in which the arterial walls become thick and lose their elasticity

arteriotomy (ar-tē-rē-OT-ō-mē)—incision of an artery

arteriovenous malformation (AVM)—condition in which there is an anastomosis between an artery and a vein, typified by tortuous and/or dilated vessels

cannulation (kan-ū-LĀ-shun)—process of introducing a tube or catheter into an organ or cavity of the body   *(continued)*

The **imaging equipment** in the special procedures laboratory must be as versatile as the radiographer working the equipment. It should have biplane capability, which enables two views to be radiographed at one time, such as AP and lateral or both obliques. **C-arm equipment** provides such versatility. The range of movement of the C-arm can help the radiologist adjust both the needle and the patient position *(Figure 18–16)*.

Many examinations require the exposure of numerous films in only a few seconds. **Biplane rapid film changers** can permit as many as six films per second to be exposed. A **shifting (stepping) tabletop** is necessary for some examinations. For example, to perform a femoral angiogram (femoral shift), the tabletop must be able to shift the patient to several different positions over the film changers.

The special procedures laboratory must also have an **automatic injector** or **pressure injector.** Although contrast medium can be injected into some vessels by hand, a pressure injector is usually needed for the majority of procedures. By use of the pressure injector, contrast medium fills the blood vessel adequately, allowing for a more accurate diagnosis. The injector permits contrast medium to be delivered in a controlled manner over a specific time, giving a specific amount at the correct flow rate. As the contrast medium is injected into the bloodstream, it is diluted by the blood. Setting the correct factors (ie, amount, flow rate, and time) ensures an adequate concentration of contrast medium in the blood vessel to visualize the needed anatomic features.

Most special procedures laboratories are equipped with **digital subtraction angiography** (DSA). A computer is used to enhance the real-time image by subtracting out unnecessary structures such as bones, leaving the vessels filled with contrast medium. The computer also allows the technologist to manipulate the window levels, contrast, and frames to compensate for any movement or other distractions. DSA can be used alone or with conventional cut films to help diagnose a patient's condition. It also allows the radiologist to use less contrast medium but still achieve diagnostic images. A special procedures laboratory is illustrated in *Figure 18–17*.

ANGIOGRAPHIC PROCEDURES

The root *angio-* refers to a "vessel," and the term *angiogram* is defined as radiographic examination of a vessel, specifically a blood vessel, after injection of contrast medium. The individual examinations are generally named according to the particular site under investigation.

Cardiac Catheterization and Coronary Angiography

Cardiac catheterization and coronary angiography are the most commonly performed angiographic examinations. They are performed in the cardiac catheterization laboratory by the cardiologist in conjunction with the radiographer and critical care nurse.

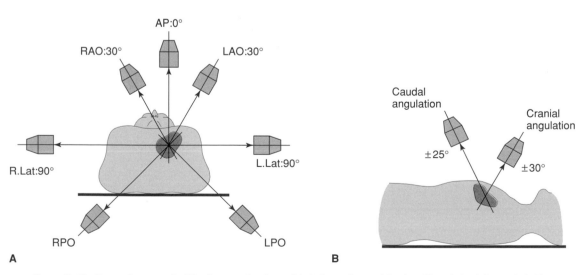

Figure 18–16. Range of movement of the C-arm makes it possible to image in a variety of positions to best demonstrate the anatomy of interest. **(A)** Rotation around short axis, **(B)** angulation along long axis (longitudinal plane).

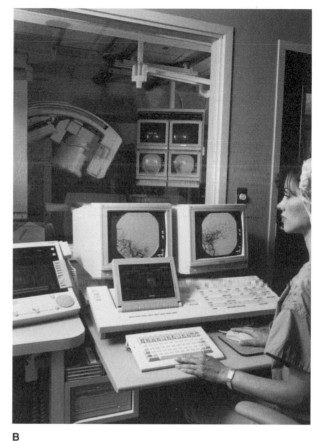

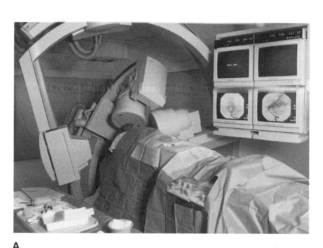

A   B

Figure 18–17. Special procedures laboratory. *(Courtesy of Philips Medical Systems.)*

Cardiac catheterization is a procedure in which a catheter is introduced directly into one of the chambers of the heart to record hemodynamic and physiologic information. **Coronary angiography** involves the placement of a catheter by the radiologist into the coronary arteries and the injection of contrast medium, with fluoroscopic images recorded by the radiographer on cine film or digital disk.

The cells of the heart muscle receive their oxygen and nutrients from blood supplied by the coronary arteries. The two major coronary arteries are the right and the left with their corresponding branches. Both arteries arise above the cusps of the aortic valve. These cusps, called the sinuses of Valsalva, are three dilations in the wall of the aorta behind the flaps of the three aortic valve leaflets. The right coronary artery (RCA) originates in the right aortic cusp, runs along the right side of the heart, and then divides into posterior descending and posterior lateral branches. The left coronary artery originates in the left aortic cusp, continues a short distance, and then divides into two major branches. The first branch, the left anterior descending (LAD), runs along the front border of the heart to the apex. The second branch, the circumflex, courses along the back side of the heart toward the inferior wall *(Figure 18–18)*.

Along with diagnosing the health of the coronary arteries, the cardiologist can study the competency of the heart valves. Four valves help in the forward flow of blood through the chambers of the heart. As previously discussed under Anatomy of the Cardiovascular System, venous blood empties into the right atrium from the body, then flows through the **tricuspid valve** into the right ventricle. It then passes through the **pulmonic valve,** through the pulmonary artery, and into the lungs, where it is circulated for reoxygenation. Oxygenated blood comes into the left atrium from the lungs, via the pulmonary veins, through the **mitral valve,** into the left ventricle which pumps blood through the **aortic valve** into systemic circulation of the body. Valves can begin to leak or to constrict over time. Both of these problems can be diagnosed during a cardiac catheterization *(Figure 18–19).*

The purpose of cardiac catheterization is to confirm suspected pathologic conditions, to define anatomic or physiologic abnormalities of the heart, and to determine the presence or absence of associated conditions. *Table 18–1* lists indications for performing coronary angiography.

Relative contraindications may postpone cardiac catheterization until a certain problem can be corrected, such as uncontrolled ventricular irritability, hypokalemia, hypertension, febrile illness, pulmonary edema, anticoagulated state, contrast allergy, and severe renal sufficiency. Years ago, it would have been

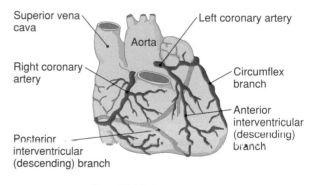

Figure 18–18. Coronary arteries.

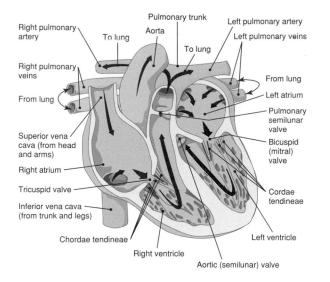

Figure 18–19. Blood flow through the heart is identified by arrows. The colored arrows on the left side of the heart denote oxygenated blood. Note the location of the four valves in the heart.

Table 18–1. Indications for Performing Coronary Angiography

Any suspected coronary artery disease
Any thrombus formation
Suspected valvular disease or cardiomyopathies
Suspected coronary spasm
Suspected anomalies (defects such as atrial septal defect and ventricular septal defect)
Atypical chest pain

---

considered too dangerous to perform cardiac catheterization in the presence of these conditions; today, however, medication can be used to control most problems, allowing the examination to be performed so that the patient can be diagnosed quickly and safely.

As with most angiography, cardiac catheterization can be performed via the brachial or femoral approach, although the femoral approach is by far the most common method. The Seldinger technique is used to access the artery. The pertinent catheter is introduced through the sheath or introducer and then directed to the heart. The patient's ECG and blood pressure are monitored continuously throughout the procedure.

During cardiac catheterization, the cardiologist threads the catheter in retrograde fashion from the femoral artery to the heart, positioning it in the ostium of the coronary artery. Once the catheter is in place, the cardiologist injects contrast medium into the artery and the radiographer records the angiogram on 35-mm film or digital disk. The radiographer rotates the C-arm around the patient to provide the cardiologist with adequate information to diagnose the patient. The C-arm can be angled cranially, caudally, RAO, or LAO to record required projections. As an artery fills with contrast medium, its contour is revealed. Arteries should have smooth borders and should naturally taper as they encircle the heart. Coronary artery disease or blockages may look as if the artery pinches down on itself, which causes the blood flow to be reduced or completely stopped. When blood flow is reduced or stopped, the patient can have chest pain or eventually a heart attack *(Figure 18–20).*

Interventions in the Cardiac Catheterization Laboratory

Once blockages are found in the coronary arteries, the cardiologist has three ways to treat the patient: medications, bypass surgery, or an interventional procedure. The following interventional procedures are performed in the cardiac catheterization laboratory.

Percutaneous Transluminal Coronary Angioplasty (PTCA). In PTCA, a balloon, mounted on a special catheter, is placed in the artery at the site of the lesion *(Figure 18–21).* By use of a controlled system, the balloon is inflated and the force of the balloon is used to try to push the blockage up against the arterial wall. By trying to remodel the lesion with the balloon, the lumen of the artery is opened. The variables that can be controlled during PTCA are balloon size, inflation time, and inflation pressure.

During PTCA, the inflated balloon applies pressure in a uniform fashion, regardless of whether the lesion is concentric or eccentric *(Figure 18–22).* As the lesion is compressed, the inner lining of the artery can crack or tear in places. Because there is the possibility that the artery may tear with PTCA and other interventional procedures, a surgical team should be on standby in the event the patient should need emergency surgery.

Directional Coronary Atherectomy (DCA). In PTCA, the lesion is remodeled, but in DCA, the lesion is actually removed from the coronary artery. The DCA catheter consists of a powerful cutting device with a balloon attached to one side of the catheter. The catheter is directed to any side of the artery where the lesion has formed to allow the device to cut away the plaque *(Figure 18–23).* As the balloon is inflated, the cutting device is embedded in the lesion. It spins at 2000 rpm to cut the blockage away from the arterial wall. The tissue that is excised is then housed at the tip of the catheter. When the catheter is removed, the collected tissue is recovered and analyzed.

Coronary Stents. A blockage can return after PTCA or DCA. Stents were introduced as a means of preventing occlusion in the blood vessel by keeping the lumen open. They are being used for first-line treatment, in restenoses, and in arterial dissections to actually hold the artery open.

Stents are stainless-steel tubes mounted on angioplasty balloons *(Figure 18–24).* When a stent is placed across an area of interest, the balloon is inflated. This causes the stent to expand fully so that it is embedded in the wall of the artery, leaving an open lumen.

► Related Terminology *(continued)*

cardiology (kar-dē-OL-ō-jē)—branch of medicine concerned with the function of the heart and diseases affecting it

coarctation (ko-ark-TĀ-shun)—constricting deformity; in the case of the aorta, the lumen of the vessel is narrow because of a deformity of the tunica media

dissection (dis-SEK-shun)—longitudinal tearing of the intima of the aorta

embolism (EM-bō-lizm)—blood clot or other foreign material (eg, fat or air bubble) that moves away from its site of formation and suddenly occludes an artery, obstructing the flow of blood to the tissues supplied by the vessel

fibrillation (fi-bril-LĀ-shun)—arrhythmic condition in which the muscles of the heart quiver and contract involuntarily

hematoma (hem-ah-TŌ-mah)—accumulation of clotted blood that leaks out of a blood vessel as the result of an injury; a bruise or contusion is a minor type of hematoma

Hodgkin's (HOJ-kinz) disease—malignant condition in which the structures of the lymphatic system progressively enlarge; characterized by fever, fatigue, and possibly night sweats; depending on the stage of the disease, it is generally treated with chemotherapy or radiation of the affected lymph nodes

hypertension (hī-per-TEN-shun)—high blood pressure

hypokalemia (hī-pō-kah-LĒ-me-ah)—condition of having an abnormally low level of potassium in the blood

infarct (IN-fark)—area of necrosed tissue resulting from a lack of blood supply

ischemia (is-KĒ-me-ah)—insufficient blood supply to an organ or structure as a result of an obstruction in a blood vessel

lymphoma (lim-FŌ-mah)—neoplastic growth or tumor in the lymphatic system that is usually malignant

malignant (mah-LIG-nant)—virulent; descriptive term usually referring to cancerous tumors *(continued)*

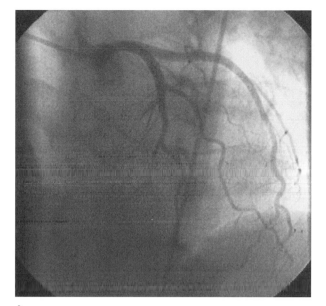

A

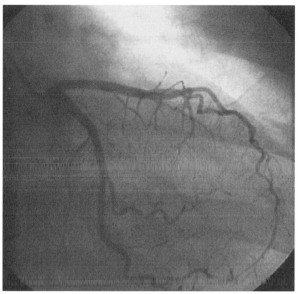

B

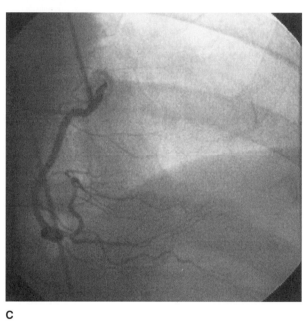

C

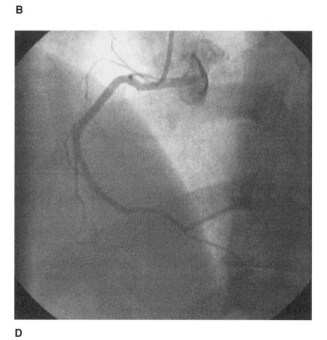

D

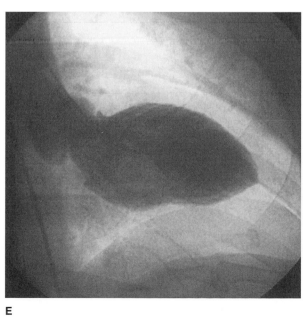

Figure 18–20. Cardiac catheterization: **(A)** left coronary artery (AP cranial), **(B)** left coronary artery (RAO), **(C)** right coronary artery (RAO), **(D)** right coronary artery (LAO), **(E)** left ventricle.

E

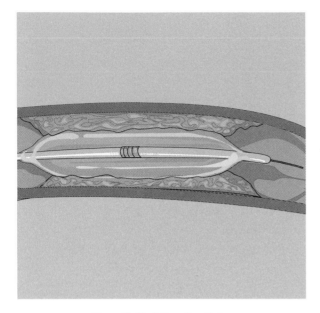

Figure 18–21. Balloon-tip catheter.

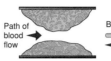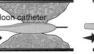

Path of blood flow

Balloon catheter

Balloon catheter expanded

Atherosclerotic plaque protrudes into lumen of artery.

Plaque is flattened against arterial wall, restoring patency to vessel.

Figure 18–22. Percutaneous transluminal coronary angioplasty.

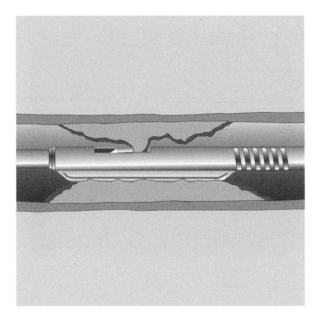

Figure 18–23. Directional coronary atherectomy.

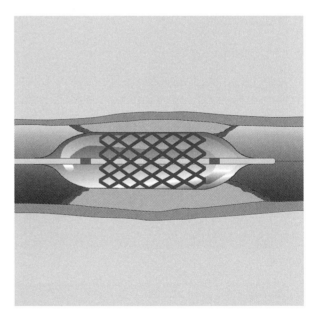

Figure 18–24. A stent demonstrated on a balloon catheter.

► Related Terminology *(continued)*

metastasis (me-TAS-tah-sis)—spread of malignant cells from one organ or area in the body to another area

patent ductus arteriosus (PĀ-tent DUK-tus ar-tē-rē-Ō-sus)—heart defect in which the ductus arteriosus between the pulmonary artery and aorta fails to close after birth, leaving an opening that may have to be surgically repaired

phlebolith (FLEB-ō-lith)—calculus in a vein   *(continued)*

Percutaneous Transluminal Coronary Rotational Ablation (PTCRA) or Rotoblator. The rotoblator removes atherosclerotic plaque by using a high-speed burr covered with diamond crystals. The burr has a tiny football-shaped tip that spins at speeds up to 190,000 rpm. The cardiologist chooses the correct burr size for the artery in question. As the cardiologist runs the spinning burr down the artery and across the lesion, the tip of the burr removes plaque by pulverizing the plaque into minute particles. Increasingly larger burr sizes are used until the desired lumen has been reached. The resulting particles are smaller than red blood cells so that they can easily be carried away in the bloodstream *(Figure 18–25)*.

Transluminal Extraction (TEC). The TEC system is a microsurgical cutting device that shaves plaque while a vacuum feature extracts the debris *(Figure 18–26)*. The TEC system, like DCA, is used to debulk the artery of clots or plaque and then remove that material from the body. The TEC catheter combines a hollow flexible tube with a cutting head on one end. The catheter and cutting end are rotated by a small motor at approximately 750 rpm. While the catheter is rotating, the cardiologist advances the catheter through the blockage. The vacuum is applied at the same time and any particles are removed from the body.

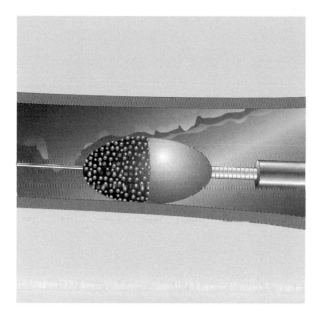

Figure 18–25. Rotoblator.

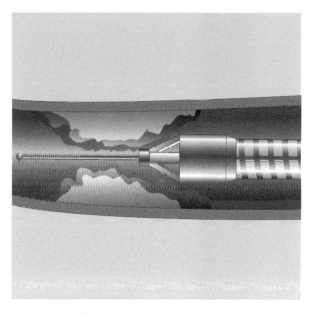

Figure 18–26. Transluminal extraction.

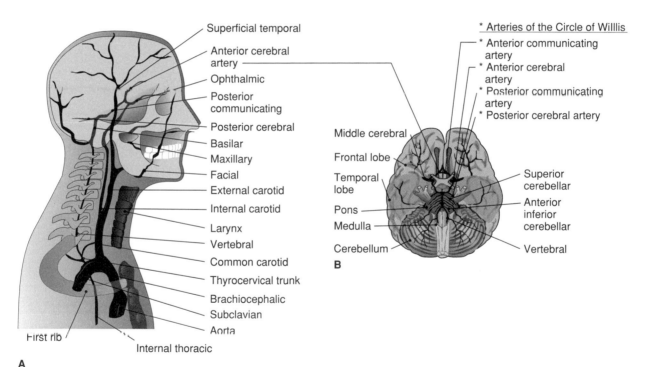
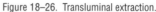

Superficial temporal

Anterior cerebral artery

Ophthalmic

Posterior communicating

Posterior cerebral

Basilar

Maxillary

Facial

External carotid

Internal carotid

Larynx

Vertebral

Common carotid

Thyrocervical trunk

Brachiocephalic

Subclavian

Aorta

First rib

Internal thoracic

A

* Arteries of the Circle of Willlis

* Anterior communicating artery

* Anterior cerebral artery

* Posterior communicating artery

* Posterior cerebral artery

Middle cerebral

Frontal lobe

Temporal lobe

Pons

Medulla

Cerebellum

Superior cerebellar

Anterior inferior cerebellar

Vertebral

B

Figure 18–27. Arteries of the neck and head: **(A)** lateral view, **(B)** inferior view.

Cerebral Angiography

The purpose of the cerebral angiogram is to visualize the blood supply to the brain. The patient may present with dizziness, headaches, transient ischemic attacks, or suspected subarachnoid hemorrhage. Even with the advent of magnetic resonance angiography, the cerebral angiogram is still widely used to diagnose the condition of the cerebral circulation, including arteriovenous malformations, thrombi, embolisms, aneurysms, arterial stenoses, and fistulas within the circulation of the brain.

The cerebrovascular circulation consists of the right and left carotid arteries and the right and left vertebral arteries. Each carotid artery bifurcates at the level of the fourth cervical vertebra into the internal and external carotid arteries. The internal carotid and its branches supply blood to the anterior portion of the brain, orbits, and forehead; the external carotid supplies the anterior neck, face, and temporal area with blood. The vertebral arteries supply blood to the posterior aspect of the brain. They travel through the cervical transverse foramina and enter the brain through the foramen magnum. Both vertebral arteries unite to form the basilar artery, which supplies the posterior portion of the brain with blood *(Figure 18–27)*.

▶ Related Terminology *(continued)*

Raynaud's disease (rā-NOZ)—condition in which an individual's fingers or toes become cyanotic and lose sensation because of spasms of the blood vessels that cause arterial insufficiency; can be triggered by stress and exposure to cold temperatures

stenosis (ste-NŌ-sis)—constriction or narrowing of a body opening, passage, or vessel (eg, renal artery)

thrombus (THROM-bus)—blood clot that may partially or completely occlude the blood vessel

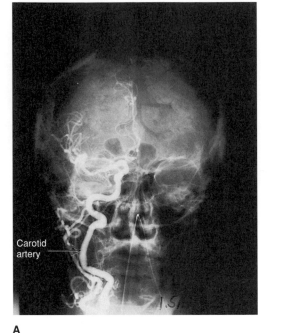
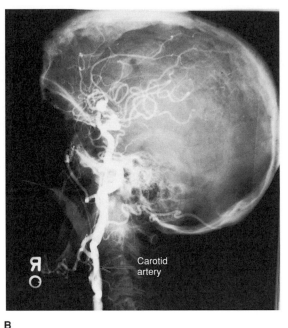

A

B

Figure 18–28. Cerebral angiogram obtained by accessing the right carotid artery: **(A)** AP, **(B)** lateral.

For a cerebral angiogram, biplane capability is necessary. Each blood vessel is subselected with a catheter and filmed in two projections as the contrast medium is being injected. AP (modified Towne) and lateral projections are most commonly taken to demonstrate the carotid arteries. If an aneurysm is suspected, both oblique projections may also be taken. Views for the vertebral angiogram include lateral and AP axial (Towne) projections to project the petrous ridges below the area of interest *(Figure 18–28)*.

Aortography

An aortogram is the study of the major blood vessel leading directly from the heart—the aorta. Beginning at the aortic valve of the heart, the aorta continues to the approximate level of L4. The thoracic portion of the aorta has four divisions. The first section, known as the **aortic bulb,** is the proximal end of the aorta which includes the three sinuses of Valsalva. The right and left coronary arteries originate in the right and left sinuses of Valsalva, respectively. Next, the **ascending** aorta extends from the bulb upward and anteriorly. At the level of the second sternocostal joint, the ascending aorta becomes the **aortic arch** to form the third division. The aortic arch travels superiorly, posteriorly, and to the left. The brachycephalic (innominate), left common carotid, and left subclavian arteries all originate from the aortic arch. It then turns inferiorly and becomes the **descending aorta** (fourth division) at the level of the fourth thoracic vertebra. The descending aorta continues on inferiorly and medially, ending at the level of L4. It is referred to as the **thoracic aorta** until it passes through the diaphragm into the abdomen *(Figure 18–29)*.

Thoracic aortography is used to diagnose many conditions, including congenital abnormalities such as patent ductus arteriosus, coarctation, and other aortic anomalies. Valvular disease such as aortic stenosis and aortic insufficiency can be diagnosed. Thoracic aortography is also performed for aortic dissections or when there is traumatic injury to the chest.

The purpose of the examination is to visualize the entire thoracic aorta from the aortic valve through the descending aorta. The most common way to perform this procedure is using the femoral approach. The radiologist positions a pigtail catheter, via the femoral artery, in the thoracic aorta just above the aortic valve. Using the power injector, the radiologist injects contrast medium into the aorta and a series of radiographs are taken.

Biplane projections are recommended for a thoracic aortagram, with the rapid film changers used to quickly radiograph the aorta. AP and lateral projections are sometimes used, but usually 30° to 45° RPO and LPO projections are used to separate structures so that information is not hidden *(Figure 18–30)*.

Thoracic aortography is not the only tool available to visualize the aorta. In many instances, CT and MRI scans are used to diagnose conditions of the aorta.

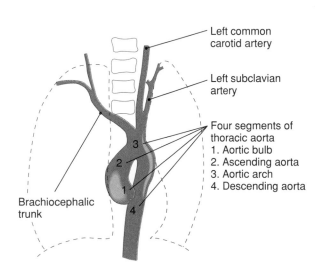

Figure 18–29. Toracic aorta.

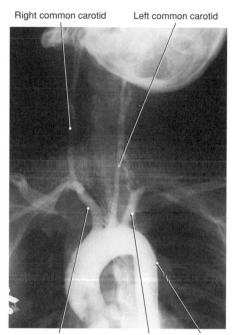

Figure 18–30. Thoracic aortogram.

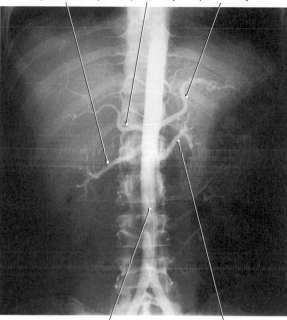

Figure 18–31. Abdominal aortogram.

Abdominal Angiography

The abdominal aorta is the continuation of the thoracic aorta. This vessel is anterior and usually slightly to the right of the spine. The abdominal aorta extends from the diaphragm to the level of L4, where it bifurcates into the right and left common iliac arteries *(Figure 18–31)*.

Abdominal angiography is performed to evaluate the presence of aneurysms, anomalies, stenoses, and trauma to the abdominal aorta. Injection of contrast medium into the abdominal aorta demonstrates its size, contour, and the location of the major branches. The radiologist can place a pigtail catheter, via the femoral, axillary, or translumbar approaches, in the aorta and inject contrast medium through the power injector to visualize all the major branches of the abdominal aorta. These major branches include the celiac axis, superior and inferior mesenteric arteries, and renal arteries.

When the femoral or axillary approach is used, the patient is positioned supine for an AP projection. The technologist should position the patient to include the area from the diaphragm to the bifurcation.

Selective Visceral Angiography

After an abdominal angiogram has been performed, the major branches of the aorta can be subselected for study *(Figure 18–32)*. The femoral approach is most commonly used when selecting particular arteries of the abdomen.

Angiography of the **celiac axis** is performed to evaluate a possible retroperitoneal tumor, aneurysm, cirrhosis of the liver, hepatitis, vascular narrowing, or trauma to the spleen. The celiac axis consists of the hepatic, splenic, and left gastric arteries, which supply blood to the liver, spleen, and stomach, respectively. The celiac artery itself is only 1 to 2 cm long and is the first major branch of the abdominal aorta. It arises on the ventral surface of the aorta at the upper margin of L1. The radiologist can select the celiac artery to visualize all three branches and can also subselect the individual branches for additional information. The patient should be positioned in the supine position for AP projections that are centered to the level of the T12–L1 intervertebral joint.

The **common hepatic artery** branches include the gastroduodenal, right, left, and middle hepatic arteries, which supply oxygenated blood to the liver, pancreas, and duodenum. When positioning for an angiogram of this vessel, the radiographer must ensure that the patient's entire right side of the abdomen will be on the radiograph. The central ray should be directed to the level of L1.

The **splenic artery** is the largest branch of the celiac artery and travels left behind the stomach to supply blood to the spleen. In a splenic angiogram, the left side of the patient's abdomen should be included on the radiograph. The central ray should be directed to the level of L1. The portal system can be demonstrated if the filming sequence is extended well past the completion of the arterial injection. Because the portal vein provides a great amount of blood flow to the liver, this phase is important for its visualization.

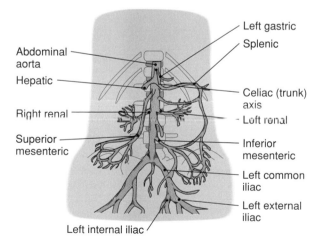

Figure 18–32. Major branches of the abdominal aorta.

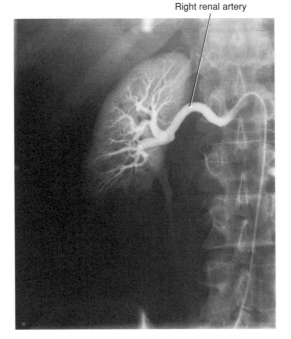

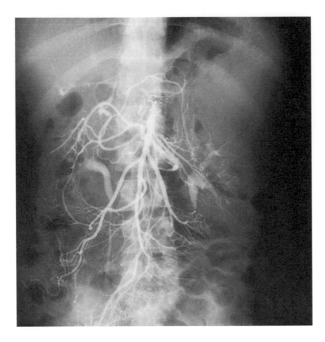

Figure 18–33. Superior mesenteric arteriogram.

Figure 18–34. Renal arteriogram.

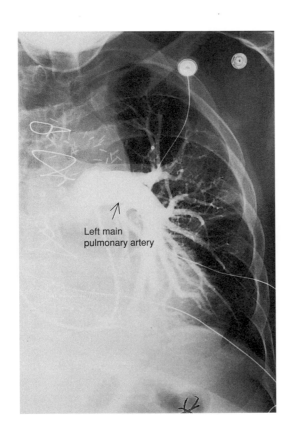

Figure 18–35. Pulmonary arteriogram.

The **superior mesenteric artery** (SMA) is the second branch of the aorta, arising at the lower border of L1. This blood vessel supplies the circulation to the small intestines with the exception of the duodenum. This artery also supplies blood to the cecum, ascending colon, and transverse colon regions of the large intestine. The superior mesenteric artery travels inferiorly from L1 to the level of the L5–S1 intervertebral joint. The patient should be in a supine position for AP projections. The central ray should be directed to the patient's midline at the level of L3 to include the main artery and its branches. A rapid series of radiographs are taken as contrast medium is injected via a power injector into a catheter *(Figure 18–33)*.

The **inferior mesenteric artery** originates on the ventral surface of the aorta at the level of L3. It travels inferiorly toward the pelvis, sending blood to the splenic flexure, descending colon, and rectosigmoid area of the large intestine. For filming, the patient should be in the supine position, with the central ray directed to the midline at the level of L5.

Either a superior mesenteric or inferior mesenteric angiogram would be performed in the case of suspected gastrointestinal bleeding or ischemic bowel.

The **renal arteries** arise on the right and left sides of the aorta below the superior mesenteric artery at the approximate level of the L1–L2 intervertebral joint. Both arteries travel out from the aorta, supplying blood to their respective kidneys. Generally, there is one right and one left renal artery. As some patients may have more than one renal artery, it is important to visualize all vessels leading to the kidney.

A renal angiogram is performed after pathology has been identified by other modalities, such as an intravenous pyelogram, CT, nuclear medicine, and/or MRI. The angiogram can help distinguish whether a mass is cystic or a vascular tumor. Other reasons to perform a renal angiogram include trauma to the area, kidney donation, uncontrolled hypertension, and suspected vascular stenosis.

An abdominal angiogram is sometimes performed first, then the renal arteries are selected for study. The patient is positioned supine, with the central ray centered to the level of L2 midway between the spine and lateral margin of the abdomen on the particular side of interest *(Figure 18–34)*. Filming can be extended to include the venous phase of the kidney circulation.

Angiographic procedures are performed to evaluate vascular structures, both arterial and venous, in many other regions of the body.

Pulmonary Angiography

Pulmonary angiography is performed to study the circulation leading from the right ventricle of the heart to the lungs. The pulmonary artery originates from the right ventricle through the pulmonic valve *(see Figure 18–6)*. The left pulmonary artery has two main branches supplying the upper and lower lobes of the left lung. The right pulmonary artery consists of the ascending branch feeding the right upper lobe and the descending branch supplying the right middle and lower lobe.

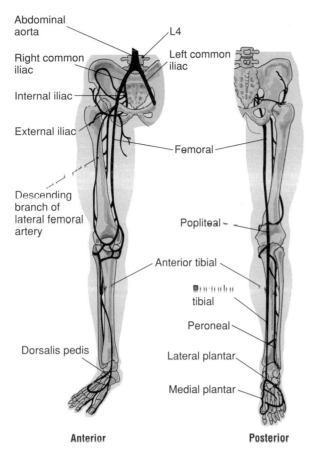

Figure 18–36. Arterial circulation of the lower limb.

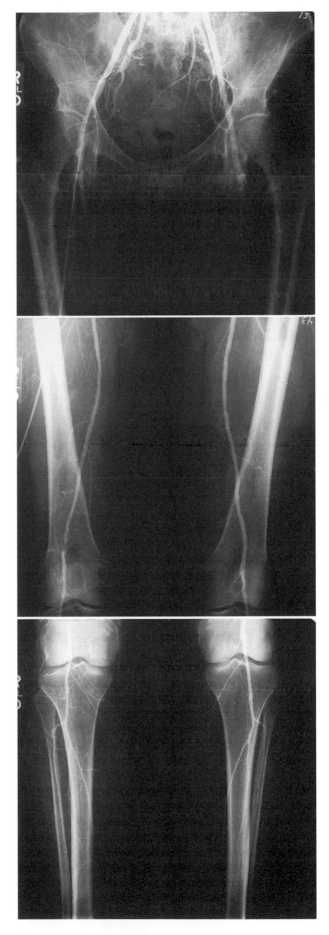

Figure 18–37. Femoral arteriogram demonstrating the upper, middle, and lower regions of the leg. Note that the legs were not internally rotated on this particular patient.

An angled pigtail catheter is most commonly used and is inserted through the femoral vein, directed retrograde up the IVC into the right atrium, through the tricuspid valve and right ventricle, and out into the pulmonary artery. The AP projection can be used as a guiding picture to assess both arteries. In the event extra views are needed, the catheter can be directed into the right or left pulmonary artery *(Figure 18–35)*. A slight 10° to 15° LPO projection can be used to demonstrate the right pulmonary artery, whereas a steeper 30° to 35° RPO projection should be used to view the left pulmonary artery.

The primary indication for performing a pulmonary angiogram on a patient is to identify pulmonary emboli. This procedure is also done in cases where vascular anomalies are suspected, including arteriovenous malformations and patent ductus arteriosus. During this examination, the patient can develop several serious complications, such as cardiac arrhythmias and cardiac arrest. For this reason, the patient is always connected to an ECG monitor with emergency equipment present in the room.

Femoral Angiography

The abdominal aorta bifurcates at L4 into the right and left common iliac arteries, with the common iliac arteries then dividing into the external and internal iliac arteries. The external iliac artery becomes the femoral artery, with its branches supplying blood all the way down the leg *(Figure 18–36)*.

A femoral angiogram is needed to study the femoral artery and its branches. The catheter is placed above the bifurcation via the femoral, axillary, or translumbar approach, and contrast medium is injected. Throughout the injection, the tabletop moves the patient over the film changer so that the area from the pelvis down to the ankles may be radiographed, if necessary. All areas of the femoral distribution will be seen if the timing sequence between injection, filming, and table movement is correct.

The patient is in the supine position for the femoral and axillary approaches, with the legs internally rotated approximately 30°. The legs should be supported to prevent motion artifacts.

Femoral angiograms are indicated for suspected vascular disease, claudication, arteriovenous malformation, tumor, embolism, ulceration, and poor circulation *(Figure 18–37)*.

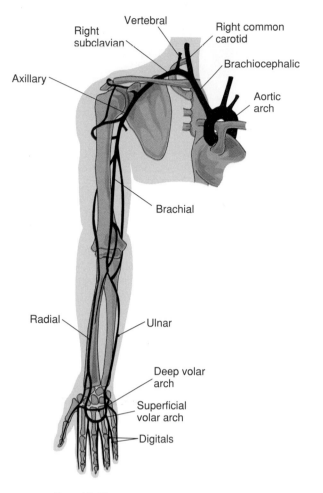

Figure 18–38. Arterial circulation of the upper limb.

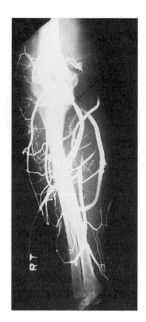

Figure 18–39. Arteriogram of the upper limb.

Upper Extremity Angiography

An upper extremity angiogram includes visualization of the subclavian, brachial, radial, and ulnar arteries *(Figure 18–38)*. The femoral approach is most commonly used, although brachial or axillary approaches are possible. The catheter is directed from the femoral artery in retrograde fashion until seated in the subclavian artery of the affected extremity. Synchronization of table movement, filming, and injection of contrast medium may be needed during the examination, depending on the area of interest *(Figure 18–39)*.

Angiograms of the upper extremity may be indicated for suspected vascular disease, arteriovenous malformation, trauma, aneurysm, embolism, and Raynaud's disease.

Venography

Venography is radiographic examination of the veins, and is defined as the study of the venous system (see *Figure 18–5*) within any area of the body. Venography is most commonly performed on the lower extremity, although studies can be done on the superior and inferior venae cavae, upper extremity, and renal veins. The primary purpose of a venogram is to rule out the presence of a thrombus. Secondary reasons include diagnosing a suspected occlusion of vessels, ruling out the presence of tumor, sampling the blood in the IVC, and evaluating traumatic injuries.

The IVC can be visualized by the femoral approach via the femoral vein or by the internal jugular approach for insertion of a vena cava filter. The radiologist accesses the femoral vein, inserts a sheath, and places the pigtail catheter in the desired position. The venous blood flow moves upward, so the catheter is positioned low, usually well below the renal veins. If there is a suspected renal tumor, an inferior vena cavagram is performed because some tumors can invade the IVC. Venous blood is sampled from the IVC and both renal veins if the patient has uncontrolled hypertension.

The patient is placed supine on the radiographic table, prepped, and draped in sterile fashion. Single-plane radiography is used, and as contrast medium is injected through the catheter, a series of radiographs are exposed using the rapid film changer *(Figure 18–40)*.

The purpose of performing a **lower leg venogram** is to rule out the presence or absence of deep vein thrombosis. In general, the lower leg extremity venogram is performed with the patient lying supine on a tilting radiographic table. The patient's unaffected leg is on a support so that the affected leg is suspended, bearing no weight. The radiologist starts an intravenous line in one of the veins of the foot, usually the dorsal pedis vein. Tourniquets are tightened around the ankle and the knee. As the contrast medium is slowly injected into the intravenous line, the tourniquets force it into the deep veins of the leg.

A series of radiographs are taken as the contrast medium is being injected. The patient is positioned partially erect at a 60° angle, and AP, oblique, and lateral projections are taken of the lower leg. The table is then lowered to 45°, and AP and lateral projections of the knees and an AP projection of the femur are taken. The table is then leveled out and an AP projection of the pelvis is taken. If the timing is correct, the contrast medium should fill the deep veins of the lower leg and the superficial femoral vein of the pelvis *(Figure 18–41)*.

For an upper extremity venogram, the patient is supine with the affected arm abducted from the body with the hand supinated. Intravenous access is obtained in a vein in the forearm. A tourniquet is placed proximal to the intravenous site and contrast medium is slowly injected. Toward the end of the injection, the tourniquet is released and radiographs are taken. AP projections of the arm and shoulder should visualize the veins of the upper extremity, including the brachial and axillary.

Lymphangiography

Lymphangiography (lim-fan-jē-OG-rah-fē) is the radiographic examination of the structures of the lymphatic system (vessels and nodes) (see *Figure 18–8*) after injection of a contrast medium. Although this procedure may still be performed at major cancer treatment centers, it has been widely displaced by CT and ultrasonography. MRI and lymphoscintigraphy are currently being studied as valuable imaging methods of the lymphatic system.

The primary indications for performing lymphangiography include suspected lymphoma (Hodgkin's disease), metastatic disease, and other malignancies, particularly of the reproductive organs. It may be used after chemotherapy to evaluate the effects of treatment on the lymph nodes or presurgically to localize nodes for biopsy. In the case of unexplained peripheral swelling, lymphangiography may be helpful in demonstrating a possible obstruction of the lymph vessels or nodes. The procedure is contraindicated if the patient has a known allergy or sensitivity to the indicator dye or iodine in the contrast medium. It is also not performed on patients currently undergoing radiation therapy to the lungs or those individuals with breathing difficulties resulting from advanced pulmonary disease.

In preparation, the patient may not have any solid food for 8 hours prior to the examination; however, clear liquids are allowed. A PA chest radiograph might be taken to evaluate the patient's lungs prior to the injection of contrast medium. An allergy history should be taken to determine if the patient has a sensitivity to iodinated contrast media.

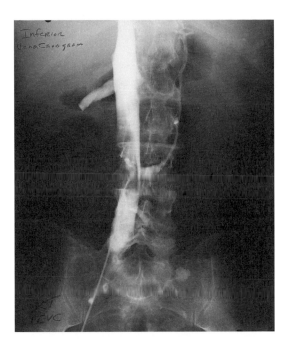

Figure 18–40. Inferior vena cavagram.

Lymphangiography is performed in a radiographic room with overhead capabilities. A sterile tray should contain the necessary supplies for cannulation of the vessel. An automatic injector is needed for the injection procedure. An iodized oil-based contrast medium (ie, Ethiodol) is injected directly into a lymphatic vessel.

The site of injection is generally the foot. Because the lymphatic vessels are difficult to find for cannulation, a blue indicator dye is first injected into the webbing between the toes. When the lymphatic vessels are visualized approximately 20 minutes later, a cutdown is performed on the dorsum of the foot. This is a minor surgical technique in which a 3-cm incision is made using sterile procedure to isolate the lymphatic vessel. The needle is placed in the vessel with its attached tubing connected to the automatic injector. The contrast medium is infused at a constant low pressure, taking approximately 1 hour to complete the injection.

Routine filming consists of the following projections: AP pelvis, AP abdomen, RPO and LPO abdomen. These sets of radiographs are first taken 1 hour after the completion of injection and then again 24 hours postinjection. The 1-hour radiographs demonstrate the lymphatic vessels, whereas the later radiographs demonstrate the nodes. As the contrast medium can remain in the nodes for several months and possibly 1 year, follow-up radiographs may be ordered periodically by the patient's physician *(Figure 18–42)*.

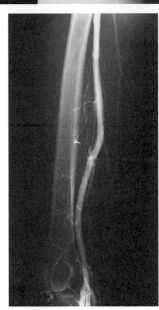

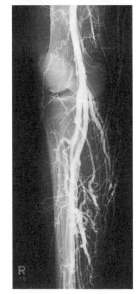

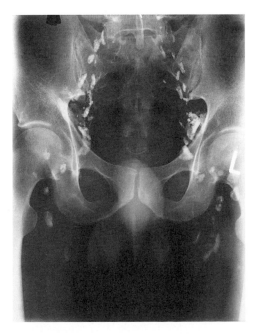

Figure 18–42. Lymphangiography: 24-hour delayed film demonstrating lymph nodes.

Figure 18–41. Lower limb venogram demonstrating the upper, middle, and lower regions of the leg. Note that the patient's leg was externally rotated on these radiographs.

SUMMARY

► The cardiovascular system is responsible for the transportation of blood to all of the organs of the body. It can be subdivided into the systemic and pulmonary circulation.

► The "pipelines" of the cardiovascular system are the arteries, arterioles, capillaries, venules, and veins.

► The exchange of oxygen and nutrients in the tissues of the body takes place in the capillary beds.

► Pulmonary arteries are the only arteries in the body to carry deoxygenated blood, whereas pulmonary veins are the only veins to carry oxygenated blood.

► Radiographic examination of blood vessels following the injection of contrast medium is known as angiography.

► Angiograms can be performed for both diagnostic and therapeutic purposes.

► The Seldinger technique is a method of accessing a blood vessel of interest. An arterial puncture is performed, followed by the introduction of a guidewire and catheter.

► An angiogram is performed under sterile conditions.

► Water-soluble, iodinated contrast medium is used to visualize the cardiovascular system.

► A selective angiographic study is performed when a branch of a main vessel (ie, the aorta) is accessed by a catheter and studied after the injection of contrast medium.

► Interventional procedures include angioplasty, atherectomy, stent placement, ablation (rotoblator), and transluminal extraction.

► Angiography can be performed therapeutically with the admission of thrombolytic agents that dissolve blood clots or placement of vena cava filters that trap blood clots.

► Venography is the study of the venous system within a specific region of the body following the injection of contrast medium.

► Equipment in a special procedures and/or cardiac catheterization laboratory may include C-arms, biplane rapid film changers, shifting tabletops, automatic pressure injectors, and digital subtraction angiography.

► The lymphatic system parallels the cardiovascular system. Lymphatic vessels and nodes are situated throughout the body.

► Lymphangiography, radiographic examination of the lymphatic system, may be performed to evaluate metastatic disease or other malignancies.

► Use of an indicator dye is required in lymphangiography as the lymphatic vessels are small and clear.

► An oil-based, iodinated contrast medium is used in lymphangiography.

► Twenty-four-hour delayed films are usually taken in lymphangiography to demonstrate the lymph nodes.

QUESTIONS FOR CRITICAL THINKING & APPLICATION

1. Discuss what is meant by a "selective" procedure with respect to angiography.

2. Explain how each of the following parameters affects the rate of delivery of contrast medium in an angiographic procedure: viscosity of the contrast medium, injector pressure, catheter length, diameter of catheter.

3. What is the purpose of using tourniquets when performing a lower extremity venogram?

4. What is the main advantage to using a catheter in an angiographic procedure? What would happen if a catheter were not used? Why does the catheter have side holes?

5. Differentiate between therapeutic and diagnostic examinations of the heart and great vessels, to include a discussion of the procedures.

6. There are a wide variety of shapes of the catheters. What is the significance of the different end tips?

7. What is the name of the technique used in angiography to cancel out all of the bony structures that are routinely demonstrated on both a preliminary (scout) radiograph and a radiograph following injection? What valuable information does the use of this technique provide?

8. A patient with testicular cancer was referred by his physician to the radiology department for a lymphangiogram after he had completed a course of chemotherapy. Explain the correlation between his diagnosis and the need for the examination.

9. Discuss the need for contrast medium in examinations of the cardiovascular system. Why is iodinated contrast medium the appropriate choice?

10. What are the advantages to using C-arm equipment in the special procedures laboratory?

FILM CRITIQUE

Identify the procedure represented by the radiograph *(Figure 18–43)*.

What are the indications for performing this exam?

What vascular anatomy is being examined? Describe the patient positioning.

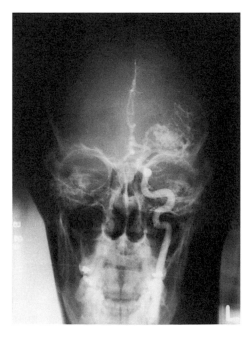

Figure 18–43

BIBLIOGRAPHY

Adler AM, Carlton RR. *Introduction to Radiography and Patient Care*. Philadelphia: WB Saunders, 1994.

Adolfini VP, Lillo SL, Willison EM. *Mammographic Imaging: A Practical Guide*. Philadelphia: JB Lippincott, 1992.

American College of Radiology. *Mammography Quality Control Manual*. Revised ed. Reston, VA: American College of Radiology, 1994.

Ballinger PW. *Merrill's Atlas of Radiographic Positions and Radiologic Procedures*. 8th ed. St. Louis: Mosby-Year Book, 1995.

Berquist T. *Diagnostic Imaging of the Acutely Injured Patient*. Baltimore: Urban & Schwarzenberg, 1985.

Bontrager KL. *Textbook of Radiographic Positioning and Related Anatomy*. 3rd ed. St. Louis: Mosby-Year Book, 1993.

Bushberg JT, Seibert JA, Leidholdt EM, Boone JM. *The Essential Physics of Medical Imaging*. Baltimore, MD: Williams & Wilkins, 1994.

Bushong S. *Radiologic Science for Radiographers*. 5th ed. St. Louis, MO: Mosby-Year Book, 1993.

Camp JD, Cilley EI. *AJR* 1931;26:905.

Carlton RR, McKenna Adler A. *Principles of Radiographic Imaging: An Art and a Science*. Albany, NY: Delmar, 1992.

Carroll QB. *Fuch's Radiographic Exposure, Processing and Quality Control*. 5th ed. Springfield, IL: Charles C Thomas, 1993.

Coons TA. MRI's role in assessing and managing breast disease. *Radiol. Technol.* 1996;67:311–336.

Cullinan AM. *Optimizing Radiographic Positioning*. Philadelphia: JB Lippincott, 1992.

Cullinan AM, Cullinan JE. *Producing Quality Radiographs*. 2nd ed. Philadelphia: JB Lippincott, 1994.

de Paredes ES. *Atlas of Film–Screen Mammography*. 2nd ed. Baltimore, MD: Williams & Wilkins, 1995.

DeVos DC. *Basic Principles of Radiographic Exposure*. 2nd ed. Baltimore: Williams & Wilkins, 1995.

Dowd SB, Wilson BG. *Encyclopedia of Radiographic Positioning*. Philadelphia: WB Saunders, 1995.

Drafke MW. *Trauma and Mobile Radiography*. Philadelphia: FA Davis, 1990.

Ehrlich RA, McCloskey ED. *Patient Care in Radiography*. 4th ed. St. Louis: Mosby-Year Book, 1993.

Eisenberg RL, Dennis CA. *Comprehensive Radiographic Pathology*. 2nd ed. St. Louis: Mosby-Year Book, 1995.

Eisenberg RL, Dennis CA, May CR. *Radiographic Positioning*. 2nd ed. Boston: Little, Brown, 1995.

Eklund GW, Cardenosa G, Parsons W. *Mammography: Positioning and Technical Considerations for Optimal Image Quality*. Minneapolis, MN: Imaging Premastering, Inc, 1994.

Francis C. Method improves consistency in L5–S1 joint space films. *Radiol. Technol.* 1992;63(5):302–305.

Garza D, Becan-McBride K. *Phlebotomy Handbook*. 2nd ed. Norwalk, CT: Appleton & Lange, 1993.

Gelman MI. *Radiology of Orthopedic Procedures, Problems, and Complications*. Saunders Monographs in Clinical Radiology, vol. 24. Philadelphia: WB Saunders, 1984.

Godderidge C. *Pediatric Imaging*. Philadelphia: WB Saunders, 1995.

Gronefeld D, Koscielicki T. Selected pathological conditions affecting the kidneys. *Sem. Radiol. Tech.* 1996; 4/3:120–135.

Guy JF. *Learning Human Anatomy*. Norwalk, CT: Appleton & Lange, 1992.

Jackson VP. The role of ultrasound in breast imaging. *Radiology*. 1990;177:305–311.

Judet R, Judet J, Letournel E. Fractures of the acetabulum: Classification and surgical approaches for open reduction. *J. Bone Joint Surg.* 1964;46A:1615–1646.

Katzberg RW (Ed). *The Contrast Media Manual*. Baltimore: Williams & Wilkins, 1992.

Kent TH, Hart MN. *Introduction to Human Disease*. 3rd ed. Norwalk, CT: Appleton & Lange, 1993.

Laudicina PF. *Applied Pathology for Radiographers*. Philadelphia: WB Saunders, 1989.

Linn-Watson, TA. *Radiographic Pathology*. Philadelphia, PA: WB Saunders, 1996.

Long E. *Intravascular X-ray Contrast Agents in the 1990s: New Issues for Pharmacists*. Philadelphia: FCG International, 1996.

Mace JD, Kowalczyk N. *Radiographic Pathology for Technologists*. 2nd ed. St. Louis: Mosby-Year Book, 1994.

Mallett M. *Handbook of Anatomy and Physiology for Students of Medical Radiation Technology*. 3rd ed. Mankato, MN: Burnell, 1981.

Marieb EN. *Human Anatomy and Physiology*. 2nd ed. Redwood City, CA: Benjamin/Cummings, 1992.

Martini F. *Fundamentals of Anatomy and Physiology*. 2nd ed. Englewood Cliffs, NJ: Prentice-Hall, 1992.

McCall RE, Tankersley CM. *Phlebotomy Essentials*. Philadelphia: JB Lippincott, 1993.

McQuillen-Martensen K. *Radiographic Critique*. Philadelphia: WB Saunders, 1996.

Mulvihill ML. *Human Diseases: A Systemic Approach*. 4th ed. Norwalk, CT: Appleton & Lange, 1995.

Prue LK. *Atlas of Mammographic Positioning*. Philadelphia: WB Saunders, 1994.

Simon R, Koenigsknecht S. *Emergency Orthopedics: The Extremities*. 3rd ed. Norwalk, CT: Appleton & Lange, 1995.

Skucas J. *Radiographic Contrast Agents*. 2nd ed. Rockville, MD: Aspen, 1989.

Snopek AM. *Fundamentals of Special Radiographic Procedures*. 3rd ed. Philadelphia: WB Saunders, 1992.

Squire LF, Novelline RA. *Fundamentals of Radiology*. 4th ed. Cambridge, MA: Harvard University Press, 1988.

Thibodeau GA. *Anatomy and Physiology*. St. Louis: Times Mirror/Mosby College, 1987.

Thibodeau GA, Patton KT. *Anatomy and Physiology*. 3rd ed. St. Louis, MO: Mosby-Year Book, 1996.

Thompson MA, Hattaway MP, Hall JD, Dowd SB. *Principles of Imaging Science and Protection*. Philadelphia: WB Saunders, 1994.

Thompson TT. *Cahoon's Formulating X-ray Techniques*. 9th ed. Durham, NC: Duke University Press, 1979.

Torres LS. *Basic Medical Techniques and Patient Care for Radiologic Technologists*. 4th ed. Philadelphia: JB Lippincott, 1993.

Tortora GJ, Grabowski SR. *Principles of Anatomy and Physiology*. 8th ed. New York: Harper Collins College, 1996.

Tortorici MR, Apfel PJ. *Advanced Radiographic and Angiographic Procedures*. Philadelphia: FA Davis, 1995.

Watkins GL, Moore TF. *Atypical Orthopedic Radiographic Procedures*. St. Louis: Mosby-Year Book, 1993.

Wentz G. *Mammography for Radiologic Technologists*. New York: McGraw-Hill, 1994.

Wojtowycz M. *Handbook of Interventional Radiology and Angiography*. St. Louis: Mosby-Year Book, 1995.

Wolbarst AB. *Physics of Radiology*. Norwalk, CT: Appleton & Lange, 1993.

Woods JJ. Amber: The next generation in chest radiography. *Journal of Kentucky Society of Radiologic Technologists*. 1992; Nov.:1–10.

INDEX

A

Abdomen, 57–80, 58f
  alternate imaging procedures for, 72
  anatomy of, 58–68
  AP, 75, 75f
  blood vessels of, 67–68, 68f
  bony structures of, 60–61
  dorsal decubitus, 78, 78f
  left lateral decubitus, 77, 77f
  location of structures in, methods of description,
    58–60
  muscles of, 61, 61f
  recumbent, evaluation criteria for, 70t
  structures of, 59t
    included in radiography, 60f
  upright AP, 76, 76f
Abdominal angiography, 541, 541f
Abdominal aorta, 541f
Abdominal cavity, 58f
Abdominal radiography
  breathing instructions for, 70
  equipment considerations in, 71
  exposure factors for, 71
  film critique, 80f
  mobile, 72, 72f
  patient preparation for, 68
  with pediatric patients, 71f, 71–72
  positioning considerations in, 68–70
  positioning for, 74–78
  procedural considerations in, 68–73
  special procedures in, 72–73
Abduction, 11f
Acanthiomeatal line, 333t
Acanthion, 331t
Accessory organs, of digestion, 447–448, 448f
Acetabulum, 173
  AP oblique, 242–243, 242f–243f
  makeup of, 220–221

PA axial oblique, 244, 244f
Acholia, 491
Acini, 490
Acromial end (extremity), 150
Acromioclavicular joint, 152, 153f, 153t
  AP
    with weights, 166–167, 166f–167f
    without weights, 166f, 166–167
Acromion, 151
Acute abdominal series, 69, 69f, 69t
Adduction, 11f
Adipose capsule, 417
Adolescents, 5
Adrenal glands, 65
Advance multiple-beam equalization radiography
    (AMBER), 40, 40f
AEC. *See* Automatic exposure control
Afferent arteriole, 418
Agenesis, 423
AIIS. *See* Anterior inferior iliac spine
Air-gap technique, 39, 39f
Ala(e), 220, 272
ALARA concept, 21
Alimentary canal, 438, 438f, 439
  layers of wall of, 439, 439f
Alveolar process
  of mandible, 361
  of maxilla, 359
Alveoli, 32, 32f
AMBER. *See* Advance multiple-beam equalization
    radiography
Amphiarthroses, 88, 89t, 90, 90f
Ampulla, of semicircular canal, 328
Anal canal, 446
Anal columns, 446
Anal sphincters, 446
Anaphylactoid reaction, 408
Anastomosis, 64, 534
Anatomical position, 12f
Anatomic terminology, 10f–11f
Aneurysm, 534

Angina, 534
Angiography
  abdominal, 541, 541f
  cerebral, 539–540, 540f
  coronary, 535
    indications for, 536t
  diagnostic, 531
  equipment considerations in, 533f, 533–534, 534f
  film critique, 547f
  patient preparation for, 532
  postprocedural care in, 533
  procedural considerations in, 531–545
  therapeutic, 531–532
Angle of Treitz, 444
Angular notch, 443
Anion, 405
Ankle
  AP, 193, 193f
  bones of, 170–172, 172f
  lateral, 196, 196f
  medial oblique, 194–195, 194f–195f
  stress views of, 178, 178f
Ankle joint, 175, 175f
  movement of, 175, 175f
Ankylosis, 92
Annulus fibrosis, 276
Anomaly, 534
Anorexia, 64
Anterior, 10f
Anterior clinoid process, 326
Anterior crest, of tibia, 172
Anterior fontanels, 329
Anterior inferior iliac spine (AIIS), 220
Anterior nasal spine, 359
Anterior semicircular canal, 328
Anterior superior iliac spine (ASIS), 220
Anterior surface, of patella, 174
Anterolateral fontanels, 330
Anteroposterior (AP) projection, 14f
Antra, 365
Anuria, 423